616.8982 21é

DATE DUE			

The American Psychiatric Publishing
Textbook of Schizophrenia

EDITORIAL BOARD

The American Psychiatric Publishing
Textbook of Schizophrenia

EDITED BY

JEFFREY A. LIEBERMAN, M.D.
T. SCOTT STROUP, M.D., M.P.H.
DIANA O. PERKINS, M.D., M.P.H.

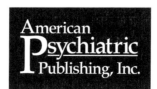

Washington, DC
London, England

Copyright © 2006 American Psychiatric Publishing, Inc.
ALL RIGHTS RESERVED

Manufactured in the United States of America on acid-free paper
10   09   08   07   06   5   4   3   2   1
First Edition

Typeset in Adobe's Frutiger and Janson Text.

American Psychiatric Publishing, Inc.
1000 Wilson Boulevard
Arlington, VA 22209-3901
www.appi.org

Library of Congress Cataloging-in-Publication Data
The American Psychiatric Publishing textbook of schizophrenia / edited by Jeffrey A. Lieberman, T. Scott Stroup, Diana O. Perkins.—1st ed.
   p. ; cm.
   Includes bibliographical references and index.
   ISBN 1-58562-191-9 (hardcover : alk. paper)
   1. Schizophrenia. I. Lieberman, Jeffrey A., 1948–. II. Stroup, T. Scott, 1960–. III. Perkins, Diana O., 1958–.
IV. American Psychiatric Publishing. V. Title: Textbook of schizophrenia. VI. Title: Schizophrenia.
   [DNLM: 1. Schizophrenia—physiopathology. 2. Schizophrenic Psychology. 3. Brain—physiopathology.
4. Schizophrenia—complications. 5. Schizophrenia—therapy. WM 203 A5123 2006]
   RC514.A442 2006
   616.89′8—dc22

                                                 2005035241

British Library Cataloguing in Publication Data
A CIP record is available from the British Library.

*To our patients for their courage and for their assistance
in the search for the causes of and cure for their illness.*

To my family in gratitude for their love, support, and patience—J.A.L.

To Thelma, Meg, Lib, and Paul—T.S.S.

*With appreciation to my husband, Clark, for his intellectual and emotional support,
and to my children, Chris, Nick, and Katie, for their tolerance and love—D.O.P.*

CONTENTS

Contributors . . . . **xi**

Foreword . . . . **xv**

David A. Lewis, M.D.

Preface . . . . **xvii**

Jeffrey A. Lieberman, M.D.
T. Scott Stroup, M.D., M.P.H.
Diana O. Perkins, M.D., M.P.H.

1 **History of Schizophrenia and Its Antecedents** **1**

Michael H. Stone, M.D.

2 **Epidemiology** **17**

William W. Eaton, Ph.D.
Chuan-Yu Chen, Ph.D.

3 **Genetics** **39**

Patrick F. Sullivan, M.D., F.R.A.N.Z.C.P.
Michael J. Owen, Ph.D., F.R.C.Psych., F.Med.Sci.
Michael C. O'Donovan, Ph.D., F.R.C.Psych.
Robert Freedman, M.D.

4 **Prenatal and Perinatal Factors** **55**

John H. Gilmore, M.D.
Robin M. Murray, M.D.

5 **Neurodevelopmental Theories** **69**

Matcheri S. Keshavan, M.D.
Andrew R. Gilbert, M.D.
Vaibhav A. Diwadkar, Ph.D.

6 **Neurochemical Theories** **85**

Daniel C. Javitt, M.D., Ph.D.
Marc Laruelle, M.D.

7   **Phospholipids in Schizophrenia** **117**

Sahebarao P. Mahadik, Ph.D.
Jeffrey K. Yao, Ph.D., F.A.C.B.

8   **Neuroprogressive Theories** **137**

L. Fredrik Jarskog, M.D.
John H. Gilmore, M.D.

9   **Neuropathology and Neural Circuits**
Implicated in Schizophrenia **151**

L. Fredrik Jarskog, M.D.
Trevor W. Robbins, Ph.D.

10   **Structural and Functional Neuroanatomy** **167**

Aysenil Belger, Ph.D.
Gabriel Dichter, Ph.D.

11   **Psychopathology** **187**

J. P. Lindenmayer, M.D.
Anzalee Khan, M.S.

12   **Co-occurring Substance Use and**
Other Psychiatric Disorders **223**

Mary F. Brunette, M.D.
Douglas L. Noordsy, M.D.
Alan I. Green, M.D.

13   **Neurocognitive Impairments** **245**

Richard S.E. Keefe, Ph.D.
Charles E. Eesley, B.S.

14   **Social Cognitive Impairments** **261**

David L. Penn, Ph.D.
Jean Addington, Ph.D.
Amy Pinkham, M.A.

15   **Social and Vocational Impairments** **275**

Kim T. Mueser, Ph.D.
Shirley M. Glynn, Ph.D.
Susan R. McGurk, Ph.D.

16   **Natural History and Predictors of Clinical Course......289**

Diana O. Perkins, M.D., M.P.H.
Lydia Miller-Andersen, M.D.
Jeffrey A. Lieberman, M.D.

17   **Pharmacotherapies 303**

T. Scott Stroup, M.D., M.P.H.
John E. Kraus, M.D., Ph.D.
Stephen R. Marder, M.D.

18   **Psychosocial Therapies 327**

Marvin S. Swartz, M.D.
John Lauriello, M.D.
Robert E. Drake, M.D., Ph.D.

19   **The Prodrome. 341**

Elizabeth M. Tully, M.D.
Thomas H. McGlashan, M.D.

20   **First Episode. 353**

Diana O. Perkins, M.D., M.P.H.
Jeffrey A. Lieberman, M.D.
Shon Lewis, M.D.

21   **Treatment of Chronic Schizophrenia 365**

Alexander L. Miller, M.D.
Joseph P. McEvoy, M.D.
Dilip V. Jeste, M.D.
Stephen R. Marder, M.D.

22   **Nonpsychiatric Comorbid Disorders 383**

Lisa Dixon, M.D., M.P.H.
Erick Messias, M.D., M.P.H., Ph.D.
Karen Wohlheiter, M.S.

23   **Treatment of Schizophrenia in the Public Sector 395**

John E. Kraus, M.D., Ph.D.
T. Scott Stroup, M.D., M.P.H.

Index. 407

CONTRIBUTORS

Jean Addington, Ph.D.
University of Toronto, Toronto, Ontario, Canada

Nancy C. Andreasen, M.D., Ph.D.
The Andrew H. Woods Chair of Psychiatry, Department of Psychiatry, University of Iowa College of Medicine, Iowa City, Iowa; Director, The MIND Institute, Albuquerque, New Mexico; Editor-in-Chief Emeritus, *The American Journal of Psychiatry*

Aysenil Belger, Ph.D.
Associate Professor, Director of Neuroimaging Research, Departments of Psychiatry and Psychology, University of North Carolina, Chapel Hill, North Carolina

Mary F. Brunette, M.D.
Assistant Professor of Psychiatry, Department of Psychiatry, Dartmouth Medical School, Lebanon, New Hampshire

William T. Carpenter Jr., M.D.
Professor of Psychiatry and Pharmacology, University of Maryland School of Medicine; Director, Maryland Psychiatric Research Center, Baltimore, Maryland

Chuan-Yu Chen, Ph.D.
Assistant Investigator, Division of Mental Health and Substance Abuse Research, National Health Research Institutes, Taipei, Taiwan

Gabriel Dichter, Ph.D.
Fellow, Neurodevelopmental Disorders Research Center, University of North Carolina, Chapel Hill, North Carolina

Vaibhav A. Diwadkar, Ph.D.
Assistant Professor, Department of Psychiatry and Behavioral Neuroscience, Wayne State University, Detroit, Michigan; Adjunct Assistant Professor, Department of Psychiatry, University of Pittsburgh School of Medicine, Pittsburgh, Pennsylvania

Lisa Dixon, M.D., M.P.H.
Professor and Director, Division of Services Research, Department of Psychiatry, University of Maryland School of Medicine; Associate Director of Research, VA Capitol Health Care Network MIRECC, Baltimore, Maryland

Robert E. Drake, M.D., Ph.D.
Professor of Psychiatry, Dartmouth Medical School, Lebanon, New Hampshire; Director, New Hampshire–Dartmouth Psychiatric Research Center, Concord, New Hampshire

William W. Eaton, Ph.D.
Professor and Chair, Department of Mental Health, Bloomberg School of Public Health, Johns Hopkins University, Baltimore, Maryland

Charles E. Eesley, B.S.
Massachusetts Institute of Technology, Cambridge, Massachusetts

Wayne S. Fenton, M.D.
Director, Division of Adult Translational Research and Treatment Development, National Institute of Mental Health, Bethesda, Maryland

Robert Freedman, M.D.
Professor, Department of Psychiatry, University of Colorado Health Sciences Center, Denver, Colorado

Andrew R. Gilbert, M.D.
Postdoctoral Research Fellow, University of Pittsburgh School of Medicine, Pittsburgh, Pennsylvania

John H. Gilmore, M.D.
Professor, Department of Psychiatry, University of North Carolina at Chapel Hill

Shirley M. Glynn, Ph.D.
VA Greater Los Angeles Healthcare System, Geffen School of Medicine, UCLA, Los Angeles, California

Alan I. Green, M.D.
Raymond Sobel Professor of Psychiatry, Professor of Pharmacology and Toxicology, and Chairman, Department of Psychiatry, Dartmouth Medical School, Lebanon, New Hampshire

Raquel Gur, M.D., Ph.D.
Karl and Linda Rickels Professor in Psychiatry, Department of Psychiatry, University of Pennsylvania School of Medicine, Philadelphia, Pennsylvania

L. Fredrik Jarskog, M.D.
Associate Professor, Department of Psychiatry, University of North Carolina—Chapel Hill, Chapel Hill, North Carolina

Daniel C. Javitt, M.D., Ph.D.
Professor of Psychiatry and Neuroscience, New York University School of Medicine, New York, New York; Director, Cognitive Neuroscience/Schizophrenia Division, Nathan Kline Institute for Psychiatric Research, Orangeburg, New York

Dilip V. Jeste, M.D.
Estelle and Edgar Levi Chair in Aging, Professor of Psychiatry and Neurosciences, and Chief, Division of Geriatric Psychiatry, University of California, San Diego/VA Medical Center, San Diego, California

Richard S. E. Keefe, Ph.D.
Associate Professor, Department of Psychiatry, Duke University Medical Center, Durham, North Carolina

Matcheri S. Keshavan, M.D.
Western Psychiatric Institute and Clinic, Pittsburgh, Pennsylvania; Wayne State University, Detroit, Michigan

Anzalee Khan, M.S.
Research Scientist, Manhattan Psychiatric Center-Nathan Kline Institute for Psychiatric Research, New York, New York; Department of Arts and Sciences, Fordham University, New York, New York

John E. Kraus, M.D., Ph.D.
Assistant Professor and Associate Director of Residency Training, Department of Psychiatry, University of North Carolina, Chapel Hill, North Carolina; Chief, Adult Admissions Psychiatry, Dorothea Dix Hospital, Raleigh, North Carolina

Marc Laruelle, M.D.
Associate Professor, Department of Psychiatry and Radiology, Columbia University College of Physicians and Surgeons, New York, New York

John Lauriello, M.D.
Associate Professor, Department of Psychiatry, University of New Mexico, Albuquerque, New Mexico

Anthony F. Lehman, M.D., M.S.P.H.
Professor and Chair, Department of Psychiatry, University of Maryland School of Medicine, Baltimore, Maryland

David A. Lewis, M.D.
Professor of Psychiatry and Neuroscience; Director, Translational Neuroscience Program; Director, Conte Center for the Neuroscience of Mental Disorders, University of Pittsburgh School of Medicine, Pittsburgh, Pennsylvania

Shon Lewis, M.D.
Professor of Adult Psychiatry, University of Manchester Education and Research Centre, School of Medicine, Wythenshawe Hospital, Manchester, England

Jeffrey A. Lieberman, M.D.
Chairman, Department of Psychiatry, College of Physicians and Surgeons of Columbia University; Director, New York State Psychiatric Institute; Director, Lieber Center for Schizophrenia Research; Psychiatrist-in-Chief, New York Presbyterian Hospital and Columbia University Medical Center, New York, New York

J. P. Lindenmayer, M.D.
Clinical Professor, Department of Psychiatry, New York University School of Medicine, New York, New York; Clinical Director, Psychopharmacology Research Unit, Manhattan Psychiatric Center–Nathan Kline Institute for Psychiatric Research, New York, New York

Sahebarao P. Mahadik, Ph.D.
Professor of Psychiatry, Department of Psychiatry and Health Behavior, Medical College of Georgia; Medical Research Service Line, VA Medical Center, Augusta, Georgia

Stephen R. Marder, M.D.
Professor, Department of Psychiatry and Biobehavioral Sciences, David Geffen School of Medicine, University of California Los Angeles; Director, Mental Illness Research, Education, and Clinical Center (MIRECC), Veterans Affairs Medical Center, Los Angeles, California

Joseph P. McEvoy, M.D.
Associate Professor, Department of Psychiatry and Behavioral Sciences, Duke University Medical Center, Durham, North Carolina; Deputy Clinical Director, John Umstead Hospital, Butner, North Carolina

Thomas H. McGlashan, M.D.
Professor of Psychiatry, Yale University School of Medicine; Director, PRIME Prodromal Research Clinic; Director, Yale Psychiatric Research at Congress Place, New Haven, Connecticut

Susan R. McGurk, Ph.D.
Assistant Professor of Psychiatry, Dartmouth Medical School, Lebanon, New Hampshire; New Hampshire-Dartmouth Psychiatric Research Center, Concord, New Hampshire

Erick Messias, M.D., M.P.H., Ph.D.
Research Professor, State University of Ceará; Director of Research, Hospital de Saúde Mental de Messejana

Alexander L. Miller, M.D.
Clinical Professor, Department of Psychiatry, The University of Texas Health Science Center at San Antonio, San Antonio, Texas

Lydia Miller-Andersen, M.D.
Assistant Professor of Psychiatry, University of North Carolina School of Medicine, Chapel Hill, North Carolina

Kim T. Mueser, Ph.D.
Professor of Psychiatry and Community and Family Medicine, Dartmouth Medical School, Lebanon, New Hampshire; New Hampshire-Dartmouth Psychiatric Research Center, Concord, New Hampshire

Robin M. Murray, M.D.
Professor of Psychiatry, Institute of Psychiatry at the Maudsley, Kings College, University of London, London, England

Douglas L. Noordsy, M.D.
Associate Professor of Psychiatry, Department of Psychiatry, Dartmouth Medical School, Lebanon, New Hampshire

Michael C. O'Donovan, Ph.D., F.R.C.Psych.
Professor of Psychiatric Genetics, Department of Psychological Medicine, Neuropsychiatric Genetics Unit, University of Wales College of Medicine, Cardiff, United Kingdom

Michael J. Owen, Ph.D., F.R.C.Psych., F.Med.Sci.
Professor, Department of Psychological Medicine, Neuropsychiatric Genetics Unit, University of Wales College of Medicine, Cardiff, United Kingdom

David L. Penn, Ph.D
Associate Professor, Department of Psychology, University of North Carolina at Chapel Hill, Chapel Hill, North Carolina

Diana O. Perkins, M.D., M.P.H.
Professor of Psychiatry, University of North Carolina School of Medicine, Chapel Hill, North Carolina

Amy Pinkham, M.A.
University of North Carolina at Chapel Hill, Chapel Hill, North Carolina

Trevor W. Robbins, Ph.D.
Professor, Department of Experimental Psychology, University of Cambridge, Cambridge, United Kingdom

Michael H. Stone, M.D.
Professor of Clinical Psychiatry, Columbia College of Physicians and Surgeons, New York, New York

T. Scott Stroup, M.D., M.P.H.
Associate Professor, Department of Psychiatry, University of North Carolina at Chapel Hill, Chapel Hill, North Carolina

Patrick F. Sullivan, M.D., F.R.A.N.Z.C.P.
Professor, Departments of Genetics, Psychiatry, and Epidemiology, University of North Carolina at Chapel Hill, Chapel Hill, North Carolina

Marvin S. Swartz, M.D.
Professor and Head, Division of Social and Community Psychiatry, Department of Psychiatry and Behavioral Sciences, Duke University Medical Center, Durham, North Carolina

Carol A. Tamminga, M.D.
Communities Foundation of Texas Inc. Chair in Brain Science, Department of Psychiatry, The University of Texas Southwestern Medical Center, Dallas, Texas

Ming T. Tsuang, M.D., Ph.D., D.Sc.
University Professor, University of California; Distinguished Professor of Psychiatry and Director, Institute of Behavioral Genomics, Department of Psychiatry, University of California, San Diego; and Director, Harvard Institute of Psychiatric Epidemiology and Genetics

Elizabeth M. Tully, M.D.
NIMH Research Fellow, Yale University School of Medicine and PRIME Prodromal Research Clinic, New Haven, Connecticut

Karen Wohlheiter, M.S.
Director of Study Management, Division of Services Research, Department of Psychiatry, University of Maryland School of Medicine, Baltimore, Maryland

Jeffrey K. Yao, Ph.D., F.A.C.B.
Research Professor of Psychiatry and Pharmaceutical Sciences, University of Pittsburgh; VA Research Career Scientist, VA Pittsburgh Healthcare System, Pittsburgh, Pennsylvania

FOREWORD

Sir William Osler famously remarked, "The physician who knows syphilis, knows medicine." The similarly complex and protean features of schizophrenia suggest the parallel aphorism that the psychiatrist who knows schizophrenia knows psychiatry. Indeed, the finding of the World Health Organization that schizophrenia is the fifth leading cause of disability and premature mortality among *all* medical disorders in market economies underlines the importance of "knowing schizophrenia." The breadth and depth of the coverage of schizophrenia in this textbook clearly adds credence to this view and provides the reader with an interesting and rewarding exploration of the many facets of this challenging clinical syndrome.

The goal of "knowing schizophrenia" is facilitated for a wide range of readers by a number of important features of this textbook. This volume comprehensively reviews the relevant bodies of information needed for a thorough understanding of our current knowledge base of schizophrenia. Many of the chapters are coauthored by experts from different institutions and frequently from different countries. This approach helps provide both a broad and an integrated perspective on different aspects of the illness. Most chapters also have easily apprehended tables and figures that crisply summarize large bodies of literature or complex models.

Just how well do we "know schizophrenia"? Certainly, much remains to be learned, but as this textbook clearly lays out, a solid (and rapidly expanding) database regarding schizophrenia currently exists. The reader is invited to explore the complex array of genetic and environmental factors that confer risk for the illness, the biological mechanisms that appear to give rise to different aspects of its clinical features, and the range of clinical interventions available to manage individuals at different phases of the illness from the prodrome through chronicity. Although the growth rate of our knowledge of schizophrenia carries the inherent risk that a textbook on the disorder will quickly become out of date, in addition to containing timely information, this textbook provides the critical background material needed to understand and interpret new research findings as they arise and at the time of its publication is the best of its kind.

The accessibility of this textbook will enable a broad readership to increase their knowledge of schizophrenia. In learning about this illness, readers will be able to see, both in the specifics regarding schizophrenia and in the way that it provides a model for other mental disorders, how "knowing schizophrenia" facilitates a broader knowledge of psychiatry. Osler was right.

David A. Lewis, M.D.

PREFACE

Of the numerous mental and behavioral disorders with which psychiatrists and mental health care providers are confronted, none is more challenging and central to their mission than schizophrenia. This brain disorder strikes persons as they are entering the prime of their life and, in many cases, runs a recurrent and ultimately chronic course that leads to substantial disability. This most devastating of mental illnesses affects the essence of what makes people human: their personality and intellect. For these reasons schizophrenia is considered the prototypic mental illness.

Schizophrenia has been widely misunderstood. Common misconceptions include the belief that schizophrenia is characterized by a split or multiple personality or that it means holding two contradictory opinions simultaneously. Another inaccurate belief is that the mental state of schizophrenia is one of heightened creativity and originality—a unique and highly idiosyncratic way of apprehending reality that is unfettered by conventional thinking.

The perpetuation of these myths reflects the relatively low level of interest and importance that our society has accorded mental illnesses in general and schizophrenia in particular. However, this most prototypic of mental illnesses is a very costly and complex one for our society to deal with. A telling example of this can be found in the deinstitutionalization movement of the 1960s and 1970s, which dramatically reduced the mental hospital inpatient population, ostensibly in the interest of providing more humane community care. However, well intended this policy may have been, it resulted in the tragedy of the homeless and untreated mentally ill that played out on the streets of urban America and that remains unresolved.

The complexity of schizophrenia as well as its care provided the motivation to devote a whole volume to this singular disorder. The topics covered represent the most essential, timely, and informative aspects of this protean condition. There are many books about schizophrenia focusing on its theories, research, diagnosis, treatment, and clinical care. However, we felt that a textbook that encompassed the current state of knowledge of its cause, nature, treatment, and services was lacking and badly needed.

To fill this gap, we invited an eminent roster of experts in a wide range of disciplines from North America and Europe to join us in creating this work by authoring specific chapters. We are enormously grateful to them for their outstanding scholarly contributions. We hope that this textbook will serve as a fount of knowledge for the generations of students, scientists, and clinicians to come, who ultimately will dispel the mystery, discover the cause, and evoke the cure for schizophrenia.

Jeffrey A. Lieberman, M.D.
T. Scott Stroup, M.D., M.P.H.
Diana O. Perkins, M.D., M.P.H.

1

HISTORY OF SCHIZOPHRENIA AND ITS ANTECEDENTS

MICHAEL H. STONE, M.D.

If by *schizophrenia* we mean only the condition, or rather the *group* of conditions, described by Eugen Bleuler in 1911, or Kraepelin's *dementia praecox,* a term that appeared for the first time in the fourth edition of his textbook (Kraepelin 1893), then our history goes back only a scant 110 years. Yet there are other starting points for a history that would not do too much violence to the modern conception of schizophrenia. The description of *démence précoce* (1860) by Bénédict Morel (1809–1873), which influenced Kraepelin's choice of a diagnostic term, could also make for a reasonable beginning. Likewise, the earlier description of James Matthew Tilly's psychosis by John Haslam (1764–1844) in his *Illustrations of Madness* (Haslam 1810) accords well with our conception of paranoid schizophrenia and would allow our history to start in the early nineteenth century. If, however, we focus more narrowly on the *term* schizophrenia—or even on the *concept,* as adumbrated in works at the turn of the last century—we would have to agree with Hoenig (1995), who warns us: "In fact there cannot be a history of pre-Kraepelinian schizophrenia, because the concept did not exist" (p. 340).

Yet if we turn our attention instead to the primordial psychodiagnostic soup out of which schizophrenia was later to evolve, we can broaden our horizon from a mere two centuries to more than two millennia. To be sure, objections have been raised in recent years to any such expansion. For example, Hare (1988) of the Bethlem Royal Hospital in London advances the hypothesis that schizophrenia is a recent disease; that descriptions of similar disorders were rare before 1800; and that while the prevalence of insanity increased during the nineteenth century, it remained low in the non-Western world until the twentieth century—as though schizophrenia were an unfortunate by-product of modern Western civilization. This is the same chord struck by Fuller-Torrey (1980), who expressed doubt as to whether schizophrenia existed before the late-eighteenth-century Industrial Revolution in Europe. The views of these two authors address not so much the radical change in the *descriptions* of mental illness that grew out of the Age of Enlightenment as the possibility that the radical social changes of that period brought into being a condition that had not heretofore existed.

But the manner of describing mental illness did change dramatically in the eighteenth century. The centuries-old habits of the traditionalists, who clung to a Graeco-Roman taxonomy based on the four elements (earth, air, fire, and water) and their corresponding temperaments (melancholic, choleric, sanguine, and phlegmatic), gave way to the views of empiricists like Wilhelm

TABLE 1–1.   Pertinent attributes of the three main types of disorder

Condition	Attributes		
	Cognitive	**Affective**	**Behavioral**
Schizophrenia (quintessential cognitive disorder)	Loosening of associations; bizarre thoughts; formal thought disorder	Inappropriate affect; blunting or flattening of affect	Eccentric behavior; abulia
Manic-depression (quintessential affective disorder)	Grandiose vs. self-deprecatory thought; flight of ideas vs. impoverishment of thought	Euphoria vs. sadness; extraversion vs. despondency	Impetuosity, pacing, great energy vs. psychomotor retardation, lethargy
Psychopathy (quintessential behavioral disorder)	Grandiosity; contemptuousness; lack of foresight	Callousness; lack of compassion, empathy, or remorse	Predatoriness; scheming; exploitativeness; viciousness; "conning"

Griesinger (1817–1868) who paid attention to detailed descriptions of symptoms—on which their nosology was based (Griesinger 1861). As for the question of whether schizophrenia existed before 1800, the way out of this conundrum is to look at schizophrenia for what it is *au fond:* a form of "madness"—or psychosis—whose most striking features involve *cognition.* In contrast, mania and melancholia are madnesses of *affect,* and our current definition of psychopathy, since the publication of Cleckley's *Mask of Sanity* (1941), also depicts a madness of *behavior.* Here we have the tripartite division of mental function—an outgrowth of what was advanced in the eighteenth century by the philosopher Immanuel Kant (1724–1804). Kant (1781/2003) wrote of disorders of experience, judgment (leading to delusion), and reason (giving way to mania). If we reformulate the division in contemporary language, we have disorders of thinking, feeling (or mood/affect), and behaving. Note that each of the paradigmatic examples of disorders in these three mental compartments is accompanied by lesser degrees of disorders in the other two. Even persons with delusional disorder (which may be unrelated to schizophrenia) of the sort described by Kendler and colleagues (Kendler and Walsh 1995) show some peculiarities of affect—namely, feelings of inferiority (Kendler and Hays 1981) and of behavior. Table 1–1 lists some of the pertinent attributes in all three spheres, as routinely found in patients with schizophrenia, manic-depression, and psychopathy—none of which is a "pure" disorder.

With this model in mind, I believe we can fairly assume, even if we cannot rigorously prove, that various forms of *primarily cognitive* madness indeed antedated the clinical vignettes of Haslam (1809, 1810). Because the ancient descriptions of *affective* madness are closer to our own descriptions of them, even 2,500 years later we feel less uncomfortable writing about the history of mania and melancholia than about the history of schizophrenia (Stone 2006). This should not be surprising. Abnormalities of mood and behavior are often more noticeable, even to medically uninformed persons, than are many disorders or peculiarities of thought. The former may be visible from a distance (wild motions, hysterical sobbing, violent fury), whereas one has actually to talk with someone to realize that he is convinced that a collection of frogs has taken up residence in his stomach (a common delusion in the sixteenth century) or that a radio embedded in a tooth is broadcasting scurrilous messages about him (as a psychiatrist in our day might hear from a patient in the emergency room). Furthermore, the distinction between strange but widely shared beliefs and delusory ideas is not always easily made, and such beliefs may be culture-bound in ways that seem "crazy" to outsiders but quite normal to members of the group or cult. This makes it difficult to assess which prophets of doom or of the "Last Days," as found in the Bible or in certain religious groups in our own day, are truly delusional and which are otherwise normal persons who entertain shared, albeit incorrect, assumptions.

Before 1800, we must content ourselves with examples of *primarily cognitive* madness, where disorder of thought outweighs whatever peculiarities of emotion and behavior are simultaneously present. This focus will not limit us to descriptions (rarely found) that mirror contemporary accounts of schizophrenia. Observers in earlier times seldom paid attention to characteristics that are now considered crucial to the diagnosis of schizophrenia, and they often paid close attention to details that we regard as irrelevant.

COGNITIVE MADNESS
IN ANCIENT TIMES

BEFORE THE GRAECO-ROMAN PERIOD

Carlsson (2003) contends that documents from old Pharaonic Egypt, from the second millennium B.C., attest to such conditions as depression, dementia, and schizophrenia. These were understood as symptoms of the heart or uterus (the latter organ being implicated in the Greek conception of "hysteria"); in short, mental diseases were varieties of physical illness. Carlsson alludes to the Ebers papyrus (ca. 1550 B.C.), but this deals with internal medicine and medications, not with vignettes of persons considered mentally ill (Alexander and Selesnick 1966). Absent detailed descriptions of the patients who suffered from these conditions, we cannot equate any of them with schizophrenia. The Egyptians believed in a four-element system, similar to what the Greeks espoused later on: earth, air, fire, and water (the supposed components of flesh, breath, heart, and body fluids, respectively). Unlike the Greeks, they did not appear to assign particular temperaments to these elements.

As for the ancient Hebrews and those with whom they interacted, there are references to "madness" in the Bible, as in Deuteronomy 28:28 and 28:34: "the Lord will strike you with madness and blindness [vehayta *m'shuga* mimareya eynekha]." But the meaning of "madness" in this context is that of ranting and carrying on wildly (Lieber 2001), perhaps more in keeping with mania than with a cognitive psychosis.

Elsewhere, the sixth-century B.C. Babylonian king Nebuchadnezzar is punished for his arrogance by the Lord with a temporary madness, in which he "was driven from men, and did eat grass as oxen, and his body was wet with the dew of heaven, till his hairs were grown like eagles' feathers, and his nails like birds' claws" (Daniel 4:33). Alexander and Selesnick (1966) interpreted this as "lycanthropy," an affliction in which people wandered about at night in deserted places and howled like wolves (of which more in the section that follows). Some persons may have shown sustained forms of cognitive madness in Biblical times, but we see little sign of it in the scriptures. And what craziness there was, was ascribed to either punishment by God or infiltration of one's soul by the Devil. Madness (which usually had an affective quality) was not an internal condition so much as something visited on one by external forces, usually on account of one's sins. An exception to this rule might be made in the case of the prophets, some of whom were regarded as "mad" because of the strange warnings and predictions that they made and because of their unconventional behavior and attire. Ezekiel, to whom the Lord spoke, enjoining him to prophesy against the Houses of Judah and Israel for their wickedness, is an example. At one point Ezekiel hears the voice of the Lord say: "And thou shall eat [thy meat] as barley cakes, and thou shall bake it with dung that cometh out of man, in their [the Israelites'] sight" (Ezekiel 4:12). Zilboorg, in his *History of Medical Psychology* (1941), takes this as evidence of Ezekiel's "coprophagia." But this is unconvincing. Either Ezekiel did no such thing, or else he did so in the kind of ecstatic state of religious fervor that was culturally syntonic in his era—and therefore not to be construed, as such an act would be in our day, as the by-product of a cognitive psychosis. Cases of primarily cognitive madness, including those that were of early onset and chronic in course, may well have existed in biblical times, but we cannot point to any in the scriptural literature.

THE GRAECO-ROMAN PERIOD

Among the Greeks in Homeric times (tenth century B.C.), and for some centuries beyond, if people became mad it was for the same reason that was accepted in biblical times: the gods had willed it. Given the link between mental illness and the powers of divinity, temples of worship seemed like the logical venue for cure. For the Greeks, it was in the temples of Aesculapeus that the priestly adepts, with their secrets of healing, did their curative work. The transition from looking to the gods to looking to human nature for the explanation of mental phenomena was slow; traditional views lingered on in the works of the great Athenian playwrights of the fifth century B.C., Sophocles and Euripides. Their contemporary during this period of enlightenment, Hippocrates of Cos (460–377 B.C.), became the father of Greek medicine. He set about demystifying mental illness, writing in *The Sacred Disease*—another name for epilepsy—that the condition was no more divine than other diseases, but arose from a natural cause like other afflictions (Hippocrates 1952). Hippocrates subscribed to the prevailing theory of the Greek philosophers concerning the four elements of nature, earth, fire, air, and water, which in bodily terms corresponded, respectively, to the four *humours*: black bile, yellow bile, blood, and phlegm (in Latin, *pituita*). To these, in turn, corresponded the four *temperaments*: melancholic, choleric, sanguine, and phlegmatic. Exaggerations of these temperaments figured in Hippocrates's taxonomy of mental diseases: black bile was present in excess in *melancholia*; yellow bile, in *mania*—whose meaning at the time was closer to wrath (the root meaning of μηνις, *manis*) than to euphoria. Hippocrates also recognized *hysteria* and *paranoia*. The latter comes closest to our conception of a deteriorating cognitive illness such as would later, in the Roman world, come under the heading of *dementia*. In contrast to *amentia*, which implied that one was born without a properly functioning mind (as in mental retardation), *dementia* was reserved for conditions where one's mind had been normal in the beginning but then deteriorated at some point later in life. In Hippocrates's time, *paranoia*, if it could be demonstrated, was grounds for being declared incompetent and for the appointment of a legal guardian (Zilboorg 1941). At least some cases of paranoia, then, may have exemplified the chronic and primarily cognitive madness that we have posited as the precursor of what was, two millennia hence, to be called "schizophrenia." Socrates (another contemporary of Hippocrates) had apparently experienced auditory hallucinations in midlife, along with trance states in which he would remain standing motionless for hours on end. But this does not accord with our notion of schizophrenia, when we consider how lucid and well-functioning Socrates was apart from these transitory symptoms.

In contrast to Hippocrates, for whom the brain was the seat of the soul (and secreted the various humours), Aristotle (384–322 B.C.) regarded the heart as the seat of the soul. Blood determined the force of the soul: if warm and mobile, the soul was strong and wise. If too moist and dense, the soul was weak and fragile. The optimal soul was likened to solar (and "masculine") light, that of the lunatic literally to lunar light, which was soft, weak, pale, moist, and "female." Persons who were "hebephrenic" were small, weak, and timid (Howells 1993). *Hebephrenia* here did not signify a subtype of schizophrenia (that would await a reuse of the term by Hecker [1871]), but rather the foolish, immature, or dull mind of a youth (ηβη, *hebe*).

According to the Stoic philosophers (who flourished from the time of Zeno, ca. 300 B.C., to that of Seneca, in the first century A.D.), melancholy arose out of sadness and anger; mania, out of hate and wrath. They spoke of an *active* principle, πνευμα (*pneuma*) or "vital breath," which is given form by being adjoined to *passive* matter. The faster, hotter, and more subtle the pneuma, the higher the psychic functions it could sustain. The "foolish" person is affected by a pneuma charged with humoural substances put into circulation by exaggerated emotional reactions. In the Stoic theory, there is still acceptance of the four humours, but a greater importance is given to the emotions themselves. A sane person was seen as having a strong and fearless soul, whereas the soul of a foolish person was "irrational" (a hint of cognitive impairment, but one that was not explicated further by clinical example). One of the major figures of the Middle Stoa was Posidonius of Apamea (135–51 B.C.), who recognized a fundamental distinction between reason and the irrational

aspects of the soul. The rules of physics, according to Posidonius, can be translated into the laws of psychology, creating the foundation for ethics and rules of conduct (Theosophy Library Online 2003).

Aesclepiades of Prusa, in the first century B.C., used *mania* in a more global sense to include paranoia (a more cognitive disorder) as well. This is reminiscent of our own tendency to speak of *madness* in everyday parlance as the general term for severe mental illnesses (psychoses)—as if being wildly and uncontrollably mad (the root meaning of μηνις, as in the *Iliad*'s "wrath of Achilles") was the quintessential form of "craziness."

Greece by this period having passed its zenith, the authors of importance stemmed either from Greek-speaking or Latin-speaking countries. Aulus Cornelius Celsus (25 B.C.–50 A.D.) described epileptic "madness," hebetude, phrenitis (which involved fever and inflammation of the brain as the primary cause of mental derangement), hysteria, melancholy, and wrathful as well as euphoric manias; in addition, he described *alienation* that might be accompanied by visual or auditory hallucinations and might be found in young persons (Celsus 1528). Here we have an intimation of dementia praecox, although without the detailed clinical descriptions that would allow us more meaningful comparison between the ancient and the modern forms of cognitive madness. Celsus also wrote of paranoid illnesses that had been called παραφροσυνη (*paraphrosune*) by Hippocrates, and later by Galen when speaking of the chronic form. The lexical meaning is that of mental *derangement*.

The physician of this early period next most famous after Hippocrates was Claudius Galen of Pergamum (129–199 A.D.). Galen is known not so much for the originality of his ideas as for his methodical collection of medical thought from the time of Hippocrates to Galen's own time, from which he created his massive compendium (Galen 1551).

Galen accepted humoural theory but applied it less strictly than had his predecessors. Black bile was still the prime factor in melancholy, but excess yellow bile was responsible for both mania and phrenitis. Galen described, under the heading of *morositas*, a deadening of the emotional life (in the absence of delirium) that shares some features with dementia praecox. Lexically, morositas conveys more the quality of peevishness or sourness. Galen divided mental life into the attributes of imagination, reason, and memory. The symptoms we associate with schizophrenia, such as catatony and paranoia (*paraphrosune*) derived supposedly from interference with the imaginative function. Behavior that departed from social custom was considered *alienation*, particularly if the behavior was bizarre. Related to this term was the label *alienist*—

current well into the nineteenth century—for physicians who treated mental illness.

Aretaeus of Cappadocia (modern Turkey), presumably a contemporary of Galen (both were in the tradition of Hippocrates), was a physician who wrote a comprehensive textbook of medicine, part of which was devoted to mental illness. He used the word *melancholy* to denote, as we still do, a depressive condition. But all other forms of "madness" he referred to as *mania*. He believed there was, indeed, one entity called *insanity*, under which heading came many other variants: paranoid delirious insanity, dysthymia (a term he used to describe "low spirits"), fanaticism (which he ascribed to excess religious devotion), catatonic or stuporous delirium, and hebetude. Some manic patients, he mentioned, are "given to extraordinary phantasies; for one is afraid that some oil-flasks might fall…and another will not drink, as fancying himself a brick, and fearing lest he should be dissolved by the liquid" (Aretaeus 1856, p. 302). Aretaeus also describes certain young persons who imagine themselves poets or philosophers. The one case he relates at some length is that of a carpenter who worked well and skillfully while working in the house he was building. But once he left his work and was out of the sight of others, he would become "completely mad"— yet if he returned to work, he quickly regained his reason (p. 302). Unfortunately, we are not given any more information about the nature of his madness. But from the above-mentioned catalog of conditions, it seems apparent that Aretaeus was aware of several types of primarily cognitive madness, such as paranoid and delusory states and fanaticism. It is not clear how the patients who exemplified these labels would be diagnosed if transported magically into our time and evaluated by current DSM criteria.

These rapid and puzzling shifts between normality and some sort of delusory state are reminiscent of a man mentioned by the poet Horace in his *Epistles* [1926, II:2]. This is the description in brief:

> Once at Argos there was a man of some rank, who used to fancy that he was listening to wonderful tragic actors, while he sat happy and applauded in the empty theater— a man who would correctly perform all other duties of life, a most worthy neighbor, an amiable host, kind to his wife….This man was cured by his kinsmen's help and care, but when he had driven out the malady…and come to himself again, he cried: "Egad, you have killed me, my friends, not saved me; for thus you have robbed me of a pleasure and taken away perforce the dearest illusion of my heart." (pp. 128–129)

Because he functioned so well in all other spheres of life, and even knew that what was so pleasurable for him was in fact an illusion, we can only say that he labored under some cognitive peculiarity (Esquirol might have called it a form of monomania), although one that was so circumscribed and nondisabling as not to resemble dementia praecox or schizophrenia.

Because the belief that the Devil could transform people into wolves (lycanthropes) was widespread in the ancient period, we cannot claim it was a *cognitive madness* to entertain such a notion. A physician of the third century, Marcellus, of whom we learn through the writings of a Galenist, Oribasius (323–400), described lycanthropy, citing cases of persons who would wander about during the night, usually in cemeteries, howling like wolves (Zilboorg 1941). It might be a less daring speculation to ascribe a primarily cognitive madness to the deluded persons who fancied themselves wolves, but even this is uncertain because we are given so few clinical hooks on which to hang such a diagnosis. Belief in lycanthropy was not to die out for another 1,500 years. During the days of the Spanish Inquisition and beyond, one could find physicians who, while doubting that the Devil could literally turn a person into a wolf, nevertheless believed that he could deceive certain persons into thinking that they had been so transformed, whereafter they behaved as wolves do (LeLoyer 1605; Sennert 1666).

In the sixth century A.D., during the height of the Byzantine empire, Aetius of Amida (527–565), who was personal physician to Emperor Justinian, wrote of dementia in young people who had previously had modest but intact minds but who subsequently appeared demented, but not delirious. That is, they showed deterioration of mental function without fever or clouding of consciousness. Galen's views on melancholia have come down to us via the works of Aetius (Zilboorg 1941).

Also in Byzantium, Alexander of Tralles (525–605) from Lydia (now Turkey) used *melancholy* as a catchall term for all forms of insanity but still ascribed the differences in the various forms to imbalances in the four humours. He spoke of more complex situations where different combinations of humoural abnormalities accounted for variations in the clinical picture. Incoherent speech and laziness in the young, for example, stemmed supposedly from abnormal amounts of both black bile and phlegm. Although we do not have sufficient information to judge how close this picture was to our dementia praecox of adolescence, Alexander did describe a syndrome characterized by emotional blunting, apathy, abulia, and negativism (refusal to answer questions) (Howells 1993). Another type of insanity was that of paranoia whose course ended in dementia. Still another was that of mystical and religious "deliria," perhaps akin to the schizophrenia-like display of paranoia and religious delusions depicted in the early nineteenth century by Karl Ideler (1841) as "religiöser Wahnsinn" ["religious madness"].

The last of the great physicians of Byzantium was Paul of Aegina (629–690) of the Alexandrian school in Egypt. He worked also in Asia Minor and is of particular importance in that he transmitted classical Graeco-Roman medical knowledge to the Arab scholars who had begun to rise to prominence in the decades following the death of Mohammad (632) and the rapid expansion of Islam. Although primarily a surgeon, he turned some attention to mental illnesses, describing such entities as catatony and demonic possession (including cases where patients felt themselves influenced by the divine and gifted with the power of prophesy). Negativistic or (as we would think of them) catatonic cases of the type mentioned by Alexander of Tralles were ascribed by Paul to damage of the phlegm in the rear ventricle of the brain. Such patients would remain immobile in whatever position they had been placed, seeming scarcely to breathe, and would refuse food.

ISLAMIC PHYSICIANS OF THE MEDIEVAL PERIOD

Having taken Alexandria in 640, the Arab armies had, by 711, conquered Egypt, Babylonia (coextensive with modern Iraq), Persia, Syria, and, in the West, the Maghreb (northern Africa) and most of Spain. Persian and Arab medicine began to supplant Graeco-Roman medicine, while having borrowed from it extensively. Although the Islamic physicians were strongly influenced by Aristotle, Hippocrates, and Galen, they added to the catalog of mental illnesses some syndromes not hitherto described. For the most part, however, they were known more for their extensive compilations and their recommendations about treatment than for originality of ideas in the domain of what would later (in the early nineteenth century) be called *psychiatry*.

Among the important physicians of this early Islamic period were Rhazes of Baghdad (860–930) and his contemporary Najab ud-din Unhammad. Najab is credited with having described some thirty diseases of the mind, subsumed under nine different headings. Most of these were variants of mania and a form of depression called "lovesickness" (*ishk* in Arabic). Among the disorders described, the closest one to the notion of a cognitive disorder is a disease in which the patient imagines himself possessed by a demon or spirit (*jinn*); this may end in a chronic form of madness (*janoon*) characterized by restlessness, taciturnity, and aggressiveness.

The most famous name among the medieval Islamic physicians is that of the Persian-born Avicenna (980–1037), whose eclecticism and industriousness as a compiler of all medical knowledge mirror those same qualities in Galen. Melancholia, for Avicenna, was still a condition of black bile, whose origin was in the area below the diaphragm (i.e., the hypo-chondria: below the rib cage), in the stomach, liver, or spleen. The supernatural played no role in Avicenna's psychology: he did not accept the notion of "demons" as playing any role in mental illness. Mania and melancholy are given more detailed treatment in Avicenna's *Canon* (1999), but there is little that suggests primarily cognitive disorders.

The last of the great Islamic physicians who influenced Western European medicine were the Spanish Moors Avenzoar of Seville (1091?–1162) and his pupil Averrhoës of Cordoba (1126–1198). Avenzoar was in contact with the French physicians of Montpellier. In his view, insanity resulted from weakening of the heat of the blood, rendering the brain cool and moist—an idea borrowed from Aristotle.

MEDIEVAL AND RENAISSANCE EUROPE

The *Reconquista*, completed by the expulsion of the Moors from Granada in 1492, put Western Europe back under Christian control and led to the resurgence of European physicians, who dominated medical thought in the succeeding centuries.

But freedom of thought was for a long time hampered by the preoccupation of the Church with heresy and with the persecution, whether as infidels or as witches, of those suspected of heretical thought. No nice distinctions were made between delusion and "improper thought," such that some were considered "mad" who were merely freethinkers or otherwise unconventional. And if such madness offended the Church, sorry fates awaited: at best, excommunication; at worst, burning at the stake. The empiricism of the Graeco-Roman and Arab physicians gave way once again to belief in external causes of madness, such as possession by demons or the work of the Devil. Thus in fifteenth-century Europe, for example, persons who saw visions or heard voices were apt to be persecuted as witches—although some of them may have exemplified the elusive cognitive madness we have been at pains to trace.

Voices of reason were still heard during this time. Bartholomaeus Anglicus in the thirteenth century expressed the view that madness came sometimes from the passions of the soul, from sorrow or dread or excessive study, or sometimes from strong drink (Howells 1993). In the early fourteenth century Bernard de Gordon (ca. 1258–1318) spoke of a juvenile *stoliditas* in which young persons mouthed empty words in sentences that trailed off, as if they did not know what they were saying. Again, the description is skimpy, so we cannot tell definitively whether this *stoliditas* overlapped significantly with our (juvenile) dementia praecox.

So long as the causes of mental illness were sought in imbalances of the humours, in demonic possession, or in abnormalities of the brain ventricles, little attention was paid to mental patients as *individuals* with life histories that may have played a role in their illness, or as persons who came from families with similar conditions. We know much more of the lives of kings and queens than we do of people in ordinary life. But now and again we get glimpses of what must be familial madness or of life stories that probably helped to launch, if not cause altogether, a case of lunacy or insanity—as psychosis would then have been called. Here we can cite the story of two fifteenth-century kings: Charles VI of France (1368–1422) and his grandson, Henry VI of England (1422–1471). Charles became ill at age 24, making silly remarks and acting in an undignified manner. He became violent when warned of treason and killed four innocent people with his own sword. He recovered and relapsed at yearly intervals, now remembering who he and his family members were, now forgetting them all, including himself (he called himself "George"), and he would run about wildly and act obscenely. He ultimately became indifferent to all, listless, and self-mutilative. Later, his pious, weak-willed grandson, Henry, went mad at age 31 and lost his memory, only to recover briefly before succumbing again, hearing voices and seeing visions. He may have lapsed into a catatonic-like stupor. Eventually he was imprisoned in the Tower of London and murdered there in 1471 by Edward IV, the son of Richard of York (Howells 1993). Although cognitive distortions were present, the recurring nature of these psychotic conditions puts one more in mind of bipolar mania. Unlike our typical manic patient, however, Henry VI was a simple and deeply religious man who hated violence and whose disposition was not stormy or volatile. Some have considered his illness as akin to our catatonic schizophrenia. As with other "mad" persons of this era, we do not have enough details to say whether Henry's illness was primarily cognitive or affective.

A century later, we encounter the extraordinary Hungarian countess Erzsébet Báthory (1560–1614) and her relatives (Penrose 1996). In a sort of midlife crisis after the death of her husband in 1604, having become worried lest her beauty decline with age, the countess took to having her servants waylay young girls from the countryside and transport them to her castle. There she would have them suspended on hooks, whereupon she would slit open their abdomens, press her body against that of the dying girls (experiencing orgasm as she did so), and then collect their blood in a tub so that she might preserve her beauty by bathing in the blood of virgins. Her moods were said to have fluctuated with the cycle of the moon; she was also given to headaches that led to "fits of possession," which have been viewed as epileptic seizures. Her uncle, Stephen Báthory, king of Poland, also had epileptic seizures. Her brother, Istvan, was "half-mad," extraordinarily cruel like his sister, and insatiable sexually ("satyriasis"). Another uncle, also named Istvan, confused summer and winter and rode around in a sleigh in July, his servants scattering white sand along his path to simulate snow. He was also known for his cruelty. A cousin, Gábor, complained of being poisoned by the Devil. And her paternal aunt, Klara, killed her first two husbands and had her lover killed, skewered, and roasted on a spit. Whether Erzsébet's madness can be assigned to epilepsy alone, for which there seemed to be a hereditary tendency, is hard to say. What seems indisputable is that there was a strong cognitive component to the madness, not only in her but in other members of her family, independent of whether the illness was primarily cognitive (hence closer to our schizophrenia) or affective (like our bipolar illness).

Johann Weyer (1515–1588), whom some consider the father of modern psychiatry (an appellation others reserve for Pinel), is important to our story not for having described a schizophrenia-like form of madness so much as for having debunked the notion of witches, sorcerers, and devils in his famous monograph *De Praestigiis Daemonum* (Weyer 1564). Fortunately, Weyer lived near the Dutch border, outside the pale of the Inquisition; otherwise, he would have paid with his life for his heretical assertions. It was Weyer's courage that paved the way for a more rational understanding of severe mental illness; gradually the burning of "witches" was replaced by the humane treatment of those mentally ill persons who were no longer regarded as instruments of the Devil. Some physicians occupied a middle position, elaborating more modern conceptions of mental illness based on their own observations yet still willing to ascribe the conditions partly to the work of the Devil. The Swiss Felix Platter (1536–1614) is an example. He felt that heredity played a role in certain disorders, and lesions of the brain in others, but he also clung to the Galenic notion of humoural imbalance as a factor. Some cases of mania he felt were caused by poisons (Platter 1602) and others by the bite of a rabid dog. He actually spent time in the dungeons where the insane were kept in his town, learning of their illnesses at first hand. Platter used the term *mentis alienatio* (alienation of the mind) in referring to the condition of certain persons interned in the dungeons.

THE SEVENTEENTH AND EIGHTEENTH CENTURIES: THE ENLIGHTENMENT

The eighteenth-century European philosophical movement known as the Enlightenment had its roots in the scientific revolution of the seventeenth century and in the ideas of Locke and Newton. Reason became the guide to all knowledge and all human concerns. The authority of the Church had grown weaker, thanks in part to the easier availability of books (after Gutenberg's press came into use in the mid-fifteenth century) and to the Protestant Reformation.

The Enlightenment gained momentum in the eighteenth century with the stimulus of Rousseau and Voltaire. The American and French revolutions gave further impetus to the ideals of freedom and liberty. The authority of the nobility also diminished; the voice of the individual, including the individual in ordinary circumstances, was heard as never before. Toward the end of the eighteenth century, the voice of the individual with mental illness was also heard for the first time.

Attachment to humoural theory was still a prominent feature of seventeenth-century medicine, dwindling only gradually with the passage of time. The physician to Louis XIV, Lazarus Riverius (1589–1655), for example, recognized an abbreviated nosology consisting of three disorders: phrenitis, mania, and melancholy (Sedler 1993). Cognitive abnormalities were present in both mania and melancholy, and thus disorders that might have approximated our concept of schizophrenia could have been grouped in either category.

The delusions associated with melancholy resemble those of our psychotic depression: some patients felt they had been changed into corn and might be eaten by hens; others, that they were made of melting wax and must avoid the fire; still others fancied themselves dead and would neither eat nor drink. There were those who tried not to urinate lest the world be drowned in a second deluge.

The Scottish physician Sir Richard Napier (1559–1634) became a celebrated healer who treated thousands of patients during his long career (Macdonald 1981). He described madness of two main types: violent and nonviolent. The latter type was subdivided into madnesses of thought, mood, and action—the classical tripartite attributes of mind. If any syndrome resembling schizophrenia were present among his cases, it would belong to his *thought-madness* category. Some of Napier's patients were frankly delusional; they might act in a frantic manner, rant incomprehensibly, laugh strangely, and at times act violently. If we try to superimpose on Napier's roster our schemata of idiopathic, genetically based schizophrenia,

with phenotypes existing alongside a proportion of "phenocopies" caused by endocrine disorders, viral infections, neurosyphilis, and frontal lobe tumors (as in the case of George Gershwin's temporal glioma—which had been treated as if "paranoid schizophrenia"), we can appreciate how difficult it is to make sense of the seventeenth-century cases. For in amongst the true cases of idiopathic cognitive madness, there must have been patients with head injury, viral brain disease, endocrine disorders, smallpox, and a host of other phenocopies, making it impossible to tease out the genuine cases (which we now acknowledge as having a biological basis) from those stemming from brains that were grossly injured or diseased. Cultural factors are another confounding element. In an age when respect for one's parents was obligatory, even if one had been grossly mistreated, someone who complained bitterly about his or her parents was considered "mad" (somewhat analogously to Russian citizens being considered "soft schizophrenics" if, before 1989, they spoke out against the Communist regime) (Jablensky 2000).

Napier's empiricism represents a refreshing change from the Galenic traditions in which physicians of the mentally ill had remained mired for so many centuries. But it was the more famous English empiricist Thomas Willis (1621–1675), discoverer of the eponymous "Circle of Willis" arterial circuit at the base of the brain, who described a clinical picture that seems familiar to us as juvenile dementia praecox. Here is the passage from his major work *De Anima Brutorum* (Willis 1672):

> There are many clear causes by which dullness may be induced in a number of formerly healthy persons. These persons, who once upon a time were clever and gifted, gradually become, without any great changes in their way of life, duller (*hebetiores*), and indeed foolish and insipid....A good number, having been to a high degree intelligent during childhood, and extremely quick to learn, end up in adolescence enfeebled and dull. Where they were handsome in aspect before, they are now without gracefulness or pleasant demeanor. (p. 509, my translation)

We would feel on more secure ground in calling such cases "schizophrenic" if Willis had added examples of delusional thinking and auditory hallucinations. But he was mainly a neurologist, attuned to the more readily discernible signs in the domains of affect and action.

Toward the end of the seventeenth century the author of the first English treatise on dermatology, Daniel Turner (1667–1741), wrote, in a book devoted to syphilis, of a married man who was convinced he had contracted this disease from a woman he had had relations with some 9 years earlier. The extract in Hunter and Macalpine (1963) shows the evolution of the man's illness as it worsened from the level of an obsession (specifically, syphilophobia) to a fixed delusional state from which no remedy available to Dr. Turner could restore him. He ended his days at the home of a relative, speaking to no one and checking himself constantly in the mirror to see that his nose had not yet fallen off from the (imaginary) disease. The distinction between severe obsessive-compulsive disorder and schizophrenia is not always easy even in our day. Without either the neuroleptics or the serotonin reuptake blockers that would become available 300 years later, this man's condition simply ran its malignant course: a primarily cognitive "madness," by all appearances—though whether schizophrenia or obsessive-compulsive disorder we cannot say for sure.

By the middle of the eighteenth century, although terms like *melancholy*, *mania*, and *lunacy* were still part of their vocabulary, physicians who treated the mentally ill no longer invoked humoural theory as explanatory. William Battie (1703–1776), who wrote the first textbook of psychiatry in the English language (Battie 1758), became the governor of Bethlem Hospital, where he instituted many reforms to improve the treatment of the insane. (A corruption of the name *Bethlem*, by the way, has given us our word *bedlam*, as a synonym for chaos and wild disorder—presumably a common state of affairs in places that housed the severely mentally ill.) Battie spoke of "deluded imagination," which for him was an essential characteristic of madness: one that "precisely discriminates this from all other animal disorders—or that man alone is properly mad, who is fully and unalterably persuaded of the existence or the appearance of any thing, which does either not exist or does not actually appear to him, and who behaves according to such erroneous persuasion" (Battie 1758, p. 6). Battie's description is that of a *primarily cognitive* madness—although in the absence of other distinguishing characteristics, the condition is compatible with either our schizophrenia or bipolar mania. Battie makes a useful discrimination between what he called *original* and *consequential* madness:

> There is reason to fear that Madness is Original, when it neither follows nor accompanies any accident, which may justly be deemed its external and remoter cause. Secondly, there is more reason to fear that, whenever this disorder is hereditary, it is Original.…Thirdly, we may affirm that Madness is Original, when it both ceases and appears afresh without any assignable cause.… Madness [that] is *consequential* to other disorders or external causes…now and then admits to relief by the removal or correction of such disorders or causes. (pp. 59–61)

Schizophrenia of insidious onset and positive family history would be classified, in Battie's schema, as a form of "original madness."

In the latter part of the eighteenth century, Thomas Arnold (1742–1816), another English physician and the owner of a large private "madhouse," is known to us primarily for his two-volume treatise on the classification of mental illnesses (Arnold 1782). His main categories—ideal insanity and notional insanity—both contain subgroups manifesting some primarily cognitive and some primarily affective or even behavioral abnormalities. By *ideal* he meant having to do with abnormal ideas and disturbances of memory; by *notional* he referred to more fully fleshed-out delusions, fancies, and whims. But abnormalities of personality that we would regard as narcissistic or psychopathic were also placed in the "notional" category. The more clearly cognitive form of madness he placed under the "delusive" type of notional insanity: "[W]ith the sound and unimpaired use, in every other respect, of the rational faculties…the Patient is under the Influence of the most Palpable, and extraordinary Delusion…such as having imagined himself to be dead" (Vol. 1, p. 135).

The Scottish physician William Cullen (1710–1790), to whom we owe the term *neurosis*, advocated the use of another term, *vesania*, for disorders of the intellectual functions (Cullen 1784). Cullen introduced the term *paranoia* into the English literature, as a by-product of his conviction that the time had come for a new nosology based on the advances in his day in both pathology and clinical observation (Hunter and Macalpine 1963). He reserved *vesania* for "lesions of the judging faculty." When these deficits occurred in the absence of fever or obtunding disorders of the brain, Cullen preferred the term *insanity*, a concept that comes close to the future descriptions of schizophrenia. Missing from Cullen's book are any illustrative clinical vignettes that would allow us to estimate the degree of concordance between his nosology and ours.

THE NINETEENTH CENTURY

The waning years of the eighteenth and the beginning years of the nineteenth century witnessed a sea change in the way the mentally ill were seen and described. These years correspond to the period of Romanticism. This movement placed the individual at the center of his or her own world and encouraged the free expression of feelings and emotion. The works of Goethe (especially his novel *The Sorrows of Young Werther*) and Byron, and in music those of Schumann and Chopin, are exemplars of Romanticism. Paralleling this change in society was the change in psychiatry, where detailed descriptions of mentally ill patients, and even of their early life histories, began to appear in the pages of the prominent authors of this new period.

The term *psychiatry* itself, originated by Johann Reil (1759–1813) in his *Rhapsodien* (1803), became accepted into common medical parlance; likewise, *alienist* gave way to *psychiatrist* as a name for the practitioner.

Arguably, the first case from the past that strikes the contemporary ear as a genuine example of schizophrenia is that of a patient in Bethlem Hospital. Confidentiality about patients' names was not yet mandatory, so we know the patient by name: James Tilly Matthews. His family had hired lawyers in hopes of having him released; he had been in Bethlem already 13 years when Haslam wrote up the case (which tells us something about the course of illness). Here are some of the comments from Haslam's lengthy description:

> Mr. Matthews insists that in some apartment near London Wall, there is a gang of villains profoundly skilled in Pneumatic Chemistry, who assail him by means of an Air Loom. The assailants of the gang use different preparations for the purposes of "assailment" [Matthews's term for the ways in which the gang harass him]: Seminal fluid, male and female—effluvia of copper—ditto of sulphur—the vapours of vitriol and aqua fortis—effluvia of dogs—stinking human breath—stench of the cesspool [the list goes on]. [The operations that the gang perform on Matthews consist of:] "*fluid locking*" by which the readiness of speech is impeded, "*cutting soul from sense*" so that the sentiments of the heart can have no communication with the operations of the intellect; "*stone-making*"—forming a calculus in the bladder of any person impregnated; "*thigh-talking*" where the gang contrives to direct their voice-sayings to the external part of the thigh, so that the organ of hearing is lodged in that situation; "*thought-making*"—while one of these villains is sucking at the brain of the person assailed, to extract his existing sentiments, another of the gang…will force into his mind a train of ideas very different from the real subject of his thoughts. …" (Haslam 1810, pp. 20–35, but the list of infernal machines goes on for many pages)

Although Schneider's "first-rank symptoms" (1959) (among them, thought withdrawal and thought broadcast; see Table 1–2) are not as "pathognomonic" of schizophrenia as Schneider had asserted (Carpenter et al. 1973), since they can occur in mania as well, Matthews's prolonged course of psychosis and the bizarre twists to his paranoid thoughts—including the "Schneiderian" abnormalities—make a powerful argument that Matthews was indeed *schizophrenic* by modern criteria.

In France, Jean Etienne Esquirol (1772–1840) may well have seen similar patients, but he still used broad terms like *mania* in ways that covered both the affective and the cognitive psychoses. He mentioned in his great 1838 text, for example, that "maniacs are remarkable for their false sensations, illusions, and hallucinations, and for the improper associations of ideas, which are reported

TABLE 1–2. "Pathognomonic" symptoms of schizophrenia, as formulated by Kurt Schneider

A. Hallucinatory

  1. Patient hears hallucinatory voices speaking his thoughts aloud.

  2. Patient experiences himself as the subject about whom hallucinatory voices are arguing or discussing.

  3. Patient hears hallucinatory voices describing his activity as it takes place.

B. Delusional

  4. A normal perception is followed by a delusional interpretation of a highly personalized significance.

C. Pertaining to ego boundary

  5. The patient is a passive and reluctant recipient of bodily sensation imposed from the outside (Somatic Passivity).

  6. The experience of one's own thoughts as though they were put in one's mind by an external force (Thought Insertion).

  7. Patient believes his thoughts are being removed from his mind by some external agency (Thought Withdrawal).

  8. The experience of one's thoughts being magically transmitted to others (Thought Broadcast).

  9. Affects experienced as controlled externally.

  10. Impulses experienced as controlled externally.

  11. Motor activity experienced as controlled externally.

Source. Schneider 1959.

with great rapidity and without order or connection" (Esquirol 1838, Vol. 2, pp. 132–133). Furthermore, mania is distinct from monomania, in that there is a disruption (*bouleversement*) of *all* the intellectual faculties, rather than just of one as in the monomanias. Esquirol also spoke of *délire* as primarily a disturbance of perception, as when a person's ideas are not in keeping with his or her perceptions—the most common cause of which is hallucinations (Berrios and Porter 1995). This notion of a *split* between different agencies of the mind is reminiscent of the split Bleuler would later speak of between thought and affect. Others used the term *délire* in a different way: for Étienne-Jean Georget (1820), it signified either a disorder of the intellect or an illness of the brain. For permanent conditions, such as that of Haslam's patient, Georget used *folie*—a term as general and vague in outline as *délire*. As Berrios and Porter point out, by the late-middle nineteenth century the notion of an *Einheitspsychose* (see Zeller 1844) had become popular; according to this notion there was but *one* psychosis, with a variety of outward differences attributable to environmental and other factors.

Zeller's position is echoed in the remarks of Heinrich Neumann (1814–1884), a contemporary of Morel and Griesinger, who in his unhappiness with the existing classificatory systems also insisted: "There is but one type of mental disturbance and we call it insanity" (Neumann 1859, p. 167). This view seems like a return to the taxonomy of Aretaeus, for whom (besides melancholy) there was only *mania* in its multiple forms.

What was becoming clear in the early part of mid-nineteenth century was that the cross-sectional view of mental illness—the display of symptoms at a given point in time—might not be the most reliable index of the underlying condition. We now begin to see increasing interest in the longitudinal view: the *onset, course*, and *outcome* of the condition in question. In Haslam's patient, for example, it was the chronic, malignant, and unvarying course of the illness that gave it the stamp of schizophrenia rather than of mania or some other psychosis. These are the features that Kraepelin would emphasize in his description of *dementia praecox* at the end of the nineteenth century.

Kraepelin's term, as noted above, derived from the *démence précoce* of Morel, for whom mental disease represented the breakdown in the unitary, coherent functioning of the three mental compartments, "feeling, understanding, and acting" (i.e., affect, thought and behavior). Morel saw mental illness as the result of hereditary weakness and drew attention to the "degeneration" observable in the forebears of his *démence précoce* patients, whose fathers were often addicted to alcoholic or narcotics (Morel 1860). The patients Morel described under this heading were generally adolescents or young adults. Influenced by Darwin, Morel looked in his young patients for physical signs of malformations and peculiarities that might represent inherited features that were associated with the early onset of mental deterioration.

For much of the second half of the nineteenth century, many of the important contributors to our understanding of schizophrenia were German. To put their ideas in perspective, it will be helpful to look at the work of their predecessor Karl Ideler (1795–1860), director of psychiatry at Berlin's Charité Hospital. Ideler was one of the first in psychiatry to show a strong interest in the psychology of his patients: the ways in which their early experience shaped the direction of their thoughts, and their illnesses, when they later succumbed to mental disorders. To this end he wrote a series of lengthy biographies of mental patients (Ideler 1841). There had been an earlier collection of such biographies during this Romantic period by a lay author, Christian Spiess (1796), but Ideler may be the first psychiatrist to give us such accounts. More remarkably, Ideler also mentions in his biographies some of the traumas suffered by his patients in their childhood—including physical abuse by a parent. His are some of the earliest such descriptions in the psychiatric literature. Case #9 of the Biographies, for example, concerns a woman, born in 1805, whose father was an alcoholic miller—physically abusive both to his wife and his daughter. The daughter leaves home at age 15 to do house-service in various homes, and later she marries a "wild drunkard" who periodically smashes glassware and throws the pieces at her. She has two children by him, endures his abuse for 4 years, and then contemplates divorce. At that point she has a religious delusion in which

> an angel in the form of a winged 12-year old boy enters her house, telling her that he has come from God in order to announce to her that she should divorce her husband, that all her sins are forgiven, and that she has been sent to all mankind to bring to them penance and conversion. Filled with joy, she is about to take the angel by the arm to caress him, when he flies out the window. (Ideler 1841, p. 184, my translation).

Remaining entrenched in this delusion for some 5 years, the woman is eventually admitted to the Charité Hospital, where she continues to have religious delusions as well as dreams in which God commands her to preach to the people. Ideler saw as the force behind her delusion the irreconcilable conflict between her sense of holiness and her feeling of sinfulness for having divorced, having been raised to believe it was God's will that a wife remain with her husband.

Because her delusion was circumscribed, not as all-encompassing as Matthews's, it might be considered a religious-type *monomanie* by Esquirol, and perhaps an "atypical schizophrenia" or "schizoaffective disorder" under current criteria.

We do not again encounter this fine sensitivity to the psychodynamics until Freud's time. For Ideler's successor at the Charité, Griesinger, mental disease was brain disease; psychiatry and neurology were one. He had no patience for what could not be observed directly; his was a psychiatry without psychology and represented a total break with the spirit of Ideler and the Romantics. Griesinger, a pupil of Ernst Zeller (1804–1877), at first recognized only affective and reversible disorders as "primary." But after hearing a lecture by Ludwig Snell in 1865 on "monomania as the primary form of mental disturbance," Griesinger found himself in agreement, and in a subsequent lecture of his own in 1867 he spoke of *primäre Verrücktheit* (primary insanity)—the same idea as Snell's (Janzarik 1987). It was at this point, a year before his death, that Griesinger gave up the traditional system of classification in favor of the newer one, where "insanity could become manifest even in the absence of (previous) melancholia or mania" (Janzarik 1987, p. 11). This new approach paved the way for Griesinger's pupil, Kraepelin, to rework the idea of a primary cognitive psychosis into his concept of dementia praecox.

The division of psychotic disorders into two broad groups, the *affective* (represented by melancholy and mania) and the *cognitive* (as dementia praecox or, later, schizophrenia), was hampered in Griesinger's day and for a few decades beyond by the way in which "mania" continued to spill over conceptually into the cognitive area (as *Wahnsinn* or madness). It took some time for psychiatry to accept the more restricted use of the terms *melancholy* and *mania* to refer only to affective psychoses—even though the groundwork had been laid in the 1850s, after Jean-Pierre Falret (with his *folie circulaire*) and Jules Baillarger (with his *folie à double forme*) had emphasized the commonality and interchangeability between the "up" and "down" forms of affective illness.

What one saw instead in the years between Griesinger and Kraepelin was the proliferation of syndromes and conditions of a primarily cognitive nature—each with its own designation. Among the names associated with these conditions are *persecutory delirium, folie raisonnante, folie lucide, sensitive Beziehungswahn,* and *paranoia*. Taking a page from Cullen, Karl Ludwig Kahlbaum (1828–1899) spoke of *vesania typica* (Kahlbaum 1863).

Later, Kahlbaum (1874) described cases of catatonia—in which mental deterioration is accompanied by muscular rigidities, peculiar attitudes and postures, and stuporous states, along with a tendency, in speech, to *verbigeration* (a term coined by Kahlbaum). The term *catatonia* was an old one, going back to ancient times; catatonic stupor without melancholia was earlier described by Louis Delasiauve in France in 1851 (Berrios and Porter 1995). Meantime, Kahlbaum's pupil Ewald Hecker (1843–1909) described *hebephrenia* (Hecker 1871), as a rapidly deteriorating form of adolescent cognitive psychosis, ending in extreme silliness and inappropriateness of thought and affect.

MOVING INTO THE TWENTIETH CENTURY

It remained for Emil Kraepelin (1855–1926) to find the red thread that ran through the myriad variants of cognitive psychosis, each with its separate label. Like his teacher, Griesinger, Kraepelin was more interested in symptoms, and in the biological abnormalities he assumed underlay them, than in the minute details of the psychological lives of the many thousands of patients and their case histories that he encountered over the course of his long career. He suggested the term *dementia praecox* (Kraepelin 1893) as the main heading of which the many diagnostic entities were only variants or subgroups. Now subsumed under the new heading were Hecker's *hebephrenia*, Kahlbaum's *catatonia*, Snell's *monomania*, Griesinger's *primary insanity*, Kretschmer's *paranoia*, and others (Sass 1987).

Later, Kraepelin included also the *folie raisonnante* (reasoning madness) of Sérieux and Capgras (1909)—although some contest the wisdom of considering this a variant of dementia praecox because of the absence of the hallucinations and other stigmata of the latter disorder. It is worth a moment's digression to give the reader a taste of the symptomatology of *folie raisonnante*, from Sérieux and Capgras's book: Having fallen ill with this condition, a certain Madame X was hospitalized by her family—for whose action she conceived a profound bitterness that made her convinced they were "against" her. As the authors described it:

> Madame X studied minutely the letter she received [from her family]. The punctuation marks, the orthographic mistakes, allowed for many interpretations. Her brother wrote her "nous désirons ta guérison" [we wish for your recovery]—to which she remarked that the period was larger than usual. This should therefore read: "nous ne désirons point ta guérison"—that is, "we don't wish for your recovery at all." (p. 21, my translation)

As for Capgras, he is of course famous for describing the subtype of paranoia in which the patient is convinced that the person before him or her (usually a close relative) is not that person at all, but a "double" who is merely impersonating the original. As it turns out, there are certain patients who, in addition to showing *folie raisonnante* or Capgras's syndrome, have additional symptoms of schizophrenia; they show *more*, that is, than mere delusional disorder (as described by Kendler) in the absence of other cognitive abnormalities. Such patients would deserve inclusion in Kraepelin's dementia praecox as he originally described it.

Besides unifying all these conditions under his *dementia praecox*, Kraepelin focused on the long-term course, rather than just on the symptoms, and expressed the view that dementia praecox had a generally downhill progression, beginning in adolescence or early adulthood and ending in chronic mental deterioration. Many dissenting voices were heard: Else Pappenheim, Sergei Korsakoff, and Ernst Meyer all objected to the gloomy conclusion to which Kraepelin's research had led him, even though he himself acknowledged that only about one patient in eight recovered without lasting defect (Zilboorg 1941).

Eugen Bleuler (1857–1939), whose famous monograph was published in 1911, agreed with Kraepelin on many points. His book was called, in deference to his colleague, *Dementia praecox, oder die Gruppe der Schizophrenieen* (Bleuler 1911). This assumes a "group" of related disorders to be placed under the new term *schizophrenia*, which he preferred to *dementia praecox* for at least two reasons. Bleuler was more optimistic about the long-term outcome of the condition and wished to find a label that was less freighted with a pessimistic prognosis. Also, schizophrenia lends itself to a descriptive adjective (*schizophrenic*) that one can then apply to the patient or the diagnosis; *dementia praecox* lacks this advantage. Bleuler is well known for regarding as primary the "four *A*s": **A**utism, **A**ssociation defect, **A**mbivalence, and **A**ffect inappropriateness. The symptoms that Kraepelin saw as primary—delusion, hallucination, formal thought disorder, and negativism—were relegated to secondary signs in Bleuler's schema. Both Kraepelin and Bleuler believed that the condition was "endogenous" (Kraepelin's term), stemming from as yet undiscovered brain abnormality. Kraepelin hired Alois Alzheimer (1864–1915) to examine the brains of schizophrenic individuals in search of the elusive abnormality—a task in which he failed, although he did discover changes in neurological architecture that underlay "Alzheimer's senile dementia."

Because the "four *A*s" can be found over a wider array of mental disorders than is the case with Kraepelin's primary symptoms—ambivalence is particularly common, for example—Bleuler's schema has been criticized as too general or nonspecific. Bleuler mentioned the illness of composer Robert Schumann in the 1911 monograph as an example of "schizophrenia." But Schumann has been rediagnosed convincingly in recent years with manic depression (we would currently call it bipolar disorder)—ending in his suicide by starvation in 1856 (Ostwald 1985).

Bleuler respected Freud and the psychoanalytic movement and was more "psychologically minded" than Kraepelin—one manifestation of which was that Bleuler spent considerable time, often on a daily basis, with the schizophrenic patients under his care at Zürich's Burghölzli Hospital. This rapprochement, coupled with Bleuler's more favorable view of schizophrenia's outcome, probably contributed to the enthusiasm during early years of the twentieth century for the psychoanalytic treatment of schizophrenic patients. Although evidence was accumulating that there was a strong genetic factor operating in schizophrenia (Rüdin 1916; Kety 1976), contrarian voices were heard to the effect that schizophrenia was merely a "reaction" (Meyer 1952) that an adverse environment could make manifest in anyone (Glover 1932).

Many of the successfully treated patients turned out, on closer examination, to be manic-depressive (Vaillant 1963). But particularly in the United States, there was no real impetus to look more closely at the diagnostic standards in common use—until the advent of the neuroleptic drugs, beginning with chlorpromazine, in the 1950s, and the antimanic drugs, beginning with lithium, a little later. Once medications became available to treat specific conditions, it made sense to look closely at the symptom display of one's patients to ascertain whether they were good candidates for one or the other class of drug.

The search for the optimal diagnostic criteria for schizophrenia did not stop with Kraepelin and Bleuler. New models were proposed in the middle years of the twentieth century by a number of investigators in Europe. The so-called Heidelberg school, which Kurt Schneider (1887–1967) directed from 1946 to 1955, was especially important—although Schneider's first-rank symptoms of schizophrenia had been annunciated earlier, in 1938 in *Nervenarzt*, when he was director of a psychiatric research group in Munich. What is striking about the Schneider criteria is that all eleven are cognitive in nature—even the last three, which have to do with affects, impulses, and motor activity being *experienced as controlled externally*. Schneider and his colleagues viewed schizophrenia as the prototypical form of what I have been calling "primarily cognitive madness," and they were convinced they were dealing with an essentially biologically based disorder. The criteria suggested a year earlier by the Norwegian investigator Gabriel Langfeldt (1937) were almost as exclusively cognitive in nature: his first two items—severe derealization and depersonalization—occur with some regularity in the affective disorders as well. Elsewhere I have provided a full listing of these and other criterion sets (Stone 1980). Eventually, even American psychiatry abandoned the Bleulerian criteria (while retaining the name *schizophrenia* because of its convenience), adopting a more neo-Kraepelinian stance. For example, in the current edition of the *Diagnostic and Statistical Manual of Mental Disorders* (DSM-IV-TR; American Psychiatric Association 2000), the main criteria are those of delusions, hallucinations, and disorganized speech (the external accompaniment of disorganized thought).

But even as we have come to rely less on his diagnostic criteria, Bleuler deserves considerable credit for emphasizing the nonhomogeneity of the condition: the "group" of schizophrenias. For just as earlier medical terms like *dropsy* and *pneumonia* turned out to cover a multiplicity of etiologies, ongoing research into the genetics, neurochemistry, and neuroimaging of schizophrenic patients is revealing not one, but a number of varieties of primarily cognitive psychosis—interrelated, overlapping, but in certain parameters distinct—that, currently at least, all seem to fit under the heading of schizophrenia.

REFERENCES

Alexander FG, Selesnick ST: The History of Psychiatry. New York, Harper & Row, 1966

American Psychiatric Association: Diagnostic and Statistical Manual of Mental Disorders, 4th Edition, Text Revison. Washington, DC, American Psychiatric Publishing, 2000

Aretaeus: The Extant Works of Aretaeus the Cappadocian, translated by Adam F. London, The Sydenham Society, 1856

Arnold T: Observations on the Nature, Kinds, Causes, and Prevention of Insanity, Lunacy, or Madness. 2 Vols. Leicester, England, Robinson & Cadell, 1782

Avicenna: Al-Qanun fi'l Tibb [The Canon of Medicine], translated by Gruner OC, Shah MH. Adapted by Bakhtiar L. Chicago, IL, KAZI, 1999

Battie W: A Treatise on Madness. London, Whiston and White, 1758

Berrios G, Porter R: A History of Clinical Psychiatry: The Origin and History of Psychiatric Disorders. New York, New York University Press, 1995

Bleuler E: Dementia praecox, oder die Gruppe der Schizophrenien [Dementia praecox, or the Group of the Schizophrenias]. Leipzig, Germany, Franz Deuticke, 1911

Carlsson LU: Schizophrenia throughout history. Human Brain Informatics, 2003. Available at: http://www.hubin.org/facts/history/history_schizophrenia_en.html.

Carpenter WT Jr, Strauss JS, Muleh S: Are there pathognomonic symptoms in schizophrenia? Arch Gen Psychiatry 28:847–852, 1973

Celsus AC: Medicina: libri VIII quam emendatissimi, graecis etiam omnibus dictionibus restitutes [Medicine: Corrected as Much as Possible and Translated From the Greek and Other Languages]. Venice, Aldine, 1528

Cleckley H: The Mask of Sanity. St. Louis, MO, CV Mosby, 1941

Cullen W: First Lines in the Practice of Physic. Edinburgh, Elliot, 1784

Esquirol J-E: Des maladies mentales [Concerning Mental Illnesses]. 2 vols. Paris, J-B Baillière, 1838

Fuller-Torrey E: Schizophrenia and Civilisation. Northvale, NJ, Jason Aronson, 1980

Galen C: Epitome Galeni Pergameni operum, in Quatuor partes digesta. Basel, M Isingrinium, 1551

Georget EJ: De la folie: considérations sur cette maladie [Concerning Madness: Considerations About This Condition]. Paris, Crevot, 1820

Glover E: Psychoanalytic approach to the classification of mental disorders. J Ment Sci 78:819–842, 1932

Griesinger W: Die Pathologie und Therapie psychischen Krankheiten für Ärzte und Studirende [The Pathology and Therapy of Psychical Illnesses–for Physicians and Students]. Brunswick, Germany, F Wreden, 1861

Hare E: Schizophrenia as a recent disease. Br J Psychiatry 153:521–531, 1988

Haslam J: Observations on Madness. London, J Callow, 1809

Haslam J: Illustrations of Madness. London, J Callow, 1810

Hecker E: Die Hebephrenie. Ein Beitrag zur klinischen Psychiatrie [A Contribution to Clinical Psychiatry]. Arch Pathol Anat Berlin 52:394–429, 1871

Hippocrates: The Sacred Disease, Vol. 2, translated by Jones WHS. Loeb Classical Library. Cambridge, MA, Harvard University Press, 1952, pp 138–183

Hoenig J: Schizophrenia, in A History of Clinical Psychiatry: The Origin and History of Psychiatric Disorders. Edited by Berrios G, Porter R. New York, New York University Press, 1995, pp 336–348

Horace: Satires, Epistles and Ars Poetica, translated by Fairclough HR. Loeb Classical Library. Cambridge, MA, Harvard University Press, 1926

Howells JG: Introduction, in The Concept of Schizophrenia. Edited by Howells JG. Washington, DC, American Psychiatric Press, 1993, pp ix–xxiv

Hunter R, Macalpine I: Three Hundred Years of Psychiatry: 1535–1860. Oxford, UK, Oxford University Press, 1963

Ideler KW: Biographieen Geisteskranker in ihrer psychologischen Entwicklung [Biographies of the Mentally Ill in Their Psychological Development]. Berlin, EH Schröder, 1841

Jablensky A: Prevalence and incidence of schizophrenia spectrum disorders: implications for prevention. Aust N Z J Psychiatry 34(suppl):S26–S34, S35–S38 (discussion), 2000

Janzarik W: The concept of schizophrenia: history and problems, in Search for the Causes of Schizophrenia. Edited by Häfner H, Gattaz WF, Janzarik W. Berlin, Springer-Verlag, 1987, pp 11–18

Kahlbaum KL: Die Gruppierungen der psychischen Krankheiten und die Einteilung der Seelenstörungen [The Grouping of Psychical Illnesses and the Partitioning of the Mental Disorders]. Danzig, 1863

Kahlbaum KL: Die Katatonie oder das Spannungsirresein: eine klinische Form psychischer Krankheit [Catatonia, or the Tension-Madness: A Clinical Form of Psychical Illness]. Berlin, Hirschwald, 1874

Kant I: Critique of Pure Reason (1781). Translated by Kemp Smith N. London, Palgrave-Macmillan 2003

Kendler KS, Hays P: Paranoid psychosis (delusional disorder) and schizophrenia: a family history study. Arch Gen Psychiatry 38:547–551, 1981

Kendler KS, Walsh D: Schizophreniform disorder, delusional disorder and psychotic disorder not otherwise specified: clinical features, outcome and familial psychopathology. Acta Psychiatr Scand 91:370–378, 1995

Kety SS: Genetic aspects of schizophrenia. Psychiatric Annals 6:11–32, 1976

Kraepelin E: Psychiatrie. 4th Ed. Ein Lehrbuch für Studirende und Ärzte [Psychiatry, 4th Edition: A Textbook for Students and Physicians]. Leipzig, Germany, Abel, 1893

Langfeldt G: The prognosis in schizophrenia and the factors influencing the course of the disease. Acta Psychiatr Scand Suppl 13, 1937

LeLoyer P: A Treatise of Specters or Strange Sights, Visions and Apparitions Appearing Sensibly Unto Men (translated from the French). London, Matthew Lownes, 1605

Lieber DL (ed): Etz Hayim: Torah and Commentary. New York, The Jewish Publication Society, 2001

Macdonald M: Mystical Bedlam: Madness, Anxiety and Healing in Seventeenth England. Cambridge, UK, Cambridge University Press, 1981

Meyer A: Collected Papers. 4 Vols. Baltimore, MD, Johns Hopkins University Press, 1952

Morel BA: Traité des maladies mentales [A Treatise on Mental Illnesses]. Paris, Victor Masson, 1860

Neumann H: Lehrbuch der Psychiatrie [Textbook of Psychiatry]. Erlangen, Germany, 1859

Ostwald P: Schumann: The Inner Voices of a Musical Genius. Boston, MA, Northeastern University Press, 1985

Penrose V: The Bloody Countess: The Crimes of Erzsébet Báthory. London, Creation Books, 1996

Platter F: Tractatus: De functionum laesionibus [Treatise on Disorders of Function]. Basel, Switzerland, Conrad Waldkirch, 1602

Reil JC: Rhapsodieen über die Anwendung der psychischen Curmethode auf Geisteszerrüttungen [Miscellaneous Essays on the Application of Psychical Methods of Cure to Disturbances of the Soul]. Halle, Germany, Curtz, 1803

Rüdin E: Zur Vererbung und Neuenstehung der Dementia Praecox [The Inheritance and Emergence of Dementia Praecox]. Berlin, Springer-Verlag, 1916

Sass H: The classification of schizophrenia in the different diagnostic systems, in Search for the Causes of Schizophrenia. Edited by Häfner H, Gattaz WF, Janzarik W. Berlin, Springer-Verlag, 1987, pp 19–28

Schneider K: Clinical Psychopathology, translated by Hamilton MW. New York, Grune & Stratton, 1959

Sedler M: Concepts of schizophrenia: 1600–1800, in The Concept of Schizophrenia. Edited by Howells JG. Washington, DC, American Psychiatric Press, 1993, pp 47–57

Sennert D: Opera omnia [Complete Works]. Paris, 1666

Sérieux P, Capgras J: Les folies raisonnantes et le délire d'interprétation [Reasoning Insanity and Interpretation-Madness]. Paris, Felix Alcan, 1909

Spiess CH: Biographieen der Wahnsinnigen [Biographies of the Mentally Ill]. Leipzig, Germany, 1796

Stone MH: The Borderline Syndromes. New York, McGraw-Hill, 1980

Stone MH: Historical aspects of mood disorders, in The American Psychiatric Association Textbook of Mood Disorders. Edited by Stein D, Kupfer D, Schatzberg A. Washington, DC, American Psychiatric Publishing, 2006, pp 3–15

Theosophy Library Online. 2003. Available at: http://theosophy.org/tlodocs/teachers/PosidoniusOfApamea.htm.

Vaillant GE: Natural history of remitting schizophrenia. Am J Psychiatry 120:367–375, 1963

Weyer J: De praestigiis daemonum et incantationibus ac veneficiis [On the Deceptions of the Demons, and on Enchantments and Magical Potions]. Basel, Switzerland, Oporinus, 1564

Willis T: De anima brutorum. Quae hominis vitalis ac sensitiva est [A Discourse Concerning the Soul of Brutes–Which Is That of the Vital and Sensitive of Man]. Oxford, UK, Richard Davis, 1672

Zeller E: Die Einheitspsychose [The Unitary Psychosis]. Allgemeine Zeitschrift für Psychiatrie 1:1–79, 1844

Zilboorg G: A History of Medical Psychology. New York, WW Norton, 1941

EPIDEMIOLOGY

WILLIAM W. EATON, PH.D.

CHUAN-YU CHEN, PH.D.

The epidemiology of schizophrenia has progressed, over the course of about a century, from bare essentials of descriptive accounts, surrounded by controversy, in the first three quarters of the twentieth century to a surge in analytic epidemiological findings over the last two decades. In this chapter, we review that history, focusing on the period since the review by Yolles and Kramer (1969) and concentrating on results that are most credible methodologically and consistent across studies, particularly the most recent developments.

METHODS

CASE IDENTIFICATION

Since the classic United States–United Kingdom studies (Kramer 1969), there has been an emphasis on careful diagnosis according to replicable methods in epidemiological work. The closest thing to a gold standard for diagnosis is a semistructured examination, such as the Present State Examination (PSE; Wing et al. 1967), Schedules for Clinical Assessment in Neuropsychiatry (SCAN; Wing et al. 1990), or Structured Clinical Inter-

view for DSM-III-R (SCID; Williams et al. 1992). In this examination modality, the interviewing clinician uses a guide that requires a certain minimum of questions to be asked but leaves the judgment as to the presence of a sign or symptom up to the examiner. The examiner can interrogate freely and cross-examine if necessary and need not follow a strict order. The examiner must necessarily have training in medicine as well as psychopathology because organic causes of signs and symptoms of schizophrenia are always possible. A disadvantage of this modality is its expense.

Since about 1980, structured psychiatric diagnostic instruments, such as the Diagnostic Interview Schedule (DIS; Robins et al. 1981) and the Composite International Diagnostic Interview (CIDI; Wittchen et al. 1991), have been developed that can be administered by individuals without clinical training. With these survey diagnostic instruments, the respondent determines whether a sign or symptom is present or absent by answering a carefully worded, standardized question posed by the interviewer. The results of this method have never been completely credible for disorders such as schizophrenia, in which lack of insight is common.

Supported by National Institute of Mental Health grant 53188.

TABLE 2–1.   Prevalence and incidence of schizophrenia per 1,000 population

Area	Date	Author	Age (y)	Prevalence		Incidence
				Type	**Rate**	
Denmark	1977	Nielsen	≥15	Lifetime	2.7	
	1972	Munk-Jorgensen	All	Annual		0.12
Baltimore, Maryland	1963	Wing	All	Annual	7.0	
	1963	Warthen	All	Annual		0.70
Camberwell, England	1963	Wing	≥15	Annual	4.4	
	1971	Hailey	All	Annual		0.11
Ireland	1973	Walsh	≥15	Point	8.3	
	1986	World Health Organization	15–54	Annual		0.22
Portogruaro, Italy	1982–1989	de Salvia et al.	≥15	Annual	2.7	
	1989	de Salvia et al.	≥15	Annual		0.19
Hampstead, England	1991–1995	Jeffreys et al.	All	Point	5.1	
	1991–1995	McNaught et al.	All	Annual		0.14

Source.   Selected from reviews by Eaton (1985, 1991), with additions of data from studies by Jeffreys et al. (1997), McNaught et al. (1997), and de Salvia et al. (1993).

CASE FINDING

Two common methods of finding cases in epidemiological studies are the survey and the register. In the *survey* approach, an entire population, or a sample thereof, is listed in some manner without regard to the presence or absence of psychiatric disorder. Each person on the roster is interviewed individually to determine whether he or she meets the criteria for schizophrenia. The advantage of the survey is that its results do not depend on whether the individual is receiving treatment for the disorder. As such, the most credible estimates for basic statistics of the disorder, such as prevalence, are determined via surveys of this sort. The disadvantage is that schizophrenia is rare in the population, which means that many individuals must be queried to locate a sufficient number of cases for the numerator of the rate. For example, if the prevalence rate of schizophrenia is about 5 per 1,000, as discussed later in this chapter, then to estimate the rate in three age groups by two gender groups, with 30 in the numerator of each of the resulting six cells, would require that 36,000 individuals be surveyed. If the survey is to be done with a medically trained interviewer, the expense is prohibitive. An incidence study requires that the population be monitored over time, an even more daunting task.

The *register* method of case finding relies on treatment facilities to organize their psychiatric admissions or outpatient files in such a way as to eliminate duplication between facilities. For registers that cover a known geographic or administrative area, the census of population forms the denominator for the prevalence rate. Register systems have less difficulty following up the population through time and are able to estimate incidence as well as prevalence. Registers rely on the diagnoses of treating clinicians, which have less reliability and validity than a research examination such as the SCAN or PSE. Furthermore, surveys have shown that 10%–50% of the persons with schizophrenia do not enter the system of psychiatric treatment and thus are omitted from the numerator of the rates (Eaton 1985). Despite these shortcomings, the most credible data on the epidemiology of schizophrenia come from registers including inpatient and outpatient facilities for an entire nation, in which the diagnosis is typically made carefully according to the standards of the *International Classification of Diseases* and in which treatment for schizophrenia in particular and health conditions in general is free.

DESCRIPTIVE EPIDEMIOLOGY

PREVALENCE

The *point prevalence* of schizophrenia is the proportion of the population at a point in time that has the disorder. The point prevalence of schizophrenia is about 5 per 1,000 population. The estimate depends on the age distribution of the population; if persons too young to be at risk are included in the denominator, for example, the estimates will be lower. Table 2–1 presents findings from areas in

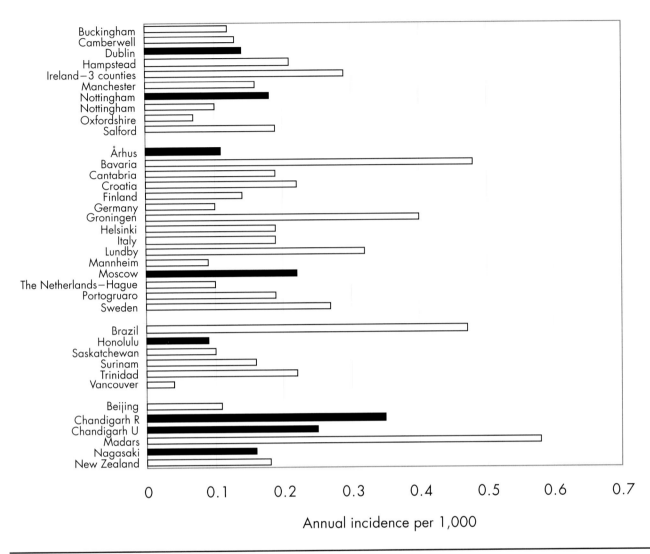

FIGURE 2–1. Incidence of schizophrenia in selected studies published after 1985.

Criteria: study focus is the general population of a defined geographic area; diagnosis is made by a psychiatrist; case finding includes inpatient and outpatient services; greater than 25,000 person-years of risk in age group studies. Dark bars represent the World Health Organization study of incidence.

which credible estimates of both prevalence and incidence are available. The range in prevalence in Table 2–1 is from 2.7 per 1,000 to 8.3 per 1,000, and this range would not be much affected if several dozen other studies, available from prior reviews, were included (Eaton 1985).

The types of prevalence estimates vary from point prevalence, which would be expected to be the smallest, to *lifetime prevalence*, which is the proportion of a population at a point in time that either has the disorder or has had it over their lifetime up to the time of the estimation—presumably yielding the largest rate for a nonfatal disorder such as schizophrenia. Lifetime prevalence has been estimated by surveys with examinations by medically trained persons, with resulting prevalence rates not too different from those shown in Table 2–1 (Eaton 1985).

INCIDENCE

The incidence of schizophrenia is about 0.20 per 1,000 per year. The incidence rates presented are all estimated for 1 year, making the comparison somewhat tighter. The range in annual incidence in Table 2–1 is from 0.11 per 1,000 to 0.70 per 1,000, and this range would not be much affected if several dozen other studies, reviewed elsewhere, were included (Eaton 1991, 1999). The presentation of prevalence and incidence figures from the same areas in juxtaposition shows that the point prevalence is usually more than 10 times the annual incidence, indicating the chronic nature of the disorder.

Considerable variation is seen in incidence rates around the world, as shown in Figure 2–1. The dark bars in this

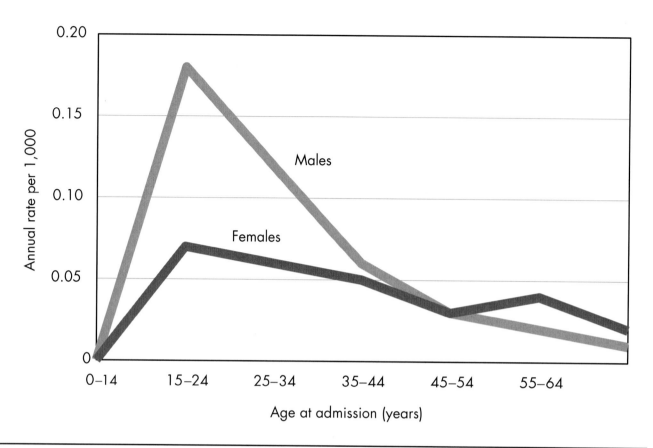

FIGURE 2–2.   Age at onset of schizophrenia (ICD-8; World Health Organization 1967), by sex: Denmark, 1970–1982.

Source.   Adapted from Munk-Jorgensen 1987.

figure represent findings from the World Health Organization study of incidence, which show a smaller variation, presumably a result of the standardization of method (Sartorius et al. 1986). The conclusion of that study suggested to some that there was little or no variation in schizophrenia around the world, which would make schizophrenia a very unusual disease indeed. Figure 2–1 shows variation greater than one order of magnitude, from a low estimate in Vancouver, British Columbia, of 0.04 per 1,000 per year to a high estimate in Madras, India, of 0.58 per 1,000 per year. Both the Vancouver (Beiser et al. 1993) and the Madras (Rajkumar 1993) studies were carefully done, and their estimates are credible.

The force of morbidity for schizophrenia, as measured by the incidence rate, peaks in young adulthood. Figure 2–2 shows estimates of incidence by age and sex for Denmark in 1970–1982 (Munk-Jorgensen 1987). The peak incidence for males and females is in the decade 15–24. The peak for young adults is more marked for males, and females have a second peak at age 55–64. This age-by-sex shape to the incidence curve is consistent in the research literature, even for a much broader diagnostic spectrum,

as in data from locations in the United States (Babigian 1985) prior to DSM-III (American Psychiatric Association 1980), which narrowed the diagnosis and made it closer to that used in Britain and Europe. Figure 2–2 suggests that males have higher lifetime risk of schizophrenia, which is borne out in a meta-analysis addressing that issue, showing that males have about 30%–40% higher lifetime risk of developing schizophrenia (Aleman et al. 2003).

NATURAL HISTORY

ONSET

The onset of schizophrenia is varied. In the classic long-term follow-up study by Ciompi (1980), about 50% had an acute onset, and 50% a long prodrome. The intensive study of the prodrome by Hafner and colleagues (1999) suggested that onset of negative symptoms tends to occur about 5 years before the initial psychotic episode, with onset of positive symptoms much closer to the time of first hospitalization.

CHILDHOOD DEVELOPMENTAL ABNORMALITIES

Many long-term follow-up studies, both retrospective and prospective, suggest that various signs, symptoms, conditions, and behaviors are associated with raised risk for schizophrenia, but none has sufficient strength or uniqueness to be useful in prediction. Work on high-risk groups showed that offspring of schizophrenic parents were more likely to have a lower IQ, poor attentional skills, thought disorder–like symptoms, poor social adjustment, and psychiatric symptoms as compared with the offspring of control subjects (for reviews, see Niemi et al. 2003; Tarrant and Jones 1999).

Although several concerns have been raised about the generalizability of high-risk findings to nonfamilial forms of schizophrenia, longitudinal studies conducted in the United Kingdom, Sweden, Finland, and New Zealand have provided evidence that individuals with schizophrenia differ from their peers even in early childhood in a variety of developmental markers, such as the age of attaining developmental milestones (Isohanni et al. 2001; Jones 1997; Jones et al. 1994), levels of cognitive functioning (David et al. 1997; Gunnell et al. 2002), educational achievement (M. Cannon et al. 1999; Done et al. 1994; Isohanni et al. 1998; Jones et al. 1994), neurological and motor development (M. Cannon et al. 2002a; T.D. Cannon et al. 1999; Leask et al. 2002), social competence (Done et al. 1994; Malmberg et al. 1998), and psychological disturbances (Malmberg et al. 1998). No common causal paths appear to link these developmental markers with schizophrenia (Jones and Tarrant 1999). Indeed, individuals who later develop schizophrenia or related disorders may have already experienced a general or pan-developmental impairment early in their childhood. For example, M. Cannon et al. (2002a), using prospectively collected data from the 1972–1973 birth cohort in New Zealand, found that schizophrenic subjects may have had a significant deficit in neuromotor, language, and cognitive development in the first decade of their lives. In addition, children who later received diagnoses of schizophreniform disorders were more likely to have experienced higher levels of emotional problems and peer rejection. The compelling evidence linking an array of childhood developmental abnormalities and schizophrenia is consistent with the hypothesis that schizophrenia is a neurodevelopmental disorder, with causes that may be traced to a defect in the early brain development (Murray 1987; Weinberger 1995).

MINOR PHYSICAL ANOMALIES

Minor physical anomalies, defined by small structural deviations observed in various parts of the body (e.g., global head, eyes, ears, mouths, hands, and feet), are elevated in individuals with schizophrenia and their siblings as compared with the rest of the population (Ismail et al. 1998, 2000; Lane et al. 1997; Schiffman et al. 2002). In one clinical comparison between schizophrenic patients with patients' siblings and nonschizophrenic subjects via the modified Waldrop scale (Waldrop et al. 1968), Ismail and colleagues (1998) found that the highest occurrence of minor physical anomalies tends to occur in those with schizophrenia, followed by their siblings and nonschizophrenic subjects accordingly. The significant odds ratios of minor physical anomalies with schizophrenia ranged from 31 for the feature of heterochromia in eyes to 3 in those with a curved fifth finger. Similar evidence was shown in one prospective population-based study in Denmark, which suggested that three or more minor physical anomalies in childhood might be associated with an estimated three to four times higher risk to develop schizophrenia spectrum disorders in adulthood (Schiffman et al. 2002).

Although there has been argument about the measurement issues of minor physical anomalies (e.g., the content validity of Waldrop scale) (McNeil et al. 2000), the higher risk associated with minor physical anomalies in schizophrenia was consistently reported even after application of other measurement instruments or a revised Waldrop scale with additional items (Ismail et al. 1998; Lane et al. 1997; Schiffman et al. 2002). One possible explanation for minor physical anomalies–related excess in schizophrenia is that minor physical anomalies may be the manifestation of prenatal developmental disruption occurring in the first or second trimester of pregnancy, a critical period of brain development. For example, because both minor physical anomalies and the central nervous system have embryonic origins from the ectoderm, it is very likely that the presence of minor physical anomalies may be an externally observed sign of abnormal brain development.

COURSE

The symptomatic course of schizophrenia is varied also. In Ciompi's (1980) study, about half had an undulating course, with partial or full remissions followed by recurrences, in an unpredictable pattern. About one-third had a relatively chronic, unremitting course with poor outcome. A small minority in that study had a steady pattern of recovery with good outcome. Follow-up studies that are not strictly prospective, such as the study by Ciompi, can be deceptive because they tend to focus on a residue of chronic cases, making the disorder appear more chronic than it actually is.

Figure 2–3 shows data on time to rehospitalization for a cohort of patients with schizophrenia in Denmark. The

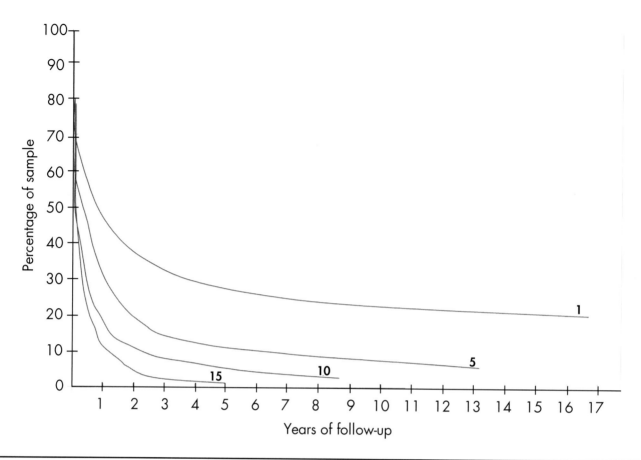

FIGURE 2–3.   Community survival in schizophrenia: Denmark.

Note.   1, 5, 10, and 15 represent the number of hospital discharges.

Source.   Adapted from Mortensen and Eaton 1994.

proportion remaining in the community without rehospitalization is shown on the vertical axis, and time is on the horizontal axis. After the initial hospitalization, about 25% are not rehospitalized, even after 15 years. For that subgroup of the cohort with 10 hospitalizations, more than 90% are rehospitalized within 3 years following the tenth episode. The occurrence of episodes could be reinforcing the illness (so-called *schubweis* [stepwise] process), or the hospitalization itself could be damaging (Eaton 1974a), but it seems more likely that the cohort is sorting itself into those with a tendency for more rather than less chronicity of disorder. This process may lead clinicians and others to overestimate the chronicity of the disorder because they see individuals in the bottom curve of Figure 2–3 about 15 times as often as individuals in the top curve (Cohen and Cohen 1984). For this reason, the natural history of schizophrenia is best studied with cohorts of first-onset patients (Ram et al. 1992).

OUTCOME

Predictors of outcome for schizophrenia remain elusive for the most part. In a review of 13 prospective studies of course in first-onset cohorts, negative symptoms predicted poor outcome in 4 studies, and gradual onset, typical of negative symptoms (as noted earlier) also predicted poor outcome in several studies (Ram et al. 1992). There is variation in the course of schizophrenia around the world, with better prognosis in so-called developing countries. Table 2–2 shows a summary of data from the World Health Organization (1979) study on this issue; we extracted the data in the rightmost columns from the publication of Leff and colleagues (1992). Those in developing countries were less likely to have been chronically psychotic over the period of follow-up and more likely to have had no residual symptoms after 5 years than were those in the developed countries. This result remains to

TABLE 2–2.   World Health Organization follow-up of schizophrenia

	Sample size	Percentage with no symptoms	Percentage with chronic psychosis
Developed countries			
London, England	50	6	40
Aarhus, Denmark	64	5	14
Moscow, Russia	66	17	21
Prague, Czechoslovakia	65	6	23
Washington, D.C., United States	51	3	23
Developing countries			
Agra, India	73	42	10
Cali, Colombia	91	11	21
Ibadan, Nigeria	68	34	10

Source.   Leff et al. 1992.

be explained. Perhaps individuals meeting criteria for schizophrenia in developing countries include a subset destined for better prognosis because of the risk factor structure in those countries—for example, more deaths of compromised fetuses or a cause connected to good prognosis, such as a parasite that is rare in developed countries. Another interpretation is that the environment of recovery in the developed world is more pernicious, involving harsher economic competition, a greater degree of stigma, and smaller family networks to share the burden of care for the patient with schizophrenia.

The course of schizophrenia, from early prodrome to later outcome, is related to social variables, including socioeconomic position and marital status, as shown by a recent study by Agerbo et al. (2004) (see Figure 2–4). Individuals who eventually receive a schizophrenia diagnosis are more likely than others to be single, even as much as 20 years prior to diagnosis, when the relative odds are about 4. The relative odds of being single, as compared with those who have never received a schizophrenia diagnosis, peak at the time of admission—at more than 15—and remain high for decades afterward. The effect is greater for males, possibly because onset of the disorder, which takes place, on average, earlier than in females, occurs during the years of formation of marriages. Likewise, individuals who eventually receive a schizophrenia diagnosis are more likely than others to be unemployed, many years before the first diagnosis of schizophrenia and many years after (Figure 2–5). Although there is a long literature on the relation of low socioeconomic position to risk for schizophrenia (1854 Massachusetts Commission on Lunacy et al. 1971; Dohrenwend et al. 1992), it seems likely that the association is a result of the effects of insidious

onset on the ability of the individual to compete in the job market. Recent studies from Scandinavia suggest that, if anything, the parents of schizophrenic patients are likely to come from a higher, not lower, social position (Byrne et al. 2004).

RISK FACTORS

A family history of schizophrenia is an important risk factor that is dealt with elsewhere in this volume (see Chapter 5, "Neurodevelopmental Theories"). In this section, we present risk factors that have been found in at least several credible studies and that were present prior to the onset of schizophrenia.

PREGNANCY AND BIRTH

For a long time, it has been known that individuals with schizophrenia are more likely to be born in the winter (Figure 2–6). This risk factor is interesting in part because it is indisputably not genetic in origin. The relative risk is small—on the order of a 10% increase for those born in the winter compared with the summer. But it has been replicated many times (possibly because it is so easy to do a study of season of birth). Methodological challenges to the finding have been made (M. S. Lewis 1989), on the basis of the way the beginning of the calendar year interacts with the shape of the onset curve for schizophrenia, but subsequent studies adjusted for the methodological difficulties and still found an effect. The effect exists in the Southern Hemisphere, with more births during the Southern Hemisphere winter season, which does not co-

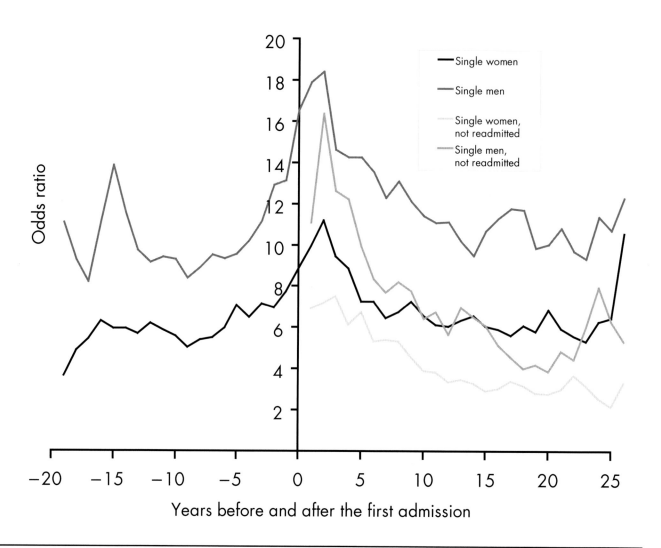

FIGURE 2–4.   Odds ratios of being single for individuals with schizophrenia compared with healthy control subjects.

Rates are adjusted for age, gender, calendar year, and labor market affiliation.

Source.   Reprinted from Agerbo E, Byrne M, Eaton W, et al.: "Marital and Labor Market Status in the Long Run in Schizophrenia." *Archives of General Psychiatry* 61:28–33, 2004. Copyright 2004, American Medical Association. Used with permission.

incide with the beginning of the calendar year. One possible explanation is that the mother is passing through the second trimester of her pregnancy in the height of the flu season and that infections during that period raise risk for schizophrenia in the offspring.

The finding regarding season of birth suggests that something about pregnancy and birth might be awry in individuals who later develop schizophrenia. Case-control studies have been available for decades on this issue, but the generally positive findings were clouded by the possibility that the mother's recall was biased. In the last 15 years, many studies have reported a relative odds of about 2 for those with a birth complication, and several meta-analyses on this topic exist (Geddes and Lawrie

1995; Geddes et al. 1999; Verdoux et al. 1997). Later analyses have begun to specify the individual type of birth complication, with the hope of elucidating the causal mechanism. Figure 2–7 selects results from a meta-analysis of eight prospective studies, in which the 95% confidence interval (CI) has 0.85 or larger as its lower bound (i.e., significant or nearly so), along with the number of studies on the left side of the figure associated with each obstetrical factor (M. Cannon et al. 2002b). This presentation facilitates assessment of consistency across studies, as well as strength and significance. For example, the relative odds for preeclampsia is not large (1.36) and does not meet conventional levels of statistical significance, but the estimate is based on six studies. The complications sug-

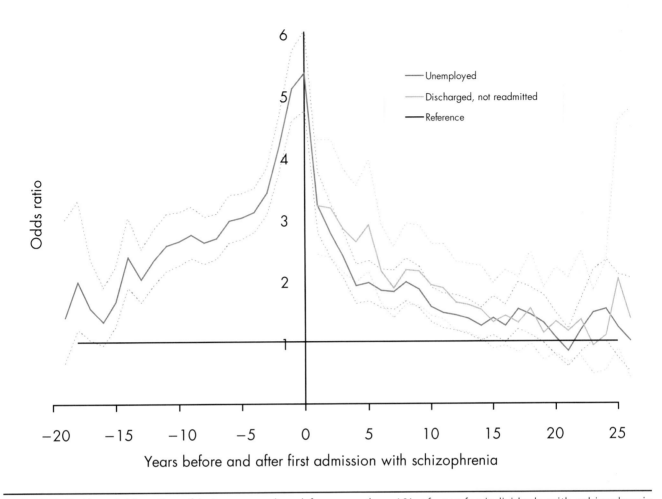

FIGURE 2–5. Odds ratios of being unemployed for more than 1% of year for individuals with schizophrenia compared with control subjects with reference to fully or self-employed individuals.
Rates are adjusted for age, gender, calendar year, and marital status. Dotted lines are 95% confidence bands.
Source. Reprinted from Agerbo E, Byrne M, Eaton W, et al.: "Marital and Labor Market Status in the Long Run in Schizophrenia." *Archives of General Psychiatry* 61:28–33, 2004. Copyright 2004, American Medical Association. Used with permission.

gest as a possible cause malnutrition (Susser and Lin 1992), extreme prematurity, and hypoxia or ischemia (Dalman et al. 1999; Rosso et al. 2000; Zornberg et al. 2000).

PARENTAL AGE

The role of advanced parental age in relation to a higher risk of schizophrenia was first proposed in the mid-twentieth century and has gained extensive scientific attention in recent years. According to the family background data of 1,000 patients in the Ontario Hospital, Canada, Gregory (1959) reported that schizophrenic patients' parents were, on average, 2–3 years older than parents in the general population. However, subsequent investigations have shown inconsistent findings (Granville-Grossman 1966; Hare and Moran 1979), and it also has been argued that observed maternal age–associated higher risk in schizo-

phrenia might be largely confounded by raised paternal age (Hare and Moran 1979; Kinnell 1983). Recently, several population-based epidemiological studies in Denmark, Israel, Sweden, and the United States have provided stronger evidence as to the role of paternal age in schizophrenia (Brown et al. 2002; Byrne et al. 2003; Dalman and Allebeck 2002; Malaspina et al. 2001; Zammit et al. 2003). For example, Malaspina and colleagues (2001) used population-based birth cohort data in Israel and found that the relative risk of schizophrenia rose monotonically in each 5-year group of paternal age, with a maximum relative risk of 2.96 (95% CI=1.60–5.47) in the group aged 55 or older in comparison with the group ages 20–24. Additionally, once paternal age is statistically adjusted, maternal age no longer is a significant predictor of schizophrenia. The evidence from one nested case–control study indicated that the paternal age–related excess in the risk of schizophrenia is generally greater in females (Byrne et al. 2003).

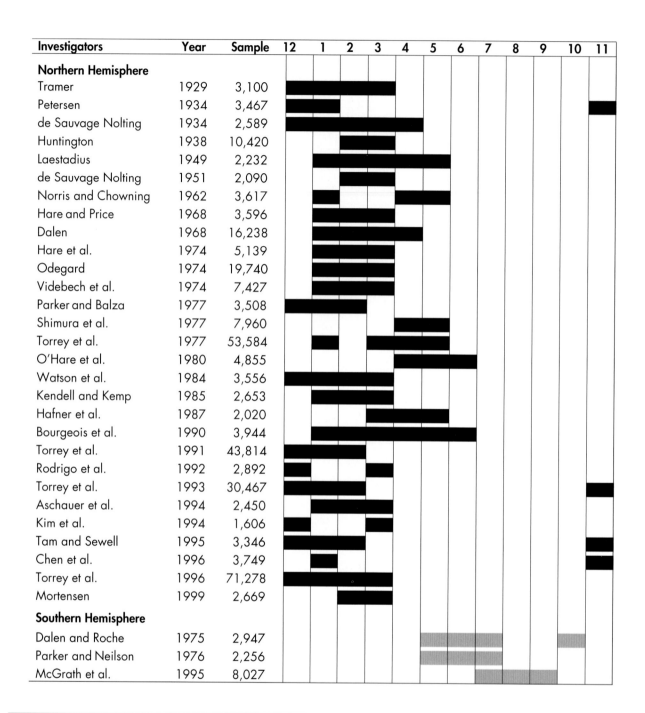

FIGURE 2–6.   Season of birth and schizophrenia.

Source.   Drawn from Torrey et al. 1997, with additions of data from studies by Mortensen et al. 1999; only studies with sample sizes larger than 1,500 are included.

Several hypotheses have been posited to explain the underlying mechanisms linking advancing paternal age to schizophrenia. Unlike females, in whom all germline cell divisions are completed before birth, males have germline cell divisions throughout their reproductive period. As a result of accumulation of mutagens, reduced fidelity of DNA replication, and inefficiency of repair mechanisms,

males with advancing age have a greater chance to produce sperm with mutations (i.e., de novo mutations; Crow 2000; Malaspina 2001; Penrose 1955). If de novo mutations explain the link between advancing paternal age and schizophrenia, then the observed association is presumably stronger in sporadic cases than in familial ones, because de novo mutations largely involve one single-base

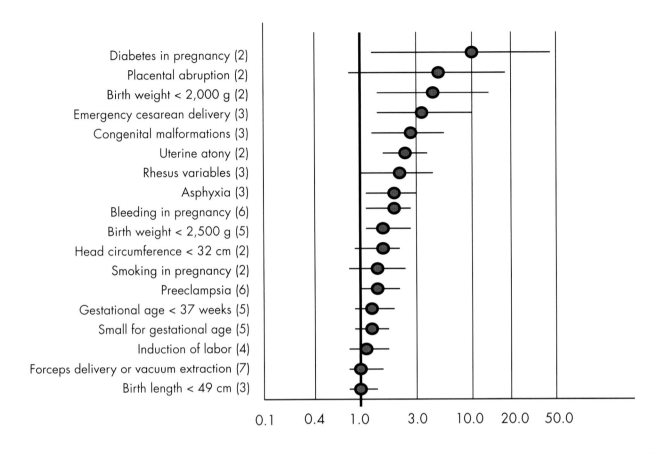

FIGURE 2–7. Pregnancy and birth complications and schizophrenia in meta-analytic review.

Number of studies for each complication is given in parentheses.

Source. Adapted from M. Cannon et al. 2002b.

substitution (Crow 2000). Another possible explanation is that certain schizophrenia-related vulnerabilities or risk factors (e.g., genetic traits, personality, or lower socioeconomic status) might impair the individual's social functions and consequently delay the age at marriage and fatherhood (Hare and Moran 1979; Kinnell 1983). A third hypothesis is that offspring of older fathers may experience more stressful life events, such as loss of father in early childhood, as compared with their peers with younger fathers.

INFECTIONS AND THE IMMUNE SYSTEM

A series of ecological studies suggested that persons whose mothers were in their second trimester of pregnancy during a flu epidemic had a higher risk for schizophrenia (e.g., see Brown and Susser 2002; Mednick et al. 1988; Munk-Jorgensen and Ewald 2001). Infection during pregnancy as a risk factor is consistent with the neurodevelopmental theory of schizophrenia (Murray 1987; Weinberger 1987). Later studies, which are more convincing,

include individual assessment of infection via either comparison of antibodies in adults with schizophrenia and nonschizophrenic individuals (Yolken and Torrey 1995) or, even more convincing, prospective studies in which the infection can be determined to have occurred during the pregnancy. Consistent evidence shows that individuals with antibodies to *Toxoplasma gondii* have higher prevalence of schizophrenia (Torrey and Yolken 2003). One study suggested a relative risk of 5.2 for individuals with documented infection by the rubella virus during fetal development (Brown et al. 2000). Another prospective study found higher risk for psychosis in individuals whose mothers had higher levels of antibodies to herpes simplex virus (Buka et al. 2001). A study in Brazil compared individuals who had meningitis during the 1971–1974 epidemic with their siblings who did not have meningitis. The study found that the prevalence of psychosis, and schizophrenia specifically, was five times higher in those who had meningitis. The finding is intriguing because the average age at infection with meningitis was 26 months (i.e., much later than prenatal infection) (Gattaz et al. 2004). If

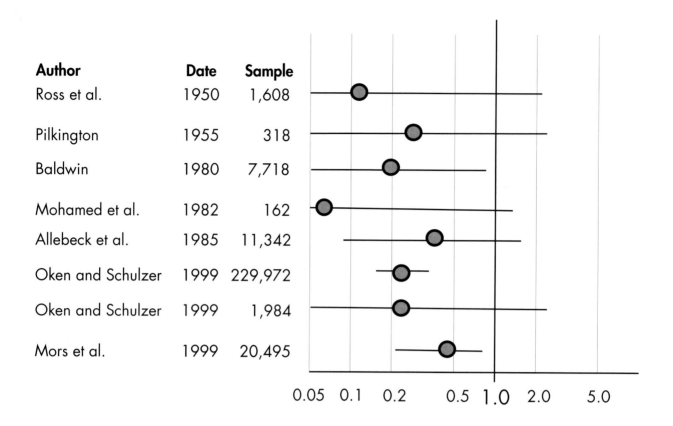

FIGURE 2–8.   Arthritis and schizophrenia: odds ratios and 95% confidence intervals in eight studies.

Source.   Eaton et al. 1992; Mors et al. 1999; Oken and Schulzer 1999.

this finding is replicated, it will have important implications for the neurodevelopmental theory of schizophrenia.

AUTOIMMUNE DISEASES

A relatively small but consistent literature indicates that persons with schizophrenia have unusual resistance or susceptibility to autoimmune diseases. Studies have consistently shown that individuals with schizophrenia are somehow less likely to have rheumatoid arthritis (Eaton et al. 1992). Figure 2–8 shows eight studies with relative odds ranging from less than 0.1 to 0.5 protective effect. Medications for schizophrenia could be protective for rheumatoid arthritis in some unknown way, but two of the studies in Figure 2–8 were conducted before neuroleptic medications became available. Other physiological consequences of schizophrenia may be protective, or a single gene could raise risk for the one disorder and protect for the other. A single small study suggested that mothers of individuals with schizophrenia have lower risk for rheumatoid arthritis, but its size and quality were not convincing (McLaughlin 1977). It is intriguing, in this regard,

that case–control studies have shown that persons taking nonsteroidal anti-inflammatory medications, which primarily treat arthritis, may be protected from dementia (Etminan et al. 2003; in 't Veld et al. 2002).

Other autoimmune disorders have been linked to schizophrenia as well (Gilvarry et al. 1996; Wright et al. 1996), including thyroid disorders (DeLisi et al. 1991), type 1 diabetes (Wright et al. 1996), and celiac disease (Eaton et al. 2004). Currently, the evidence is strongest for thyroid disorders and celiac disease. In a study from the Danish population registers, persons whose parents had celiac disease were three times more likely to receive schizophrenia diagnoses later. Celiac disease is an immune reaction to wheat gluten. One possible explanation is that the increased permeability of the intestine brought about by celiac disease increases the level of antigen exposure, which increases the risk for autoimmune response. Also, gluten proteins may be broken down into psychoactive peptides (Dohan 1980).

The results linking schizophrenia to autoimmune disease are paralleled by the clinical and laboratory study of autoimmune processes in schizophrenia. There are apparently abnormalities of the immune system in schizophre-

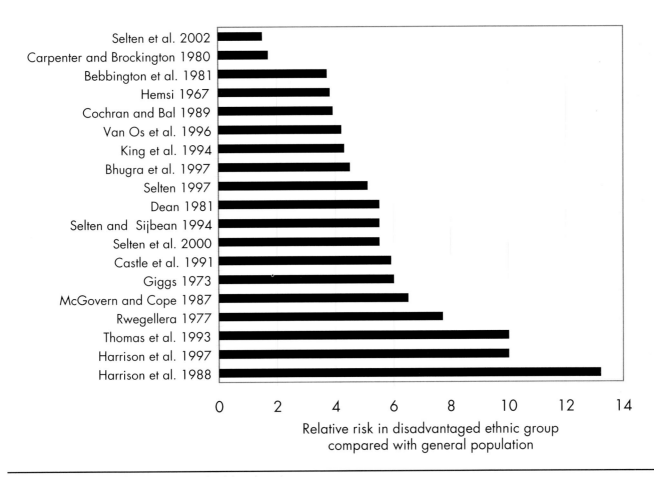

FIGURE 2–9. Ethnic status and schizophrenia.

Incidence studies since 1967.

Source. Eaton and Harrison 2000; Selten et al. 2001, 2002.

nia, but it is not clear whether these are a cause or a consequence of schizophrenia or its treatment (Ganguli et al. 1993, 1994). A single weakness in the immune system in schizophrenic patients may explain both the data on infections and the results on autoimmune disorders, but this remains to be proven (Rothermundt et al. 2001). Clinical trials of anti-inflammatory (Muller et al. 2002) and antibiotic (Dickerson et al. 2003) agents for schizophrenia are ongoing.

ETHNICITY

Ethnic status is a relatively easy-to-identify characteristic of an individual that indicates a shared history with others. Markers of ethnic status include race, country of origin, and religion. Country of origin has proven to be a consistent risk factor for schizophrenia in the United Kingdom and the Netherlands. In the United Kingdom, those immigrating from Africa or the Caribbean, and their second-generation offspring, have rates of schizophrenia up to 10 times higher than those in the general population

(Eaton and Harrison 2000) (Figure 2–9). Because immigrant groups who do not have black skin do not have higher rates, and because the second generation is affected, the stresses of immigration are unlikely to explain this finding. Rates in the countries of origin are not elevated, so the higher rates are unlikely to reflect a genetic difference between races. The cause appears to be the psychological conditions associated with being black in England or being from Surinam in Holland. Discrimination, or a more subtle form of difficulty associated with planning one's life when the future is as uncertain as it is for racial groups at the structural bottom of society, could be a factor (Eaton and Harrison 2001).

CANNABIS

Numerous case–control studies have shown that persons with schizophrenia are more likely to have taken, or be using, cannabis (Hall and Degenhardt 2000). Prospective studies done in Sweden, the Netherlands, New Zealand, and Israel showed higher risk, ranging from 2 to 25 (Arse-

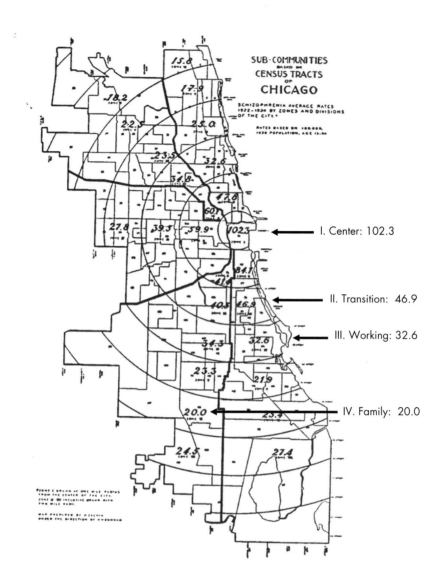

I. Center: 102.3

II. Transition: 46.9

III. Working: 32.6

IV. Family: 20.0

FIGURE 2–10. Urban residence and schizophrenia: rates of schizophrenia by distance from the center of the city. *Source.* Original drawing from Faris and Dunham 1939.

nault et al. 2002; van Os et al. 2002; Weiser et al. 2003; Zammit et al. 2002). Individuals in the premorbid phase of schizophrenia may respond to initial, mild symptoms of schizophrenia by using drugs, even though these studies have attempted to control for premorbid conditions. In contrast, cannabis could precipitate, or even cause, an episode of schizophrenia.

URBAN RESIDENCE

In the 1930s, Faris and Dunham (1939) showed that although the addresses of patients with first admissions for manic-depressive illness were distributed more or less randomly throughout Chicago, Illinois, admissions for

schizophrenia tended to come from the center of the city, with decreasing rates as one moved outward into zones of transition, working class, and family. Figure 2–10 shows an original drawing from their study, with rates and pointers inserted by us to clarify the result. This finding and other similar findings (Eaton 1974b) were interpreted as a result of the selection into the city of individuals who would develop schizophrenia. But later studies from Europe were strictly prospective, with the cohort defined in late adolescence, well prior to onset (G. Lewis et al. 1992), or even at birth (Marcelis et al. 1998).

The relative risk is about two to four times higher for those born in urban areas. The difficulty is identifying the plausible biological process associated with urban resi-

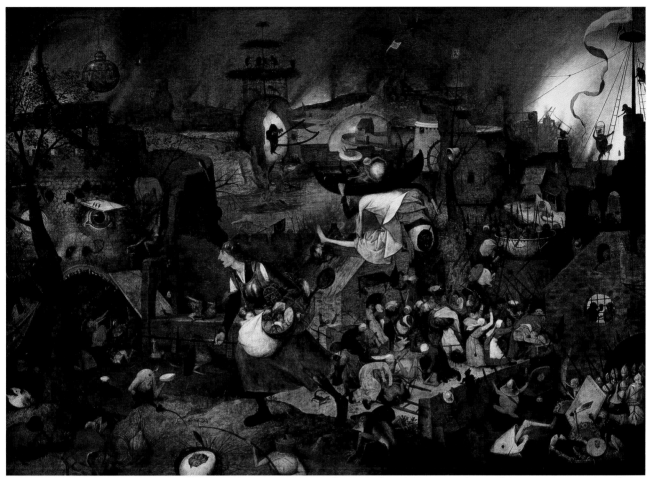

The Art Archive / Mayer van der Bergh Museum Antwerp / Dagli Orti

FIGURE 2–11. *Mad Meg (Dulle Griet)* (1562), by Pieter Bruegel the Elder (ca. 1525–1569).

dence. It could include differences in the physical environment, such as the higher concentration of lead in the soil and air in cities; differences in the cultural environment, such as the expectation to leave the family of origin and define a new life plan (Eaton and Harrison 2001); differences in birth practices, such as breast-feeding (McCreadie 1997); crowding, which might permit spread of infections (Torrey and Yolken 1998); and, as discussed below, differences in the manner in which animals are, or are not, brought into the household (Torrey and Yolken 1995).

MODERNIZATION

A body of evidence suggests that schizophrenia is a disease of relatively recent origin. Studying this possibility requires a more creative approach to data than is general in epidemiology because the relevant observations must necessarily be made before the beginnings of the disci-

pline. Hare (1988) observed that it is difficult to find a precise clinical description of a patient with schizophrenia prior to the beginning of the nineteenth century. Foucault (1979)—departing perhaps most strongly from a strict epidemiological method—puts the date in the seventeenth century, with the beginnings of the *Hôpital Général* in France in 1656. Recognizable descriptions of bipolar disorder in the period of Galenic medicine were made by Aretaus (Mora 1985), but the descriptions that might be related to the occurrence of schizophrenia are more vague and very rare (Roccatagliata 1991). The comparison is surprising, because schizophrenia is more common and more dramatic, especially in its consequences for the individual. Until Shakespeare, Western and non-Western literature apparently was devoid of references to anyone resembling a person with schizophrenia. Shakespeare provides a description of Ophelia (*Hamlet* 4.5), which suggests he must have been aware of psychosis:

She speaks much of her father; says she hears there's tricks in the world, and hems, and beats her heart, spurns enviously at straws, speaks things in doubt that carry but half sense. Her speech is nothing, yet the unshaped use of it doth move the hearers to collection. They aim at it and botch the words up fit to their own thoughts; which, as her winks and nods and gestures yield them, indeed would make one think there would be thought, though nothing sure, yet much unhappily.

During the same epoch as Shakespeare, Breughel produced the remarkable painting entitled *Mad Meg* (Figure 2–11). Although little is known about Breughel's personal life, his three dozen surviving paintings show that he liked to paint unusual but realistic scenes, such as dancing epidemics, crippled people, and blind people. It is clear that this particular painting was important to him because he painted it twice in its entirety. Some observers believe that he met and interacted with a person who had schizophrenia and attempted to paint her entire world, including her symptomatology (cacophony of voices in the milling crowd), ambiguous sexuality (effeminate body topped by very masculine face holding up a boat), and religious imagery (large face with gateway to hell on the left side) (Panse and Schmidt 1967). The painting makes reference to earlier works by Bosch, which include the theme of madness (the shape of the boat resembles Bosch's *Ship of Fools*; the upturned funnel as a hat may refer to Bosch's *Extraction of the Stone of Madness*). The figure of Meg is deliberately askew in various ways: one leg is longer than the other; and she carries various bizarre implements such as the chest, frying pan, and sword. If this interpretation is true, then the painting of Mad Meg can be said to be the first deliberate representation of schizophrenia to have been made.

Data more typical of epidemiological research are available beginning in the nineteenth century, with statistics from asylums. Torrey and Miller (2001) collected data from four separate areas: England, Ireland, Atlantic Canada, and the United States. In each of these regions, the number, and the proportion, of individuals in asylums increased—from fewer than 1 in 1,000 to more than 5 in 1,000 (incidentally, the current estimate for the prevalence of schizophrenia, discussed earlier). Most of these individuals are presumed to be psychotic, and possibly a majority, or at least a substantial proportion, would be given diagnoses of schizophrenia. Figure 2–12 shows the data for the United States, to which we have made additions. The data produced by Torrey and Miller exaggerate the trend for the United States somewhat because the data collection ended with the beginning of the era of neuroleptics and deinstitutionalization. We have added data points from the National Reporting System of the National

Institute of Mental Health, and it is clear that the trend is downward after 1960. (Although the more recent downward trend has been the subject of some discussion [see Allardyce et al. 2000; Jablensky 1995; Oldehinkel and Giel 1995; Suvisaari et al. 1999], it seems likely to be explained by the combination of diagnostic narrowing and deinstitutionalization [Allardyce et al. 2000].) Nevertheless, even with the new, later data points, there appears to be an upward trend over two centuries, with a doubling or quadrupling of the prevalence. Likewise, adding to the figure the carefully collected data from the classic study of Goldhammer and Marshall (1953) suggests an upward trend as well (contrary to the conclusion of the authors).

There is a large range of suspected causes of a rise in the prevalence of schizophrenia in the modern era—that is, since about 1600. For example, there has been an explosion in the number of new chemicals created during the last 400 years, which somehow could be neurotoxic. Many of the possible explanations for the rise in prevalence of schizophrenia with modernization parallel the explanations for the higher risk in urban areas: animals in the household, crowding in cities, and difficulty formulating a life plan when the future is uncertain.

CONCLUSION

What has been accomplished over the last several decades, and what are prospects for future progress? Even as late as a quarter century ago, the epidemiology of schizophrenia was nearly a blank page. There was even argumentation about the value of the concept itself. The only risk factors that seemed strong and consistent were the conditions of lower social class life and the family history of schizophrenia. Since that time, there has been considerable progress delineating a more or less consistent picture of the descriptive epidemiology and the natural history of schizophrenia. Research in analytic epidemiology has generated a series of heretofore unsuspected risk factors, as described earlier. In general, the risk factors have been considered in the context of theories of how schizophrenia might actually be developing in the psychological and physiological life of the individual—even if the linkage is sometimes speculative. These developments are healthy.

In the future, concerted efforts will be made to study risk factors in combination. This process has begun already. For example, Mortensen et al. (1999) have studied the combined effects of season of birth, urbanization of birthplace, and family history of schizophrenia. The combination is informative in evaluating the importance of the risk factors. Although the relative risk for urban birth

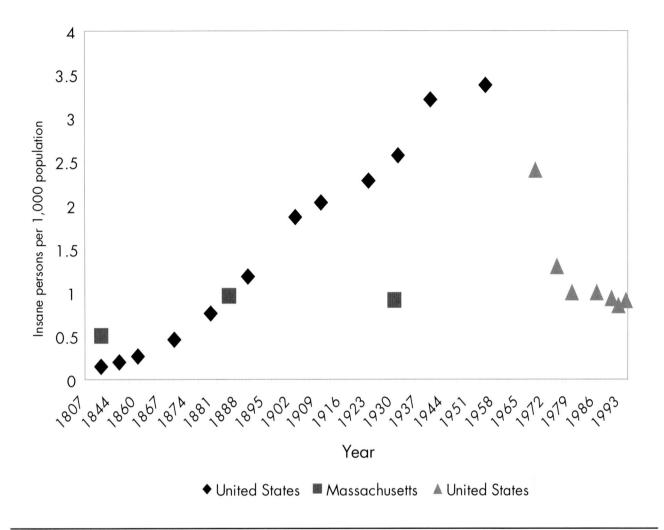

FIGURE 2–12. Modernization and schizophrenia: insanity in the United States, 1807–1994.
Source. United States, 1840–1955 (Torrey and Miller 2001); Massachusetts, 1844–1930 (Goldhammer and Marshall 1953, as organized in Eaton 2001); United States, 1969–1994 (Witkin et al. 1998).

is much smaller than the risk associated with having a parent who is schizophrenic, the importance of urban birth is greater because a much larger proportion of the population is born in urban areas compared with the proportion with parents who have schizophrenia—the situation of relative versus population-attributable risk (Mortensen et al. 1999). If the causal path connected to urban birth could be identified, the prospects for prevention would be much stronger.

The combination of risk factors will facilitate prospective studies of high-risk individuals, in which the high risk is not simply the result of family history, as in earlier high-risk studies. Furthermore, combination of risk factors will raise the positive predictive value of the risk formulation, to the point at which it may be ethically feasible to approach the individual, identify the risk, and begin efforts

to protect him or her from the catastrophic effects of the first episode of schizophrenia. Studies such as these have begun, albeit very cautiously (McGorry et al. 1996; Tsuang et al. 1999; Woods et al. 2003). In general, epidemiological research has built a strong knowledge base over the past quarter century, and this knowledge base will continue to contribute to public health efforts in prevention of schizophrenia in the coming decades.

REFERENCES

1854 Massachusetts Commission on Lunacy, Edward Jarvis, Massachusetts, et al: Insanity and Idiocy in Massachusetts: Report of the Commission on Lunacy. Boston, MA, Harvard University Press, 1971

Agerbo E, Byrne M, Eaton W, et al: Marital and labor market status in the long run in schizophrenia. Arch Gen Psychiatry 61:28–33, 2004

Aleman A, Kahn RS, Selten J-P: Sex differences in the risk of schizophrenia: evidence from a meta-analysis. Arch Gen Psychiatry 60:565–571, 2003

Allardyce J, Morrison G, Van Os J, et al: Schizophrenia is not disappearing in south-west Scotland. Br J Psychiatry 177:38–41, 2000

American Psychiatric Association: Diagnostic and Statistical Manual of Mental Disorders, 3rd Edition. Washington, DC, American Psychiatric Association, 1980

Arsenault L, Cannon M, Poulton R, et al: Cannabis use in adolescence and risk for adult psychosis: longitudinal prospective study. BMJ 325:1212–1213, 2002

Babigian HM: Schizophrenia: epidemiology, in Comprehensive Textbook of Psychiatry/IV. Edited by Kaplan HI, Sadock BJ. Baltimore, MD, Williams & Wilkins, 1985, pp 643–650

Beiser M, Erickson D, Fleming JAE, et al: Establishing the onset of psychotic illness. Am J Psychiatry 150:1349–1354, 1993

Brown AS, Susser ES: In utero infection and adult schizophrenia. Ment Retard Dev Disabil Res Rev 8:51–57, 2002

Brown AS, Cohen P, Greenwald S, et al: Nonaffective psychosis after prenatal exposure to rubella. Am J Psychiatry 157:438–443, 2000

Brown AS, Schaefer CA, Wyatt RJ, et al: Paternal age and risk of schizophrenia in adult offspring. Am J Psychiatry 159:1528–1533, 2002

Buka SL, Tsuang MT, Torrey EF, et al: Maternal infections and subsequent psychosis among offspring. Arch Gen Psychiatry 58:1032–1037, 2001

Byrne M, Agerbo E, Ewald H, et al: Parental age and risk of schizophrenia: a case-control study. Arch Gen Psychiatry 60:673–678, 2003

Byrne M, Agerbo E, Eaton W, et al: Parental socio-economic status and risk for first admission with schizophrenia: a Danish national register based study. Soc Psychiatry Psychiatr Epidemiol 39:87–96, 2004

Cannon M, Jones P, Huttunen MO, et al: School performance in Finnish children and later development of schizophrenia: a population-based longitudinal study. Arch Gen Psychiatry 56:457–463, 1999

Cannon M, Caspi A, Moffitt TE, et al: Evidence for early childhood, pan-developmental impairment specific to schizophreniform disorder: results from a longitudinal birth cohort. Arch Gen Psychiatry 59:449–456, 2002a

Cannon M, Jones PB, Murray RM: Obstetric complications and schizophrenia: historical and meta-analytic review. Am J Psychiatry 159:1080–1092, 2002b

Cannon TD, Rosso IM, Bearden CE, et al: A prospective cohort study of neurodevelopmental processes in the genesis and epigenesis of schizophrenia. Dev Psychopathol 11:467–485, 1999

Ciompi L: The natural history of schizophrenia in the long term. Br J Psychiatry 136:413–420, 1980

Cohen P, Cohen J: The clinician's illusion. Arch Gen Psychiatry 41:1178–1182, 1984

Crow JF: The origins, patterns and implications of human spontaneous mutation. Nat Rev Genet 1:40–47, 2000

Dalman C, Allebeck P: Paternal age and schizophrenia: further support for an association. Am J Psychiatry 159:1591–1592, 2002

Dalman C, Allebeck P, Cullberg J, et al: Obstetric complications and the risk of schizophrenia: a longitudinal study of a national birth cohort. Arch Gen Psychiatry 56:234–240, 1999

David AS, Malmberg A, Brandt L, et al: IQ and risk for schizophrenia: a population-based cohort study. Psychol Med 27:1311–1323, 1997

de Salvia D, Barbato A, Salvo P, et al: Prevalence and incidence of schizophrenic disorders in Portogruaro: an Italian case register study. J Nerv Ment Dis 181:275–282, 1993

DeLisi LE, Boccio AM, Riordan H, et al: Familial thyroid disease and delayed language development in first admission patients with schizophrenia. Psychiatry Res 38:39–50, 1991

Dickerson FB, Boronow JJ, Stallings CR, et al: Reduction of symptoms by valacyclovir in cytomegalovirus-seropositive individuals with schizophrenia. Am J Psychiatry 160:2234–2236, 2003

Dohan F: Hypothesis: genes and neuroactive peptides from food as cause of schizophrenia. Adv Biochem Psychopharmacol 22:535–547, 1980

Dohrenwend BP, Levav I, Shrout PE, et al: Socioeconomic status and psychiatric disorders: the causation-selection issue. Science 255:946–952, 1992

Done DJ, Crow TJ, Johnstone EC, et al: Childhood antecedents of schizophrenia and affective illness: social adjustment at ages 7 and 11. BMJ 309:699–703, 1994

Eaton WW: Mental hospitalization as a reinforcement process. Am Sociol Rev 39:252–260, 1974a

Eaton WW: Residence, social class, and schizophrenia. J Health Soc Behav 15:289–299, 1974b

Eaton W: The epidemiology of schizophrenia. Epidemiol Rev 7:105–126, 1985

Eaton WW: Update on the epidemiology of schizophrenia. Epidemiol Rev 13:320–328, 1991

Eaton WW: Evidence for universality and uniformity of schizophrenia around the world: assessment and implications, in Search for the Causes of Schizophrenia, IV: Balance of the Century. Edited by Gattaz WF, Hafner H. Darmstadt, Germany, Steinkopf, 1999, pp 21–33

Eaton W: The Sociology of Mental Disorders. Westport, CT, Praeger, 2001

Eaton WW, Harrison G: Ethnic disadvantage and schizophrenia. Acta Psychiatr Scand 102 (suppl):38–43, 2000

Eaton WW, Harrison G: Life chances, life planning, and schizophrenia: a review and interpretation of research on social deprivation. Int J Ment Health 30:58–81, 2001

Eaton W, Hayward C, Ram R: Schizophrenia and rheumatoid arthritis: a review. Schizophr Res 6:181–192, 1992

Eaton W, Mortensen PB, Mors O, et al: Celiac disease and schizophrenia: a Danish national register-based study. BMJ 328:438–439, 2004

Etminan M, Gill S, Samii A: Effect of non-steroidal anti-inflammatory drugs on risk of Alzheimer's disease: systematic review and meta-analysis of observational studies. BMJ 327:128, 2003

Faris RE, Dunham W: Mental Disorders in Urban Areas. Chicago, IL, University of Chicago Press, 1939

Foucault M: Discipline and Punish: The Birth of the Prison. New York, Vintage, 1979

Ganguli R, Brar J, Chengappa K, et al: Autoimmunity in schizophrenia: a review of recent findings. Ann Med 25:489–496, 1993

Ganguli R, Brar J, Rabin B: Immune abnormalities in schizophrenia: evidence for the autoimmune hypothesis. Harv Rev Psychiatry 2:70–83, 1994

Gattaz WF, Abrahao AL, Foccacia R: Childhood meningitis, brain maturation and the risk of psychosis. Eur Arch Psychiatry Clin Neurosci 254:23–26, 2004

Geddes JR, Lawrie SM: Obstetric complications and schizophrenia: a meta-analysis. Br J Psychiatry 167:786–793, 1995

Geddes JR, Verdoux H, Takei N, et al: Schizophrenia and complications of pregnancy and labor: an individual patient data meta-analysis. Schizophr Bull 25:413–423, 1999

Gilvarry CM, Sham PC, Jones PB, et al: Family history of autoimmune diseases in psychosis. Schizophr Res 19:33–40, 1996

Goldhammer H, Marshall AW: Psychosis and Civilization: Two Studies in the Frequency of Mental Disease. New York, Free Press, 1953

Granville-Grossman KL: Parental age and schizophrenia. Br J Psychiatry 112:899–905, 1966

Gregory I: Factors influencing first admission rates to Canadian mental hospitals, III: an analysis by education, marital status, country of birth, religion and rural-urban residence, 1950–1952. Can Psychiatr Assoc J 4:133–151, 1959

Gunnell D, Harrison G, Rasmussen F, et al: Associations between premorbid intellectual performance, early life exposures and early onset schizophrenia: cohort study. Br J Psychiatry 181:298–305, 2002

Hafner H, Maurer K, Loffler W, et al: Onset and prodromal phase as determinants of the course, in Search for the Causes of Schizophrenia, IV: Balance of the Century. Edited by Gattaz WF, Hafner H. Darmstadt, Germany, Steinkopf, 1999, pp 35–58

Hall W, Degenhardt L: Cannabis use and psychosis: a review of clinical and epidemiological evidence. Aust N Z J Psychiatry 34:26–34, 2000

Hare E: Schizophrenia as a recent disease. Br J Psychiatry 153:521–531, 1988

Hare EH, Moran PA: Raised parental age in psychiatric patients: evidence for the constitutional hypothesis. Br J Psychiatry 134:169–177, 1979

in 't Veld BA, Launer LJ, Breteler MM, et al: Pharmacologic agents associated with a preventive effect on Alzheimer's disease: a review of the epidemiologic evidence. Epidemiol Rev 24:248–268, 2002

Ismail B, Cantor-Graae E, McNeil TF: Minor physical anomalies in schizophrenic patients and their siblings. Am J Psychiatry 155:1695–1702, 1998

Ismail B, Cantor-Graae E, McNeil TF: Minor physical anomalies in schizophrenia: cognitive, neurological and other clinical correlates. J Psychiatr Res 34:45–56, 2000

Isohanni I, Jarvelin MR, Nieminen P, et al: School performance as a predictor of psychiatric hospitalization in adult life: a 28-year follow-up in the Northern Finland 1966 Birth Cohort. Psychol Med 28:967–974, 1998

Isohanni M, Jones PB, Moilanen K, et al: Early developmental milestones in adult schizophrenia and other psychoses: a 31-year follow-up of the Northern Finland 1966 Birth Cohort. Schizophr Res 52:1–19, 2001

Jablensky A: Schizophrenia: recent epidemiologic issues. Epidemiol Rev 17:10–20, 1995

Jeffreys SE, Harvey CA, McNaught AS, et al: The Hampstead Schizophrenia Survey 1991, I: prevalence and service use comparisons in an inner London health authority, 1986–1991. Br J Psychiatry 170:301–306, 1997

Jones P: The early origins of schizophrenia. Br Med Bull 53:135–155, 1997

Jones PB, Tarrant CJ: Specificity of developmental precursors to schizophrenia and affective disorders. Schizophr Res 39:121–125, 1999

Jones P, Rodgers B, Murray R, et al: Child developmental risk factors for adult schizophrenia in the British 1946 birth cohort. Lancet 344:1398–1402, 1994

Kinnell HG: Parental age in schizophrenia. Br J Psychiatry 142:204, 1983

Kramer M: Cross-national study of diagnosis of the mental disorders: origin of the problem. Am J Psychiatry 125:1–11, 1969

Lane A, Kinsella A, Murphy P, et al: The anthropometric assessment of dysmorphic features in schizophrenia as an index of its developmental origins. Psychol Med 27:1155–1164, 1997

Leask SJ, Done DJ, Crow TJ: Adult psychosis, common childhood infections and neurological soft signs in a national birth cohort. Br J Psychiatry 181:387–392, 2002

Leff J, Sartorius N, Jablensky A, et al: The International Pilot Study of Schizophrenia: five-year follow-up findings. Psychol Med 22:131–145, 1992

Lewis G, David A, Andreasson SAP: Schizophrenia and city life. Lancet 340:137–140, 1992

Lewis MS: Age incidence and schizophrenia, part I: the season of birth controversy. Schizophr Bull 15:59–73, 1989

Malaspina D: Paternal factors and schizophrenia risk: de novo mutations and imprinting. Schizophr Bull 27:379–393, 2001

Malaspina D, Harlap S, Fennig S, et al: Advancing paternal age and the risk of schizophrenia. Arch Gen Psychiatry 58:361–367, 2001

Malmberg A, Lewis G, David A, et al: Premorbid adjustment and personality in people with schizophrenia. Br J Psychiatry 172:308–313, 1998

Marcelis M, Navarro-Mateu F, Murray R, et al: Urbanization and psychosis: a study of 1942–1978 birth cohorts in the Netherlands. Psychol Med 28:871–879, 1998

McCreadie RG: The Nithsdale Schizophrenia Surveys 16: breast-feeding and schizophrenia: preliminary results and hypotheses. Br J Psychiatry 170:334–337, 1997

McGorry PD, Edwards J, Mihalopoulos C, et al: EPPIC: an evolving system of early detection and optimal management. Schizophr Bull 22:305–326, 1996

McLaughlin D: Racial and Sex Differences in Length of Hospitalization of Schizophrenics. Honolulu, HI, 1977

McNaught AS, Jeffreys SE, Harvey CA, et al: The Hampstead Schizophrenia Survey 1991, II: incidence and migration in inner London. Br J Psychiatry 170:307–311, 1997

McNeil TF, Cantor-Graae E, Ismail B: Obstetric complications and congenital malformation in schizophrenia. Brain Res Brain Res Rev 31:166–178, 2000

Mednick S, Machon RA, Huttunen MO, et al: Adult schizophrenia following prenatal exposure to an influenza epidemic. Arch Gen Psychiatry 45:189–192, 1988

Mora G: History of psychiatry, in Comprehensive Textbook of Psychiatry/IV. Edited by Kaplan HI, Sadock. BJ. Baltimore, MD, Williams & Wilkins, 1985, pp 2034–2054

Mors O, Mortensen PB, Ewald H: A population-based register study of the association between schizophrenia and rheumatoid arthritis. Schizophr Res 40:67–74, 1999

Mortensen PB, Eaton WW: Predictors for readmission risk in schizophrenia. Psychol Med 24:223–232, 1994

Mortensen PB, Pedersen CB, Westergaard T, et al: Familial and non-familial risk factors for schizophrenia: a population-based study. N Engl J Med 340:603–608, 1999

Muller N, Riedel M, Scheppach C, et al: Beneficial antipsychotic effects of celecoxib add-on therapy compared to risperidone alone in schizophrenia. Am J Psychiatry 159:1029–1034, 2002

Munk-Jorgensen P: First-admission rates and marital status of schizophrenics. Acta Psychiatr Scand 76:210–216, 1987

Munk-Jorgensen P, Ewald H: Epidemiology in neurobiological research: exemplified by the influenza-schizophrenia theory. Br J Psychiatry 40 (suppl):30–32, 2001

Murray RM: Is schizophrenia a neurodevelopmental disorder? BMJ 295:681–682, 1987

Niemi LT, Suvisaari JM, Tuulio-Henriksson A, et al: Childhood developmental abnormalities in schizophrenia: evidence from high-risk studies. Schizophr Res 60:239–258, 2003

Oken RJ, Schulzer M: At issue: schizophrenia and rheumatoid arthritis: the negative association revisited. Schizophr Bull 25:625–638, 1999

Oldehinkel AJ, Giel R: Time trends in the care-based incidence of schizophrenia. Br J Psychiatry 167:777–782, 1995

Panse F, Schmidt HJ: Pieter Bruegels Dulle Griet: Bildnis einer psychisch kranken. Bayer Lehrerkursen, 1967

Penrose LS: Parental age and mutation. Lancet 269:312–313, 1955

Rajkumar SRPRTMSM: Incidence of schizophrenia in an urban community in Madras. Indian J Psychiatry 35:18–21, 1993

Ram R, Bromet EJ, Eaton WW, et al: The natural course of schizophrenia: a review of first admission studies. Schizophr Bull 18:185–207, 1992

Robins LN, Helzer JE, Croughan J, et al: National Institute of Mental Health Diagnostic Interview Schedule: its history, characteristics, and validity. Arch Gen Psychiatry 38:381–389, 1981

Roccatagliata G: Classical concepts of schizophrenia, in The Concept of Schizophrenia: Historical Perspectives. Edited by Howells JG. Washington, DC, American Psychiatric Press, 1991, pp 1–27

Rosso IM, Cannon TD, Huttunen T, et al: Obstetric risk factors for early onset schizophrenia in a Finnish birth cohort. Am J Psychiatry 157:801–807, 2000

Rothermundt M, Arolt V, Bayer TA: Review of immunological and immunopathological findings in schizophrenia. Brain Behav Immun 15:319–339, 2001

Sartorius N, Jablensky A, Korten A, et al: Early manifestations and first-contact incidence of schizophrenia in different cultures. Psychol Med 16:909–928, 1986

Schiffman J, Ekstrom M, LaBrie J, et al: Minor physical anomalies and schizophrenia spectrum disorders: a prospective investigation. Am J Psychiatry 159:238–243, 2002

Selten JP, Veen N, Feller W, et al: Incidence of psychotic disorders in immigrant groups to the Netherlands. Br J Psychiatry 178:367–372, 2001

Selten JP, Cantor-Graae E, Slaets J, et al: Odegaard's selection hypothesis revisited: schizophrenia in Surinamese immigrants to the Netherlands. Am J Psychiatry 159:669–671, 2002

Susser ES, Lin SP: Schizophrenia after prenatal exposure to the Dutch hunger winter of 1944–1945. Arch Gen Psychiatry 49:983–988, 1992

Suvisaari JM, Haukka JK, Tanskanen AJ, et al: Decline in the incidence of schizophrenia in Finnish cohorts born from 1954 to 1965. Arch Gen Psychiatry 56:733–740, 1999

Tarrant CJ, Jones PB: Precursors to schizophrenia: do biological markers have specificity? Can J Psychiatry 44:335–349, 1999

Torrey EF, Miller J: The Invisible Plague: The Rise of Mental Illness From 1750 to the Present. New Brunswick, NJ, Rutgers University Press, 2001

Torrey E, Yolken R: At issue: could schizophrenia be a viral zoonosis transmitted from house cats? Schizophr Bull 21:167–171, 1995

Torrey EF, Yolken RH: Is household crowding a risk factor for schizophrenia? Ninth Biennial Winter Workshop on Schizophrenia, 1998

Torrey EF, Yolken RH: Toxoplasma gondii and schizophrenia. Emerg Infect Dis 9:1375–1380, 2003

Torrey EF, Miller J, Rawlings R, et al: Seasonality of births in schizophrenia and bipolar disorder: a review of the literature. Schizophr Res 7:1–38, 1997

Tsuang MT, Stone WS, Seidman LJ, et al: Treatment of nonpsychotic relatives of patients with schizophrenia: four case studies. Biol Psychiatry 45:1412–1418, 1999

van Os J, Bak M, Hanssen M, et al: Cannabis use and psychosis: a longitudinal population-based study. Am J Epidemiol 156:319–327, 2002

Verdoux H, Geddes JR, Takei N, et al: Obstetric complications and age at onset in schizophrenia: an international collaborative meta-analysis of individual patient data. Am J Psychiatry 154:1220–1227, 1997

Waldrop MF, Pedersen FA, Bell RQ: Minor physical anomalies and behavior in preschool children. Child Dev 39:391–400, 1968

Weinberger DR: Implications of normal brain development for the pathogenesis of schizophrenia. Arch Gen Psychiatry 44:660–669, 1987

Weinberger DR: From neuropathology to neurodevelopment. Lancet 346:552–557, 1995

Weiser M, Reichenberg A, Rabinowitz J, et al: Self-reported drug abuse in male adolescents with behavioral disturbances, and follow-up for future schizophrenia. Biol Psychiatry 54:655–660, 2003

Williams JBW, Gibbon M, First MB, et al: The Structured Clinical Interview for DSM-III-R (SCID), II: multisite test-retest reliability. Arch Gen Psychiatry 49:630–636, 1992

Wing J, Birley J, Cooper J, et al: Reliability of a procedure for measuring and classifying "present psychiatric state." Br J Psychiatry 113:499–515, 1967

Wing JK, Babor T, Brugha T, et al: SCAN: Schedules for Clinical Assessment in Neuropsychiatry. Arch Gen Psychiatry 47:589–593, 1990

Witkin MJ, Atay JE, Manderscheid RW, et al: Highlights of organized mental health services in 1994 and major national and state trends, in Mental Health, United States, 1998. Edited by Manderscheid RW, Henderson MJ. Rockville, MD, U.S. Department of Health and Human Services, 1998, pp 143–175

Wittchen HU, Robins LN, Cottler LB, et al: Cross-cultural feasibility, reliability and sources of variance of the Composite International Diagnostic Interview (CIDI). Br J Psychiatry 159:645–653, 1991

Woods SW, Breier A, Zipursky RB, et al: Randomized trial of olanzapine versus placebo in the symptomatic acute treatment of the schizophrenic prodrome. Biol Psychiatry 54:453–464, 2003

World Health Organization: International Classification of Diseases, 8th Revision. Geneva, World Health Organization, 1967

World Health Organization: Schizophrenia: An International Follow-up Study. New York, Wiley, 1979

Wright P, Sham PC, Gilvarry CM, et al: Autoimmune diseases in the pedigrees of schizophrenic and control subjects. Schizophr Res 20:261–267, 1996

Yolken RH, Torrey EF: Viruses, schizophrenia, and bipolar disorder. Clin Microbiol Rev 8:131–145, 1995

Yolles SF, Kramer M: Vital statistics, in The Schizophrenic Syndrome. Edited by Bellak L. New York, Grune & Stratton, 1969

Zammit S, Allebeck P, Andreasson S, et al: Self-reported cannabis use as risk factor for schizophrenia in Swedish conscripts of 1969: historical cohort study. BMJ 325:1199–2004, 2002

Zammit S, Allebeck P, Dalman C, et al: Paternal age and risk for schizophrenia. Br J Psychiatry 183:405–408, 2003

Zornberg GL, Buka SL, Tsuang MT: Hypoxic-ischemia-related fetal/neonatal complications and risk of schizophrenia and other nonaffective psychoses: a 19-year longitudinal study. Am J Psychiatry 157:196–202, 2000

GENETICS

PATRICK F. SULLIVAN, M.D., F.R.A.N.Z.C.P.

MICHAEL J. OWEN, PH.D., F.R.C.PSYCH., F.MED.SCI.

MICHAEL C. O'DONOVAN, PH.D., F.R.C.PSYCH.

ROBERT FREEDMAN, M.D.

In this chapter, we review current knowledge about the genetics of schizophrenia. The diverse approaches that fall within the rubric of genetics have been a focus of intense interest and, as with any prominent approach, are not without controversy, false leads, and informed dissension. However, since the completion of the draft sequence of the human genome in 2001, this rapidly evolving field has become quite exciting, and the prospect of real progress is evident.

On a conceptual level, genetics can serve three broad purposes in regard to schizophrenia research. First, and most common, genetic approaches can help clinicians understand the etiology of schizophrenia. Second, pharmacogenetic approaches can assist in the quest for individualized treatments, optimizing the chance of treatment response and minimizing the chance of important side effects. Finally, genetic approaches can help clinicians understand the enormous clinical heterogeneity of schizophrenia. In this chapter, we cover the major developments in these areas.

From the perspective of a group of individuals with schizophrenia, it is critical to view schizophrenia as a complex trait. On average, at a group level, schizophrenia results from a mixture of genetic and environmental influences. For schizophrenia, "nature versus nurture" is a false dichotomy because it is always "nature *and* nurture." Schizophrenia is likely to be complex for a second reason. At the individual level, the pathophysiology of schizophrenia is not uniform, and any sample of individuals with clinically defined schizophrenia is likely to contain several different "types" of illness. Some proportion of individuals would have a highly genetic form of schizophrenia, some would have a highly environmental variant, and some would have schizophrenia that resulted from interactions between genetic and environmental influences.

These features of schizophrenia are distinct from prototypic genetic disorders. Table 3–1 compares and contrasts examples of single-gene disorders with complex traits such as schizophrenia. Unlike single-gene disorders such as Huntington's disease and cystic fibrosis (OMIM—Online Mendelian Inheritance in Man; available at: http://www.ncbi.nlm.nih.gov/entrez/query.fcgi?db=OMIM), complex traits such as schizophrenia are far more common and carry enormous societal burden. A person who carries a predisposing genotype for a single-gene disorder has a virtually 100% risk of developing the disorder; the link between genotype and clinical trait is essentially deterministic. For a complex trait, the link between genotype and phenotype is more subtle, and genotype risks are

TABLE 3–1.   Single-gene disorders compared with complex traits

	Single-gene disorder	Complex trait
Examples	Huntington's disease Cystic fibrosis	Schizophrenia Types 1 and 2 diabetes mellitus
Prevalence	Rare (<0.001%)	Common (~1%–25%)
Societal burden	Low	Very high
Gene→trait	Deterministic	Probabilistic
Number of genes	1	Many
Allele frequencies	Usually rare	Both common and rare
Etiology	Homogeneous	Heterogeneous
Interactions (gene×gene, gene×environment)	Not typical	Likely

probabilistic. For example, a relatively strong genetic risk factor for schizophrenia might increase its lifetime risk from 0.8% to 1.2%. Schizophrenia is thus dissimilar to those rare medical disorders that usually are associated with the word *genetic*.

Following the main themes in the field, the largest part of this chapter is devoted to work on the etiology of schizophrenia. First, we discuss the phenotype of schizophrenia. We then summarize the evidence that led us to believe that genetic factors predispose to schizophrenia. We review the evidence about the etiology of schizophrenia from genomic studies. Finally, we cover briefly the pharmacogenetics of schizophrenia.

PHENOTYPE OF SCHIZOPHRENIA

The pathogenesis of schizophrenia is unknown, and no compelling biological markers of sufficient sensitivity and specificity exist. As such, a diagnosis of schizophrenia is effectively syndromic and based on signs and symptoms with reference to a clinically derived definition of illness. In view of the extensive clinical heterogeneity, many largely unsuccessful attempts have been made to delineate etiologically distinct subgroups. Nevertheless, the use of structured and semistructured interviews together with explicit operational diagnostic criteria allows high degrees of diagnostic reliability to be achieved. It is plausible that *schizophrenia* as currently defined may include several heterogeneous disease processes.

Family, adoption, and twin studies have shown that the phenotype extends beyond the core diagnosis of schizophrenia to include a spectrum of disorders, such as "poor outcome" or schizophrenic schizoaffective disorder and schizotypal personality disorder (Farmer et al. 1987;

Kendler et al. 1995). The definitional boundaries of this spectrum are uncertain. Although it is clear that individual differences in liability to schizophrenia are substantially genetic, we have no clear idea what form this "liability" actually takes. We are as yet unable conclusively to identify endophenotypes that are intermediate between genetic predisposition and the ultimate clinical phenotype (Gottesman and Gould 2003).

For example, one plausible endophenotype for schizophrenia is a failure in inhibitory neuronal dysfunction characterized by decreased inhibition of the P50 evoked response to the second of paired auditory stimuli 0.5 seconds apart, which has been replicated by multiple investigators (Freedman et al. 2000). Diminished P50 inhibition is found in other clinical contexts (e.g., mania, stimulant abuse, and alcohol withdrawal) but appears to be a trait deficit in schizophrenia alone. Preliminary investigations suggest that the inheritance of this putative endophenotype for schizophrenia may be Mendelian and substantially influenced by variation in the α7 nicotinic acetylcholine receptor subunit gene (*CHRNA7*) (Freedman et al. 1997; Leonard et al. 1998). Mutation screening of *CHRNA7* has identified a series of polymorphisms in the core promoter region of the gene, which diminish function of the promoter in vitro and are associated with both schizophrenia and diminished P50 inhibition in nonschizophrenic subjects (Leonard et al. 2002).

However, despite the persisting uncertainties about the definition of schizophrenia and the difficulties that arise from this fundamental problem, schizophrenia is a compelling candidate for studies aimed at identifying disease genes. Notwithstanding recent advances in imaging, transcriptomics, and proteomics, the human brain remains very difficult to study directly, and interpretation of cause and effect is problematic.

GENETIC EPIDEMIOLOGY OF SCHIZOPHRENIA

The field of genetic epidemiology encompasses a diverse set of conceptual, methodological, and analytical approaches that have in common the attempt to understand the etiology of a behavioral trait or biomedical disorder (Kendler 1993; Plomin et al. 1997). In humans, much of the work in this area has focused on etiology, with one of three main types of studies.

Family studies can be conceptualized as a type of case–control study, as described in detail elsewhere (Weissman et al. 1986). In these studies, *cases* are probands with schizophrenia, and *control subjects* have no history of schizophrenia and usually are matched for confounding variables such as age and gender. The outcome of interest is the prevalence of schizophrenia in biological relatives (usually first-degree relatives). These studies can detect the familiality of schizophrenia (i.e., whether it "runs" in families) but cannot disentangle genetic influences from environmental influences to which members of a family are exposed. Adoption and twin studies are the two principal approaches to delineating genetic and environmental effects in humans. *Adoption studies* are a social quasi experiment in which the offspring of one set of parents is reared from early in life by unrelated strangers. *Twin studies* are a biological quasi-experiment that contrasts pairs of monozygotic twins with dizygotic twins.

These types of studies have been a focus of considerable interest in schizophrenia research. Their results need to be interpreted in the context of two issues. First, these studies make numerous assumptions. For example, twin studies assume that monozygotic twins share all of their genes and dizygotic twins share half of their genes identical by descent. This assumption is only approximately true. The existence of congruent results across different study designs with differing assumptions supports the strength of the conclusions. Second, these studies provide only broad and approximate information about the etiology of schizophrenia. They can tell us whether a trait is familial and the approximate extent to which familial traits aggregate for genetic or environmental reasons. These studies—many of which date to the pregenomic era—carry little or no information about the specific etiology of a trait. However, these studies provide critical information about the rationality of searching for genes that underlie schizophrenia.

FAMILY STUDIES

Since 1980, 11 "modern" family studies of schizophrenia have been published (Kendler 2000). Several dozen family studies were published before 1980, but these "ancient" studies lacked design features now viewed as critical (control groups, direct interviews, blinded diagnoses, and the use of systematic diagnostic criteria). These studies yield an odds ratio of the risk of schizophrenia in the first-degree relatives (i.e., parents, siblings, children) of patients with schizophrenia compared with control subjects.

Figure 3–1 shows the results of a meta-analysis conducted for this chapter on the basis of a published summary of the modern family studies of schizophrenia (Kendler 2000). (Meta-analysis is the "analysis of analyses" and is a means of quantitatively summarizing a literature.) The odds ratios from these studies were homogeneous ($\chi^2_{10} = 4.25$, $P = 0.94$). The meta-analytic summation of these 11 studies in a random-effects model yielded highly significant evidence for increased familial risk to first-degree relatives ($\chi^2_1 = 138.6$, $P < 0.001$) and an odds ratio of 9.77. This suggests that the first-degree relatives of individuals with schizophrenia are nearly 10 times more likely to be affected with schizophrenia than are comparison subjects. The precision of this estimate is shown by its 95% confidence interval (CI) of 6.16–15.50. Thus, this meta-analysis of "modern" family studies provided strong and consistent evidence of the familiality of schizophrenia. Notably, the direction and magnitude of this conclusion are remarkably similar to the results from the "ancient" family studies of schizophrenia.

ADOPTION STUDIES

Five primary adoption studies of schizophrenia have been done (Kendler 2000), and the number and quality of these reports make it difficult to conduct meta-analytic procedures, and most investigated the schizophrenia spectrum. Briefly, variants of the basic adoption design can be used to test two key hypotheses about schizophrenia. First, by investigating the adoptive relatives of adoptees with and without schizophrenia, researchers can assess the contribution of postnatal environmental factors. The two relevant studies had a summary odds ratio estimate that did not differ significantly from unity ($\chi^2_1 = 0.76$, $P = 0.38$). Thus, environmental factors that occur after the age at adoption are not etiologically important for schizophrenia. Second, there are two ways in which to assess the effect of genetic etiological factors. The stronger approach is to compare the biological relatives of adoptees with and without schizophrenia. The summary odds ratio for this comparison was significant ($\chi^2_1 = 21.5$, $P < 0.001$) and was estimated at 4.98 (95% CI=2.38–10.4). In addition, one can compare the offspring of parents with schizophrenia who were adopted with the adopted offspring of control parents. This comparison was significant ($\chi^2_1 = 17.7$, $P <$

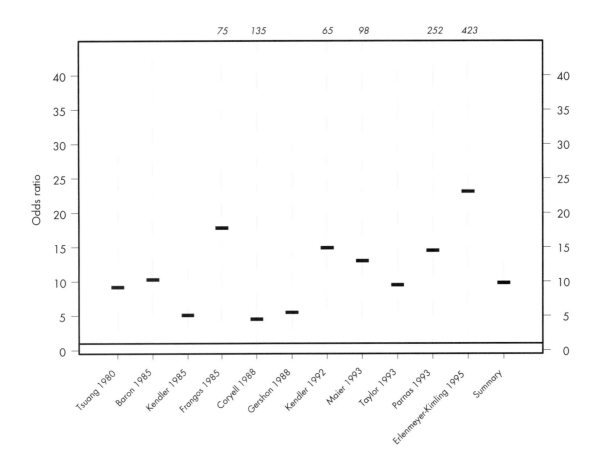

FIGURE 3–1.   Family studies of schizophrenia.

Odds ratios refer to the risk of schizophrenia in the first-degree relatives of patients with schizophrenia compared with the risk in the first-degree relatives of control subjects. The 11 "modern" family studies of schizophrenia are depicted on the x-axis. The y-axis shows the odds ratios for each individual study, with the point estimate given by horizontal bars and 95% confidence intervals (CIs) given by vertical lines. The upper bounds for 6 studies were large and are truncated at 45. The meta-analytic summary odds ratio was 9.8 (95% CI=6.2–15.5).

See Kendler 2000 for review of and citations for studies cited in this figure.

0.001), and the summary odds ratio was estimated at 3.48 (95% CI=1.90–6.40). The adoption literature suggests that postnatal environmental effects are not important in the etiology of schizophrenia, whereas genetic effects are significant. These conclusions are qualified by the relatively small sample sizes of these studies.

TWIN STUDIES

A meta-analysis of twin studies of schizophrenia was recently published (Sullivan et al. 2003). After a structured literature review, 12 twin studies of schizophrenia that met inclusion criteria for meta-analysis were identified, and the results were summarized with a meta-analytic approach (Figure 3–2).

One principal result of this meta-analysis of 12 published twin studies of schizophrenia was expected, and the other was quite surprising. Consistent with prior summaries of the twin literature on schizophrenia, the meta-analytic summary estimate of its heritability was very high, estimated at 81% (95% CI=73%–90%), and this result may provide a useful summary of a diverse literature. However, we also identified small but significant common environmental effects on liability to schizophrenia (point estimate=11%; 95% CI=3%–19%).

The high heritability of schizophrenia is consistent with prior summaries of this literature. Critically, this estimate is quite high and supports the rationality of searching for the genetic determinants of schizophrenia. However, it was notable that there was a nonzero contribution

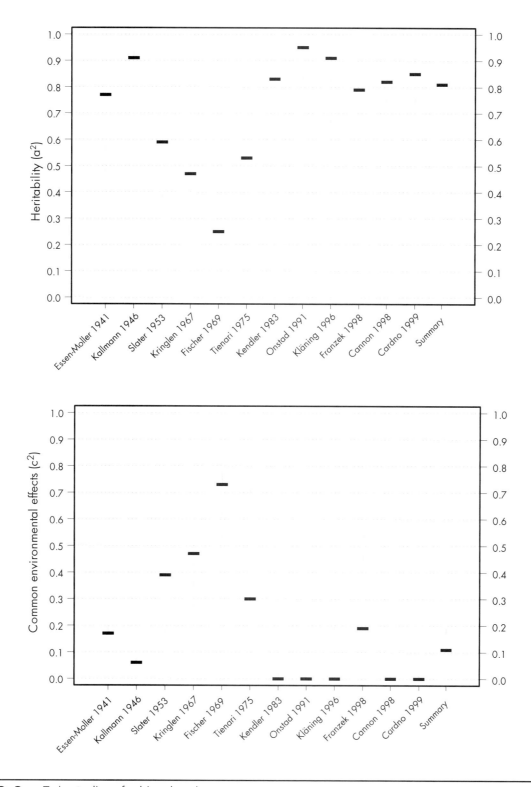

FIGURE 3–2.   Twin studies of schizophrenia.

Heritability (a²) **(top)** and common or shared environmental effects (c²) **(bottom).** The 12 twin studies meeting inclusion criteria are on the x-axes. The y-axes show the proportion of variance *(horizontal bar)* and the 95% confidence intervals on the estimate *(vertical line)*.

See Sullivan et al. 2003 for review of and citations for studies cited in this figure.

of environmental influences shared by members of a twin pair. This finding is ironic because it is unusual to find a behavioral trait or disorder with significant common environmental influences (Goldsmith et al. 1987) and because schizophrenia is usually considered one of the "more genetic" psychiatric disorders. The magnitude of the finding suggests that these influences have a modest effect on liability to schizophrenia. When considering this surprising finding further, we discovered that significant common environmental effects for schizophrenia actually have been reported previously (McGue et al. 1983; Rao et al. 1981). When these prior reports were published in the early 1980s, there was a sharp division within psychiatry as to whether schizophrenia resulted from biological/genetic factors or environmental factors such as an adverse maternal–child relationship. These perspectives often were framed as mutually exclusive ("nature *or* nurture"). The stronger genetic component to schizophrenia was the more strongly emphasized result. Our rediscovery of subtle but nontrivial common environmental effects on schizophrenia is likely to be interpreted differently now than in the 1980s. It is important to note that the traditional phrases *common environment* and *shared environment* are misnomers in that they generally evoke risk factors such as parental rearing behavior and traumatic life events. In the context of twin analyses, *common environment* refers to any process that makes members of a twin pair similar regardless of zygosity. These processes include the classic pre- and postnatal environmental factors noted earlier but also encompass profoundly biological processes such as exposure to infectious agents; macro- or micronutrient dietary characteristics; and exposure to environmental toxins, teratogens, and other intrauterine factors. They can even include profoundly genomic processes such as the establishment of DNA methylation patterns and retrotransposon activity in early stages of individual development.

SUMMARY

These quantitative summaries of the published literature on the genetic epidemiology of schizophrenia support several important conclusions that set the stage for the work described in the remainder of this chapter. Schizophrenia is a highly familial disorder that is strongly affected by genetic influences. However, the small but significant importance of common environmental factors underscores schizophrenia's identity as a complex trait. Nonetheless, the genetic epidemiological data suggest that it is rational to search for genes that underlie susceptibility to schizophrenia.

GENOMIC APPROACHES TO THE ETIOLOGY OF SCHIZOPHRENIA

MODE OF TRANSMISSION

Studies of different classes of relatives clearly indicate that schizophrenia cannot be caused by a single-gene disorder or a collection of single-gene disorders, even when incomplete penetrance is taken into account. Rather, the mode of transmission is complex and non-Mendelian. Critically, the number of susceptibility loci, the disease risk conferred by each locus, the extent of genetic heterogeneity, and the degree of interaction among loci all remain unknown. The predicted lack of simple one-to-one relations between genotype and phenotype makes the task of identifying susceptibility genes difficult and clearly implies the need for large sample sizes for both initial findings and replication (Owen et al. 2000).

CHROMOSOMAL ABNORMALITIES

Numerous investigations have attempted to identify chromosomal abnormalities in individuals with schizophrenia, reasoning that genes predisposing to schizophrenia could be localized to the disrupted genomic regions. Cytogenetic anomalies (e.g., translocations and deletions) may be pathogenic through several mechanisms: direct disruption of a gene, formation of a new gene by fusing two spatially separated genes, indirect disruption of the function of neighboring genes by a position effect, or alteration of the copy number for a gene (deletions, duplications, and unbalanced translocations). A single incidence of a cytogenetic abnormality is insufficient to suggest causality. Of the many reports (Bassett et al. 2000), the evidence is compelling for two regions.

First, a balanced reciprocal translocation between chromosome 1q42 and 11q14.3 has been shown to cosegregate with schizophrenia in several studies. No genes appear to be disrupted by the chromosome 11 breakpoint, whereas two genes are disrupted in the chromosome 1q42 region. These two genes have been named *DISC1* and *DISC2* (**d**isrupted **in sc**hizophrenia), and several lines of evidence suggest their potential importance in schizophrenia (Owen et al. 2004).

Second, there is an association between a 1.5 megabase deletion on 22q11 and schizophrenia (McDermid and Morrow 2002; Owen et al. 2004). Deletions in this region are associated with velocardiofacial syndrome (VCFS). VCFS occurs in about 1 in 4,000 live births (Murphy 2002). Its phenotype is variable but includes cleft palate, cardiac anomalies, typical facies, and learning

TABLE 3–2. Schematic of steps in conducting a genome scan for schizophrenia

Step	Description	Reason	Output
1. Sample collection	Ascertain family pedigrees in which multiple individuals are affected with schizophrenia. Diagnosis should be confident. The minimum size is an affected relative pair (e.g., two affected siblings), and the maximum size could include dozens of relatives and multiple generations.	Studying "multiplex" pedigrees increases the chance that one or more genes are causal.	N individuals from K pedigrees
2. Genome scan	Genotype all individuals for many polymorphic genetic markers (varies across studies; range=250–1,000). These markers are approximately evenly scattered across the genome. The genomic location of each marker is known.	Which markers are used and the number per study are variable (250–1,000 markers). This is an essential step in attempting to find genes for schizophrenia. Quality control is critical.	N individuals with G genotypes per individual, sorted by the position of the marker in the genome
3. Linkage analysis	Complex computer algorithms are used to analyze the data: • Compute the linkage evidence for each family at the location of each marker. Each element in the matrix is the linkage evidence of the ith family at the jth marker. • Summarize the overall evidence via a weighted sum across all families.	Determine the regions of the genome that show evidence for "linkage" between schizophrenia and markers at known locations.	• K families $\times$ G markers at known locations • $1 \times G$ matrix
4. Follow-up	Which regions replicate across studies? Which genes in these regions are likely positional candidate genes for schizophrenia?	Numerous significance tests have been conducted. With a high chance of type I error and (usually) limited statistical power, what do we believe?	Qualitative or quantitative analytic summary

disabilities. A bidirectional association with schizophrenia is seen because individuals with VCFS have an elevated lifetime risk of a psychotic disorder reminiscent of schizophrenia (18%), and approximately 2% of individuals with schizophrenia have a deletion in the relevant area of 22q11 (Murphy 2002). Further support is provided by schizophrenia linkage studies implicating 22q (see next subsection) and the observation that mice with an orthologous deletion have sensorimotor gating impairments reminiscent of schizophrenia (Paylor et al. 2001).

LINKAGE STUDIES

The purpose of a linkage study for a complex trait such as schizophrenia is to identify the genomic regions that might harbor predisposing or protective genes. In essence, linkage is a "discovery science" tool that does not require a priori assumptions about the nature and locations of genes involved in the etiology of schizophrenia

(Cardon and Bell 2001; Sham 1998). A full discussion of the conceptual and statistical basis of linkage studies is beyond the scope of this chapter. The steps in conducting a linkage study are shown in Table 3–2.

The general steps are sample collection, genotyping for a "genome scan," linkage analysis, and follow-up. For schizophrenia, more than 20 genome scans have been conducted whose intention was to discover genes that might be involved in the etiology of schizophrenia. The findings of these studies are complex and difficult to summarize even with a qualitative "box score" approach. Moreover, a quantitative summary is required in order to detect subtle effects for which individual studies possess low statistical power.

Recently, Lewis et al. (2003) completed a meta-analysis of 20 genome scans for schizophrenia. Although this approach has several important weaknesses and caveats (Levinson et al. 2003), it has the important advantage of being able to summarize an unwieldy literature. This anal-

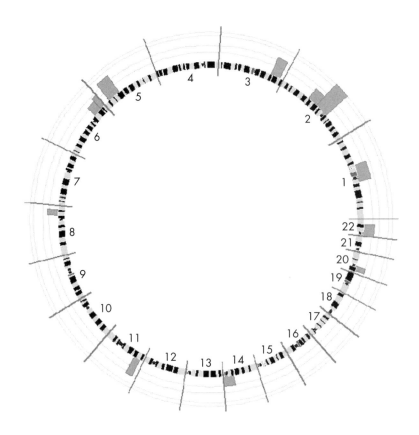

FIGURE 3–3.   Results from a meta-analysis of 20 genome scans for schizophrenia.

The human genome is depicted as a circle from the beginning of the short arm of chromosome 1 and moving counterclockwise to the end of the short arm of chromosome 22. The major Giemsa stain bands are overlaid. The darker solid bars show the locations of the 12 nominally significant regions from the meta-analysis. The height of the bars is proportional to the $-\log 10$ of its *P* value. The light concentric circles depict significance levels of 0.05, 0.01, 0.001, and 0.000417 (the genomewide significance).
Source.   Based on data from Lewis et al. 2003.

ysis is likely to be an important but imprecise tool—the regions highlighted by this analysis may well contain genes critical to the etiology of schizophrenia, but etiologically important genes may lie in regions not highlighted.

The results of this meta-analysis are depicted graphically in Figure 3–3. Twelve genomic regions reached nominal statistical significance, and a region on chromosome 2 was significant even after adjustment for multiple comparisons. In effect, this analysis suggests that the search space for loci that are likely to contain susceptibility genes for schizophrenia has been narrowed considerably: the 12 regions highlighted by the meta-analysis contain 2,181 known genes (13.8% of all known genes) and 320 million base pairs (11.2% of the genome).

The genome scan approach can identify candidate genes based on their position under a linkage peak and can provide statistical support. Linkage is an imperfect tool:

some of these regions are likely false positives and some false negatives. Other approaches are required to prove the involvement of a given gene in schizophrenia.

ASSOCIATION STUDIES

Association studies are essentially case–control studies that use one or more genetic markers as risk factors. The features, strengths, and weaknesses of these studies are described elsewhere (Sullivan et al. 2001). Findings from more than 500 association studies of schizophrenia have been published. As a body of work, these studies have numerous methodological difficulties, including small sample sizes, poorly matched control subjects, and type I errors. These critical difficulties render interpretation of many studies difficult. Nonetheless, these studies have proven informative and, if done well, can provide crucial information.

TABLE 3–3.   Evidence supporting variation in specific genes in the etiology of schizophrenia

Gene	Gene product or effect	Location	Linkage evidence, bin (of 120)	Association evidence, box score	Other evidence
NRG1	Neuregulin 1	8p12	55	6 of 7 samples	Altered expression in dorsal lateral prefrontal cortex in schizophrenia, known to be involved in the developing nervous system
DTNBP1	Dystrobrevin binding protein 1	6p22.3	10	6 of 8 samples	Involved in multiple neuronal functions (e.g., synapse formation and maintenance); colocalizes with postsynaptic γ-aminobutyric acid receptors
G72 and *G30*	Produces *PLG72*	13q33.2	62	1 sample	Protein product not yet well characterized; expressed in brain and interacts with D-amino acid oxidase (DAO), which is independently associated with schizophrenia; association of *G72* and *G30* with bipolar disorder replicated in several samples
RGS4	Regulator of G-protein signaling 4	1q23.3	14	2 of 3 samples	Altered brain expression in schizophrenia via microarray studies of postmortem samples
COMT	Catechol-*O*-methyl-transferase	22q11.21	9	Inconsistent	Deletion associated with schizophrenia; functional variant implicated in schizophrenia by neuroimaging and neuropsychological testing
PRODH	Proline dehydrogenase	22q11.21	9	1 of 4 samples	Deletion associated with schizophrenia; mouse model suggests its importance as an endophenotype
DISC1 and *DISC2*	Disrupted in schizophrenia 1 and 2	1q42.2	38		Balanced translocation associated with schizophrenia
HTR2A	Serotonin$_{2A}$ receptor	13q14.2	81	Meta-analytic support	Target for multiple antipsychotic drugs
DRD3	Dopamine$_3$ receptor	3q13.31	68	Meta-analytic support	Implicated via dopaminergic theory of schizophrenia

BEST CURRENT CANDIDATE GENES FOR SCHIZOPHRENIA

The literature on the molecular genetics of schizophrenia appears to be moving rapidly, and any review of this area is quickly outdated. At the same time, evidence is beginning to amass to suggest the potential importance of several genes in the etiology of schizophrenia. The genes that appear to be front-runners and for which published data are available from independent groups as of January 2004 are shown in Table 3–3.

Neuregulin 1 (NRG1)

The neuregulin 1 gene (*NRG1*) is in a bin that ranked 55th of 120 in the Lewis meta-analysis (Lewis et al. 2003) but is relatively close to the proximal bin that ranked 12th. Despite the modest linkage evidence, the same haplotype of markers in *NRG1* has shown notably consistent association evidence across two Icelandic (Stefansson et al. 2002) and two United Kingdom samples (Stefansson et al. 2003; N.M. Williams et al. 2003). Positive data implicating different haplotypes have also emerged from two Chinese samples (Tang et al. 2004; Yang et al. 2003) and an Irish sample (Corvin et al. 2004), but were not found in a Japanese sample (Iwata et al. 2004). In addition, some evidence indicates that *NRG1* isoforms are differentially expressed in dorsolateral prefrontal cortex of individuals with schizophrenia (Hashimoto et al. 2004).

These studies provide strong statistical evidence that variation in *NRG1* confers susceptibility to schizophrenia. At present, the specific risk alleles and pathogenetic mechanisms are unknown. However, a sizable literature supports the contention that *NRG1* isoforms play critical roles in the developing nervous system and brain as well as in oncogenesis (Falls 2003). It has been proposed that *NRG1* might influence disease susceptibility by altering the expression and activities of a broad range of neuroreceptors, particular nicotinic acetylcholinergic and *N*-methyl-D-aspartate (NMDA) glutamatergic receptors. *NRG1* is also an important regulator of glial cells and myelination.

Dystrobrevin Binding Protein 1 (DTNBP1)

The dystrobrevin binding protein 1 (*DTNBP1*) is located in a meta-analytic bin that received substantial linkage support as well as in multiple individual studies. Further work on this linkage peak in an Irish sample suggested the potential importance of *DTNBP1* (Straub et al. 2002; van den Oord et al. 2003). Significant evidence for association was found with several single nucleotide polymorphisms (SNPs) and haplotypes, a finding that remained after a conservative analysis that included only a single affected person from each nuclear family ($P=0.008–0.0001$ for three-marker haplotypes). Straub and colleagues were unable to identify the specific susceptibility variants.

Despite a modest number of studies, the evidence for *DTNBP1* as a susceptibility gene for schizophrenia is now strong. The first replication study—in German and Israeli families showing evidence for linkage to 6p—gave evidence of association in both samples (Schwab et al. 2003). A *DTNBP1* haplotype was also significantly associated in a Chinese sample (Tang et al. 2003) and in a Swedish sample (particularly in subjects with a family history of schizophrenia) (Van Den Bogaert et al. 2003), but not in additional Irish (Morris et al. 2003) and German and Polish samples (Van Den Bogaert et al. 2003). In addition, a large United Kingdom case–control study initially failed to find evidence of association for the markers used in other studies, but when novel SNPs (particularly one in the most 5′ promoter) were included with markers from the original study, highly significant evidence for association was obtained ($P=0.00005$) (N.M. Williams et al. 2004a). When the same markers were examined in a previously negative Irish sample (Morris et al. 2003), the specific risk haplotype observed was significantly more common in the patient sample.

Taken together, the data from these samples studied by multiple independent groups provide compelling evidence that variation in *DTNBP1*, or a neighboring gene, confers susceptibility for schizophrenia. Individual markers that directly increase disease susceptibility have not yet been found. The Cardiff, United Kingdom, and Dublin, Ireland, samples had identical risk haplotypes, but these differed from those in the other studies. The differences likely reflect allelic heterogeneity at the *DTNBP1* locus. The true susceptibility variants remain unidentified.

G72 *and* G30

The third gene was identified within a region of 13q22–34 initially implicated in a linkage study. Evidence from the Lewis meta-analysis was not impressive, but this region had linkage support in some studies. The Genset group in France obtained single-point association evidence after examining a 5-million base pair region with 191 SNP markers in approximately 200 French-Canadian schizophrenic patients and control subjects (Chumakov et al. 2002). Examination of haplotypes showed much stronger evidence for association ($P=3 \times 10^{-6}$, even after correction for multiple comparisons). The authors identified two possible genes (which were overlapping but located on opposite DNA strands) in the associated region that might account for the finding and designated them *G72* and *G30*. No known homologs for either gene were found, and sequence analysis did not show any likely function. Both were expressed in brain (and other tissues), but only *G72* gave a product after in vitro translation, designated *PLG72*. On this basis, *G72/PLG72* was selected for further functional analysis, which showed a possible interaction with D-amino acid oxidase (DAO). By genotyping eight SNPs across the *DAO* gene, Chumakov and colleagues (2002) were then able to report that four intronic SNPs also were associated with schizophrenia ($P=0.001$) in the French-Canadians. Although the function of *DAO* is largely unknown, it appears to modulate the level of D-serine in brain. D-Serine may modulate NMDA glutamatergic receptors, suggesting that the *G72* and *DAO* associations support the long-standing hypothesis of abnormal glutamatergic transmission in schizophrenia.

The statistical evidence for association between *G72* and *G30* and schizophrenia is impressive, as is the additional finding of association with the interacting gene *DAO*. These findings are as-yet unreplicated. However, polymorphisms in *G72* and *G30* have been associated with bipolar disorder (Chen et al. 2004; Hattori et al. 2003). Given the clear possibility of partial overlap between the etiology of schizophrenia and bipolar disorder, these findings may have relevance to both disorders.

Regulator of G-Protein Signaling 4 (RGS4)

Unlike *NRG1*, *DTNBP1*, and *G30* and *G72*, which were identified by positional genetic approaches, the gene for regulator of G-protein signaling 4 (*RGS4*) was identified from differential expression data from postmortem brain tissue (Mirnics et al. 2001b). Microarray studies of global gene expression, subsequently confirmed by single-gene expression analysis, reported that *RGS4* expression was downregulated in the brains of patients with schizophrenia (Mirnics et al. 2001a, 2001b). In addition, *RGS4* maps to 1q21–q22, a region previously implicated by linkage in schizophrenia.

Chowdari and colleagues (2002) investigated two proband–parent trio samples from the United States and from India, as well as a third small sample recruited by the National Institute of Mental Health Collaborative Genetics Initiative. Significant associations were independently obtained in each of the United States samples for haplotypes encompassing four SNPs in the 5′ flanking sequence and the first intron of *RGS4*. As for *DTNBP1*, different alleles in different samples defined the risk haplotype. Significant association was not obtained for the larger Indian sample, but the overall evidence for association was significant across all three samples (*P*=0.0027). Two other groups have recently reported positive findings with this gene (Morris et al. 2004; N.M. Williams et al. 2004b). Although these findings are encouraging, *RGS4* does not yet enjoy the same depth of support as does *DTNBP1* or *NRG1*.

Catechol-*O*-Methyltransferase (COMT)

The catechol-*O*-methyltransferase gene (*COMT*) is a candidate for involvement in schizophrenia because of its location in the region of 22q11 deleted in VCFS and because it encodes a key dopamine catabolic enzyme. The COMT protein occurs as two distinct forms: a soluble form found in the cell cytoplasm (S-COMT) and a longer, membrane-bound form (MB-COMT). In most tissues, the S-COMT form predominates, but the MB-COMT form is the more prevalent species in brain. *COMT* contains a valine-to-methionine substitution at codon 108 of S-COMT and codon 158 of MB-COMT. The valine variant of S-COMT is reported to have greater activity and thermostability than the methionine variant, but the effects on MB-COMT are unknown. The valine variant has been associated with reduced executive frontal lobe function, suggesting a mechanism by which *COMT* might act as a susceptibility or modifying locus for schizophrenia (Egan et al. 2001).

Despite the plausibility of this association, the accumulated evidence to date is inconsistent. Intriguingly, the largest study to date suggested that variation in *COMT* other than the valine-methionine polymorphism is strongly associated with schizophrenia (Shifman et al. 2002). At the time of this writing, the issue of whether variation in *COMT* contributes to susceptibility to schizophrenia remains a matter of considerable controversy.

Proline Dehydrogenase (PRODH)

The proline dehydrogenase gene (*PRODH*), also located in the VCFS-deleted region on 22q11, is a candidate for involvement in schizophrenia according to linkage findings and because mice with an inactivated *PRODH* gene have abnormalities of sensorimotor gating reminiscent of those that may be a trait marker for schizophrenia (Gogos et al. 1999). An initial study that showed a complex pattern of association with schizophrenia (Liu et al. 2002) was not replicated in several samples.

Disrupted in Schizophrenia 1 and 2 (DISC1 *and* DISC2)

A reciprocal translocation between 1q42 and 11q14.3 was found in a large Scottish family cosegregated with schizophrenia (lod score=3.6) and other psychiatric disorders (lod score=7.1) (Blackwood et al. 2001). This translocation has been reported to disrupt two genes on chromosome 1: *DISC1* and *DISC2* (Millar et al. 2000). *DISC2* may regulate *DISC1* expression via antisense RNA (Millar et al. 2000). The DISC1 protein may regulate cytoskeletal function, and DISC1 truncation might contribute to schizophrenia by affecting neuronal functions dependent on cytoskeletal regulation (e.g., neuronal migration, neurite architecture, and intracellular transport). Some support for a general pathogenic role for at least one of these genes was provided by a study by Hennah et al. (2003), in which haplotypes at *DISC1* were associated with schizophrenia in an isolated Finnish population. This finding, if confirmed, suggests that the putative link between abnormal *DISC1* function and schizophrenia might not be specific to the unique family segregating the translocation. Results from other samples are required to determine whether the latter finding gains more general support.

Serotonin$_{2A}$ Receptor (HTR2A)

Serotonin receptor$_{2A}$ (*HTR2A*) is a therapeutic target for several antipsychotic drugs. Multiple association studies of a T-to-C polymorphism in *HTR2A* have been published with conflicting results. However, two meta-analytic summaries (Lohmueller et al. 2003; J. Williams et al. 1997) found a weak but strongly significant association. Notably, the effect size of this polymorphism was quite modest—a 7%–20% increase in risk for schizophrenia—which necessitates very large sample sizes to reliably detect its effect. These findings suggest that variation in *HTR2A* confers at most a very small effect on disease susceptibility. Another possibility is that variation at this locus modifies the disease phenotype rather than conferring disease susceptibility per se.

Dopamine₃ Receptor (DRD3)

The notion of dopaminergic hyperfunction in schizophrenia has been a historically important hypothesis. This hypothesis has received support from studies of the dopamine₃ receptor gene (*DRD3*). Most association studies have focused on a serine-to-glycine polymorphism in exon 1 of *DRD3*. As with *HTR2A*, the results of individual studies are inconsistent, but two meta-analyses (Lohmueller et al. 2003; J. Williams et al. 1998) presented evidence for a small but significant effect. The magnitude of the effect suggested a modest 10%–20% increase in the risk for schizophrenia.

SUMMARY

The genes discussed in this section are a snapshot taken in January 2004 of what appear to be the major current contenders for etiological risk factors for schizophrenia. The accumulated evidence at the time of this writing is variable—from strong (*NRG1, DTNBP1*) through intermediate (*RGS4, G72/G30/DAO, HTR2A, DRD3*) to weak (*COMT, PRODH*). None of these genes is certain to be involved in the etiology of schizophrenia. On the basis of the history of psychiatric genetics, it is critical to adopt a long view of this area of research. The key is not the excitement generated by a single highly publicized study but rather the weight of the evidence from multiple studies and lines of inquiry.

A second reason to be cautious in the interpretation of these studies is that the results of linkage and association studies—the traditional molecular genetic study designs in humans—yield only *statistical support* for candidate genes for schizophrenia. These studies alone cannot "prove" the etiological importance of a gene. However, schizophrenia research now has multiple attractive targets whose significance is now being investigated via an array of other techniques. The polymorphisms in most of the genes in Table 3–3 are not obvious "smoking guns": the mechanisms underlying the functional significance of most of these polymorphisms are obscure and may involve very subtle alterations in protein production and function.

PHARMACOGENETICS

One of the most striking features of modern medicines is how often they fail to work. Even when they do work, they are often associated with serious adverse reactions. (Goldstein 2003, p. 553)

Most individuals with schizophrenia benefit from long-term pharmacotherapy. However, the benefits of antipsychotic treatment are inconsistent, incomplete, and often countered by significant side effects—relatively rare, life-threatening conditions (e.g., agranulocytosis, sudden cardiac death), side effects associated with long-term physical morbidity (e.g., tardive dyskinesia, increased body mass, impaired glucose metabolism), and subjectively unpleasant states associated with nonadherence (e.g., akathisia). Although most individuals respond to treatment, poor or partial response is common, and many patients require trials of multiple medications.

Currently, our capacity to predict these phenomena—therapeutic response and clinically significant side effects—is limited. Given the relatively poor understanding of individual differences in the beneficial effects and side effects of these medications, there are no effective means by which to match individual patients with schizophrenia to treatments that maximize the probability of favorable treatment response and/or minimize the probability of important side effects. The ability to use the numerous antipsychotic medications more precisely through a scientifically based pharmacotherapy that is individualized to specific patients is an unrealized goal.

Interindividual differences in the therapeutic benefits and adverse drug reactions are likely influenced to a significant degree by genetic variation (Evans and McLeod 2003; Vesell 1989). Serious adverse drug reactions are common in hospitalized patients (incidence=6.7%) (Lazarou et al. 1998) and cause substantial morbidity, mortality, and cost (Griffin 1997). Phillips et al. (2001) conducted a systematic review and determined that 16 of 27 (59%) drugs that are commonly associated with adverse drug reactions are metabolized by one or more enzymes that have variant alleles associated with poor metabolism. Thus, it is likely that adverse drug reactions are at least partly a result of individual differences in drug metabolism.

The term *pharmacogenetics* is often used to refer to efforts to dissect the genetic contributions to individual variation in therapeutic drug response or liability to adverse effects. In psychiatry, attention has focused mostly on the hepatic enzymes that metabolize antipsychotic medications (cytochrome P450 1A2 [CYP1A2], CYP2D6, CYP3A4) or that are the known molecular targets of these medications (*DRD2, DRD3, HTR2A*). As examples of the potential explanatory power of this approach, the dosage of warfarin and risk of bleeding complications are strongly influenced by inactivating genetic variations in its metabolic pathway (principally CYP2C9) (Daly and King 2003), and the risk of venous thromboembolism associated with oral contraceptive use appears to be strongly influenced by the factor V Leiden and factor II G20210A mutations (Emmerich et al. 2001).

The literature on the pharmacogenetics of antipsychotic therapeutic response and side-effect liability is large and unwieldy and is based on relatively few studies. However, some tenable hypotheses arise from this literature. First, a few hypothesized associations are supported by a preponderance of evidence (e.g., *DRD3* and risk of tardive dyskinesia). Second, hypothesized associations with both positive and negative results are found in the literature (e.g., *HTR2A* and treatment response). Third, tenable hypothesized associations have been investigated in only one or a few studies (e.g., *DRD1* and treatment response). Fourth, tenable hypotheses based on molecular pharmacokinetic and pharmacodynamic data are essentially unstudied.

The best-supported current finding in the pharmacogenetic literature on antipsychotics is probably the association of a serine-to-glycine change in *DRD3* with tardive dyskinesia. A recent meta-analysis supported this association, with a pooled odds ratio of 1.52 (95% CI=1.08–1.68) (Lerer et al. 2002). This polymorphism also has been associated with schizophrenia itself (Lohmueller et al. 2003; J. Williams et al. 1998), particularly in treatment responders (Shaikh et al. 1996).

CONCLUSION

Schizophrenia has historically proven to be highly resistant to attempts to discern its etiology, and few hard facts exist about the origins of this often-devastating neuropsychiatric illness. Application of molecular genetic strategies in schizophrenia is rational, and it was widely anticipated that these techniques would lead to very rapid advances. It is not surprising that this proved to be an inflated hope that led to pronouncements that "linkage has failed," a critique that also went too far.

As shown in Table 3–3, there are several logical candidate genes for schizophrenia, a few of which have unprecedented empirical support. It is likely that some of the genes in Table 3–3 will prove to be false leads, and this result should be anticipated. However, it would be a monumental advance for schizophrenia research if even *one* of these genes (or a gene network to which it belongs) proves to be involved in the etiology of schizophrenia. It is essential to take a long view of this body of work and to weigh the accumulated evidence rather than single, perhaps highly publicized, studies.

REFERENCES

Bassett AS, Chow EW, Weksberg R: Chromosomal abnormalities and schizophrenia. Am J Med Genet 97:45–51, 2000

Blackwood DH, Fordyce A, Walker MT, et al: Schizophrenia and affective disorders—cosegregation with a translocation at chromosome 1q42 that directly disrupts brain-expressed genes: clinical and P300 findings in a family. Am J Hum Genet 69:428–433, 2001

Cardon LR, Bell JI: Association study designs for complex diseases. Nat Rev Genet 2:91–99, 2001

Chen YS, Akula N, Detera-Wadleigh SD, et al: Findings in an independent sample support an association between bipolar affective disorder and the G72/G30 locus on chromosome 13q33. Mol Psychiatry 9:87–92, 2004

Chowdari KV, Mirnics K, Semwal P, et al: Association and linkage analyses of RGS4 polymorphisms in schizophrenia. Hum Mol Genet 11:1373–1380, 2002

Chumakov I, Blumenfeld M, Guerassimenko O, et al: Genetic and physiological data implicating the new human gene G72 and the gene for D-amino acid oxidase in schizophrenia. Proc Natl Acad Sci U S A 99:13675–13680, 2002

Corvin AP, Morris DW, McGhee K, et al: Confirmation and refinement of an "at-risk" haplotype for schizophrenia suggests the EST cluster, Hs.97362, as a potential susceptibility gene at the Neuregulin-1 locus. Mol Psychiatry 9(2):208–213, 2004

Daly AK, King BP: Pharmacogenetics of oral anticoagulants. Pharmacogenetics 13:247–252, 2003

Egan M, Goldberg T, Kolachana B, et al: Effect of COMT Val108/158 Met genotype on frontal lobe function and risk for schizophrenia. Proc Natl Acad Sci U S A 98:6917–6922, 2001

Emmerich J, Rosendaal FR, Cattaneo M, et al: Combined effect of factor V Leiden and prothrombin 20210A on the risk of venous thromboembolism—pooled analysis of 8 case-control studies including 2310 cases and 3204 controls. Study Group for Pooled-Analysis in Venous Thromboembolism [published erratum appears in Thromb Haemost 86:1598, 2001]. Thromb Haemost 86:809–816, 2001

Evans WE, McLeod HL: Pharmacogenomics—drug disposition, drug targets, and side effects. N Engl J Med 348:538–549, 2003

Falls DL: Neuregulins: functions, forms, and signaling strategies. Exp Cell Res 284:14–30, 2003

Farmer AE, McGuffin P, Gottesman II: Twin concordance for DSM-III schizophrenia: scrutinizing the validity of the definition. Arch Gen Psychiatry 44:634–641, 1987

Freedman R, Coon H, Myles-Worsley M, et al: Linkage of a neurophysiological deficit in schizophrenia to a chromosome 15 locus. Proc Natl Acad Sci U S A 94:587–592, 1997

Freedman R, Adams CE, Adler LE, et al: Inhibitory neurophysiological deficit as a phenotype for genetic investigation of schizophrenia. Am J Med Genet 97:58–64, 2000

Gogos JA, Santha M, Takacs Z, et al: The gene encoding proline dehydrogenase modulates sensorimotor gating in mice. Nat Genet 21:434–439, 1999

Goldsmith HH, Buss AH, Plonim R, et al: Roundtable: what is temperament? Child Dev 58:505–529, 1987

Goldstein DB: Pharmacogenetics in the laboratory and the clinic. N Engl J Med 348:553–556, 2003

Gottesman II, Gould TD: The endophenotype concept in psychiatry: etymology and strategic intentions. Am J Psychiatry 160:636–645, 2003

Griffin JP: The cost of adverse drug reactions. Adverse Drug React Toxicol Rev 16:75–78, 1997

Hashimoto R, Straub RE, Weickert CS, et al: Expression analysis of neuregulin-1 in the dorsolateral prefrontal cortex in schizophrenia. Mol Psychiatry 9:299–307, 2004

Hattori E, Liu C, Badner JA, et al: Polymorphisms at the G72/G30 gene locus, on 13q33, are associated with bipolar disorder in two independent pedigree series. Am J Hum Genet 72:1131–1140, 2003

Hennah W, Varilo T, Kestila M, et al: Haplotype transmission analysis provides evidence of association for DISC1 to schizophrenia and suggests sex-dependent effects. Hum Mol Genet 12:3151–3159, 2003

Iwata N, Suzuki T, Ikeda M, et al: No association with the neuregulin 1 haplotype to Japanese schizophrenia. Mol Psychiatry 9:126–127, 2004

Kendler KS: Twin studies of psychiatric illness: current status and future directions. Arch Gen Psychiatry 50:905–915, 1993

Kendler KS: Schizophrenia: genetics, in Comprehensive Textbook of Psychiatry. Edited by Sadock BJ, Kaplan VA. Philadelphia, PA, Lippincott Williams & Wilkins, 2000, pp 1147–1159

Kendler KS, Neale MC, Walsh D: Evaluating the spectrum concept of schizophrenia in the Roscommon Family Study. Am J Psychiatry 152:749–754, 1995

Lazarou J, Pomeranz BH, Corey PN: Incidence of adverse drug reactions in hospitalized patients: a meta-analysis of prospective studies. JAMA 279:1200–1205, 1998

Leonard S, Gault J, Moore T, et al: Further investigation of a chromosome 15 locus in schizophrenia: analysis of affected sibpairs from the NIMH Genetics Initiative. Am J Med Genet 81:308–312, 1998

Leonard S, Gault J, Hopkins J, et al: Association of promoter variants in the alpha7 nicotinic acetylcholine receptor subunit gene with an inhibitory deficit found in schizophrenia. Arch Gen Psychiatry 59:1085–1096, 2002

Lerer B, Segman RH, Fangerau H, et al: Pharmacogenetics of tardive dyskinesia: combined analysis of 780 patients supports association with dopamine D3 receptor gene Ser9Gly polymorphism. Neuropsychopharmacology 27:105–119, 2002

Levinson DF, Levinson MD, Segurado R, et al: Genome scan meta-analysis of schizophrenia and bipolar disorder, part I: methods and power analysis. Am J Hum Genet 73:17–33, 2003

Lewis CM, Levinson DF, Wise LH, et al: Genome scan meta-analysis of schizophrenia and bipolar disorder, part II: schizophrenia. Am J Hum Genet 73:34–48, 2003

Liu H, Heath SC, Sobin C, et al: Genetic variation at the 22q11 PRODH2/DGCR6 locus presents an unusual pattern and increases susceptibility to schizophrenia. Proc Natl Acad Sci U S A 99:3717–3722, 2002

Lohmueller KE, Pearce CL, Pike M, et al: Meta-analysis of genetic association studies supports a contribution of common variants to susceptibility to common disease. Nat Genet 33:177–182, 2003

McDermid HE, Morrow BE: Genomic disorders on 22q11. Am J Hum Genet 70:1077–1088, 2002

McGue M, Gottesman II, Rao DC: The transmission of schizophrenia under a multifactorial threshold model. Am J Hum Genet 35:1161–1178, 1983

Millar JK, Wilson-Annan JC, Anderson S, et al: Disruption of two novel genes by a translocation co-segregating with schizophrenia. Hum Mol Genet 9:1415–1423, 2000

Mirnics K, Middleton FA, Lewis DA, et al: Analysis of complex brain disorders with gene expression microarrays: schizophrenia as a disease of the synapse. Trends Neurosci 24:479–486, 2001a

Mirnics K, Middleton FA, Stanwood GD, et al: Disease-specific changes in regulator of G-protein signaling 4 (RGS4) expression in schizophrenia. Mol Psychiatry 6:293–301, 2001b

Morris DW, McGhee KA, Schwaiger S, et al: No evidence for association of the dysbindin gene [DTNBP1] with schizophrenia in an Irish population-based study. Schizophr Res 60:167–172, 2003

Morris DW, Rodgers A, McGhee KA, et al: Confirming RGS4 as a susceptibility gene for schizophrenia. Am J Med Genet 125B:50–53, 2004

Murphy KC: Schizophrenia and velo-cardio-facial syndrome. Lancet 359:426–430, 2002

Murphy KC, Jones RG, Griffiths E, et al: Chromosome 22qII deletions: an under-recognised cause of idiopathic learning disability. Br J Psychiatry 172:180–183, 1998

Owen MJ, Cardno AG, O'Donovan MC: Psychiatric genetics: back to the future. Mol Psychiatry 5:22–31, 2000

Owen MJ, Williams NM, O'Donovan MC: The molecular genetics of schizophrenia: new findings promise new insights. Mol Psychiatry 9:14–27, 2004

Paylor R, McIlwain KL, McAninch R, et al: Mice deleted for the DiGeorge/velocardiofacial syndrome region show abnormal sensorimotor gating and learning and memory impairments. Hum Mol Genet 10:2645–2650, 2001

Phillips KA, Veenstra DL, Oren E, et al: Potential role of pharmacogenomics in reducing adverse drug reactions: a systematic review. JAMA 286:2270–2279, 2001

Plomin R, DeFries JC, McClearn GE, et al: Behavioral Genetics, 3rd Edition. New York, WH Freeman, 1997

Rao DC, Morton NE, Gottesman II, et al: Path analysis of qualitative data on pairs of relatives: application to schizophrenia. Hum Hered 31:325–333, 1981

Schwab S, Knapp M, Mondabon S, et al: Support for association of schizophrenia with genetic variation in the 6p22.3 gene, dysbindin, in sib-pair families with linkage and in an additional sample of triad families. Am J Hum Genet 72:185–190, 2003

Shaikh S, Collier DA, Sham PC, et al: Allelic association between a Ser-9-Gly polymorphism in the dopamine D3 receptor gene and schizophrenia. Hum Genet 97:714–719, 1996

Sham PC: Statistics in Human Genetics. New York, Wiley, 1998

Shifman S, Bronstein M, Sternfeld M, et al: A highly significant association between a COMT haplotype and schizophrenia. Am J Hum Genet 71:1296–1302, 2002

Stefansson H, Sigurdsson E, Steinthorsdottir V, et al: Neuregulin 1 and susceptibility to schizophrenia. Am J Hum Genet 71: 877–892, 2002

Stefansson H, Sarginson J, Kong A, et al: Association of neuregulin 1 with schizophrenia confirmed in a Scottish population. Am J Hum Genet 72:83–87, 2003

Straub RE, Jiang Y, MacLean CJ, et al: Genetic variation in the 6p22.3 gene DTNBP1, the human ortholog of the mouse Dysbindin gene, is associated with schizophrenia [published erratum appears in Am J Hum Genet 72:1007, 2002]. Am J Hum Genet 71:337–348, 2002

Sullivan PF, Eaves LJ, Kendler KS, et al: Genetic case-control association studies in neuropsychiatry. Arch Gen Psychiatry 58:1015–1024, 2001

Sullivan PF, Kendler KS, Neale MC: Schizophrenia as a complex trait: evidence from a meta-analysis of twin studies. Arch Gen Psychiatry 60:1187–1192, 2003

Tang JX, Zhou J, Fan JB, et al: Family based association study of DTNBP1 in 6p22.3 and schizophrenia. Mol Psychiatry 8:717–718, 2003

Tang JX, Chen WY, He G, et al: Polymorphisms within 5´ end of neuregulin 1 gene are genetically associated with schizophrenia in the Chinese population. Mol Psychiatry 9:11–12, 2004

Van Den Bogaert A, Schumacher J, Schulze TG, et al: The DTNBP1 (dysbindin) gene contributes to schizophrenia, depending on family history of the disease. Am J Hum Genet 73:1438–1443, 2003

van den Oord EJ, Sullivan PF, Jiang Y, et al: Identification of a high-risk haplotype for the dystrobrevin binding protein 1 (DTNBP1) gene in the Irish study of high-density schizophrenia families. Mol Psychiatry 8:499–510, 2003

Vesell ES: Pharmacogenetic perspectives gained from twin and family studies. Pharmacol Ther 41:535–552, 1989

Weissman MM, Merikangas KR, John K, et al: Family genetic studies of psychiatric disorders: developing technologies. Arch Gen Psychiatry 43:1104–1116, 1986

Williams J, McGuffin P, Nothen M, et al: Meta-analysis of association between the 5-HT2a receptor T102C polymorphism and schizophrenia. EMASS Collaborative Group. European Multicentre Association Study of Schizophrenia. Lancet 349:1221, 1997

Williams J, Spurlock G, Holmans P, et al: A meta-analysis and transmission disequilibrium study of association between the dopamine D3 receptor gene and schizophrenia [published erratum appears in Mol Psychiatry 3:458, 1998]. Mol Psychiatry 3:141–149, 1998

Williams NM, Preece A, Spurlock G, et al: Support for genetic variation in neuregulin 1 and susceptibility to schizophrenia. Mol Psychiatry 8:485–487, 2003

Williams NM, Preece A, Morris DW, et al: Identification in two independent samples of a novel schizophrenia risk haplotype of the dystrobrevin binding protein gene (DTNBP1). Arch Gen Psychiatry 61(4):336–344, 2004a

Williams NM, Preece A, Spurlock G, et al: Support for RGS4 as a susceptibility gene for schizophrenia. Biol Psychiatry 55:192–195, 2004b

Yang JZ, Si TM, Ruan Y, et al: Association study of neuregulin 1 gene with schizophrenia. Mol Psychiatry 8:706–709, 2003

PRENATAL AND PERINATAL FACTORS

John H. Gilmore, M.D.

Robin M. Murray, M.D.

Strong evidence indicates that genetic factors are important in the etiology of schizophrenia (see Chapter 3, "Genetics," this volume). However, it is clear that environmental factors also play a critical role. In this chapter, we review what is known about the relative contribution of early environmental factors to the etiology of schizophrenia and which early environmental factors have been implicated. We also explore the potential mechanisms through which early environmental risk factors act on the developing brain and increase the risk for schizophrenia. We do not discuss environmental factors such as drug abuse and social stress, which may operate closer to the onset of the disorder.

ROLE OF ENVIRONMENTAL FACTORS IN ETIOLOGY OF SCHIZOPHRENIA

Twin studies estimate the heritability of schizophrenia to be approximately 80%, with environmental factors accounting for the remaining 20% of liability (Cardno et al. 1999; Sullivan et al. 2003). Heritability estimates derived from twin studies are based on a comparison of concordances for schizophrenia between monozygotic (MZ) and dizygotic (DZ) twins.

The twin methodology itself has two major limitations that may overestimate the genetic contribution and underestimate the environmental contribution to schizophrenia. First, heritability estimates assume additive effects of genes and environment and do not take into account the possibility of gene–environment interactions; this issue is discussed in detail by Van Os and Sham (2004).

Second, twin methodology is based on the equal environment assumption (i.e., that MZ and DZ twins share similar prenatal environments). However, it has become increasingly obvious that the prenatal environment of MZ twins is significantly different from that of DZ twins, mainly because most MZ twins share a placenta, whereas DZ twins have separate placentas. In extreme cases, monochorionic placentation and twin–twin transfusion syndrome can lead to large size differences between twins; in general, however, MZ twins have lower birth weights, higher rates of premature birth, and more adverse perinatal outcomes than do DZ twins (Dube et al. 2002). These same pre-and perinatal environmental risk factors also may increase risk for schizophrenia and could therefore lead to higher concordance rates in MZ twins that would be falsely attributed to genetic factors. A shared placenta also may result in concordant exposure to infec-

TABLE 4–1.   Relative contributions of environmental risk factors and genes to risk for schizophrenia

		Odds ratio/ Relative risk	Study
Obstetrical complications	Gestational age< 37 weeks	2.44	Geddes et al. 1999
	Premature rupture of membranes	3.11	Geddes et al. 1999
	Low birth weight (<2,500 g)	1.51	Geddes et al. 1999
	Incubator or resuscitation	2.21	Geddes et al. 1999
	Diabetes in pregnancy	7.76	M. Cannon et al. 2002
	Placental abruption	4.02	M. Cannon et al. 2002
	Birth weight< 2,000 g	3.89	M. Cannon et al. 2002
	Birth weight< 2,500 g	1.67	M. Cannon et al. 2002
	Emergency cesarean delivery	3.24	M. Cannon et al. 2002
	Uterine atony	2.29	M. Cannon et al. 2002
	Rhesus factor variables	2.00	M. Cannon et al. 2002
	Asphyxia	1.74	M. Cannon et al. 2002
	Bleeding in pregnancy	1.69	M. Cannon et al. 2002
	Preeclampsia	1.36	M. Cannon et al. 2002
	Hypoxia-ischemia related	4.56	Zornberg et al. 2000
Other environmental factors	Respiratory infection	2.13	Brown et al. 2000b
	Influenza	3.0	Brown et al. 2004a
	Malnutrition	2.0	Susser and Lin 1992
	Urban birth	2.4	Mortensen et al. 1999
	Season of birth	1.11	Mortensen et al. 1999
Genes	Dysbindin	1.14–1.87	Schwab et al. 2003
	Neuregulin	1.25–2.20	Stefansson et al. 2002, 2003; Williams et al. 2003
	Catechol-*O*-methyltransferase	1.59	Egan et al. 2001; Wonodi et al. 2003

tion or placental pathology, whereas dichorionic DZ twins would be more likely to have discordant exposures. In a comment on the twin method, Phillips (1993) concluded that "the results of twin studies may be especially misleading in disorders in which the prenatal environment is thought to play a part in their etiology" (p. 1009). The latter is likely to be the case with schizophrenia. It is not clear, however, if being a twin increases the risk of developing schizophrenia because studies addressing this question have yielded conflicting results (Kendler et al. 1996; Klaning et al. 1996).

The overall contribution of genes for liability for schizophrenia may be large, whereas the contribution of individual genes appears to be small. Odds ratios (ORs) for recently reported susceptibility genes are less than 2.0 (see Table 4–1). For example, the neuregulin "at-risk hap-

lotype" is present in only 9.5%–15.4% of patients and in 5.9%–7.5% of control subjects, giving ORs in the 1.25–2.20 range (Stefansson et al. 2003; Williams et al. 2003). For catechol-*O*-methyltransferase (COMT), the OR for the risk genotype is 1.59 at maximum (Egan et al. 2001; Wonodi et al. 2003); for dysbindin, the OR is 1.14–1.87 (Schwab et al. 2003). In a similar fashion, studies of the dysbindin gene find the risk haplotype present in only 6% of patients (van den Oord et al. 2003).

The picture emerges that genetic background is necessary but may not be sufficient to cause schizophrenia and that the contribution of individual genes to risk for schizophrenia is small. Perhaps the most obvious indication of the important role environmental factors play in schizophrenia is the observation that concordance rates in MZ twins are only in the 40%–45% range (Cardno et al.

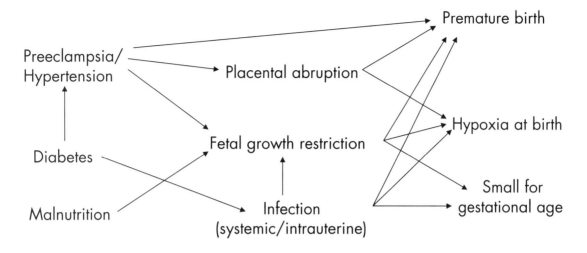

FIGURE 4–1. Interrelations between pre- and perinatal risk factors for schizophrenia.

1999; Tsuang et al. 2001). Furthermore, the ORs for several early environmental risk factors are of about the same order as those for individual risk genes (see Table 4–1). Therefore, it is critically important to improve our ability to define accurately environmental risk factors and to delineate mechanisms of action, to understand not only the etiology of schizophrenia but also the pathophysiology that underlies clinical symptomatology.

In the following section, we review the pre- and perinatal factors associated with increased risk for schizophrenia with a focus on potential mechanisms of action and what is known about their effect on brain development and neurodevelopmental outcome.

PRENATAL AND PERINATAL COMPLICATIONS

Considerable evidence shows that pre- and perinatal obstetrical complications increase risk for schizophrenia. Three meta-analyses have been performed. Geddes and Lawrie (1995) found that the presence of any obstetrical complication, broadly defined, increased risk for schizophrenia with an OR of 2.0. Subsequent studies attempted to understand the contribution of individual complications to risk for schizophrenia. Geddes et al. (1999) analyzed a set of studies that used the same Lewis–Murray scale for assessing obstetrical complications and found that premature rupture of the membranes, gestational age less than 37 weeks at birth, and the use of resuscitation or an incubator after birth increased the risk for schizophrenia. However, many of the studies included in these two meta-analyses were limited by methodological factors,

including selection and potential publication biases (Geddes and Lawrie 1995), nonspecific and sometimes retrospective definitions of complications, varying definitions across studies, and a lack of severity indicators.

In response to these methodological issues, M. Cannon et al. (2002) performed a meta-analysis on more recent prospective population-based studies; they found that several types of complications increased risk for schizophrenia, including low birth weight (<2,500 g), bleeding in pregnancy, diabetes in pregnancy, preeclampsia, rhesus incompatibility, asphyxia, and emergency cesarean delivery. ORs for individual complications in these meta-analyses ranged from 1.36 for preeclampsia to 7.76 for gestational diabetes (Table 4–1). A more recent study further suggested that maternal hypertension and treatment with a diuretic increased the risk for schizophrenia (OR=4.9; Sorensen et al. 2003).

The variety of obstetrical complications associated with increased risk of schizophrenia at first suggests that there may be multiple potential mechanisms underlying the associations. In addition, it is difficult to determine whether a true association with each factor exists or whether the observed association is a marker for other factors. However, a careful review of the many prenatal and perinatal complications that increase risk for schizophrenia, their causes, and their relations to one another allows the identification of some likely common mechanisms (see Figure 4–1).

Hypoxia-Ischemia

Many studies have focused on "hypoxic-ischemic–related" complications and have found that these increase the risk for schizophrenia with an OR of up to 4.5 (Zornberg et al. 2000). Others have found that hypoxic-ischemic complications increase risk of early-onset schizophrenia but not later-onset schizophrenia (T.D. Cannon et al. 2000; Rosso et al. 2000). What is considered a hypoxic-ischemic complication varies from study to study, and it is open to argument whether some of the complications are actually associated with hypoxia or with ischemia. Quantitative assessments of oxygenation status are lacking. It is also clear that a chronic hypoxia associated with hypertension during pregnancy (including preeclampsia) and acute hypoxia during delivery would likely have very different effects on brain development and thus should be differentiated.

FETAL GROWTH RESTRICTION

A second focus has been on abnormal growth. Many studies indicate that low birth weight is a risk factor for schizophrenia; in some studies, the association with low birth weight is found in the context of premature birth, and in other studies, it is not. Infants who are born small for gestational age typically have experienced fetal growth restriction. Clinically, fetal growth restriction is present in 3%–10% of pregnancies and is subtyped as symmetrical and asymmetrical. Symmetrical growth restriction involves a proportional lag of body and head size, whereas asymmetrical growth restriction refers to a decreased body size with a relatively normal head size. Asymmetrical growth restriction is due to a "brain-sparing effect" by which nutrients and oxygen are delivered to the developing brain at the expense of the rest of the body (Leveno et al. 2003). Some evidence suggests that this brain-sparing effect may be relevant to schizophrenia; Wahlbeck et al. (2001) found that birth weight and birth length were significantly smaller but head circumference was not in children who went on to develop schizophrenia. Future studies should distinguish fetal growth restriction as symmetrical or asymmetrical.

About 20% of fetal growth restriction is due to chromosomal disorders and other congenital malformation (Resnik 2002). Maternal vascular disease, especially early-onset severe preeclampsia and chronic hypertension, accounts for another 20%–30%. Other causes include disorders that cause thrombosis in the placenta, malnutrition, infection, smoking and other substance use, and multiple gestations. Fetal growth restriction is associated with fetal demise, premature birth, meconium aspiration, hypoxia, hypoglycemia, and acidosis during delivery. However, it is important to note that many cases of fetal growth restriction may actually represent a constitutionally small but otherwise normal fetus (Lin and Santolaya-Forgas 1998a).

Thus, fetal growth restriction represents a wide range of pathology (and, indeed, nonpathology) that includes abnormal blood flow and subsequent hypoxia, as well as hypoglycemia and acidosis in a subset of cases. Currently, blood flow can be measured in the umbilical artery and even in the fetal cerebral circulation, allowing a better determination of whether blood flow and oxygenation abnormalities actually exist in a specific fetus with fetal growth restriction (Lin and Santolaya-Forgas 1998b; Pardi et al. 2002).

Fetal growth restriction has a significant effect on brain development and ultimate neurodevelopmental outcome. Infants with fetal growth restriction and abnormal umbilical artery blood flow are more likely to be born prematurely and to have impaired intellectual development, mental retardation, and severe motor impairment (Vossbeck et al. 2001; Wienerroither et al. 2001). Term infants with fetal growth restriction have small but significant decreases in IQ when studied in adolescence (Paz et al. 2001).

PREMATURE BIRTH

Birth before 37 weeks' gestation is relatively common and occurs in 11% of the population. About 50% of preterm births are considered idiopathic, and 30%–40% are caused by an infection of some kind, especially intrauterine infection, which is often chronic and clinically unrecognized prior to delivery (Haram et al. 2003). Other causes of preterm birth include immunological disorders; cervical incompetence; uterine abnormalities; and maternal factors, such as preeclampsia, drug use, cigarette smoking, and poor nutrition (Leveno et al. 2003). Depending on its magnitude and cause, prematurity can be associated with postnatal complications, including infection, hypoxia, and cerebral damage in the form of intraventricular hemorrhage and periventricular leukomalacia.

Children born prematurely or with very low birth weight have poor neurodevelopmental outcomes, including mental retardation, learning disorders, and behavior problems (Saigal 2000; Wolke 1998). Studies suggest that these abnormalities persist into adolescence and adult life (Stewart et al. 1999). Individuals born very preterm are less likely than their full-term counterparts to take risks or drugs in adolescence or to be involved in criminal behavior (Hack et al. 2002). It is not clear whether these individuals' conventional behavior is a result of their recognition of their own limitations or whether it is a consequence of their parents having kept a particularly close eye on them. Structural brain abnormalities, consistent with structural abnormalities found in patients with schizophrenia, including reduced cortical gray matter and hippocampal volumes and enlarged lateral ventricle volumes, are observed in childhood and adolescence in children born very preterm or of low very birth weight (Allin et al. 2004; Isaacs et al. 2000; Nosarti et al. 2002, 2003; Peterson et al. 2000). Other outcomes common both to such individuals and to people with schizophrenia are an excess of neurological soft signs and abnormalities of language lateralization (Rushe et al. 2004).

PREMATURE RUPTURE OF MEMBRANES

Premature rupture of membranes is a major cause of preterm birth and is itself associated with amniotic fluid infection, multiple fetuses, abruptio placentae, and a previous preterm birth (Leveno et al. 2003).

PREECLAMPSIA AND HYPERTENSION

Hypertension complicates about 3.7% of pregnancies and is the most common medical complication of pregnancy. Preeclampsia, one of the hypertensive disorders of pregnancy, is characterized by reduced organ perfusion due to vasospasm (Leveno et al. 2003). Other hypertensive disorders include eclampsia, gestational hypertension, chronic hypertension, and preeclampsia superimposed on chronic hypertension.

The cause of preeclampsia is unknown, but preeclampsia is thought to be primarily a disorder of endothelial cell injury resulting from an excessive maternal inflammatory response to pregnancy (Redman et al. 1999). Preeclampsia is associated with abnormalities of the spiral arteries of the placenta that result in decreased placental blood flow and ischemia. Vasospasm can lead to infarction and reperfusion, resulting in hypoxia and the activation of inflammatory cytokines within the placenta (Henriksen 1998). Preeclampsia is associated with low birth weight, preterm birth, and fetal growth restriction in severe cases. Maternal hypertension does not appear to cause poorer neurodevelopmental outcome apart from those associated with complications of prematurity (Gray et al. 1998), although a recent study did find mild developmental delay at age 2 years, independent of associated complications (Cheng et al. 2004).

PLACENTAL ABRUPTION AND BLEEDING

Premature separation of the placenta occurs in 1 in 200 pregnancies (Leveno et al. 2003). Placental abruption has an infant mortality rate of approximately 20%–25% and is associated with preterm birth and fetal growth restriction (Ananth et al. 1999). Approximately 14% of infant survivors have significant neurological deficits (Abdella et al.

1984). Placental abruption is associated with increased maternal age and parity, preeclampsia and chronic hypertension, and preterm rupture of the membranes.

DIABETES IN PREGNANCY

In the meta-analysis by M. Cannon et al. (2002), diabetes in pregnancy was associated with increased risk for schizophrenia, although it is not clear from the studies reviewed whether this was gestational diabetes or diabetes that was present before pregnancy. Diabetes of either type is present in 2.6% of pregnancies that result in a live birth. Diabetes is associated with macrosomia, which can be associated with delivery complications resulting from cephalopelvic disproportion (Leveno et al. 2003). Preexisting diabetes is associated with fetal demise, congenital abnormalities such as central nervous system abnormalities, preeclampsia, and preterm birth. Mothers with diabetes are also at high risk for infections, with 80% developing at least one infection during pregnancy compared with 25% of nondiabetic mothers (Leveno et al. 2003). Evidence indicates that the offspring of mothers with diabetes have normal IQ; however, those children who experienced neonatal hypoglycemia have abnormalities of attention, motor control, and perception (Stenninger et al. 1998).

Little is known about the mechanisms through which maternal diabetes acts on the developing fetal brain. Mature rats born to diabetic mothers have significant decreases in synaptic length and dendritic spines of cerebellar Purkinje's neurons (Yamano et al. 1986). The developing fetal brain also has an enhanced inflammatory response to teratogens in diabetic mice (Lian et al. 2004). Diabetes in pregnancy also causes an increase in reactive oxygen species and peroxide production in the neonatal brain (Raza and John 2004). These studies suggest that maternal diabetes may make the developing brain more sensitive to additional insults.

UTERINE ATONY

Uterine atony is a common cause of postpartum hemorrhage that, by itself, would not be expected to have an effect on brain development. However, uterine atony is associated with prolonged labor and chorioamnionitis (Leveno et al. 2003), which would have an effect on the developing brain.

RHESUS FACTOR INCOMPATIBILITY

Rhesus (Rh) factor incompatibility as a risk factor for schizophrenia was first described by Hollister et al. (1996) and confirmed in studies that were part of the M. Cannon et al. (2002) meta-analysis. Recently, genetic approaches also have found that maternal–fetal genotype incompatibility at the *RHD* locus increases risk of schizophrenia (OR=1.7 and 2.6) (Kraft et al. 2004; C.G.S. Palmer et al. 2002). Rh factor incompatibility can lead to hypoxia as well as high levels of bilirubin, which could have a deleterious effect on the developing brain, including apoptosis of neurons and astrocytes (Shapiro 2003). In addition, inflammatory cytokines are increased in the setting of Rh factor incompatibility, which would have an adverse effect on the developing brain (Davenport 1994).

PRENATAL EXPOSURE TO MATERNAL INFECTION

Most research on prenatal exposure to infection and schizophrenia has focused on a specific viral infection—that of influenza. The findings are inconsistent, but most published studies indicate that maternal influenza infection during pregnancy is associated with a higher incidence of schizophrenia in offspring (Bagalkote et al. 2000; McGrath et al. 1995); whether this reflects reality or publication bias remains to be seen. Some have implicated infections other than influenza, including pneumonia and diphtheria (Watson et al. 1984), measles, varicella-zoster, polio (Torrey et al. 1988), bronchopneumonia (O'Callaghan et al. 1994), and poliovirus (Suvisaari et al. 1999).

Recent studies have moved beyond ecological association to studies that link infections in an individual mother with schizophrenia in her child. Respiratory infections, broadly defined, in the second trimester have been found to increase risk for schizophrenia (relative risk=2.13; Brown et al. 2000b). In this same cohort, serological evidence of maternal exposure to influenza in the first half of pregnancy increased risk for schizophrenia (OR=3.0; Brown et al. 2004b). Rubella infections during pregnancy also have been linked to increased risk for schizophrenia (relative risk=5.2; Brown et al. 2000a). Finally, the offspring of mothers with elevated levels of immunoglobulin G (IgG) and IgM, as well as antibodies to herpes simplex virus type 2, during pregnancy have an increased risk for schizophrenia (Buka et al. 2001b).

SEASON OF BIRTH AND PLACE OF BIRTH

The excess of late winter to early spring births is one of the more consistent epidemiological findings in schizophrenia (Torrey et al. 1997). In a large population-based study, season of birth had an OR of 1.11 and accounted for 10.5% of the population attributable risk (Mortensen et al. 1999). Curiously, one report suggested an excess of summer births in patients with the deficit subtype of schizophrenia, should the latter exist as a distinct entity (Kirkpatrick et al. 2002). Many factors have been postulated to underlie the excess of late winter to early spring births in schizophrenia, including infections, nutritional deficiency, toxic exposures, and meteorological factors such as light and temperature (Tochigi et al. 2004; Torrey et al. 1997).

Urban birth also increases risk for schizophrenia, with an OR of 1.4–2.4 and a population attributable fraction in Holland and Denmark of approximately 30% (Marcelis et al. 1998; Mortensen et al. 1999). It is not clear at what stage of life urban birth produces its effect, but possible underlying factors include infection, diet, toxic exposures, and stress.

NUTRITION

Maternal malnutrition has been reported to increase the risk of schizophrenia in offspring. Children born to mothers with severe food deprivation in the Dutch Hunger Winter had higher rates of schizophrenia (relative risk= 2.0; Susser and Lin 1992; Susser et al. 1996). This exposure also was reported to be associated with increased risk of schizoid personality disorder (Hoek et al. 1996) and affective disorder (Brown et al. 2000c). Patients with schizophrenia exposed to the prenatal famine were found to have decreased intracranial volumes and more white matter hyperintensities compared with patients without exposure (Hulshoff Pol et al. 2000). For obvious reasons, it has been difficult to find a sample on which to replicate the findings of the Dutch Hunger Winter.

STRESS

Some reports indicate that maternal stress during pregnancy and in the first year of life can increase the risk for schizophrenic offspring. For example, children whose fathers died during the mother's pregnancy were more likely to develop schizophrenia than were control subjects (Huttunen and Niskanen 1978). Mothers with an unwanted pregnancy also were more likely to have a child who went on to develop schizophrenia (Myhrman et al. 1996). However, other studies failed to find increased risk after prenatal exposure to a Dutch flood disaster (Selten et al. 1999) or a war in Israel (Selten et al. 2003). Although maternal stress can influence fetal brain development, the case for a specific link to risk for schizophrenia is weak.

MECHANISMS OF ENVIRONMENTAL RISK FACTORS

Various obstetrical and other prenatal environmental risk factors appear to contribute to risk for schizophrenia. The different pre- and perinatal risk factors are often associated with one another, and one type of complication can cause another. In addition, one kind of complication, such as diabetes, malnutrition, or infection, may make the developing brain more vulnerable to a subsequent insult, such as hypoxia. Furthermore, early risk factors for schizophrenia that might initially be considered environmental for the fetus, such as preeclampsia and gestational hypertension, have genetic components (Nilsson et al. 2004).

Progress in understanding how these environmental factors increase risk for schizophrenia requires a better understanding of the mechanisms of action—how they affect early brain development. At first glance, the long list of seemingly diverse pre- and perinatal factors that increase risk for schizophrenia makes this appear to be a daunting task. However, review of the risk factors, their causes, and their effects on the developing brain, as well as their relation to one another, allows us to focus on potential mechanisms.

We propose that four major mechanisms of action—hypoxia-ischemia, inflammation and infection (inflammatory cytokines), malnutrition, and stress responses—underlie these early risk factors for schizophrenia. As outlined in the following subsections, the four major mechanisms of action we propose can each alter brain development in a manner consistent with the neuropathology of schizophrenia (see Chapter 9, "Neuropathology and Neural Circuits Implicated in Schizophrenia," this volume). An improved understanding of the basic mechanisms that underlie early risk factors for schizophrenia will make it possible to focus future research, both in the laboratory and in the clinic, by making the assessment of these risk factors more precise and quantitative.

HYPOXIA-ISCHEMIA

Chronic ischemia during fetal development can occur in some cases of fetal growth restriction, as well as in preeclampsia and chronic hypertension. Acute hypoxia may be present in, or caused by, many birth complications linked to risk for schizophrenia, including fetal growth restriction, placental abruption, intrauterine infection, emergency cesarean delivery, asphyxia, and resuscitation. Hypoxia is also often present during the postnatal period after preterm birth.

Hypoxia-ischemia can cause a wide variety of abnormalities in the developing brain related to excitotoxic injury and cell death (Johnston et al. 2001). Relevant to the more subtle neuropathology that underlies schizophrenia, moderate postnatal hypoxia in rats can cause abnormal development of synapses in the hippocampus and cortex, as well as abnormal myelination of the corpus callosum and other pathways (Curristin et al. 2002). Neonatal hypoxia-ischemia also causes premature death of subplate neurons, which would affect the activity-dependent refinement of cortical connections (McQuillen et al. 2003). Indeed, cesarean birth and anoxia have been reported to cause long-lasting abnormalities in dopamine functioning and abnormal prepulse inhibition in guinea pigs and rats (Vaillancourt and Boska 2000) and dopamine hypofunction in the medial prefrontal cortex of rats (Brake et al. 2000).

As we noted earlier, fetal growth restriction likely is the result of multiple mechanisms, including hypoxia, malnutrition, and inflammation. A few studies have attempted to understand the effect of fetal growth restriction on the developing brain. Fetal growth restriction due to placental embolization in sheep is associated with cerebral white matter damage (Duncan et al. 2000). Fetal growth restriction resulting from unilateral uterine artery ligation in guinea pigs causes delayed myelination (Nitsos and Rees 1990), ventriculomegaly and reduced hippocampal volume (E.C. Mallard et al. 1999), and decreased neuron number in the hippocampus and cerebellum (C. Mallard et al. 2000) and altered dendritic morphology in the hippocampus (Dieni and Rees 2003). These models indicate that fetal growth restriction caused by compromised placental blood flow has a significant long-term effect on brain development consistent with the known neuropathology of schizophrenia. The range of neuropathological effects observed in these models, from subtle alterations of dendritic morphology to gross white matter damage, is consistent with the range of outcomes described clinically, from subtle decreases in IQ to cerebral palsy.

INFECTION AND INFLAMMATION

Many of the perinatal complications associated with schizophrenia can be caused by infection (Bergstrom 2003). As reviewed earlier, 30%–40% of preterm births are due to infection (Goldenberg et al. 2000; Haram et al. 2003). Infection, either intrauterine or systemic, is also a risk factor for fetal growth restriction (Beckmann et al. 1993), preeclampsia (Hsu and Witter 1995), and premature rupture of the membranes (Leveno et al. 2003). In addition, the signs of birth asphyxia such as low Apgar scores and neonatal seizures are often secondary to maternal infection (Grether and Nelson 1997). Finally, maternal diabetes significantly increases the incidence of infections during pregnancy (Leveno et al. 2003).

Several animal models indicate that prenatal exposure to maternal infection can cause long-lasting behavior changes consistent with those found in schizophrenia. Maternal infection with human influenza virus in mice results in abnormalities in prepulse inhibition (Shi et al. 2003). Maternal exposure to poly I:C, a synthetic double-stranded RNA that stimulates a cytokine response, causes prepulse inhibition abnormalities (Shi et al. 2003) and disrupted latent inhibition (Zuckerman and Weiner 2003; Zuckerman et al. 2003). Maternal exposure to *Escherichia coli* lipopolysaccharide, a cell wall endotoxin, also disrupts sensorimotor gating in the offspring (Borrell et al. 2002). Maternal exposure to influenza can cause defective corticogenesis (Fatemi et al. 1999) and increased cortical pyramidal cell density (Fatemi et al. 2002).

Hypotheses about the role of infection in the etiology of schizophrenia have focused on direct infection of the developing fetus (Yolken and Torrey 1995) or the generation of antibodies that cross-react with neuronal antigens (Wright et al. 1993). Because various infections are associated with increased risk of schizophrenia, a feature common to all infections would be a likely candidate mechanism. Such a common mechanism may be that cytokines, generated in response to maternal infection, alter early brain development and increase risk for schizophrenia (Gilmore and Jarskog 1997). Interleukin-1β (IL-1β), interleukin-6 (IL-6), and tumor necrosis factor–α (TNF-α) are elevated in the maternal–fetal unit after maternal infection in human pregnancies (Hillier et al. 1993; Yoon et al. 1996) and in animal models (Fidel et al. 1994; Urakubo et al. 2001). Cytokines decrease survival of serotoninergic and dopaminergic neurons (Jarskog et al. 1997), hippocampal neurons (Araujo and Cotman 1995), and cortical neurons (Marx et al. 2001). Prenatal exposure to maternal infection alters neurotrophic factor expression in the fetal and neonatal brain (Gilmore et al. 2003). Finally, IL-1β, IL-6, and TNF-α also can decrease the dendritic complexity of developing cortical neurons (Gilmore et al. 2004).

Recent studies give some support to this hypothesis by reporting increased blood levels of TNF-α (Buka et al. 2001a) and IL-8 (Brown et al. 2004a) in pregnant mothers whose children went on to develop schizophrenia. In addition, associations between schizophrenia and polymorphisms of cytokine genes increase cytokine production, including TNF-α (Boin et al. 2001; Jun et al. 2003; Meira-Lima et al. 2003) and IL-1β (Katila et al. 1999). Furthermore, associations are found between polymorphisms for IL-1β (Meisenzahl et al. 2001) and the TNF receptor–II (Wassink et al. 2000) and abnormal brain morphology in patients with schizophrenia, including lat-

eral ventricle enlargement and cortical gray matter and white matter reductions. Genes that increase the inflammatory response to perinatal infection or hypoxia would increase risk for schizophrenia through cytokine actions on the developing brain, an example of a possible gene–environment interaction.

Inflammatory cytokines also have been implicated in hypoxic-ischemic injury to the developing brain. IL-6 and TNF-α are elevated in the cerebrospinal fluid and cord blood of infants with hypoxic-ischemic encephalopathy and asphyxia (Chiesa et al. 2003; Silveira and Procianoy 2003). Hypoxia-ischemia increases the expression of cytokines in the brain, and mounting evidence indicates that these inflammatory cytokines play a critical role in neuronal injury after hypoxia and other perinatal insults (Saliba and Henrot 2001; Silverstein et al. 1997). Cytokines play a major role in the pathophysiology of both infectious and hypoxic-ischemic complications and offer a unifying mechanism of action for these risk factors for schizophrenia.

MALNUTRITION

Poor nutrition can result in fetal growth restriction and preterm delivery, each of which can have an adverse effect on brain development. In addition, evidence shows that prenatal nutritional deprivation alone can cause long-lasting changes in aspects of brain development that are relevant to schizophrenia (Brown et al. 1996; Butler et al. 1994). Prenatal protein restriction causes abnormal synaptic function in the corpus callosum (Soto-Moyano et al. 1998), decreased mossy fiber plexus in the hippocampus (Fiacco et al. 2003), and abnormal prepulse inhibition (A.A. Palmer et al. 2004). Prenatal vitamin B$_6$ restriction decreases dendrite complexity and synaptic density in the cortex (Groziak and Kirksey 1990). Malnutrition also makes the developing brain more susceptible to subsequent excitotoxic injury (Guo-Ross et al. 2002). Finally, increasing evidence indicates that prenatal diet plays an important role in epigenetic gene regulation, including DNA methylation (Poirier 2002; Waterland and Jirtle 2003). Environmental factors such as diet can increase or decrease the methylation of DNA in the promoter regions of specific genes, causing permanent changes in the rate at which these genes are expressed.

STRESS HORMONES

Even though the evidence that maternal psychological stress can increase risk for schizophrenia is weak, the stress response to hypoxia, infection, and other pre- and perinatal complications must be considered as a potential mechanism (Koenig et al. 2002). Prenatal maternal stress, acting through corticosteroids, results in a variety of abnormalities in the developing brain (Edwards and Burnham 2001; Matthews 2000). Of particular relevance to schizophrenia, prenatal stress results in decreased synaptophysin immunoreactivity in the cortex and hippocampus of adult animals (Hayashi et al. 1998; Koo et al. 2003) and alterations in pre- and postsynaptic gene expression in frontal cortex (Kinnunen et al. 2003). Neurogenesis in the hippocampus is also inhibited by prenatal stress (Coe et al. 2003; Lemaire et al. 2000). Finally, prenatal corticosterone exposure also alters hippocampal γ-aminobutyric acid systems (Stone et al. 2001), and prenatal exposure to stress causes long-lasting changes in the neuroendocrine response to stress in animals, which also could contribute to ongoing central nervous system damage (Edwards and Burnham 2001; Matthews 2000).

CONCLUSION

Studies of early environmental risk factors often have relied on imprecise methods of identifying ill-defined factors though epidemiological studies. By comparison, molecular genetic studies offer the advantage of precision. However, our improving understanding of the mechanisms that underlie early environmental risk factors now also allows the use of more precise, quantitative measures of such risk factors in individual pregnancies. Examples of such measures are prenatal ultrasound measures of brain growth and structure, placental size, and umbilical artery and even middle cerebral artery blood flow in the developing fetus. Also, inflammatory and stress mediators can be measured in maternal and fetal cord blood, placental pathology can be assessed objectively, and oxygenation at the time of birth can be assessed quantitatively. As the assessment of individual environmental risk factors becomes more precise, we will be better able to identify pathological mechanisms that contribute to risk for schizophrenia.

Indeed, our understanding of the etiopathophysiology of schizophrenia will remain incomplete without a better knowledge of the mechanisms through which early environmental risk factors act. Multiple genes in the population likely each convey a small risk for schizophrenia, acting in combination with one another and with environmental factors. These susceptibility genes cannot be altered. However, environmental factors, which also play a critical role in ultimate development of schizophrenia, offer our best hope for the prevention of the illness. Psychiatric research has embraced the complex methodology and the large, expensive studies that are needed to delin-

eate the small contributions of individual genes to overall risk for schizophrenia. In a similar way, new methodologies will be needed to determine the early environmental factors that increase risk for schizophrenia. This will require building collaborations with obstetricians, maternal-fetal medicine specialists, neonatologists, and pediatricians. It also will require the development of animal models that will allow a more precise determination of the effect of these early environmental risk factors on relevant neurodevelopmental processes.

Perhaps just as important, it is critical to develop and apply methodologies to study gene–environment interactions, both in the clinic and in the laboratory. This would include clinical studies that combine genetic and epidemiological approaches (e.g., Caspi et al. 2003; Clayton and McKeigue 2001) aimed at ascertaining whether the action of certain genes is to render the individual particularly vulnerable to certain early environmental hazards such as hypoxia and infection. It also would include the development of animal models that allow the study of interactions between genes of risk and environmental risk factors and their effect on brain development. We are optimistic that such approaches will provide important advances in understanding the causes of schizophrenia.

REFERENCES

Abdella TN, Sibai BM, Hays JM Jr, et al: Relationship of hypertensive disease to abruptio placentae. Obstet Gynecol 63:365–370, 1984

Allin M, Henderson M, Suckling J, et al: Effects of very low birthweight on brain structure in adulthood. Dev Med Child Neurol 46:46–53, 2004

Ananth CV, Berkowitz GS, Savitz DA, et al: Placental abruption and adverse perinatal outcomes. JAMA 282:1646–1651, 1999

Araujo DM, Cotman CW: Differential effects of interleukin-1b and interleukin-2 on glia and hippocampal neurons in culture. Int J Dev Neurosci 13:201–212, 1995

Bagalkote H, Pang D, Jones PB: Maternal influenza and schizophrenia in the offspring. Int J Ment Health 29:3–21, 2000

Beckmann I, Meisel-Mikolajczyk F, Leszczynski P, et al: Endotoxin-induced fetal growth retardation in the pregnant guinea pig. Am J Obstet Gynecol 168:714–718, 1993

Bergstrom S: Infection-related morbidities in the mother, fetus and neonate. J Nutr 133:1656S–1660S, 2003

Boin F, Zanardini R, Pioli R, et al: Association between –G308A tumor necrosis factor alpha gene polymorphism and schizophrenia. Mol Psychiatry 6:79–82, 2001

Borrell J, Vela JM, Arevalo-Martin A, et al: Prenatal immune challenge disrupts sensorimotor gating in adult rats: implications for the etiopathogenesis of schizophrenia. Neuropsychopharmacology 26:204–215, 2002

Brake WG, Sullivan RM, Alain Gratton A: Perinatal distress leads to lateralized medial prefrontal cortical dopamine hypofunction in adult rats. J Neurosci 20:5538–5543, 2000

Brown AS, Susser ES, Butler PD, et al: Neurobiological plausibility of prenatal nutritional deprivation as a risk factor for schizophrenia. J Nerv Ment Dis 184:71–85, 1996

Brown AS, Cohen P, Greenwald S, et al: Nonaffective psychosis after prenatal exposure to rubella. Am J Psychiatry 157:438–443, 2000a

Brown AS, Schaefer CA, Wyatt RJ, et al: Maternal exposure to respiratory infections and adult schizophrenia spectrum disorders: a prospective birth cohort study. Schizophr Bull 26:287–295, 2000b

Brown AS, van Os J, Driessens C, et al: Further evidence of relation between prenatal famine and major affective disorder. Am J Psychiatry 157:190–195, 2000c

Brown AS, Begg M, Gravenstein S, et al: Serologic evidence of prenatal influenza in the etiology of schizophrenia. Arch Gen Psychiatry 61:774–780, 2004a

Brown AS, Hooten J, Schaefer CA, et al: Elevated maternal interleukin-8 levels and risk of schizophrenia in adult offspring. Am J Psychiatry 161:889–895, 2004b

Buka SL, Tsuang MT, Torrey EF, et al: Maternal cytokine levels during pregnancy and adult psychosis. Brain Behav Immun 15:411–420, 2001a

Buka SL, Tsuang MT, Torrey EF, et al: Maternal infections and subsequent psychosis among offspring. Arch Gen Psychiatry 58:1032–1037, 2001b

Butler PD, Susser ES, Brown AS, et al: Prenatal nutritional deprivation as a risk factor in schizophrenia: preclinical evidence. Neuropsychopharmacology 11:227–235, 1994

Cannon M, Jones PB, Murray RM: Obstetric complications and schizophrenia: historical and meta-analytic review. Am J Psychiatry 159:1080–1092, 2002

Cannon TD, Rosso IM, Hollister JM, et al: A prospective cohort study of genetic and perinatal influences in the etiology of schizophrenia. Schizophr Bull 26:351–366, 2000

Cardno AG, Marshall EJ, Coid B, et al: Heritability estimates for psychotic disorders: the Maudsley twin psychosis series. Arch Gen Psychiatry 56:162–168, 1999

Caspi A, Sugden K, Moffitt TE, et al: Influence of life stress on depression: moderation by a polymorphism in the 5-HTT gene. Science 301:386–389, 2003

Cheng SW, Chou HC, Tsou KI, et al: Delivery before 32 weeks of gestation for maternal pre-eclampsia: neonatal outcome and 2-year developmental outcome. Early Hum Dev 76:39–46, 2004

Chiesa C, Pellegrini G, Panero A, et al: Umbilical cord interleukin-6 levels are elevated in term neonates with perinatal asphyxia. Eur J Clin Invest 33:352–358, 2003

Clayton D, McKeigue PM: Epidemiological methods for studying genes and environmental factors in complex diseases. Lancet 358:1356–1360, 2001

Coe CL, Kramer M, Czeh B, et al: Prenatal stress diminishes neurogenesis in the dentate gyrus of juvenile rhesus monkeys. Biol Psychiatry 54:1025–1034, 2003

Curristin SM, Cao A, Stewart WB, et al: Disrupted synaptic development in the hypoxic newborn brain. Proc Natl Acad Sci U S A 99:15729–15734, 2002

Davenport R: Cytokines and erythrocyte incompatibility. Curr Opin Hematol 1:452–456, 1994

Dieni S, Rees S: Dendritic morphology is altered in hippocampal neurons following prenatal compromise. J Neurobiol 55:41–52, 2003

Dube J, Dodds L, Armson BA: Does chorionicity or zygosity predict adverse perinatal outcomes in twins? Am J Obstet Gynecol 186:579–583, 2002

Duncan JR, Cock ML, Harding R, et al: Relation between damage to the placenta and the fetal brain after late-gestation placental embolization and fetal growth restriction in sheep. Am J Obstet Gynecol 183:1013–1022, 2000

Edwards HE, Burnham WM: The impact of corticosteroids on the developing animal. Pediatr Res 50:433–440, 2001

Egan MF, Goldberg TE, Kolachana BS, et al: Effect of COMT Val[108/158]Met genotype on frontal lobe function and risk for schizophrenia. Proc Natl Acad Sci U S A 98:6917–6922, 2001

Fatemi SH, Emamian ES, Kist D, et al: Defective corticogenesis and reduction in reelin immunoreactivity in cortex and hippocampus of prenatally infected neonatal mice. Mol Psychiatry 4:145–154, 1999

Fatemi SH, Earle J, Kanodia R, et al: Prenatal viral infection leads to pyramidal cell atrophy and macrocephaly in adulthood: implications for the genesis of autism and schizophrenia. Cell Mol Neurobiol 22:25–33, 2002

Fiacco TA, Rosene DL, Galler JR, et al: Increased density of hippocampal kainate receptors but normal density of NMDA and AMPA receptors in a rat model of prenatal protein malnutrition. J Comp Neurol 456:350–360, 2003

Fidel PL Jr, Romero R, Wolf N, et al: Systemic and local cytokine profiles in endotoxin-induced preterm parturition in mice. Am J Obstet Gynecol 170:1467–1475, 1994

Geddes JR, Lawrie SM: Obstetric complications and schizophrenia: a meta-analysis. Br J Psychiatry 167:786–793, 1995

Geddes JR, Verdoux H, Takei N, et al: Schizophrenia and complications of pregnancy and labor: an individual patient data meta-analysis. Schizophr Bull 25:413–423, 1999

Gilmore JH, Jarskog LF: Exposure to infection and brain development: cytokines in the pathogenesis of schizophrenia. Schizophr Res 24:365–367, 1997

Gilmore JH, Jarskog LF, Vadlamudi S: Maternal infection regulates BDNF and NGF expression in fetal and neonatal brain and maternal-fetal unit of the rat. J Neuroimmunol 138:49–55, 2003

Gilmore JH, Fredrik Jarskog L, Vadlamudi S, et al: Prenatal infection and risk for schizophrenia: IL-1β, IL-6, and TNFα inhibit cortical neuron dendrite development. Neuropsychopharmacology 29:1221–1229, 2004

Goldenberg RL, Hauth JC, Andrews WW: Intrauterine infection and preterm delivery. N Engl J Med 342:1500–1507, 2000

Gray PH, O'Callaghan MJ, Mohay HA, et al: Maternal hypertension and neurodevelopmental outcome in very preterm infants. Arch Dis Child Fetal Neonatal Ed 79:F88–F93, 1998

Grether JK, Nelson KB: Maternal infection and cerebral palsy in infants of normal birth weight. JAMA 278:207–211, 1997

Groziak SM, Kirksey A: Effects of maternal restriction in vitamin B-6 on neocortex development in rats: neuron differentiation and synaptogenesis. J Nutr 120:485–492, 1990

Guo-Ross SX, Clark S, Montoya DA, et al: Prenatal choline supplementation protects against postnatal neurotoxicity. J Neurosci 22:RC195, 2002

Hack M, Flannery DJ, Schluchter M, et al: Outcomes in young adulthood for very-low-birth-weight infants. N Engl J Med 346:149–157, 2002

Haram K, Mortensen JH, Wollen AL: Preterm delivery: an overview. Acta Obstet Gynecol Scand 82:687–704, 2003

Hayashi A, Nagaoka M, Yamada K, et al: Maternal stress induces synaptic loss and developmental disabilities of offspring. Int J Dev Neurosci 16:209–216, 1998

Henriksen T: Hypertension in pregnancy and preeclampsia—diagnosis and treatment. Scand J Rheumatol Suppl 107:86–91, 1998

Hillier SL, Witkin SS, Krohn MA, et al: The relationship of amniotic fluid cytokines and preterm delivery, amniotic fluid infection, histologic chorioamnionitis, and chorioamnion infection. Obstet Gynecol 81:941–948, 1993

Hoek HW, Susser E, Buck KA, et al: Schizoid personality disorder after prenatal exposure to famine. Am J Psychiatry 153:1637–1639, 1996

Hollister JM, Laing P, Mednick SA: Rhesus incompatibility as a risk factor for schizophrenia in male adults. Arch Gen Psychiatry 53:19–24, 1996

Hsu CD, Witter FR: Urogenital infection in preeclampsia. Int J Gynecol Obstet 49:271–275, 1995

Hulshoff Pol HE, Hoek HW, Susser E, et al: Prenatal exposure to famine and brain morphology in schizophrenia. Am J Psychiatry 157:1170–1172, 2000

Huttunen MO, Niskanen P: Prenatal loss of father and psychiatric disorders. Arch Gen Psychiatry 35:429–431, 1978

Isaacs EB, Lucas A, Chong WK, et al: Hippocampal volume and everyday memory in children of very low birth weight. Pediatr Res 47:713–720, 2000

Jarskog LF, Xiao H, Wilkie MB, et al: Cytokine regulation of embryonic rat dopamine and serotonin neuronal survival in vitro. Int J Dev Neurosci 15:711–716, 1997

Johnston MV, Trescher WH, Ishida A, et al: Neurobiology of hypoxic-ischemic injury in the developing brain. Pediatr Res 49:735–741, 2001

Jun TY, Pae CU, Chae JH, et al: TNFβ polymorphism may be associated with schizophrenia in the Korean population. Schizophr Res 61:39–45, 2003

Katila H, Hanninen K, Hurme M: Polymorphisms of the interleukin-1 gene complex in schizophrenia. Mol Psychiatry 4:179–181, 1999

Kendler KS, Pedersen NL, Farahmand BY, et al: The treated incidence of psychotic and affective illness in twins compared with population expectation: a study in the Swedish Twin and Psychiatric Registries. Psychol Med 26:1135–1144, 1996

Kinnunen AK, Koenig JI, Bilbe G: Repeated variable prenatal stress alters pre- and postsynaptic gene expression in the rat frontal pole. J Neurochem 86:736–748, 2003

Kirkpatrick B, Tek C, Allardyce J, et al: Summer birth and deficit schizophrenia in Dumfries and Galloway, Southwestern Scotland. Am J Psychiatry 159:1382–1387, 2002

Klaning U, Mortensen PB, Kyvik KO: Increased occurrence of schizophrenia and other psychiatric illnesses among twins. Br J Psychiatry 168:688–692, 1996

Koenig JI, Kirkpatrick B, Lee P: Glucocorticoid hormones and early brain development in schizophrenia. Neuropsychopharmacology 27:309–318, 2002

Koo JW, Park CH, Choi SH, et al: The postnatal environment can counteract prenatal effects on cognitive ability, cell proliferation, and synaptic protein expression. FASEB J 17:1556–1558, 2003

Kraft P, Palmer CG, Woodward AJ, et al: RHD maternal-fetal genotype incompatibility and schizophrenia: extending the MFG test to include multiple siblings and birth order. Eur J Hum Genet 12:192–198, 2004

Lemaire V, Koehl M, Le Moal M, et al: Prenatal stress produces learning deficits associated with an inhibition of neurogenesis in the hippocampus. Proc Natl Acad Sci U S A 97:11032–11037, 2000

Leveno KJ, Cunningham FG, Gant NF, et al: Williams Manual of Obstetrics, 21st ed. New York, McGraw-Hill, 2003

Lian Q, Dheen ST, Liao D, et al: Enhanced inflammatory response in neural tubes of embryos derived from diabetic mice exposed to a teratogen. J Neurosci Res 75:554–564, 2004

Lin CC, Santolaya-Forgas J: Current concepts of fetal growth restriction, part I: causes, classification, and pathophysiology. Obstet Gynecol 92:1044–1055, 1998a

Lin CC, Santolaya-Forgas J: Current concepts of fetal growth restriction, part II: diagnosis and management. Obstet Gynecol 92:1044–1055, 1998b

Mallard C, Loeliger M, Copolov D, et al: Reduced number of neurons in the hippocampus and the cerebellum in the postnatal guinea-pig following intrauterine growth restriction. Neuroscience 100:327–333, 2000

Mallard EC, Rehn A, Rees S, et al: Ventriculomegaly and reduced hippocampal volume following intrauterine growth-restriction: implications for the aetiology of schizophrenia. Schizophr Res 40:11–21, 1999

Marcelis M, Navarro-Mateu F, Murray R, et al: Urbanization and psychosis: a study of 1942–1978 birth cohorts in the Netherlands. Psychol Med 28:871–879, 1998

Marx CE, Jarskog LF, Lauder JM, et al: Cytokine effects on cortical neuron MAP-2 immunoreactivity: implications for schizophrenia. Biol Psychiatry 50:743–749, 2001

Matthews SG: Antenatal glucocorticoids and programming of the developing CNS. Pediatr Res 47:291–300, 2000

McGrath J, Castle D, Murray RM: How can we judge whether or not prenatal exposure to influenza causes schizophrenia? in Neural Development and Schizophrenia: Theory and Research. Edited by Mednick SA, Hollister JM. New York, Plenum, 1995, pp 203–214

McQuillen PS, Sheldon RA, Shatz CJ, et al: Selective vulnerability of subplate neurons after neonatal hypoxia-ischemia. J Neurosci 23:3308–3315, 2003

Meira-Lima IV, Pereira AC, Mota GF, et al: Analysis of a polymorphism in the promoter region of the tumor necrosis factor alpha gene in schizophrenia and bipolar disorder: further support for an association with schizophrenia. Mol Psychiatry 8:718–720, 2003

Meisenzahl EM, Rujescu D, Kirner A, et al: Association of an interleukin-1β genetic polymorphism with altered brain structure in patients with schizophrenia. Am J Psychiatry 158:1316–1319, 2001

Mortensen PB, Pedersen CB, Westergaard T, et al: Effects of family history and place and season of birth on the risk of schizophrenia. N Engl J Med 340:603–608, 1999

Myhrman A, Rantakallio P, Ishohanni M, et al: Unwantedness of a pregnancy and schizophrenia in the child. Br J Psychiatry 169:637–640, 1996

Nilsson E, Salonen RH, Cnattingius S, et al: The importance of genetic and environmental effects for pre-eclampsia and gestational hypertension: a family study. BJOG 111:200–206, 2004

Nitsos I, Rees S: The effects of intrauterine growth retardation on the development of neuroglia in fetal guinea pigs. An immunohistochemical and ultrastructural study. Int J Dev Neurosci 8:233–244, 1990

Nosarti C, Al-Asady MH, Frangou S, et al: Adolescents who were born very preterm have decreased brain volumes. Brain 125:1616–1623, 2002

Nosarti C, Rifkin L, Murray RM: The neurodevelopmental consequences of very preterm birth: brain plasticity and its limits, in Neurodevelopmental Mechanisms in the Genesis and Epigenesis of Psychopathology. Edited by Cicchetti D, Walker E. Cambridge, UK, Cambridge University Press, 2003, pp 34–62

O'Callaghan E, Sham PC, Takei N, et al: The relationship of schizophrenic births to 16 infectious diseases. Br J Psychiatry 165:353–356, 1994

Palmer AA, Printz DJ, Butler PD, et al: Prenatal protein deprivation in rats induces changes in prepulse inhibition and NMDA receptor binding. Brain Res 996:193–201, 2004

Palmer CGS, Turunen JA, Sinsheimer JS, et al: *RHD* maternal-fetal genotype incompatibility increases schizophrenia susceptibility. Am J Hum Genet 71:1312–1319, 2002

Pardi G, Marconi AM, Cetin I: Placental-fetal interrelationship in IUGR fetuses—a review. Placenta 23 (suppl A):S136–S141, 2002

Paz I, Laor A, Gale R, et al: Term infants with fetal growth restriction are not at increased risk for low intelligence scores at 17 years. J Pediatr 138:87–91, 2001

Peterson BS, Vohr B, Staib LH, et al: Regional brain volume abnormalities and long-term cognitive outcome in preterm infants. JAMA 284:1939–1947, 2000

Phillips DI: Twin studies in medical research: can they tell us whether diseases are genetically determined? Lancet 341:1008–1009, 1993

Poirier LA: The effects of diet, genetics, and chemicals on toxicity and aberrant DNA methylation: an introduction. J Nutr 132:2336S–2339S, 2002

Raza H, John A: Glutathione metabolism and oxidative stress in neonatal rat tissues from streptozotocin-induced diabetic mothers. Diabetes Metab Res Rev 20:72–78, 2004

Redman CW, Sacks GP, Sargent IL: Preeclampsia: an excessive maternal inflammatory response to pregnancy. Am J Obstet Gynecol 180:499–506, 1999

Resnik R: Intrauterine growth restriction. Obstet Gynecol 99:490–496, 2002

Rushe TM, Temple CM, Rifkin L, et al: Lateralisation of language function in young adults born very preterm. Arch Dis Child Fetal Neonatal Ed 89:F112–F118, 2004

Rosso IM, Cannon TD, Huttunen T, et al: Obstetric risk factors for early onset schizophrenia in a Finnish birth cohort. Am J Psychiatry 157:801–807, 2000

Saigal S: Follow-up of very low birthweight babies to adolescence. Semin Neonatol 5:107–118, 2000

Saliba E, Henrot A: Inflammatory mediators and neonatal brain damage. Biol Neonate 79:224–227, 2001

Schwab SG, Knapp M, Mondabon S, et al: Support for association of schizophrenia with genetic variation in the 6p22.3 gene, dysbindin, in sib-pair families with linkage and in an additional sample of triad families. Am J Hum Genet 72:185–190, 2003

Selten J-P, van der Graaf Y, van Duursen R, et al: Psychotic illness after prenatal exposure to the 1953 Dutch Flood Disaster. Schizophr Res 35:243–245, 1999

Selten J-P, Cantor-Graae E, Nahon D, et al: No relationship between risk of schizophrenia and prenatal exposure to stress during the Six-Day War or Yom Kippur War in Israel. Schizophr Res 63:131–135, 2003

Shapiro SM: Bilirubin toxicity in the developing nervous system. Pediatr Neurol 29:410–421, 2003

Shi L, Fatemi SH, Sidwell RW, et al: Maternal influenza infection causes marked behavioral and pharmacological changes in the offspring. J Neurosci 23:297–302, 2003

Silveira RC, Procianoy RS: Interleukin-6 and tumor necrosis factor-alpha levels in plasma and cerebrospinal fluid of term newborn infants with hypoxic-ischemic encephalopathy. J Pediatr 143:625–629, 2003

Silverstein FS, Barks JD, Hagan P, et al: Cytokines and perinatal brain injury. Neurochem Int 30:375–383, 1997

Sorensen HJ, Mortensen EL, Reinisch JM, et al: Do hypertension and diuretic treatment in pregnancy increase the risk of schizophrenia in offspring? Am J Psychiatry 160:464–468, 2003

Soto-Moyano R, Alarcon S, Belmar J, et al: Prenatal protein restriction alters synaptic mechanisms of callosal connections in the rat visual cortex. Int J Dev Neurosci 16:75–84, 1998

Stefansson H, Sigurdsson E, Steinthorsdottir V, et al: Neuregulin 1 and susceptibility to schizophrenia. Am J Hum Genet 71:877–892, 2002

Stefansson H, Sarginson J, Kong A, et al: Association of neuregulin 1 with schizophrenia confirmed in a Scottish population. Am J Hum Genet 72:83–87, 2003

Stenninger E, Flink R, Eriksson B, et al: Long-term neurological dysfunction and neonatal hypoglycaemia after diabetic pregnancy. Arch Dis Child Fetal Neonatal Ed 79:F174–F179, 1998

Stewart A, Rifkin L, Amess PN, et al: Brain structure and neurocognitive and behavioural function in adolescents who were born very preterm. Lancet 353:1653–1657, 1999

Stone DJ, Walsh JP, Sebro R, et al: Effects of pre- and postnatal corticosterone exposure on the rat hippocampal GABA system. Hippocampus 11:492–507, 2001

Sullivan PF, Kendler KS, Neale MC: Schizophrenia as a complex trait: evidence from a meta-analysis of twin studies. Arch Gen Psychiatry 60:1187–1192, 2003

Susser ES, Lin SP: Schizophrenia after prenatal exposure to the Dutch Hunger Winter of 1944–1945. Arch Gen Psychiatry 49:983–998, 1992

Susser E, Neugebauer R, Hoek HW, et al: Schizophrenia after prenatal famine: further evidence. Arch Gen Psychiatry 53:25–31, 1996

Suvisaari J, Haukka J, Tanskanen A, et al: Association between prenatal exposure to poliovirus infection and adult schizophrenia. Am J Psychiatry 156:1100–1102, 1999

Tochigi M, Okazaki Y, Kato N, et al: What causes the seasonality of birth in schizophrenia? Neurosci Res 48:1–11, 2004

Torrey EF, Rawlings R, Waldman IN: Schizophrenic births and viral diseases in two states. Schizophr Res 1:73–77, 1988

Torrey EF, Miller J, Rawlings R, et al: Seasonality of births in schizophrenia and bipolar disorder: a review of the literature. Schizophr Res 28:1–38, 1997

Tsuang MT, Stone WS, Faraone SV: Genes, environment and schizophrenia. Br J Psychiatry 187 (suppl 40):S18–S24, 2001

Urakubo A, Jarskog LF, Lieberman JA, et al: Prenatal exposure to maternal infection alters cytokine expression in the placenta, amniotic fluid, and fetal brain. Schizophr Res 47:27–36, 2001

Vaillancourt C, Boksa P: Birth insult alters dopamine-mediated behavior in a precocial species, the guinea pig: implications for schizophrenia. Neuropsychopharmacology 23:654–666, 2000

van den Oord EJ, Sullivan PF, Jiang Y, et al: Identification of a high-risk haplotype for the dystrobrevin binding protein 1 (*DTNBP1*) gene in the Irish Study of High-Density Schizophrenia families. Mol Psychiatry 8:499–510, 2003

Van Os J, Sham P: Gene-environmental correlation and interaction in schizophrenia, in The Epidemiology of Schizophrenia. Edited by Murray RM, Jones PB, Susser E, et al. Cambridge, UK, Cambridge University Press, 2004, pp 235–253

Vossbeck S, de Camargo OK, Grab D, et al: Neonatal and neurodevelopmental outcome in infants born before 30 weeks of gestation with absent or reversed end-diastolic flow velocities in the umbilical artery. Eur J Pediatr 160:128–134, 2001

Wahlbeck K, Forsen T, Osmond C, et al: Association of schizophrenia with low maternal body mass index, small size at birth, and thinness during childhood. Arch Gen Psychiatry 58:48–52, 2001

Wassink TH, Crowe RR, Andreasen NC: Tumor necrosis factor receptor-II: heritability and effect on brain morphology in schizophrenia. Mol Psychiatry 5:678–682, 2000

Waterland RA, Jirtle RL: Transposable elements: targets for early nutritional effects on epigenetic gene regulation. Mol Cell Biol 23:5293–5300, 2003

Watson CG, Kucala T, Tilleskjor C, et al: Schizophrenic birth seasonality in relation to the incidence of infectious diseases and temperature extremes. Arch Gen Psychiatry 41:85–90, 1984

Wienerroither H, Steiner H, Tomaselli J, et al: Intrauterine blood flow and long-term intellectual, neurologic, and social development. Obstet Gynecol 97:449–453, 2001

Williams NM, Preece A, Spurlock G, et al: Support for genetic variation in neuregulin 1 and susceptibility to schizophrenia. Mol Psychiatry 8:485–487, 2003

Wolke D: Psychological development of prematurely born children. Arch Dis Child 78:567–570, 1998

Wonodi I, Stine OC, Mitchell BD, et al: Association between Val[108/158] Met polymorphism of the COMT gene and schizophrenia. Am J Med Genet B Neuropsychiatr Genet 120:47–50, 2003

Wright P, Gill M, Murray RM: Schizophrenia: genetics and the maternal immune response to viral infection. Am J Med Genet 48:40–46, 1993

Yamano T, Shimada M, Fujizeki Y, et al: Quantitative synaptic changes on Purkinje cell dendritic spines of rats born from streptozotocin-induced diabetic mothers. Brain Dev 8:269–273, 1986

Yolken RH, Torrey EF: Viruses, schizophrenia, and bipolar disorder. Clin Microbiol Rev 8:131–145, 1995

Yoon BH, Romero R, Yang SH, et al: Interleukin-6 concentrations in umbilical cord plasma are elevated in neonates with white matter lesions associated with periventricular leukomalacia. Am J Obstet Gynecol 174:1433–1440, 1996

Zornberg GL, Buka SL, Tsuang MT: Hypoxic-ischemic-related fetal/neonatal complications and risk of schizophrenia and other nonaffective psychoses: a 19-year longitudinal study. Am J Psychiatry 157:196–202, 2000

Zuckerman L, Weiner I: Post-pubertal emergence of disrupted latent inhibition following prenatal immune activation. Psychopharmacology 169:308–313, 2003

Zuckerman L, Rehavi M, Nachman R, et al: Immune activation during pregnancy in rats leads to a postpubertal emergence of disrupted latent inhibition, dopaminergic hyperfunction, and altered limbic morphology in the offspring: a novel neurodevelopmental model of schizophrenia. Neuropsychopharmacology 28:1778–1789, 2003

NEURODEVELOPMENTAL THEORIES

MATCHERI S. KESHAVAN, M.D.

ANDREW R. GILBERT, M.D.

VAIBHAV A. DIWADKAR, PH.D.

The dominant model of schizophrenia during the past century has been the Kraepelinian concept of a degenerative disease, captured in the term *dementia praecox*. However, the view that abnormal neurodevelopment may underlie schizophrenia has been gaining acceptance in recent years. This idea is not new and dates to the earliest modern conceptions of the illness. For example, deficits in social interaction as well as premorbid signs in childhood were noted by both Bleuler and Kraepelin (see Malmberg et al. 1998; Marenco and Weinberger 2001). During the late nineteenth century, Thomas Clouston (1891) observed developmental dysmorphic abnormalities, such as high arched palate, in patients he considered as having "adolescent insanity." Early twentieth-century neuropathologists such as Southard observed brain changes in schizophrenia that were attributed to developmental deviations (Casanova 1995). Bender (1953) and subsequently Fish and Hagin (1972) argued that schizophrenia might reflect a developmental "encephalopathy."

Over the past two decades, at least three developmental formulations have been proposed: those that posit altered pre- or perinatal brain development, those proposing peri-adolescent developmental abnormalities, and those that argue for progressive neuroregressive processes after illness onset. In this chapter, we review and attempt to integrate these models. We first examine *whether* the clinical manifestations of schizophrenia reflect a neurodevelopmental diathesis. Second, we examine *where* in the brain—in other words, which neuronal structures or networks may explain the developmental manifestations of the illness. Third, we address *what* the microscopic and neurochemical underpinnings of the developmental brain changes are. Fourth, we examine *when* during development the disease related processes might begin. Fifth, we review the question of *why* they occur—in other words, the etiology of brain developmental alterations, with reference to the genetic and environmental determinants of the illness and their interaction. Finally, we develop a po-

This work was supported in part by National Institute of Mental Health grants MH45156, MH68680, and MH45203 and a National Alliance for Research on Schizophrenia and Depression Established Investigator Award.

tential integrative model of this illness and outline future directions of research.

DOES DISORDERED BRAIN DEVELOPMENT MEDIATE SCHIZOPHRENIA?

Although a large literature has accumulated pertaining to abnormalities in brain development in schizophrenia, the evidence thus far has remained circumstantial. The strongest, albeit indirect, evidence of disordered neurodevelopment stems from observations of premorbid behavioral, neurocognitive, and minor physical anomalies as well as evidence of risk factors leading to brain adversity before the clinical manifestations of the illness. These factors include subtle impairments in general intellectual ability as well as selective deficits in a variety of cognitive functions known to characterize schizophrenia (i.e., attention and executive functions, psychomotor abilities, language, and memory). Minor physical anomalies, indicating disordered early development, are also seen. These data have emerged from prospective general population cohort studies, studies of persons with increased risk for schizophrenia ("high-risk" studies) (Keshavan 2004), and studies of previously collected data on individuals with already manifest illness (archival-observational studies) (Walker et al. 1994).

Working memory—the ability to maintain memories temporarily online to permit further cognitive processing (Goldman-Rakic 1999)—is thought to rely on the tonic activity of neurons in the prefrontal cortex (Leung et al. 2002). Schizophrenia is marked by impaired spatial and verbal working memory (Goldman-Rakic 1999), suggesting that this cognitive domain may be compromised in individuals early in the illness as well as in those at risk for the illness. Several studies have demonstrated that first-episode schizophrenia patients show impairments in spatial and verbal working memory (maintaining spatial or verbal information online) compared with healthy control subjects (Elvevag and Goldberg 2000).

Impairments in attentional processing and executive function have also been observed in high-risk offspring of schizophrenia patients (Cornblatt et al. 1999). First-degree relatives have decreased speed of performance on the Stroop color-naming task and the Wisconsin Card Sorting Test, which are measures of executive function; the performance of relatives is in general intermediate between that of healthy control subjects and schizophrenia patients. Deficits in performance have also been observed in tasks in which decisions must be based on contextual

information. In such continuous performance tasks (e.g., the "AX" version of the Continuous Performance Test [AX-CPT]), subjects must respond to targets in a sequence only if they are preceded by particular items (e.g., *A* followed by an *X*) but not others. As with first-episode and chronic schizophrenia patients, first-degree relatives show processing deficits in such tasks (MacDonald et al. 2003). Attentional impairment is trait related, stable over time, and related to genetic vulnerability (Michie et al. 2000).

Archival observational studies (Walker et al. 1994), as well as population cohort studies (Rosso et al. 2000a), point to an association between motor coordination problems and/or delayed motor milestones and later schizophrenia. Fish (1984) originally observed neuromotor deviations in about a half of the offspring subjects in her infant and children study, a pattern she termed *pandysmaturation*. Similar neuromotor dysfunctions have been observed in other studies (Erlenmeyer-Kimling 2000) and may predict affective flattening in adolescence (Dworkin et al. 1993).

Other premorbid impairments involve memory and language difficulties. Short-term verbal memory was impaired in 83% of offspring who later developed schizophrenia in the New York High-Risk Project (NYHRP) study (Erlenmeyer-Kimling 2000), showing a high sensitivity but with relatively high false-positive rates (28%). By contrast, attentional impairments had lower sensitivity (58%) and lower false-positive rates (18%). Premorbid language impairments, including decreased speech intelligibility, have been observed in population cohort studies (Bearden et al. 2000). The presence of receptive language difficulties appears to be associated with a significant increase in risk for later schizophrenia (M. Cannon et al. 2002).

Minor physical anomalies (MPAs), such as malformations of the ear and palate and facial dysmorphology, may provide important clues to understanding schizophrenia spectrum disorders from a neurodevelopmental perspective. Such anomalies reflect possible irregularities in the development of the ectoderm and may give clues to the timing of the pathology. Offspring of schizophrenia parents with a high number of minor physical anomalies have been found to develop schizophrenia spectrum disorders more often than other psychopathology (Dworkin et al. 1993). In the Edinburgh High-Risk Study, MPAs were elevated in the high-risk subjects compared with control subjects but did not predict psychotic symptoms (Lawrie et al. 2001).

In summary, premorbid clinical and neurobehavioral data point to developmental brain pathology in schizophrenia. However, such data do not tell where in the brain such pathology might emerge. Answers to such questions need to be derived from careful in vivo imaging and electrophysiological and neuropathological studies, as is discussed in the following sections.

WHERE IN THE BRAIN ARE THE DEVELOPMENTAL ABNORMALITIES THAT UNDERLIE SCHIZOPHRENIA?

The generalized nature of the premorbid alterations, which is reviewed in the preceding section, has suggested that schizophrenia may not be characterized by a focal "lesion" but could more likely be associated with widespread corticocortical disconnection. The neurocognitive deficits, such as working memory, language, and executive processing deficits, identified in patients may reflect disordered connectivity in the heteromodal association cortices. However, critical regions of the brain such as the prefrontal cortex may be particularly vulnerable to abnormal neurodevelopment in schizophrenia (Lewis 1997; Weinberger et al. 2001). Over the past two decades neuroimaging techniques have been valuable in characterizing the structural and functional neuroanatomy of these neuronal network abnormalities.

The development and application of in vivo neuroimaging techniques have helped identify regions of morphometric changes in schizophrenia that are consistent with the pathophysiological alterations mentioned previously. Studies of first-episode schizophrenia patients compared with age-matched healthy control subjects have reported significant reductions in gray matter volume in the heteromodal association cortex, thalamus, cerebellum, and basal ganglia (McCarley et al. 1999; Shenton et al. 2001). These findings suggest that brain structural alterations are present early in the illness and potentially may precede its clinical manifestations.

Assessing volumetric abnormalities in individuals at risk for schizophrenia assumes particular importance, given that magnetic resonance imaging (MRI) measurements of brain volume are sensitive to normal development (Giedd et al. 1999). Several studies have assessed first-degree relative samples in an attempt to identify premorbid structural alterations in brain morphometry. These studies have uncovered gray matter reductions in structures such as the prefrontal cortex, temporal cortex (e.g., amygdala and hippocampi), and thalamus. Other findings include ventricular enlargement, lack of cerebral asymmetry, and reductions in whole-brain white matter volume (Lawrie 2004). These anatomic alterations are generally located in brain areas that subserve cognitive domains such as spatial and verbal working memory, executive function, and language (Mesulam 1998); these are the domains in which relatives appear to show cognitive impairment. Clearly, structural neuroimaging studies converge to suggest that risk for and abnormalities in

schizophrenia may partly result from prolonged abnormal neurodevelopmental processes that precede the onset of psychosis (Keshavan 1997).

Functional MRI (fMRI) studies allow us to glean insights into the functional neuroanatomy of developmental brain changes underlying schizophrenia. fMRI studies in first-episode patients suggest significant impairments in prefrontal function, termed *hypofrontality* (Andreasen et al. 1977; Barch et al. 2001). Few fMRI studies exist in the child and adolescent high-risk population, and therefore the functional correlates of these cognitive abnormalities have not been well identified. Preliminary studies have indicated differences in fMRI-measured activation in the prefrontal cortex during spatial working memory (Keshavan et al. 2002). Similar functional alterations are also seen in adult nonpsychotic relatives (Callicott et al. 2003). However, demonstrations of hypo- or hyperactivation in schizophrenia remain difficult to interpret (Manoach 2003).

In summary, available evidence indicates that premorbid abnormalities in brain development might lead to anatomical and physiological alterations in widely distributed cortical and subcortical networks. An understanding of the microstructural and neurochemical underpinnings of such deficits is critical for our efforts to determine the causative factors that determine their emergence.

WHAT NEURODEVELOPMENTAL ALTERATIONS OCCUR AT THE MICROSCOPIC AND MOLECULAR LEVELS?

As discussed previously, studies of first-episode schizophrenia patients and of young at-risk relatives have revealed significant abnormalities in brain structure and function before illness onset and thus may reflect a primary disease process. Such brain changes in schizophrenia may reflect several neuropathological processes, including neuronal and glial cell abnormalities, synaptic dysfunction, and cellular disarray (Cho et al. 2003), and may lead to neurochemical alterations underlying the emergence of psychopathology.

NEUROPATHOLOGY

Postmortem studies have reported a 5%–10% reduction in cortical thickness in the dorsal prefrontal cortex of subjects with schizophrenia (Harrison and Lewis 2001). Interestingly, the "cortical thinning" in schizophrenia corresponds with an increase in cell packing density but no change in total neuron number. The increase in cell packing density may reflect a decrease in the number of axon terminals, distal dendrites, and dendritic spines that represent the principal components of cortical synapses. A reduction in neuronal size may also contribute to the findings of reduced cortical thickness (Pierri et al. 2001; Rajkowska et al. 1998).

Abnormalities in specific neuronal subtypes, such as the reduction in pyramidal neuron size in the cortex of patients with schizophrenia, may result from aberrant thalamocortical projections that arise during development. The reduction in somal size, as well as the decreased dendritic spine density reported in several studies of schizophrenic brains (Pierri et al. 2001; Rajkowska et al. 1998), may be explained by a loss of afferent inputs to the cortex. Abnormalities in cortical inhibitory neurons in schizophrenia may contribute to aberrant thalamocortical connectivity in individuals with schizophrenia (Harrison and Lewis 2001).

Recently, glial cells have been recognized as essential components of information processing and synaptic integration. Historically, the absence of gliosis in schizophrenia was considered supportive of an early neurodevelopmental origin of the illness and as evidence against a neurodegenerative process. However, the developmental onset of the glial response remains to be understood and therefore cannot be used to estimate the timing of brain alterations in schizophrenia (Lewis and Levitt 2002). Furthermore, because neuronal injury and apoptosis do not always result in gliosis, the absence of gliosis does not rule out a neurodegenerative process (Cho et al. 2003). Interestingly, evidence of reduced numbers of glial cells in the orbitofrontal cortex, anterior cingulate, and primary motor cortices may reflect regionally specific glial cell abnormalities in schizophrenia (Benes et al. 1986, 1991; Cotter et al. 2001; Rajkowska et al. 1999). Continued studies of glial cell function and the role of these cells during development may reveal a more pivotal role in schizophrenia and neurodevelopmental theories of schizophrenia.

Studies reporting disordered arrangements of neurons in schizophrenia brains suggest that neuronal disarray may be associated with the development of this illness. Normal neuronal arrangement and cortical development require several processes, including subplate formation, neuronal migration toward cortical layer formation, and neuronal orientation. Disordered subplate neurons in cortical and temporal lobes in schizophrenic patients and in a subset of schizophrenic patients have been reported (Akbarian et al. 1993, 1996). Other reports of abnormal neuronal distribution in entorhinal regions of schizophrenic patients may suggest that a process of aberrant neuronal migration occurs during development in schizophrenia (Falkai et al. 2000).

Evidence suggestive of neurobiological abnormalities in schizophrenia may reflect insults and disturbances that occur throughout early and late neurodevelopment. Although there are clear cortical disturbances in patients with schizophrenia, evident on both a macroscopic and microscopic level, their influence on phenotypic features of the illness, and the timing of these insults remain to be clearly elucidated.

NEUROTRANSMITTER MECHANISMS

Although the classical dopaminergic theory has long held center stage in neurochemical theories of schizophrenia, considerable evidence of dysfunctional glutamatergic and γ-aminobutyric acid (GABA) systems in this illness has emerged over the past two decades. These neurotransmitters play vital roles in early brain development, postnatal plasticity, and brain degeneration. Attempts at effective treatments for schizophrenia frequently target these specific systems. Therefore, these neurotransmitters are good candidates to be considered in neurodevelopmental theories of schizophrenia.

Accumulating evidence over the past decade has challenged prior hypotheses of dopaminergic system hyperfunction in schizophrenia (Lewis and Lieberman 2000). A greater understanding of more complex interactions of the dopaminergic system with other neurotransmitter systems, variable dopamine (DA) regulation in different brain regions, and multiple DA receptor types has led to a more complex and broader understanding of DA's role in schizophrenia. In his 1987 landmark paper, Weinberger proposed that schizophrenia may be related to deficits in the mesocortical dopaminergic system, leading to mesolimbic dopaminergic system overactivity (Weinberger 1987). Grace (1991) proposed a deficit in tonic DA drive and an exaggeration of the phasic DA release in response to stress. Several studies have revealed neurobiological alterations related to dopaminergic neurotransmission that support its dysregulation underlying disordered development of schizophrenia. For example, positron emission tomography studies of patients with schizophrenia have revealed aberrant presynaptic storage, release, reuptake, and metabolic mechanisms in dopaminergic mesolimbic systems (Laruelle 2000). Recent reports of reduced density of cortical DA axons and specific DA regulatory proteins, as well as cortical dopamine D_1 receptor upregulation may both reflect and contribute to working memory deficits, a common feature of schizophrenia (Abi-Dargham et al. 2002; Akil et al. 1999; Albert et al. 2002; Goldman-Rakic 1994).

Glutamate, the predominant excitatory neurotransmitter in the mammalian brain, is critical for neuronal migration and neuronal survival during early development, for neuronal plasticity during adolescence, and for neuronal excitability and viability throughout life. Glutamate is therefore well positioned as a potential candidate for a pathophysiological role in a disorder such as schizophrenia in which processes of development, neuronal regulation, and neurotoxicity may all be involved. The glutamatergic hypothesis of schizophrenia arose from observations of similarities between the clinical manifestations of schizophrenia and psychosis caused by phencyclidine, an *N*-methyl-D-asparate (NMDA) receptor antagonist (Coyle 1996; Javitt and Zukin 1991; Tamminga 1998), and reductions in cerebrospinal fluid glutamate levels (Kim et al. 1980). This model has been supported by observations of altered glutamate metabolism in schizophrenia (Tsai and Coyle 1995) and altered gene expression for NMDA receptor subunits (Akbarian et al. 1996).

The observations of psychotic symptoms resulting from drugs affecting serotonergic systems, such as lysergic acid diethylamide (LSD) and psilocybin, suggest involvement of this neurotransmitter in schizophrenia. Alterations in binding properties of serotonin (5-HT) and mutations in 5-HT–related genes have been variably reported. Though on balance there is relatively little direct evidence for the serotonergic hypothesis, the therapeutic role of 5-HT–DA antagonists in the past decade has rekindled a possible etiopathogenic role for 5-HT.

GABA, the major inhibitory neurotransmitter in the central nervous system, has also been implicated in schizophrenia. Postmortem observations of decreased expression of glutamic acid decarboxylase (an enzyme involved in GABA synthesis) in cortical brain regions (Volk et al. 2000) suggest involvement of this neurotransmitter in the pathophysiology of schizophrenia. These findings are consistent with the findings of $GABA_A$ receptor upregulation in frontolimbic regions (Benes et al. 1996). GABAergic neurons, which are largely interneurons, are thought to be critical for regulating pyramidal cell activity and may play an important role in cognitive operations. The role of GABA in schizophrenia has also been of interest in relation to expression of reelin, an extracellular matrix protein. Reelin-deficient animals have been used as an animal model for schizophrenia (Costa et al. 2001). Abnormalities in cortical GABA and pyramidal neurons have been described in both schizophrenic brains as well as in reelin-deficient rodent brains (Liu et al. 2001).

MEMBRANE AND NEURONAL INTEGRITY

The integrity of neuronal cell membranes, largely comprising phospholipids, is critical for optimum functioning of neurotransmitter receptors, ion channels, and signal transduction. Several in vivo imaging techniques, such as magnetic resonance spectroscopy (MRS), allow for the investigation of abnormal membrane physiology and neurochemistry in psychiatric illness and in at-risk populations. Physiological events in neurodevelopment, such as neuritic sprouting and neuronal membrane loss, are expressed by changes in concentration of MRS-measurable metabolites, such as phosphomonoesters (PMEs) and phosphodiesters (PDE), among others (Pettegrew et al. 1993; Stanley 2002). Higher free-PME levels are observed at the time and site of neuritic sprouting, and higher free-PDE levels are observed at the site and time of neuronal membrane breakdown. Reported reductions in PME levels in the prefrontal cortex of young relatives of schizophrenia patients (Keshavan et al. 2003) reflect a possible reduction in neuritic sprouting. A reduction in the ratio of PME to PDE in the same population may reflect an alteration in the membrane phospholipid turnover (Keshavan et al. 2003; Klemm et al. 2001); increases in PDE levels have also been observed (Rzanny et al. 2003).

Proton MRS studies can quantify levels of *N*-acetyl aspartate (NAA), which is considered to be a general marker of neuronal integrity. Alterations in the estimated concentrations of these metabolites in patient or at-risk populations are suggestive of premorbid physiologic abnormalities. Emerging studies have documented reductions in this metabolite in young relatives of patients, and the directions of these alterations are consistent with those observed in individuals with schizophrenia. Reductions in NAA (expressed as NAA:choline ratios) in the anterior cingulate have been observed in offspring of patients (Keshavan et al. 1997). NAA:creatine ratio reductions in the hippocampus have also been observed in adult relatives (Callicott et al. 1998).

Taken together, in vivo and postmortem neuropathological studies suggest microstuctural and neurochemical alterations that may predate illness onset and may reflect aberrant brain maturational processes. Alterations in the glutamatergic, GABAergic, and dopaminergic systems may be developmentally mediated and precede illness onset. Given the typical onset of illness during adolescence or early adulthood, the questions of when such abnormalities begin and how they evolve over time assume importance.

WHEN MIGHT ABNORMAL BRAIN DEVELOPMENT BEGIN?

An understanding of the clinical facts of schizophrenia can help us identify potential "windows" into the timing of developmental pathophysiology in this illness (Wyatt et al. 1988). Certain clinical observations consistently characterize the course of schizophrenia: 1) premorbid deficits, discussed previously that date back to early development in many cases (Done et al. 1994; Jones and Cannon 1998); 2) characteristic onset in adolescence (Hafner et al. 1993); 3) deterioration during the early course of schizophrenia, at least in a subgroup of patients (McGlashan and Fenton 1993). These observations have led to three proposed models for the timing of pathophysiological processes in schizophrenia.

THE EARLY DEVELOPMENTAL MODEL

The observed premorbid brain abnormalities in schizophrenia primarily point to one or several causal factors intra- or perinatally, perhaps during the second half of gestation. In these "early" neurodevelopmental models (Murray and Lewis 1987; Weinberger 1987), a fixed lesion from early life interacts with normal brain maturation occurring later. This view is supported by neuropathological observations suggesting altered cytoarchitecture indicative of possible errors in the early developmental phenomena of neural genesis or migration in schizophrenia, and epidemiological data suggesting associations between early neurobehavioral deficits and subsequent emergence of schizophrenia, as discussed earlier.

If such an early developmental derailment occurs, it is unlikely to involve the earliest steps of neurogenesis; defects of neural tube formation (i.e., midline cysts, spina bifida) are not associated with increased incidence of schizophrenia. Cell death by necrosis is also unlikely, because necrosis is typically followed by glial proliferation, and reactive gliosis is not seen in schizophrenia (Kotrla et al. 1997). However, as discussed earlier, this issue is by no means resolved. The processes of programmed cell death, neural migration, and/or synaptic proliferation that begin during the second trimester of pregnancy are more likely to be involved. Regardless of the process involved, these abnormalities can explain premorbid behavioral precursors of schizophrenia (Fish 1987; Watt 1978). However, the "early" theory falls short of providing a complete explanation for the fact that the characteristic signs and symptoms of schizophrenia do not begin till adolescence or early adulthood.

THE LATE DEVELOPMENTAL MODEL

On the basis of the typical adolescent onset of schizophrenic illness, it has been proposed, alternatively, that the pathophysiology of this disorder has its onset in postnatal life. From data indicating substantial changes in brain biology during adolescence, Feinberg initially proposed that schizophrenia may result from an abnormality in peri-adolescent synaptic pruning (Feinberg 1982–1983, 1990). This model, however, did not clarify whether too much, too little, or the wrong synapses were being pruned.

Adolescence is characterized by substantive changes in several in vivo neurobiological measures that may indirectly reflect changes in synapse density. Delta sleep, which represents the summed postsynaptic potentials in large assemblies of cortical and subcortical axons and dendrites, dramatically decreases during adolescence (Feinberg 1982–1983). Peri-adolescent reductions are also seen in the synthesis of membrane phospholipids, as measured by phosphorus MRS studies (Pettegrew et al. 1991), as well as in cortical gray matter volumes, as measured by structural MRI (Jernigan and Tallal 1990). Furthermore, regional prefrontal metabolism also decreases during peri-adolescence (Chugani et al. 1987). In patients with schizophrenia, relative to healthy control subjects, similar but more pronounced decrements are seen in delta sleep (Keshavan et al. 1998b), membrane synthesis (Pettegrew et al. 1991), gray matter volume (Zipursky 1992), and prefrontal metabolism (Andreasen et al. 1992). These observations suggest indirectly the possibility of an exaggeration of the normative process of synaptic pruning in certain brain regions such as prefrontal cortex in schizophrenia (Keshavan et al. 1994; Pettegrew et al. 1997). Neural network modeling studies also support the view that schizophrenia may be associated with synaptic or axonal pruning but not neuronal cell death (Hoffman and McGlashan 1997; McGlashan and Hoffman 2000). Neuropathological studies show reduction in the synapse-rich neuropil and a consequent increase in cortical neuron density (Selemon et al. 1995); reductions have also been reported in the expression of synaptophysin, a synaptic marker (Eastwood and Harrison 1995; Glantz and Lewis 1997), and in the density of dendritic spines (Garey et al. 1994). These observations suggest an overall reduction of cortical synapse-rich neuropil in schizophrenia, leading to reduced neuronal plasticity. The net effect of these reductions may ultimately be manifested by a reduction of neuronal modulatory capacity to handle the normative academic, familial, and interpersonal demands of adolescence. When a critical threshold of such neuropil loss is exceeded, symptoms and signs of schizophrenia may appear.

THE POST-ILLNESS PROGRESSION MODEL

The "early" and "late" developmental models discussed previously do not satisfactorily account for the observations that some, though not all, schizophrenia patients may have a deteriorating rather than static course, at least during the first few years of their illness (Loebel et al. 1992; McGlashan and Fenton 1993). Patients appear to take longer to recover and show less complete recovery over successive episodes of this illness (Lieberman et al. 1996). Prolonged untreated illness predicts a poorer outcome, suggesting a possible "neurotoxic" effect of psychosis (Lieberman 1993). Progressive structural alterations may be seen in the brains of schizophrenia patients in some (DeLisi 1995; Keshavan et al. 1998a; Thompson et al. 2001), although some studies show no change (Jaskiw et al. 1994). Alterations in neurophysiological indices, such as evoked-response potentials (P300), are also consistent with ongoing cerebral degeneration in a significant subgroup of schizophrenia patients (Mathalon et al. 2000).

A potential mechanism for such progressive change is that of neurochemical sensitization, which may result from repeated exposure to neurochemical stressors (Lieberman et al. 1997). Stimulants such as amphetamine and cocaine only rarely produce psychosis in healthy humans during acute administration, but intermittent administration appears to lead to paranoid forms of psychosis. Psychostimulants also display cross-sensitization (i.e., repeated administration leading to increased sensitivity to other drugs or environmental stressors). Such sensitization is associated with increased stimulant-induced dopamine release and appears to be a glutamate-dependent process with the involvement of both NMDA and non-NMDA glutamate receptors (Kalivas and Duffy 1995). There is also some evidence that genetic factors may influence the susceptibility to stimulant sensitization. Furthermore, the view that schizophrenia patients may have an enhanced dopaminergic sensitivity is supported by neuroimaging studies, reporting increased striatal amphetamine-induced dopamine release in patients (Laruelle et al. 1996). Glutamatergic and GABAergic systems in cortico-thalamo-striatal circuits are integrated, with GABA providing the inhibitory input and glutamate providing the excitory inputs; dopamine exerts an important modulatory effect on both of these systems (Krystal et al. 1999). Thus, disturbances in any one of the neurochemical systems may impart effects on all of the systems under consideration.

The three views of the timing of schizophrenia pathogenesis, although they may seem conflicting, may not necessarily be mutually exclusive. It may be that an early brain maturational derailment predisposes the individual to a later developmental aberrance and perhaps to post-illness neurotoxic processes. Accordingly, a "three-hit" model has been proposed (Keshavan 1999). The precise etiological mechanisms that might lead to the emergence (or otherwise) of such a cascade of pathogenesis remain to be determined and will be discussed in the next section.

WHY MIGHT BRAIN DEVELOPMENT BE DERAILED?

As is the case with other common disorders in medicine, such as coronary artery disease and diabetes, schizophrenia is best viewed as a complex disorder with multiple, interactive etiological factors. It is likely that several genetic susceptibility loci and a variety of environmental factors are involved.

GENETIC FACTORS

Although the specific mechanisms of genetic susceptibility in schizophrenia remain to be elucidated, inheritance clearly contributes to the etiopathogenesis of the disorder. Risk for schizophrenia increases with the percentage of shared genes (Gottesman 1991). Schizophrenia occurs in approximately 2% of third-degree relatives, in 2%–6% of second-degree relatives, and in 6%–17% of the first-degree relatives of an affected individual. Twin studies estimate that if one twin is affected, the risk of schizophrenia in the unaffected twin is approximately 17% for dizygotic twins and approaches 50% for monozygotic twins (Cardno and Gottesman 2000). Interestingly, adoption studies have demonstrated that shared environmental factors do not account for the familial features of schizophrenia (Lewis and Levitt 2002). Thus, neither genetic liability nor nongenetic factors alone can account for the clinical manifestations of the disorder.

Despite overwhelming evidence of a genetic etiological component, specific susceptibility genes remain to be identified in schizophrenia. Several chromosomal loci have been found to be associated with schizophrenia; the genetic liability appears to be transmitted in a polygenic, non-Mendelian pattern. These potential "candidate genes," interacting with environmental stressors, may play important roles in the development of schizophrenia. Genes involved in normal development as well as in other neurodevelopmental disorders have been of particular interest. The phenotype of all neurons is controlled by a specific set of genes expressed within the cell, contributing to functional specialization. The influence of individual transcription factors may be carried through multiple cell divisions and persist beyond the growth of a specific cell lineage. The coordinated boundaries of expression of these factors may dictate morphological boundaries and impart organization to the adult brain. Gene expression contributes to several domains of neural development, including cellular segmentation, adhesion, and survival. Recent studies have focused attention on the genes that coordinate these specific biological activities, contributing to neuronal connectivity and advanced cognitive function. A better understanding of their function and impact on neurodevelopment has allowed for their consideration in the development of neuropsychiatric disorders such as schizophrenia.

Several functional areas of neurodevelopment have emerged as important sites in the search for schizophrenia candidate genes. Transcriptional regulatory proteins influence cell migration and differentiation and have become an important area of research in schizophrenia. Cell adhesion molecules (CAMs) play an important role in morphogenesis, differentiation, and migration of neurons as well as the regulation of axonal growth in the developing brain (Klempan et al. 2004). Further, studies suggest that CAMs may influence learning and memory and brain development in response to environmental stimuli (Fields and Itoh 1996). Neurotrophins, important molecular regulators of neuronal survival and differentiation (Thoenen 1995), are of great interest both in expression studies and in molecular association and linkage studies. Alterations in brain-derived neurotrophic factor (BDNF) have been reported in postmortem studies of patients with schizophrenia; these findings, as well as recent evidence of a relationship between a BDNF polymorphism and episodic memory deficits, support BDNF as a putative schizophrenia susceptibility factor (Egan et al. 2003; Muglia et al. 2003) .

There is accumulating evidence of a relationship between schizophrenia susceptibility and allelic variations in genes whose protein products may contribute to the regulation of neurotransmission and synaptic activity (see Chapter 3, "Genetics"). A number of convincing susceptibility genes have recently been identified in schizophrenia. Several lines of evidence suggest that allelic variations in catechol-O-methyltransferase (COMT), a major enzyme involved in dopamine degradation, may contribute to the liability to schizophrenia (Riley and McGuffin 2000). Genetic association and microarray studies have reported that the gene for RGS4 (regulator of G-protein signaling 4), a member of the family of regulators of G-protein signaling proteins, is another strong schizophrenia susceptibility candidate, particularly in light of its importance in neurotransmission and cellular signaling (Lewis and Levitt 2002). RGS4 negatively regulates G-protein signaling, in particular the mGlu5 (metabotropic glutamate receptor 5) receptor, which is colocalized with and stimulates NMDA receptor function. Significant associations between variations in the gene for DTNBP1 (dystrobrevin-binding protein 1, or dysbindin) and schizophrenia and related phenotypes recently have been reported (Straub et al. 2002). Dysbindin regulates nitric oxide synthase, which in turn affects NMDA receptor function (Moghaddam 2002). Dysbin-

din's role in both synaptic activity and GABA receptor modulation makes it a strong candidate as a susceptibility locus that may influence the risk of schizophrenia. Another gene associated with neurotransmission (in this case, glutamate receptor activity), NRG1 (neuregulin 1), has also been identified as a strong candidate gene for schizophrenia (Stefansson et al. 2002).

Although these genes may subserve some other functions as well, they share in common their effects on neurotransmitter function, notably glutamate, GABA, and dopamine. It has also been suggested that impaired cortical glutamate neurotransmission can predispose to pathologically enhanced, stress-activated, monoaminergic neurotransmission leading to psychosis (Billingslea et al. 2003; Moghaddam 2002). Thus, diverse genetic factors might interact with environmental factors to result in a common phenotypic manifestation of schizophrenia. It is possible that together these candidate genes may induce schizophrenia susceptibility through common neurochemical pathways or that a combination of allelic variations in each of these genes contributes liability for different phenotypic features of the illness. The altered patterns of gene expression may be influenced by environmental events occurring during sensitive periods of neurodevelopment, such as the prenatal, perinatal, and adolescence time frames (Lewis and Levitt 2002).

ENVIRONMENTAL RISK FACTORS

Studies of monozygotic twins showing phenotypic discordance have generally been interpreted as supporting the role of environmental factors. Longitudinal studies of general population samples have revealed a wealth of information on developmental risk factors for early brain adversity in schizophrenia. Case–control and large-scale epidemiological data point to an increased frequency of obstetric and perinatal complications (Cannon et al. 2000; Dalman et al. 1999; Rosso et al. 2000b). Population-based cohort studies have also revealed valuable information about other potential etiological variables. The north Finland birth cohort (Rantakallio et al. 1997) and the U.K. National Child Development Study (Leask et al. 2002) revealed associations between childhood infections and later schizophrenia. Risk for schizophrenia has been associated in birth cohort studies with urban place of birth (Harrison and Owen 2003), migration (Cantor-Graae et al. 2003), paternal age (Brown et al. 2002), birth order (Kemppainen et al. 2001), exposure to prenatal rubella (Brown et al. 2001), and low maternal and birth weights (Wahlbeck et al. 2001). It has been suggested that risk factors occurring during the second or third trimester of pregnancy may be particularly associated with the susceptibility to schizophrenia. Later, biological environmental factors such as substance abuse have been implicated in contributing to schizophrenia risk. Although the role of psychosocial stress is still entertained, little evidence now exists for a causative role by psychodynamic factors.

EPIGENETIC FACTORS

The sequential emergence of biological and psychopathological manifestations of schizophrenia during the protracted period of postnatal development suggests that genetic as well as epigenetic factors must be considered. Genetic research in psychiatry has been dominated by a preoccupation with finding DNA sequence variation among causes of schizophrenia. However, recent interest has focused on the role of variation in DNA expression (epigenetics) during development (Petronis 2001). The differentiation of ectoderm into neurons and keratocytes involves epigenetic factors influencing pluripotent and undifferentiated embryonic cells to become highly specialized (Holliday 1994; Slack 2002). During embryonic development, the genome is subjected to major changes in epigenetic regulation (Reik et al. 2001). Studies using gene knockout mice have revealed that alterations in genes encoding epigenetic regulators may result in developmental defects. In human studies, mutations of MECP2, a methyl CpG-binding protein involved in DNA and chromatin modification, have been found to contribute to Rett's syndrome, a neurodevelopmental disorder (Van den Veyver and Zoghbi 2001). Epigenetic inactivation of *FMR1* (fragile X mental retardation-1) has been described as an important etiopathogenic factor in the development of fragile X syndrome, with evidence of abnormal synaptic plasticity in both human studies and *FMR1* knockout mice studies (El-Osta 2002).

Evidence of a relationship between epigenetic dysregulation and teratogenic effects during embryogenesis may better inform our understanding of gene-environment effects on neurodevelopment. For example, the teratogen valproic acid likely induces developmental defects through its epigenetic effects on histones (Phiel et al. 2001). An epigenetic role in the development of schizophrenia may explain the 50% discordance rates of monozygotic twins. Although the twins contain the same DNA sequence in the majority of somatic cells, epigenetic differences may accumulate over cell divisions throughout development. Potential differences in epigenetic regulation of candidate genes could result in the phenotypic expression of the disorder in only one twin (Torrey et al. 1999).

TOWARD AN INTEGRATION: A UNITARY GENETIC-DEVELOPMENTAL PERSPECTIVE

It is clear from the previous discussion that any one deterministic model is unlikely to explain the complex syndrome of schizophrenia. The schizophrenia syndrome is better understood as resulting from the cumulative effects of genetic and environmental factors unfolding during critical periods of development (Figure 5–1). The premorbid vulnerability to schizophrenia may be caused by multiple genetic and environmental factors interacting to affect early brain development. The adolescent onset of the disorder may be determined by late brain maturational processes as well as the stressors unique to adolescence. The interaction between genetic and environmental influences in determining the onset of schizophrenia was conceptualized by Waddington (1957) in the "canalization" model. In this model, normal development over time is represented by a ball traveling on a groove or valley initially specified by the genome on a model surface. Multiple causative factors, including genetic influences and environmental factors, may lead development to progress (or "canalize") along trajectories that cross thresholds for expression of psychopathology. Genetic and environmental risk factors early in life may influence the direction of the developmental trajectory. The slopes of the valley may be shallow early in life so that the trajectory can be pushed beyond the threshold for psychopathology even with mild degrees of adverse risk factors. The valley might get steeper later as development continues and plasticity diminishes, leading either to resilience and normalcy or to persistent psychopathology (Grossman et al. 2003; Woolf 1997).

The canals in which development proceeds are also determined by the complex epigenetic "landscape" as discussed previously. Epigenetic effects on the developing brain may be inherited through the germline, secondary to environmental factors, and may also be random events. Epigenetic effects may result in varying degrees of morphological and functional brain changes during development. The temporal delay of schizophrenia onset may result from a combination of inherited and acquired epimutations. The impact of epigenetic effects may remain below the threshold of phenotypic expression until 1) the effects are unmasked via completion of normal or accelerated neurodevelopmental processes such as synaptic pruning, and/or 2) an inflation of environmental stressors triggers a "break."

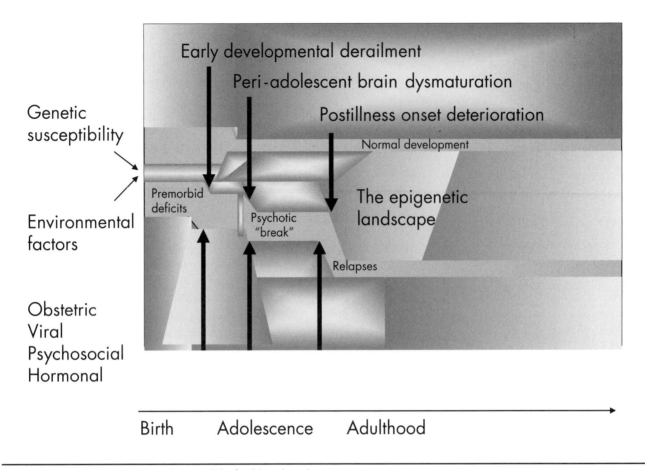

FIGURE 5–1.   An integrative model of schizophrenia.

The iterative interactions between the genome and the "envirome" have cellular and molecular consequences. It is likely that early brain developmental defects (e.g., neuromigrational errors or defective neuronal proliferation) predispose to excessive postnatal synaptic pruning and/or neuronal apoptosis leading to the schizophrenic endophenotype. Excitotoxic neuronal loss interacting with genetic factors may result from early brain adversity (viruses, malnutrition, perinatal trauma), leading to selective loss of NMDA receptor–bearing glutamatergic neurons in cortical and subcortical structures. This would account for the premorbid neurocognitive abnormalities seen among children and adolescents at risk for schizophrenia. The normative synaptic pruning process that sets in around late childhood and adolescence may interact with the state of reduced tonic glutamatergic neurotransmission, perhaps acting via NMDA receptors, to result in a net excess of synapse elimination in the cortical and subcortical structures. The glutamatergic and possibly GABAergic dysfunctions might lead to dysregulation of the dopaminergic system—a system that matures later, closer to adolescence. This dysregulation could underlie the typical adolescent onset of psychotic symptoms. The development of a defi-cit state and of persistent psychopathology after illness onset may be determined by the possible neurotoxic effect of continuing psychotic illness, perhaps as a result of progressive neurochemical sensitization.

CONCLUSION

From a unitary genetic-neurodevelopmental perspective, schizophrenia likely results from genetically mediated alterations in early and late maturational processes of brain development, interacting with environmental factors and downstream epigenetic effects on molecular systems. Continued studies investigating gene–environment and gene–gene interactions should significantly improve our understanding of the complex genetic factors that contribute to schizophrenia development. The creation of unitary models, integrating genetic, environmental, and developmental factors and exploring common themes such as glutamatergic dysfunction, should prove useful in elucidating the etiopathogenesis of this disorder. We need models to simplify and analyze problems that are otherwise intractable. Neurodevelopmental models offer considerable explanatory power and point to several lines of future research.

First, the strength of any explanatory model lies in its ability to generate testable hypotheses, which can then be examined using appropriate animal models. The developmental origins of schizophrenia can be examined by three types of heuristic animal models (Lipska et al. 2003). The first, the disrupted neurogenesis model, is exemplified by the neonatal ventral hippocampal lesion model, which was derived from early developmental lesion theories. The second approach is to use pharmacological models in a developmental perspective. Well-known pharmacological models, such as the NMDA receptor blockade in adult animals (Moghaddam 2003), have only rarely used a developmental perspective. Early lesions in the glutamatergic system may inform investigation of the integrative neurochemical models proposed in this chapter. A third strategy involves conditional transgenic models that seek to selectively reduce or enhance expression of genes involved in critical periods of development. An example of such models is the heterozygous reeler mouse, which expresses 50% of the brain reeler content of the wild-type mouse. This animal model expresses many neurobiological characteristics of the schizophrenia phenotype (Liu et al. 2001). Other molecular targets for manipulation studies in animal models include genes involved in glutamatergic and dopaminergic neurotransmission that have been recently identified as associated with schizophrenia. The apparent multifactorial (multiple genes and environmental factors) etiology of schizophrenia makes such efforts extremely challenging.

Second, individuals at risk for schizophrenia, such as young relatives of schizophrenia patients, offer an important opportunity to study the etiopathogenesis of the illness. The nature, timing, and causative factors underlying neurodevelopmental deviations predisposing to schizophrenia may be related in prospective studies of this at-risk population. Noninvasive in vivo neuroimaging techniques such as proton MRS (Stanley et al. 2000) may be able to address these questions. Using high-field magnets (i.e., 3 Tesla or higher), it may be possible to reliably delineate the GABA, glutamate, and glutamine signals with proton MRS. These approaches will also allow neurobiological prediction of the emergence of psychopathology during the critical development phases of adolescence and early adulthood as well as help us examine the neurobiology of transition from the premorbid to the prodrome and then the psychotic phases of the schizophrenic illness.

Finally, an important test of the value of neurodevelopmental models is whether they can generate hypotheses about novel preventive and therapeutic interventions. It is clear from the above discussion that although schizophrenia begins in late adolescence or early adulthood, its seeds are planted early. A long-term neurodevelopmental process occurs, eventually leading to deviant brain functioning. It is also evident that multiple and sequential etiological factors may interact and additively contribute to the emergence of the illness. This view suggests that preventive treatments may be tailored to the evolutionary stage of the disease process in individuals predisposed to the disorder. An improved understanding and definition of this target population is essential. The identification of risk factors is critical for accurate selection of those individuals at risk who are most appropriate for preventive treatment. Considerable ongoing research is currently devoted to the identification and validation of such risk factors.

REFERENCES

Abi-Dargham A, Mawlawi O, Lombardo I, et al: Prefrontal dopamine D1 receptors and working memory in schizophrenia. J Neurosci 22:3708–3719, 2002

Akbarian S, Bunney WE, Potkin SG, et al: Altered distribution of nicotamine-adenine dinucleotide phosphate-diaphorase cells in frontal lobe of schizophrenics implies disturbances of cortical development. Arch Gen Psychiatry 50:169–177, 1993

Akbarian S, Sucher NJ, Bradley D, et al: Selective alterations in gene expression for NMDA receptor subunits in prefrontal cortex of schizophrenics. J Neurosci 16:19–30, 1996

Akil M, Pierri JN, Whitehead RE, et al: Lamina-specific alterations in the dopamine innervation of the prefrontal cortex in schizophrenic subjects. Am J Psychiatry 156:1580–1589, 1999

Albert KA, Hemmings HC Jr, Adamo AI, et al: Evidence for decreased DARPP-32 in the prefrontal cortex of patients with schizophrenia. Arch Gen Psychiatry 59:705–712, 2002

Andreasen NC, Endicott J, Spitzer RL, et al: The family history method using diagnostic criteria: reliability and validity. Arch Gen Psychiatry 34:1229–1235, 1977

Andreasen NC, Rezzi K, Alliger R, et al: Hypofrontality in neuroleptic-naive patients and in patients with chronic schizophrenia. Arch Gen Psychiatry 49:943–958, 1992

Barch DM, Carter CS, Braver TS, et al: Selective deficits in prefrontal cortex function in medication-naive patients with schizophrenia. Arch Gen Psychiatry 58:280–288, 2001

Bearden CE, Rosso IM, Hollister JM, et al: A prospective cohort study of childhood behavioral deviance and language abnormalities as predictors of adult schizophrenia. Schizophr Bull 26:395–410, 2000

Bender L: Childhood schizophrenia. Psychiatr Q 27:663–681, 1953

Benes FM, Davidson J, Bird ED: Quantitative cytoarchitectural studies of the cerebral cortex of schizophrenics. Arch Gen Psychiatry 43:31–35, 1986

Benes FM, McSparren J, Bird ED, et al: Deficits in small interneurons in prefrontal and cingulate cortices of schizophrenic and schizoaffective patients. Arch Gen Psychiatry 48:996–1001, 1991

Benes FM, Vincent SL, Marie A, et al: Up-regulation of GABAA receptor binding on neurons of the prefrontal cortex in schizophrenic subjects. Neuroscience 75:1021–1031, 1996

Billingslea EN, Mastropaolo J, Rosse RB, et al: Interaction of stress and strain on glutamatergic neurotransmission: relevance to schizophrenia. Pharmacol Biochem Behav 74:351–356, 2003

Brown AS, Schaefer CA, Wyatt RJ, et al: Paternal age and risk of schizophrenia in adult offspring. Am J Psychiatry 159:1528–1533, 2002

Brown RT, Freeman WS, Perrin JM, et al: Prevalence and assessment of attention-deficit/hyperactivity disorder in primary care settings (electronic article). Pediatrics 107:E43, 2001. Available at: http://pediatrics.aappublications.org/cgi/content/full/107/3/e43. Accessed May 9, 2005.

Callicott JH, Egan MF, Bertolino A, et al: Hippocampal N-acetyl aspartate in unaffected siblings of patients with schizophrenia: a possible intermediate neurobiological phenotype. Biol Psychiatry 44:941–950, 1998

Callicott JH, Egan MF, Mattay VS, et al: Abnormal fMRI response of the dorsolateral prefrontal cortex in cognitively intact siblings of patients with schizophrenia. Am J Psychiatry 160:709–719, 2003

Cannon M, Caspi A, Moffitt TE, et al: Evidence for early childhood, pan-developmental impairment specific to schizophreniform disorder: results from a longitudinal birth cohort. Arch Gen Psychiatry 59:449–456, 2002

Cannon TD, Rosso IM, Hollister JM, et al: A prospective cohort study of genetic and perinatal influences in the etiology of schizophrenia. Schizophr Bull 26:351–366, 2000

Cantor-Graae E, Pedersen CB, McNeil TF, et al: Migration as a risk factor for schizophrenia: a Danish population-based cohort study. Br J Psychiatry 182:117–122, 2003

Cardno AG, Gottesman II: Twin studies of schizophrenia: from bow-and-arrow concordances to star wars Mx and functional genomics. Am J Med Genet 97:12–17, 2000

Casanova MF: Elmer Ernest Southard 1876–1920. Biol Psychiatry 38:71–73, 1995

Cho R, Gilbert A, Lewis DA: The neurobiology of schizophrenia, in The Neurobiology of Mental Disorders. Edited by Charney DS. New York, Oxford University Press, 2003, pp 299–310

Chugani HT, Phelps ME, Mazziotta JC: Positron-emission tomography study of human brain functional development. Ann Neurol 22:487–497, 1987

Clouston TS: Neuroses of Development: The Morrison Lectures for 1890. Edinburgh, Scotland, Oliver & Boyd, 1891

Cornblatt B, Obuchowski M, Roberts S, et al: Cognitive and behavioral precursors of schizophrenia. Dev Psychopathol 11:487–508, 1999

Costa E, Davis J, Grayson DR, et al: Dendritic spine hypoplasticity and downregulation of reelin and GABAergic tone in schizophrenia vulnerability. Neurobiol Dis 8:723–742, 2001

Cotter DR, Pariante CM, Everall IP: Glial cell abnormalities in major psychiatric disorders: the evidence and implications. Brain Res Bull 55:585–595, 2001

Coyle JT: The glutamatergic dysfunction hypothesis for schizophrenia. Harv Rev Psychiatry 3:241–253, 1996

Dalman C, Allebeck P, Cullberg J, et al: Obstetric complications and the risk of schizophrenia: a longitudinal study of a national birth cohort. Arch Gen Psychiatry 56:234–240, 1999

DeLisi LE: A prospective follow-up study of brain morphology and cognition in first-episode schizophrenic patients: preliminary findings. Biol Psychiatry 38:349–360, 1995

Done DJ, Crow TJ, Johnstone EC, et al: Childhood antecedents of schizophrenia and affective illness: social adjustments at ages 7 and 11. BMJ 309:699–703, 1994

Dworkin RH, Cornblatt BA, Friedmann R, et al: Childhood precursors of affective vs. social deficits in adolescents at risk for schizophrenia. Schizophr Bull 19:563–577, 1993

Eastwood SL, Harrison PJ: Decreased synaptophysin in the medical temporal lobe in schizophrenia demonstrated using immunoautoradiography. Neuroscience 69:339–343, 1995

Egan MF, Kojima M, Callicott JH, et al: The BDNF val66met polymorphism affects activity-dependent secretion of BDNF and human memory and hippocampal function. Cell 112:257–269, 2003

El-Osta A: FMR1 silencing and the signals to chromatin: a unified model of transcriptional regulation. Biochem Biophys Res Commun 295:575–581, 2002

Elvevag B, Goldberg TE: Cognitive impairment in schizophrenia is the core of the disorder. Crit Rev Neurobiol 14:1–21, 2000

Erlenmeyer-Kimling L: Neurobehavioral deficits in offspring of schizophrenic parents: liability indicators and predictors of illness. Am J Med Genet 97:65–71, 2000

Falkai P, Schneider-Axmann T, Honer WG: Entorhinal cortex pre-alpha cell clusters in schizophrenia: quantitative evidence of a developmental abnormality. Biol Psychiatry 47:937–943, 2000

Feinberg I: Schizophrenia: caused by a fault in programmed synaptic elimination during adolescence? J Psychiatr Res 17:319–334, 1982–1983

Feinberg I: Cortical pruning and the development of schizophrenia. Schizophr Bull 16:567–570, 1990

Fields RD, Itoh K: Neural cell adhesion molecules in activity-dependent development and synaptic plasticity. Trends Neurosci 19:473–480, 1996

Fish B: Characteristics and sequelae of the neurointegrative disorder in infants at risk for schizophrenia: 1952–1982, in Children at Risk for Schizophrenia: A Longitudinal Perspective. Watt NF, Anthony EJ, Wynne LC, et al. New York, Cambridge University Press, 1984, pp 423–439

Fish B: Infant predictors of the longitudinal course of schizophrenic development. Schizophr Bull 13:395–409, 1987

Fish B, Hagin R: Visual-motor disorders in infants at risk for schizophrenia. Arch Gen Psychiatry 27:594–598, 1972

Garey LJ, Patel T, Ong WY: Loss on dendritic spines from cortical pyramidal cells in schizophrenia. Schizophr Res 11:137, 1994

Giedd JN, Blumenthal J, Jeffries NO, et al: Brain development during childhood and adolescence: a longitudinal MRI study. Nat Neurosci 2:861–863, 1999

Glantz LA, Lewis DA: Reduction of synaptophysin immunoreactivity in the prefrontal cortex of subjects with schizophrenia: regional and diagnostic specificity. Arch Gen Psychiatry 54:943–952, 1997

Goldman-Rakic PS: Working memory dysfunction in schizophrenia. J Neuropsychiatry Clin Neurosci 6:348–357, 1994

Goldman-Rakic PS: The physiological approach: functional architecture of working memory and disordered cognition in schizophrenia. Biol Psychiatry 46:650–661, 1999

Gottesman II: Schizophrenia Genesis: The Origins of Madness. New York, WH Freeman, 1991

Grace AA: Phasic versus tonic dopamine release and the modulation of dopamine system responsivity: a hypothesis for the etiology of schizophrenia. Neuroscience 41:1–24, 1991

Grossman AW, Churchill JD, McKinney BC, et al: Experience effects on brain development: possible contributions to psychopathology. J Child Psychol Psychiatry 44:33–63, 2003

Hafner H, Maurer K, Loffler W, et al: The influence of age and sex on the onset and early course of schizophrenia. Br J Psychiatry 162:80–86, 1993

Harrison P, Lewis D: Neuropathology in schizophrenia, in Schizophrenia. Edited by Hirsch S, Weinberger DR. Oxford, UK, Blackwell Science, 2001

Harrison PJ, Owen MJ: Genes for schizophrenia? Recent findings and their pathophysiological implications. Lancet 361:417–419, 2003

Hoffman RE, McGlashan TH: Synaptic elimination, neurodevelopment, and the mechanism of hallucinated "voices" in schizophrenia. Am J Psychiatry 154:1683–1689, 1997

Holliday R: Epigenetics: an overview. Dev Genet 15:453–457, 1994

Jaskiw GE, Juliano DM, Goldberg TE, et al: Cerebral ventricular enlargement in schizophreniform disorder does not progress: a 7-year follow-up study. Schizophr Res 14:23–28, 1994

Javitt DC, Zukin SR: Recent advances in the phencyclidine model of schizophrenia. Am J Psychiatry 148:1301–1308, 1991

Jernigan TL, Tallal P: Late childhood changes in brain morphology observable with MRI. Dev Med Child Neurol 32:379–385, 1990

Jones P, Cannon M: The new epidemiology of schizophrenia. Psychiatr Clin North Am 21:1–25, 1998

Kalivas PW, Duffy P: D1 receptors modulate glutamate transmission in the ventral tegmental area. J Neurosci 15:5379–5388, 1995

Kemppainen L, Veijola J, Jokelainen J, et al: Birth order and risk for schizophrenia: a 31-year follow-up of the Northern Finland 1966 Birth Cohort. Acta Psychiatr Scand 104:148–152, 2001

Keshavan MS: Neurodevelopment and schizophrenia: quo vadis? in Neurodevelopment and Adult Psychopathology. Edited by Keshavan MS, Murray RM. New York, Cambridge University Press, 1997, pp 267–277

Keshavan MS: Development, disease and degeneration in schizophrenia: a unitary pathophysiological model. J Psychiatr Res 33:513–521, 1999

Keshavan MS: High risk studies, brain development and schizophrenia, in Neurodevelopment and Schizophrenia. Edited by Keshavan MS, Kennedy JL, Murray RM. London, Cambridge University Press, 2004, pp 432–454

Keshavan MS, Anderson S, Pettegrew JW: Is schizophrenia due to excessive synaptic pruning in the prefrontal cortex? J Psychiatr Res 28:239–265, 1994

Keshavan MS, Montrose DM, Pierri JN, et al: Magnetic resonance imaging and spectroscopy in offspring at risk for schizophrenia: preliminary studies. Prog Neuropsychopharmacol Biol Psychiatry 21:1285–1295, 1997

Keshavan MS, Haas GL, Kahn CE, et al: Superior temporal gyrus and the course of early schizophrenia: progressive, static, or reversible? J Psychiatr Res 32:161–167, 1998a

Keshavan MS, Reynolds CF, Miewald JM, et al: Delta sleep deficits in schizophrenia: evidence from automated analyses of sleep data. Arch Gen Psychiatry 55:443–448, 1998b

Keshavan MS, Diwadkar VA, Spencer SM, et al: A preliminary functional magnetic resonance imaging study in offspring of schizophrenic parents. Prog Neuropsychopharmacol Biol Psychiatry 26:1143–1149, 2002

Keshavan MS, Stanley JA, Montrose DM, et al: Prefrontal membrane phospholipid metabolism of child and adolescent offspring at risk for schizophrenia or schizoaffective disorder: an in vivo 31P MRS study. Mol Psychiatry 8:316–323, 2003

Kim JS, Kornhuber HH, Schmid-Burgk W, et al: Low cerebrospinal fluid glutamate in schizophrenic patients and a new hypothesis on schizophrenia. Neurosci Lett 20:379–382, 1980

Klemm S, Rzanny R, Riehemann S, et al: Cerebral phosphate metabolism in first-degree relatives of patients with schizophrenia. Am J Psychiatry 158:958–960, 2001

Klempan TA, Muglia P, Kennedy JL: Genes and brain development, in Neurodevelopment and Schizophrenia. Edited by Keshavan MS, Kennedy JL, Murray RM. London, Cambridge University Press, 2004, pp 3–34

Kotrla KJ, Sater AK, Weinberger DR: Neuropathology, neurodevelopment, and schizophrenia, in Neurodevelopment and Adult Psychopatholgy. Edited by Keshavan MS, Murray RM. New York, Cambridge University Press, 1997, pp 187–198

Krystal JH, D'Souza DC, Petrakis IL, et al: NMDA agonists and antagonists as probes of glutamatergic dysfunction and pharmacotherapies in neuropsychiatric disorders. Harv Rev Psychiatry 7:125–143, 1999

Laruelle M: The role of endogenous sensitization in the pathophysiology of schizophrenia: implications from recent brain imaging studies. Brain Res Brain Res Rev 31:371–384, 2000

Laruelle M, Abi-Dargham A, van Dyck CH, et al: Single photon emission computerized tomography imaging of amphetamine-induced dopamine release in drug-free schizophrenic subjects. Proc Natl Acad Sci U S A 93:9235–9240, 1996

Lawrie SM: Premorbid structural abnormalities in schizophrenia, in Neurodevelopment and Schizophrenia. Edited by Keshavan MS, Kennedy JL, Murray RM. London, Cambridge University Press, 2004, pp 347–372

Lawrie SM, Byrne M, Miller P, et al: Neurodevelopmental indices and the development of psychotic symptoms in subjects at high risk of schizophrenia. Br J Psychiatry 178:524–530, 2001

Leask SJ, Done DJ, Crow TJ: Adult psychosis, common childhood infections and neurological soft signs in a national birth cohort. Br J Psychiatry 181:387–392, 2002

Leung HC, Gore JC, Goldman-Rakic PS: Sustained mnemonic response in the human middle frontal gyrus during on-line storage of spatial memoranda. J Cogn Neurosci 14:659–671, 2002

Lewis DA: Development of the prefrontal cortex during adolescence: insights into vulnerable neural circuits in schizophrenia. Neuropsychopharmacology 16:385–398, 1997

Lewis DA, Levitt P: Schizophrenia as a disorder of neurodevelopment. Ann Rev Neurosci 25:409–432, 2002

Lewis DA, Lieberman JA: Catching up on schizophrenia: natural history and neurobiology. Neuron 28:325–334, 2000

Lieberman J: Prediction of outcome in first-episode schizophrenia. J Clin Psychiatry 54 (3, suppl):13–17, 1993

Lieberman J, Koreen A, Chakos M, et al: Factors influencing treatment response and outcome of first-episode schizophrenia: implications for understanding the pathophysiology of schizophrenia. J Clin Psychiatry 9:5–9, 1996

Lieberman J, Sheitman BB, Kinon BJ: Neurochemical sensitization in the pathophysiology of schizophrenia: deficits and dysfunction in neuronal regulation and plasticity. Neuropsychopharmacology 17:205–229, 1997

Lipska BK, Lerman DN, Khaing ZZ, et al: The neonatal ventral hippocampal lesion model of schizophrenia: effects on dopamine and GABA mRNA markers in the rat midbrain. Eur J Neurosci 18:3097–3104, 2003

Liu WS, Pesold C, Rodriguez MA, et al: Down-regulation of dendritic spine and glutamic acid decarboxylase 67 expressions in the reelin haploinsufficient heterozygous reeler mouse. Proc Natl Acad Sci U S A 98:3477–3482, 2001

Loebel AD, Lieberman JA, Alvir JM, et al: Duration of psychosis and outcome in first-episode schizophrenia. Am J Psychiatry 149:1183–1188, 1992

MacDonald AW, Pogue-Geile MF, Johnson MK, et al: A specific deficit in context processing in the unaffected siblings of patients with schizophrenia. Arch Gen Psychiatry 60:57–65, 2003

Malmberg A, Lewis G, David A, et al: Premorbid adjustment and personality in people with schizophrenia. Br J Psychiatry 172:308–313, 1998

Manoach DS: Prefrontal cortex dysfunction during working memory performance in schizophrenia: reconciling discrepant findings. Schizophr Res 60:285–298, 2003

Marenco S, Weinberger DR: The neurodevelopmental hypothesis of schizophrenia: following a trail of evidence from cradle to grave. Dev Psychopathol 12:501–527, 2001

Mathalon DH, Ford JM, Rosenbloom M, et al: P300 reduction and prolongation with illness duration in schizophrenia. Biol Psychiatry 47:413–427, 2000

McCarley RW, Wible CG, Frumin M, et al: MRI anatomy of schizophrenia. Biol Psychiatry 45:1099–1119, 1999

McGlashan TH, Fenton WS: Subtype progression and pathophysiologic deterioration in early schizophrenia. Schizophr Bull 19:71–84, 1993

McGlashan TH, Hoffman RE: Schizophrenia as a disorder of developmentally reduced synaptic connectivity. Arch Gen Psychiatry 57:637–648, 2000

Mesulam MM: From sensation to cognition. Brain 121:1013–1052, 1998

Michie PT, Kent A, Stienstra R, et al: Phenotypic markers as risk factors in schizophrenia: neurocognitive functions. Aust N Z J Psychiatry 34 (suppl 2):S74–S85, 2000

Moghaddam B: Stress activation of glutamate neurotransmission in the prefrontal cortex: implications for dopamine-associated psychiatric disorders. Biol Psychiatry 51:775–787, 2002

Moghaddam B: Bringing order to the glutamate chaos in schizophrenia. Neuron 40:881–884, 2003

Muglia P, Vicente AM, Verga M, et al: Association between the BDNF gene and schizophrenia. Mol Psychiatry 8:146–147, 2003

Murray RM, Lewis SW: Is schizophrenia a neurodevelopmental disorder? Br Med J (Clin Res Ed) 295:681–682, 1987

Petronis A: Human morbid genetics revisited: relevance of epigenetics. Trends Genet 17:142–146, 2001

Pettegrew JW, Keshavan MS, Panchalingam K, et al: Alterations in brain high-energy phosphate and membrane phospholipid metabolism in first-episode, drug-naive schizophrenics: a pilot study of the dorsal prefrontal cortex by in vivo phosphorus-31 nuclear magnetic resonance spectroscopy. Arch Gen Psychiatry 48:563–568, 1991

Pettegrew JW, Keshavan MS, Minshew NJ: [31]P nuclear magnetic resonance spectroscopy: neurodevelopment and schizophrenia. Schizophr Bull 19:35–53, 1993

Pettegrew JW, McClure RJ, Keshavan MS, et al: [31]P magnetic resonance spectroscopy studies of developing brain, in Neurodevelopement and Adult Psychopathology. Edited by Keshavan MS, Murray RM. New York, Cambridge University Press 1997, pp 71–92

Phiel CJ, Zhang F, Huang EY, et al: Histone deacetylase is a direct target of valproic acid, a potent anticonvulsant, mood stabilizer, and teratogen. J Biol Chem 276:36734–36741, 2001

Pierri JN, Volk CL, Auh S, et al: Decreased somal size of deep layer 3 pyramidal neurons in the prefrontal cortex of subjects with schizophrenia. Arch Gen Psychiatry 58:466–473, 2001

Rajkowska G, Selemon LD, Goldman-Rakic PS: Neuronal and glial somal size in the prefrontal cortex: a postmortem morphometric study of schizophrenia and Huntington disease. Arch Gen Psychiatry 55:215–224, 1998

Rajkowska G, Miguel-Hidalgo JJ, Wei J, et al: Morphometric evidence for neuronal and glial prefrontal cell pathology in major depression. Biol Psychiatry 45:1085–1098, 1999

Rantakallio P, Jones PB, Moring J, et al: Association between central nervous system infections during childhood and adult onset schizophrenia and other psychoses: a 28-year follow-up. Int J Epidemiol 26:837–843, 1997

Reik W, Dean W, Walter J: Epigenetic reprogramming in mammalian development. Science 293:1089–1093, 2001

Riley BP, McGuffin P: Linkage and associated studies of schizophrenia. Am J Med Genet 97:23–44, 2000

Rosso IM, Bearden CE, Hollister JM, et al: Childhood neuromotor dysfunction in schizophrenia patients and their unaffected siblings: a prospective cohort study. Schizophr Bull 26:367–378, 2000a

Rosso IM, Cannon TD, Huttunen T, et al: Obstetric risk factors for early onset schizophrenia in a Finnish birth cohort. Am J Psychiatry 157:801–807, 2000b

Rzanny R, Klemm S, Reichenbach JR, et al: 31P-MR spectroscopy in children and adolescents with a familial risk of schizophrenia. Eur Radiol 13:763–770, 2003

Selemon LD, Rajkowska G, Goldman-Rakic PS: Abnormally high neuronal density in the schizophrenic cortex: a morphometric analysis of prefrontal area 9 and occipital area 17. Arch Gen Psychiatry 52:805–818, 1995

Shenton ME, Dickey CC, Frumin M, et al: A review of MRI findings in schizophrenia. Schizophr Res 49:1–52, 2001

Slack JM: Conrad Hal Waddington: the last Renaissance biologist? Nat Rev Genet 3:889–895, 2002

Stanley JA: In vivo magnetic resonance spectroscopy and its application to neuropsychiatric disorders. Can J Psychiatry 47:315–326, 2002

Stanley JA, Pettegrew JW, Keshavan MS: Magnetic resonance spectroscopy in schizophrenia: methodological issues and findings: part I. Biol Psychiatry 48:357–368, 2000

Stefansson H, Sigurdsson E, Steinthorsdottir V, et al: Neuregulin 1 and susceptibility to schizophrenia. Am J Hum Genet 71:877–892, 2002

Straub RE, Jiang Y, MacLean CJ, et al: Genetic variation in the 6p22.3 gene DTNBP1, the human ortholog of the mouse dysbindin gene, is associated with schizophrenia. Am J Hum Genet 71:337–348, 2002

Tamminga CA: Schizophrenia and glutamatergic transmission. Crit Rev Neurobiol 12:21–36, 1998

Thoenen H: Neurotrophins and neuronal plasticity. Science 270:593–598, 1995

Thompson PM, Vidal C, Giedd JN, et al: Mapping adolescent brain change reveals dynamic wave of accelerated gray matter loss in very early onset schizophrenia. Proc Natl Acad Sci U S A 98:11650–11655, 2001

Torrey EF, Bowler AE, Taylor EH, et al: Schizophrenia and Manic Depressive Disorder: The Biological Roots of Mental Illness as Revealed by the Landmark Study of Identical Twins. New York, Basic Books, 1999

Tsai G, Coyle JT: N-acetylaspartate in neuropsychiatric disorders. Prog Neurobiol 46:531–540, 1995

Van den Veyver IB, Zoghbi HY: Mutations in the gene encoding methyl-CpG-binding protein 2 cause Rett syndrome. Brain Dev 23 (suppl 1):S147–S151, 2001

Volk DW, Austin MC, Pierri JN, et al: Decreased glutamic acid decarboxylase67 messenger RNA expression in a subset of prefrontal cortical gamma-aminobutyric acid neurons in subjects with schizophrenia. Arch Gen Psychiatry 57:237–245, 2000

Waddington CH: The Strategy of the Genes. London, Allen & Unwin, 1957

Wahlbeck K, Forsen T, Osmond C, et al: Association of schizophrenia with low maternal body mass index, small size at birth, and thinness during childhood. Arch Gen Psychiatry 58:48–52, 2001

Walker EF, Savoie T, Davis D: Neuromotor precursors of schizophrenia. Schizophr Bull 20:441–451, 1994

Watt NF: Patterns of childhood social development in adult schizophrenics. Arch Gen Psychiatry 35:160–165, 1978

Weinberger DR: Implications of normal brain development for the pathogenesis of schizophrenia. Arch Gen Psychiatry 44:660–669, 1987

Weinberger DR, Egan MF, Bertolino A, et al: Prefrontal neurons and the genetics of schizophrenia. Biol Psychiatry 50:825–844, 2001

Woolf CM: Does the genotype for schizophrenia often remain unexpressed because of canalization and stochastic events during development? Psychol Med 27:659–668, 1997

Wyatt RJ, Alexander RC, Egan MF, et al: Schizophrenia, just the facts: what do we know, how well do we know it? Schizophr Res 1:3–18, 1988

Zipursky RO: Widespread cerebral gray matter volume deficits in schizophrenia. Arch Gen Psychiatry 49:195–205, 1992

NEUROCHEMICAL THEORIES

DANIEL C. JAVITT, M.D., PH.D.

MARC LARUELLE, M.D.

Schizophrenia is a severe and chronic mental illness (or group of illnesses) with high prevalence (occurring in about 0.5%–1% of the population). Symptoms of schizophrenia usually emerge during adolescence or early adulthood. Psychotic symptoms include hallucinations, typically auditory, and delusions, which frequently involve persecution and/or megalomania. Psychotic symptoms and severe thought disorganization are often grouped under the term *positive symptoms*. Deficit symptoms, also commonly referred to as *negative symptoms*, manifest themselves in many dimensions, such as affect (affect flattening), volition (apathy), speech (poverty), pleasure (anhedonia), and social life (withdrawal).

The etiology and fundamental pathology of schizophrenia remain unclear, but a large body of evidence suggests that alterations in several neurotransmitter systems are involved in the pathophysiological processes of the illness. Among these transmitters, dopamine (DA) and glutamate (GLU) have received the most attention, although other systems, such as the γ-aminobutyric acid (GABA)–ergic, serotonergic, cholinergic, and opioidergic systems, also have been implicated.

The putative role of dopaminergic systems in the pathophysiology and treatment of schizophrenia has been the subject of intense research efforts over the last 50 years. The first formulation of the DA hypothesis of schizophrenia proposed that hyperactivity of DA transmission was responsible for the positive symptoms observed in the disorder (Carlsson and Lindqvist 1963; van Rossum 1966). This hypothesis was based on the recognition that antipsychotic drugs were dopamine$_2$ (D$_2$) receptor antagonists (Carlsson and Lindqvist 1963; Creese et al. 1976; Seeman and Lee 1975) and that DA-enhancing drugs were psychotogenic (for review, see Angrist and van Kammen 1984; Lieberman et al. 1987a). Because D$_2$ receptors are expressed mainly in the striatum, several investigators proposed that hyperactivity of dopaminergic systems in the limbic striatum was associated with the emergence of psychosis (Matthysse

The authors would like to thank Stephanie Reeder for expert editorial assistance. Supported by the Public Health Service (Conte Center for Schizophrenia Research, National Institute of Mental Health 5 P50 MH066171-02, K02-MH01603-01, K02 MH01439), the Lieber Center for Schizophrenia Research at Columbia University, the Program in Cognitive Neuroscience and Schizophrenia at Nathan Kline Institute, and the New York State Office of Mental Health.

1974; Snyder 1973; Stevens 1973). Because D_2 receptor antagonists are most effective in treating positive symptoms, the classical DA hypothesis of schizophrenia provided a putative base for the positive symptoms but failed to account for the persistent negative and cognitive symptoms.

More recently, an increasing awareness of the importance of negative and cognitive symptoms in schizophrenia and their resistance to D_2 receptor antagonism has led to a reformulation of the classical DA hypothesis. Functional brain imaging studies suggested that these symptoms might arise from altered function in the prefrontal cortex (PFC) (for review, see Knable and Weinberger 1997). A wealth of preclinical studies emerged documenting the importance of the prefrontal DA transmission at dopamine$_1$ (D_1) receptors (the main DA receptor in the neocortex) for optimal cognitive functions subserved by the PFC (for review, see Goldman-Rakic et al. 2000). These observations led to the hypothesis that a deficit in DA transmission at the D_1 receptors in the PFC might be implicated in the cognitive impairments of schizophrenia (Davis et al. 1991; Weinberger 1987). The coexistence of an imbalance between an excess of subcortical DA and a deficit of prefrontal DA in schizophrenia has emerged as the "revised" DA hypothesis of schizophrenia (Davis et al. 1991).

Other than the DA theory, several lines of evidence support the hypothesis that schizophrenia might be associated with a persistent dysfunction of GLU transmission involving N-methyl-D-aspartate (NMDA) receptors (for reviews, see Goff and Coyle 2001; Javitt and Zukin 1991; Jentsch and Roth 1999; Olney and Farber 1995; Tamminga et al. 1995). This hypothesis stems essentially from the recognition that exposure to drugs that impair NMDA transmission induces, in healthy subjects, a constellation of clinical and cognitive symptoms that mirrors the full spectrum of signs and systems of schizophrenia. Thus, as opposed to the classical DA hypothesis that accounts mostly for positive symptoms, the NMDA hypothesis claims to explain positive, negative, and cognitive symptoms.

Both the NMDA hypofunction and the DA imbalance theories of schizophrenia have evolved for years as competing models, but more recent data suggest that both sets of alterations might be intimately related. Preclinical and clinical imaging data now show that an alteration in NMDA transmission induces the DA endophenotype potentially associated with schizophrenia (excess stimulation of subcortical D_2 receptors, insufficient stimulation of cortical D_1 receptors). Conversely, an increased understanding of the modulatory role of DA on GLU transmission has suggested a mechanism that might explain how alterations of DA function in schizophrenia affect NMDA transmission. Thus, the NMDA and DA models are evolving from competing to complementary theories.

In this chapter, we review the evidence supporting both DA and GLU models of schizophrenia. Following this review is a presentation of the salient features of the interactions between these neurotransmitter systems that provide avenues to bridge both DA and GLU theories into one disease model.

DOPAMINE RECEPTORS

OVERVIEW OF DOPAMINE TRANSMISSION

Dopaminergic projections are divided among nigrostriatal, mesolimbic, and mesocortical systems (Lindvall and Björklund 1983). The nigrostriatal system projects from the substantia nigra to the dorsal striatum and is involved in cognitive integration, habituation, sensorimotor coordination, and initiation of movement. The mesolimbic system projects from the ventral tegmental area (VTA) to limbic structures such as the ventral striatum, hippocampus, and amygdala. The mesocortical system projects from the VTA to cortical regions. The mesolimbic and the mesocortical systems are involved in the regulation of motivation, attention, and reward (Mogenson et al. 1980).

DA receptors were originally classified into two types: D_1 receptors, which stimulate adenylate cyclase, and D_2 receptors, which are neither coupled to nor inhibit this effector (Kebabian and Calne 1979). The advent of molecular biology techniques in the late 1980s enabled the cloning of these two receptors (Bunzow et al. 1988; Dearry et al. 1990; Monsma et al. 1990; Zhou et al. 1990), as well as three newer DA receptors—D_3, D_4, and D_5 (Sokoloff et al. 1990; Sunahara et al. 1991; Tiberi et al. 1991; Van Tol et al. 1991). The pharmacological characterization of these receptors indicated that D_1 and D_5 share similar properties, whereas the pharmacological profiles of D_3 and D_4 are similar to that of D_2. Therefore, the D_1–D_2 classification of the DA receptors has been elaborated on to consist of a D_1-like family (D_1 and D_5 receptors) and a D_2-like family (D_2, D_3, and D_4 receptors) (for review, see Missale et al. 1998; Palermo-Neto 1997).

DA receptors differ in their regional localization in the human brain (for reviews, see Joyce and Meador-Woodruff 1997; Meador-Woodruff et al. 1996; Seeman 1992). D_1 receptors show a widespread neocortical distribution, including the PFC, and are also present in high concentration in the striatum. D_5 receptors are concentrated in the hippocampus and the entorhinal cortex. D_2 receptors are concentrated in the striatum, with low concentration in the medial temporal structures (hippocampus, entorhinal cortex, amygdala) and the thalamus. The concentration of D_2 receptors in the PFC is extremely low. D_3 receptors are present in the striatum, with a particularly high concentration in the ventral striatum. D_4 receptors are present in the PFC and the hippocampus but are undetected in the striatum.

Unlike the classically understood definition of the "fast" transmitters such as GLU, DA does not directly gate ion channels; rather, the stimulation of a G protein linked to the DA receptor induces a cascade of intracellular signaling events that modify the response of the cell to other transmitters. DA is neither "inhibitory" nor "excitatory." DA action depends on the state of the neurons at the time of the stimulation and the type of receptor involved (Yang et al. 1999). In the striatum, DA modulates the response of the GABAergic medium spiny neurons to the glutamatergic drive. In this structure, it has been proposed that DA is "reinforcing" (i.e., it augments the inhibition of neurons that are unstimulated and the excitatory response of neurons that are excited) (Wickens 2000). In this manner, DA acts to gate glutamatergic inputs by increasing their signal-to-noise ratio. In the PFC, DA modulates pyramidal cell excitability, both directly and through GABAergic interneurons (Mrzljak et al. 1996; Smiley et al. 1994; Yang et al. 1999). Here again, it has been proposed that DA increases the signal-to-noise ratio of glutamatergic afferents (i.e., augmenting the response of neurons stimulated by GLU and silencing the neurons not stimulated by GLU) (Seamans et al. 2001b).

EVIDENCE SUPPORTING INCREASED DOPAMINE ACTIVITY AT STRIATAL D_2 RECEPTORS

Pharmacological Evidence

Aversive pharmacological effects. The psychotogenic effect of amphetamine and other DA-enhancing drugs such as methylphenidate and L-dopa is a cornerstone of the classical DA hypothesis of schizophrenia. Two sets of observations are relevant to this issue. First, repeated exposure to high doses of psychostimulants in nonschizophrenic subjects might gradually induce paranoid psychosis. This well-documented observation shows that sustained increase in DA activity is psychotogenic. Second, low doses of psychostimulants that are not psychotogenic in healthy subjects might induce or worsen psychotic symptoms in patients with schizophrenia. This observation indicates that patients with schizophrenia have an increased vulnerability to the psychotogenic effects of DA-enhancing drugs.

Amphetamine-induced psychosis in nonschizophrenic subjects. Although mentioned in 1938 (Young and Scoville 1938), amphetamine-induced psychosis was not clearly recognized as a possible consequence of chronic amphetamine use until 1958, when a 42-case monograph by Connell (1958) was published. In this monograph, Connell provided the "classical" definition of amphetamine psychosis as "a paranoid psychosis with ideas of references, delusions of persecution, auditory and visual hallucinations in the setting of a clear sensorium" and concluded that "the mental picture may be indistinguishable from acute or chronic paranoid schizophrenia."

In the early 1970s, several studies experimentally induced amphetamine psychosis in nonschizophrenic amphetamine abusers to better document the clinical pattern of this syndrome (Angrist and Gershon 1970; Bell 1973; Griffith et al. 1968). These experiments formally established that sustained psychostimulant exposure can produce paranoid psychosis in nonschizophrenic individuals. This reaction does not occur in the context of a delirium because subjects maintain a clear sensorium during the episode and are able to recollect the episode after its resolution. Because these studies were performed before the conceptualization of the symptoms of schizophrenia into positive and negative (Crow 1980), they did not formally assess negative symptoms. These articles included only anecdotal reports of emotional blunting, withdrawal, or alogia, thereby suggesting that sustained and excessive stimulation of DA systems does not consistently induce what are now defined as the "negative" symptoms of schizophrenia.

Ellinwood (1967; Ellinwood et al. 1973) provided one of the most insightful descriptions of amphetamine-induced psychosis by conceptualizing the condition as a continuum that evolves from the gradual onset of paranoid tendencies to delusional paranoia. The first step is characterized by stimulation of interpretative mental activities (great attention to details, intense feeling of curiosity, repetitive searching and sorting behavior). Ellinwood saw in Sherlock Holmes, a regular cocaine user, a prototypical example of the endless search for meanings ("*my mind rebels at stagnation*"). With increased exposure, these paranoid tendencies and interests for the minutiae develop into an intermediate stage, which is characterized by marked enhancement of perceptual acuity, sustained "pleasurable" suspiciousness, and compulsive probing behavior. Finally, this inquisitive behavior is reversed and projected to others (persecution), leading to paranoia and ideas of references. The "enhancement of sensitive acuity" develops into hallucinations, initially auditory and then visual and tactile. The sensorium remains clear until toxic delirium is reached. Thought disorders might manifest toward the end of the continuum near the toxic stage. Kapur (2003) recently reformulated and modernized the Ellinwood "Sherlock Holmes" theory by defining schizophrenia psychosis as a state of "aberrant salience," in which abnormal importance and meaning are assigned to elements of an individual's experience.

Another important property of psychostimulants is their ability to induce reverse tolerance or "sensitization" (Kalivas et al. 1993; Robinson and Becker 1986). Long-term sensitization to psychostimulants is a process whereby repeated exposure to these drugs results in an enhanced response after subsequent exposures. The relevance of this process for the pathophysiology of schizophrenia has been reviewed elsewhere (Laruelle 2000b; Lieberman et al. 1997). Subjects who abused psychostimulants and experienced stimulant-induced psychotic episodes were reported to remain vulnerable to low doses of psychostimulants (Connell 1958; Ellinwood et al. 1973; Sato et al. 1983). In these subjects, exposure to psychostimulants at doses that do not normally produce psychotic symptoms can trigger a recurrence of these symptoms. The similarity between these patients and the patients with schizophrenia in terms of vulnerability to the psychotogenic effects of psychostimulants has led to the theorization that schizophrenia might be associated with an "endogenous" sensitization process (Glenthoj and Hemmingsen 1997; Laruelle 2000b; Lieberman et al. 1990).

Considerable research efforts have been devoted to the identification of neuronal substrates involved in sensitization. Several studies have shown that sensitization is associated with increased stimulant-induced DA release in the axonal terminal fields (for references, see Laruelle 2000b). A recent brain imaging study confirmed that in humans, sensitization to the effects of amphetamine involves increased amphetamine-induced DA release (Boileau et al. 2003). The imaging studies reviewed later in this section show that patients with schizophrenia have an enhanced amphetamine-induced DA release, supporting the notion of an endogenous sensitization process of the subcortical DA system in schizophrenia.

Psychotogenic effects of amphetamine in schizophrenic patients. Several studies reviewed by Lieberman et al. (1987b) provided evidence that patients with schizophrenia, as a group, have increased sensitivity to the psychotogenic effects of acute psychostimulant administration. In other words, some, but not all, patients with schizophrenia present with emergence or worsening of psychotic symptoms after acute exposure to psychostimulants at doses that do not induce psychosis in healthy subjects. The psychotic response appears to be state dependent. First, patients who responded with a psychotic reaction to a psychostimulant challenge during an acute episode failed to show such a response when they were in remission. Second, the propensity to present a psychotic

reaction to a psychostimulant challenge is predictive of relapse on antipsychotic discontinuation. Thus, the clinical response to stimulants might "expose" an active phase of the illness that is not readily identifiable by the clinical symptomatology in the absence of a psychostimulant administration.

Therapeutic pharmacological effects.   Since the recognition in 1952 of the antipsychotic properties of chlorpromazine (Delay et al. 1952), antipsychotic medications have fundamentally altered the course and the prognosis of schizophrenia. They have proven effective in reducing the severity of symptoms and preventing episodes of illness exacerbation. To date, D_2 receptor antagonism is the only pharmacological property shared by all antipsychotic drugs. The clinical dose of these drugs is related to their affinity for D_2 receptors. D_2 receptor antagonism appears both necessary and sufficient for antipsychotic action (as shown by the effect of selective D_2 receptor antagonist amisulpride). The fact that patients with schizophrenia improve following administration of D_2 receptor antagonists is one of the few irrefutable pieces of evidence in schizophrenia (Weinberger 1987).

D_2 receptor blockade by antipsychotic drugs has been confirmed by numerous imaging studies (reviewed in Talbot and Laruelle 2002). In general, these studies failed to observe a relation between the degree of D_2 receptor occupancy and the quality of the clinical response. However, most studies reported doses achieving more than 50% occupancy. The minimum occupancy required for a therapeutic response remains somewhat uncertain. Two studies performed with low doses of relatively selective D_2 receptor antagonists (haloperidol and raclopride) suggest that a minimum of 50% occupancy is required to observe a rapid clinical response (Kapur et al. 2000; Nordstrom et al. 1993). Imaging studies have repeatedly confirmed the existence of a striatal D_2 receptor occupancy threshold (about 80%) above which extrapyramidal symptoms (EPS) are likely to occur (Farde et al. 1992). Thus, these data suggest the existence of a therapeutic window between 50% and 80% striatal D_2 receptor occupancy. Within this window, the relation between occupancy and response is unclear, presumably because of the variability in endogenous DA (Frankle et al. 2004). Furthermore, the occupancy threshold required for therapeutic effects may differ among drugs.

The introduction of second-generation antipsychotic drugs since the early 1990s has not fundamentally altered the prominence of D_2 receptor antagonism in the current treatment of schizophrenia. Most second-generation antipsychotic drugs also potently interact with other receptors, such as the serotonin$_{2A}$ (5-HT$_{2A}$) receptors, but the possibility to achieve an "atypical" profile with a pure D_2 receptor antagonist such as amisulpride indicates that serotonin pharmacological effects are not absolutely required to produce this effect.

However, imaging studies generally have reported lower occupancies of striatal D_2 receptors at therapeutic doses of second-generation antipsychotic drugs compared with first-generation antipsychotic drugs. This seems to be especially true for amisulpride, clozapine, and quetiapine, which provide 50%–60% D_2 receptor occupancy at clinically effective doses (for review and references, see Abi-Dargham and Laruelle 2005). In contrast, studies with first-generation antipsychotic drugs often report occupancies exceeding 75%. Thus, a parsimonious hypothesis to account for possible second-generation antipsychotic advantages is that, in general, clinical results obtained after moderate occupancies (50%–75%) are better than those obtained after high occupancies (75%–100%) and that, for a variety of reasons, second-generation antipsychotic drugs tend to maintain lower occupancies than do first-generation antipsychotic drugs. The alternative hypothesis is that the D_2 receptor occupancy required for therapeutic effects is lower in second-generation antipsychotic drugs than in first-generation antipsychotic drugs. Should the alternative hypothesis be true, the mechanisms responsible for the gain in the occupancy–efficacy relation of second-generation antipsychotic drugs remain to be fully elucidated.

A potentially important synergistic effect of 5-HT$_{2A}$ and D_2 receptor antagonism is to increase prefrontal DA, an effect not observed with selective D_2 or 5-HT$_{2A}$ receptor antagonists administered alone (Gessa et al. 2000; Ichikawa et al. 2001; Melis et al. 1999; Pehek and Yamamoto 1994; Youngren et al. 1999). This effect might be mediated by the stimulation of 5-HT$_{1A}$ receptors: it is blocked by 5-HT$_{1A}$ antagonists and is also observed following the combination of 5-HT$_{1A}$ receptor agonism and D_2 receptor antagonism (Ichikawa et al. 2001; Rollema et al. 2000). Aripiprazole, clozapine, quetiapine, and ziprasidone are also 5-HT$_{1A}$ partial agonists, and this additional property also might contribute to their ability to increase prefrontal DA. As discussed later, a decreased prefrontal DA function might contribute to the cognitive deficits present in patients with schizophrenia, and an increase in prefrontal DA induced by second-generation antipsychotics might mediate some of the modest cognitive improvements induced by these drugs (Keefe et al. 1999). Yet it is unclear whether this increase in prefrontal DA, documented as an acute response in animal studies, is sustained during the course of treatment in patients with schizophrenia.

Postmortem Evidence

The discovery of the antipsychotic effect of D_2 receptor blockade inspired decades of postmortem research seeking to determine whether schizophrenia was associated with alterations of DA transmission parameters. This large body of research has so far failed to provide definitive answers, in part, because of the confounding effect of antemortem antipsychotic treatment.

Tissue DA and homovanillic acid. Direct measures of the tissue content of DA and its metabolites failed to detect consistent and reproducible abnormalities (for review, see Cross et al. 1981; Davis et al. 1991; Reynolds 1989). Note, however, that some studies reported higher DA tissue levels in the samples from patients with schizophrenia compared with the samples from control subjects in the subcortical regions such as the caudate (Owen et al. 1978), the accumbens (Mackay et al. 1982), and the amygdala (Reynolds 1983) and that no studies reported lower DA content in these regions in the patients compared with the control subjects.

D_1 receptors. Several studies have reported that striatal D_1 receptors are unaltered in schizophrenia (Joyce et al. 1988; Pimoule et al. 1985; Reynolds and Czudek 1988; Seeman et al. 1987), although one study reported decreased density (Hess et al. 1987).

D_2 receptors. Increased density of striatal D_2 receptors in patients with schizophrenia measured with tritium spiperone and other tritium neuroleptic drugs has been a consistent finding in many postmortem studies (Cross et al. 1983; Hess et al. 1987; Joyce et al. 1988; Lee et al. 1978; Mackay et al. 1982; Mita et al. 1986; Owen et al. 1978; Reynolds et al. 1987; Seeman et al. 1984, 1987). However, chronic neuroleptic administration upregulates D_2 receptor density (Burt et al. 1977), making it unclear if these postmortem findings are related to prior neuroleptic exposure or to the disease process per se.

D_3 receptors. Gurevich et al. (1997) reported a significant increase (almost twofold) in the D_3 receptor number in postmortem samples of ventral striatum from patients with schizophrenia who were not taking neuroleptics at the time of death. In contrast, the D_3 receptor binding was normal in patients taking neuroleptics at the time of death, suggesting that treatment might normalize these receptors. However, these interesting findings have not yet been replicated, and D_3 receptor messenger ribonucleic acid (mRNA) levels were reported to be normal in the accumbens (Meador-Woodruff et al. 1997).

D4 receptors. Several studies that used ligand subtraction techniques reported an increase in striatal D_4-like receptors in schizophrenia (Marzella et al. 1997; Murray et al. 1995; Seeman et al. 1993; Sumiyoshi et al. 1995). These findings, combined with the higher affinity of clozapine for D_4 relative to other DA receptors, prompted the hypothesis that D_4 receptors might play a critical role in the pathophysiology of the illness (Seeman et al. 1995). Yet the elevation of D_4-like receptors in the striatum in patients with schizophrenia was neither confirmed by other studies that used the same subtraction technique (Lahti et al. 1996b; Reynolds and Mason 1994) nor found in one study that used the selective D_4 ligand tritium NGD 94-1 (Lahti et al. 1996a).

DA transporters. Many postmortem studies report unaltered DA transporter density in the striatum of patients with schizophrenia (Chinaglia et al. 1992; Czudek and Reynolds 1989; Hirai et al. 1988; Joyce et al. 1988; Knable et al. 1994; Pearce et al. 1990).

In conclusion, postmortem measurements of the indices of DA transmission generated two consistent observations:

1. The binding of the radioligand to D_2-like receptors in the striatum of patients with schizophrenia is increased, but it has been difficult to exclude the contribution of the premortem antipsychotic exposure in this set of findings.
2. Striatal DA transporter and D_1 receptor densities are unaffected in schizophrenia.

Imaging Evidence

DA receptors and transporters. Striatal D_2 receptor density in schizophrenia has been extensively studied with positron emission tomography (PET) and single photon emission computed tomography (SPECT) imaging, and these studies have been reviewed elsewhere (Laruelle 1998, 2003). The vast majority of these studies have had negative findings, but a meta-analysis of the results found a nonrandom distribution of the results consistent with a modest elevation of D_2 receptors in schizophrenia. Interestingly, studies performed with radiolabeled spiperone (^{11}C-labeled NMSP; $N=7$) reported elevated D_2 receptor binding in the striatum of patients with schizophrenia, whereas studies performed with radiolabeled benzamides (such as [^{11}C]raclopride and ^{123}I-labeled IBZM did not. To explain this discrepancy, Seeman (1988; Seeman et al. 1989) noted that the in vivo binding of benzamide is affected by competition with endogenous DA, but the binding of [^{11}C]-

NMSP is not. It follows that if endogenous DA levels are elevated in schizophrenia, then D_2 receptor density measured in vivo with [^{11}C]-raclopride and [^{123}I]-IBZM would be "underestimated" to a greater extent in patients with schizophrenia than in control subjects.

Several PET studies reported no alteration in D_1 transporters in the striatum of patients with schizophrenia, a finding consistent with postmortem studies (Abi-Dargham et al. 2002; Karlsson et al. 2002; Okubo et al. 1997). Also consistent with postmortem findings are the results of imaging studies reporting unaltered levels of DA transporter and of the vesicular transporters in schizophrenia (Laakso et al. 2000; Laruelle et al. 2000; Lavalaye et al. 2001; Taylor et al. 2000), although one study reported decreased levels of DA transporter in chronically ill patients (Laakso et al. 2001).

Striatal dopa decarboxylase activity. Seven studies have reported dopa accumulation in patients with schizophrenia via ^{18}F-labeled dopa (Dao-Castellana et al. 1997; Hietala et al. 1995, 1999; McGowan et al. 2004; Meyer-Lindenberg et al. 2002; Reith et al. 1994) or ^{11}C-labeled dopa (Lindstrom et al. 1999). Six of seven studies reported an increased accumulation of dopa in the striatum of patients with schizophrenia. Several studies reported high dopa accumulation in psychotic paranoid patients. Although the relation between dopa decarboxylase and the rate of DA synthesis is unclear (dopa decarboxylase is not the rate-limiting step of DA synthesis), these observations are compatible with findings of higher DA synthesis activity in patients experiencing psychotic symptoms.

Striatal amphetamine-induced DA release. The decrease in [^{11}C]raclopride and [^{123}I]-IBZM in vivo binding following acute amphetamine challenge has been well validated as a measure of the change in D_2 receptor stimulation by DA due to amphetamine-induced DA release (Breier et al. 1997; Laruelle 2000a; Laruelle et al. 1997b; Piccini et al. 2003; Villemagne et al. 1999). Of three studies examining amphetamine-induced decreases in [^{11}C]raclopride or [^{123}I]-IBZM binding in untreated patients with schizophrenia compared with well-matched control subjects (Abi-Dargham et al. 1998; Breier et al. 1997; Laruelle et al. 1996), all three reported that the decrease was larger in the untreated patients with schizophrenia (Figure 6–1). A significant relation was observed between magnitude of DA release and the transient induction or worsening of positive symptoms (Figure 6–2). The increased amphetamine-induced DA release was observed in both first-episode/drug-naive patients and patients who had previously taken antipsychotic drugs and were scanned during an episode of illness exacerbation but not in patients who were

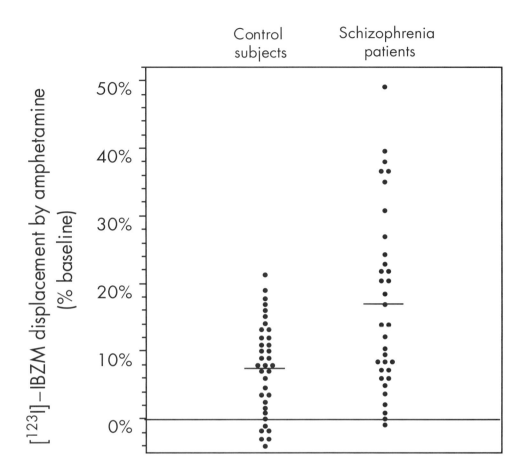

FIGURE 6–1. Effect of amphetamine (0.3 mg/kg) on ^{123}I-labeled IBZM binding in healthy control subjects and untreated patients with schizophrenia.

The y-axis shows the percentage decrease in [123I]-IBZM binding potential induced by amphetamine, which is a measure of the increased occupancy of dopamine$_2$ (D$_2$) receptors by dopamine following the challenge.

scanned during a remission phase (Laruelle et al. 1999). Thus, just like the enhanced vulnerability to the psychotogenic effects of stimulants (Lieberman et al. 1987b), the enhanced DA response to stimulants in schizophrenia appears to be state-dependent.

The increase in amphetamine-induced DA release was larger in patients experiencing an episode of illness exacerbation compared with patients in remission at the time of the scan (Laruelle et al. 1999). This exaggerated response of the dopaminergic system to amphetamine exposure did not appear to be a nonspecific effect of stress because elevated anxiety before the experiment was not associated with a larger amphetamine effect. Furthermore, nonpsychotic subjects with unipolar depression, who reported levels of anxiety similar to those of the schizophrenic patients at the time of the scan, showed normal amphetamine-induced displacement of [123I]-IBZM (Parsey et al. 2001).

These findings generally were interpreted as reflecting a larger DA release following amphetamine in the schizophrenic group. Another interpretation of these observations would be that schizophrenia is associated with increased affinity of D$_2$ receptors for DA. The development of D$_2$ receptor imaging with radiolabeled agonists is needed to settle this issue (Hwang et al. 2000; Narendran et al. 2004). Another limitation of this paradigm is that it measures change in synaptic DA transmission following a nonphysiological challenge (i.e., amphetamine) and does not provide any information about synaptic DA levels at baseline (i.e., in the unchallenged state).

Baseline occupancy of striatal D$_2$ receptors by DA. In rodents, acute depletion of synaptic DA is associated with an acute increase in the in vivo binding of [11C]raclopride or [123I]-IBZM to D$_2$ receptors (for review, see Laruelle 2000a). The increased binding is observed in vivo

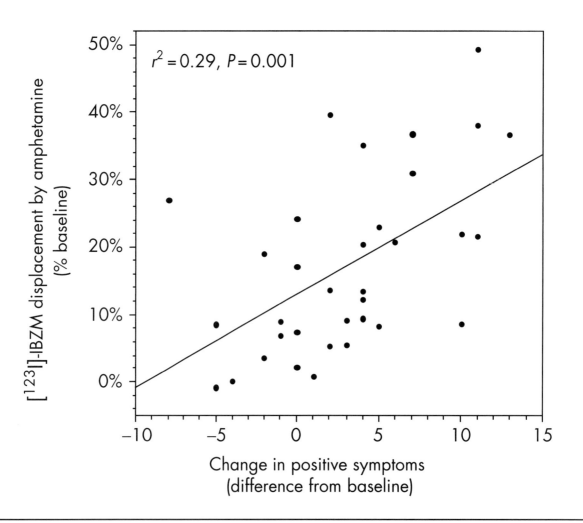

FIGURE 6–2.   Relation between striatal amphetamine-induced dopamine release (y-axis) and amphetamine-induced changes in positive symptoms measured with the positive subscale of the Positive and Negative Syndrome Scale for Schizophrenia (PANSS) in patients with schizophrenia.

Stimulation of dopamine₂ (D₂) receptors was associated with emergence or worsening of positive symptoms and accounted for about 30% of the variance in this behavioral response.

but not in vitro, indicating that it is not due to receptor upregulation but to the removal of endogenous DA and the unmasking of D_2 receptors previously occupied by DA. The acute DA depletion technique was developed in humans by using α-methyl-p-tyrosine to assess the degree of occupancy of D_2 receptors by DA (Fujita et al. 2000; Laruelle et al. 1997a; Verhoeff et al. 2001, 2002). Using this technique, investigators reported a higher occupancy of D_2 receptors by DA in patients with schizophrenia experiencing an episode of illness exacerbation compared with healthy control subjects (Abi-Dargham et al. 2000b). Again, assuming normal affinity of D_2 receptors for DA, the data are consistent with higher DA synaptic levels in patients with schizophrenia. A higher occupancy of D_2 receptors by DA in patients with schizophrenia was pre-

dictive of a good therapeutic response of these symptoms following 6 weeks of treatment with atypical antipsychotic medications. The fact that high levels of synaptic DA at baseline predicted a better or faster response to atypical antipsychotic drugs suggested that the D_2 receptor blockade induced by these drugs remains a key component in their initial mode of action.

Conclusion

Of the three alleged alterations of neurotransmission associated with schizophrenia discussed in this chapter (increased subcortical DA activity at D_2 receptors, decreased cortical DA activity at D_1 receptor, decreased GLU transmission at NMDA receptors), the first is by far

TABLE 6–1. Weight of evidence for the three putative imbalances in neurotransmission associated with schizophrenia

Type of evidence			Increase in subcortical DA	Decrease in cortical DA	NMDA deficit
Preclinical evidence (animal models)			+++	+++	+++
Clinical evidence	Indirect (pharmacological)	Adverse	+++[a]	+[b]	+++[c]
		Therapeutic	+++	—	+
	Direct	Postmortem	+	+	+
		Imaging	+++	++	—

Note. DA=dopamine; NMDA=*N*-methyl-D-aspartate; +++=strong evidence; ++=moderate evidence; +=emerging or ambiguous evidence; —=no evidence.
[a]Positive symptoms.
[b]Cognitive deficits (Parkinson's disease).
[c]Positive, negative, and cognitive symptoms.

the best established (Table 6–1). The hypothesis of increased subcortical DA activity at D_2 receptors rests both on solid pharmacological ground (repeated exposure to DA-enhancing drugs induces psychosis, blocking D_2 receptors alleviates psychosis) and on a growing body of direct imaging evidence that documented that, at least during an episode of illness exacerbation, schizophrenia is associated with increases in activity of DA neurons projecting to the striatum. The main limitation of this hypothesis is that it accounts for only one component of the clinical presentation (positive symptoms).

EVIDENCE SUPPORTING DECREASED DOPAMINE ACTIVITY AT CORTICAL D_1 RECEPTORS

Preclinical Evidence

A large body of evidence indicates that prefrontal DA activity is intimately involved in cognitive processes subserved by the dorsolateral PFC and its connections, such as tasks involving working memory. In 1979, Brozowski et al. reported, in a seminal paper, that selective DA depletion in the dorsolateral PFC in monkeys markedly impaired spatial working memory performance. The impairment was restored after treatment with DA agonists. These observations prompted numerous pharmacological studies of the role of prefrontal D_1 receptors in cognition. These studies documented that local intracerebral and systemic injections of selective D_1 receptor antagonists impaired working memory performance (Arnsten et al. 1994; Sawaguchi and Goldman-Rakic 1991, 1994; Seamans et al. 1998). Conversely, D_1 receptor agonists have beneficial effects on working memory in animals with im-

paired prefrontal DA function (Cai and Arnsten 1997; Castner et al. 2000; Schneider et al. 1994). In humans, the importance of DA for cognitive function is supported by cognitive impairment presented by patients with Parkinson's disease (Bowen et al. 1975; Stern and Langston 1985). Recent studies of the functional consequences of a polymorphism of the catechol-*O*-methyltransferase (COMT) gene also strongly support the involvement of cortical DA in working memory tasks in healthy humans (Egan et al. 2001). Together, these data generated the hypothesis that alterations in working memory and executive tasks presented by patients with schizophrenia might be the result of a deficiency in prefrontal dopaminergic systems.

Postmortem Evidence

Relatively few postmortem studies have assessed the integrity of DA markers in the dorsolateral PFC of patients with schizophrenia. With regard to the D_1 receptors, the predominant form of DA receptors in the cortex, one study reported no change (Laruelle et al. 1990), and one study reported a nonsignificant increase (Knable et al. 1996). D_1 receptor mRNA levels were reported unchanged in the PFC (Meador-Woodruff et al. 1997).

Decreased tyrosine hydroxylase–labeled axons have been reported in layer III and VI of the entorhinal cortex and in layer VI of the PFC in patients with schizophrenia—a finding that suggests that schizophrenia might be associated with a deficit in DA transmission in the entorhinal cortex and the PFC (Akil et al. 1999, 2000). This finding was clearly unrelated to premortem neuroleptic exposure. In contrast, Benes et al. (1997) observed no sig-

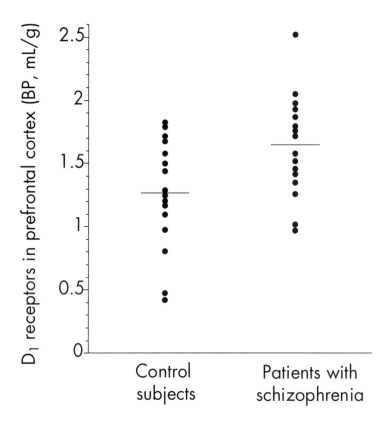

FIGURE 6–3. Distribution of ^{11}C-labeled NNC-112 binding potential (BP) in dorsolateral prefrontal cortex of healthy control subjects ($n=16$) and patients with schizophrenia ($n=16$).

Patients with schizophrenia had increased dopamine₁ (D_1) receptor availability compared with control subjects ($P=0.02$). This significant upregulation was detected in the dorsolateral prefrontal cortex but not in other regions investigated.

nificant changes in tyrosine hydroxylase–positive varicosities in the dorsolateral PFC.

Imaging Evidence

The only index of DA transmission that is currently quantifiable with noninvasive in vivo imaging is D_1 receptor availability. The first PET radiotracer for the D_1 receptor to be introduced was ^{11}C-SCH 23390 (Halldin et al. 1986). Despite the lower density of D_1 receptors in the PFC compared with the striatum (Hall et al. 1994), a test/ retest study recently reported appropriate reproducibility of the measurement of ^{11}C-SCH 23390 binding potential in the human PFC (Hirvonen et al. 2001). More recently, ^{11}C-NNC-112 was developed as a superior PET D_1 receptor radiotracer (Andersen et al. 1992; Halldin et al. 1998). In humans, ^{11}C-NNC-112 provides higher specific-to-nonspecific ratios compared with ^{11}C-SCH 23390 (Abi-Dargham et al. 1999; Halldin et al. 1998) and exquisite visualization of D_1 receptors, even

in the neocortex. The reproducibility of measurement of ^{11}C-NNC-112 binding potential in the human PFC has been established (Abi-Dargham et al. 2000a).

Three PET studies of prefrontal D_1 receptor availability in patients with schizophrenia have been published. Two studies were performed with ^{11}C-SCH 23390. The first reported decreased ^{11}C-SCH 23390 binding potential in the PFC (Okubo et al. 1997), and the other reported no change (Karlsson et al. 2002). One study was performed with ^{11}C-NNC-112 (Abi-Dargham et al. 2002) and reported increased ^{11}C-NNC-112 binding potential in the dorsolateral PFC (Figure 6–3). Upregulated D_1 receptor binding in the dorsolateral PFC of patients with schizophrenia was associated with impaired performance on the n-back test, a test relying on working memory (Figure 6–4).

Many factors, including patient heterogeneity and differences in the boundaries of the sampled regions, might potentially account for the discrepancies between the three imaging studies. However, the severity of deficits in

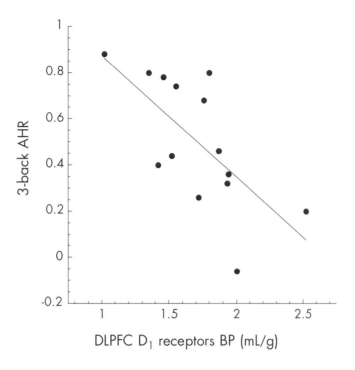

FIGURE 6–4. Relation between upregulation of dopamine$_1$ (D$_1$) receptors in the dorsolateral prefrontal cortex (DLPFC) of untreated patients with schizophrenia and performance on working memory task (3-back adjusted hit rate [AHR], lower values represent poorer performance).

tasks involving working memory was reported to be associated with both decreased PFC [^{11}C]-SCH 23390 binding potential (Okubo et al. 1997) and increased PFC [^{11}C]-NNC-112 binding potential (Abi-Dargham et al. 2002), suggesting that both alterations might reflect a common underlying deficit.

Because of the prevalent view that schizophrenia is associated with a deficit in prefrontal DA activity, the effect of chronic DA depletion on the in vivo binding of [^{11}C]-SCH 23390 and [^{11}C]-NNC-112 was investigated (Guo et al. 2001). Chronic DA depletion is associated with an increase in in vivo [^{11}C]-NNC-112 binding, presumably reflecting a compensatory upregulation of D$_1$ receptors, but no change in [^{11}C]-SCH 23390 in vivo binding. The reason that [^{11}C]-SCH 23390 binding is unaltered following chronic DA depletion remains to be elucidated, but the underlying process, when determined, might explain part of the discrepancies between the imaging studies.

Conclusion

Decreased cortical DA activity at D$_1$ receptors remains an intriguing but as yet unproven mechanism for the cognitive deficits presented by patients with schizophrenia (Ta-

ble 6–1). Although the role of prefrontal DA in cognition is well established in both animals and humans, definitive evidence that cognitive deficits in patients with schizophrenia result from deficient prefrontal DA function is lacking. This hypothesis is supported by one postmortem study that still awaits replication and extension and a few imaging studies that remain to be fully conciliated and interpreted. As discussed earlier, the modest improvement in cognition associated with second-generation antipsychotics that increase prefrontal DA supports a role for DA in these symptoms. However, it is unclear whether this prefrontal DA response is sustained over the course of treatment. The absence of adequate D$_1$ receptor agonists available for human use has precluded a more definitive clinical testing of this hypothesis. Some of these agents are currently under development, and proof of concepts studies should be available in the near future.

GLUTAMATE AND NMDA RECEPTORS

Although dopaminergic theories continue to command the greatest scientific attention, glutamatergic theories have become increasingly popular over recent years. The

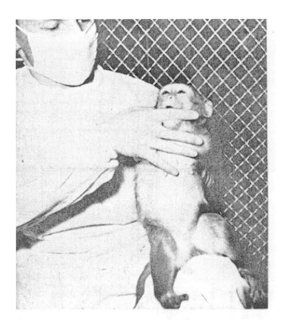
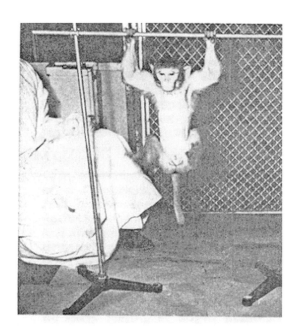

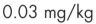

0.03 mg/kg   1.0 mg/kg

FIGURE 6–5.   Behavioral effects of the dissociative anesthetic phencyclidine (PCP) in monkeys.

At lower doses *(left)*, PCP induces a syndrome characterized by behavioral withdrawal and apathy ("dissociation"), reminiscent of negative symptoms of schizophrenia. At higher doses, PCP induces a catatonic-like syndrome *(right)*, including features such as waxy flexibility typically seen in catatonic schizophrenia, especially in the preneuroleptic era.

Source.   Reprinted from Chen GM, Weston JK: "The Analgesic and Anesthetic Effects of 1-(1-Phenylcyclohexyl)-Piperidine HCl on the Monkey." *Anesthesia and Analgesia* 39:132–137, 1960. Used with permission.

origins of glutamatergic theories date to the late 1950s with the discovery of the novel anesthetic agents phencyclidine (PCP) and ketamine. Initial primate testing (Chen and Weston 1960) showed that these agents produce a unique profile of activity, in which animals were awake but seemingly dissociated from the environment (Figure 6–5), leading them to be designated *dissociative anesthetics*. At higher doses, these agents produced rigid catatonia, similar to that observed in schizophrenia. Furthermore, in initial clinical trials, individuals exposed to these agents often developed schizophrenia-like symptoms on emerging from the anesthesia. The similarity of these emerging symptoms to the symptoms of schizophrenia led to the proposal that these agents might produce a heuristically valuable neurochemical model of schizophrenia.

Although studies with PCP and ketamine were conducted throughout the 1960s and 1970s, the primary binding site for PCP and ketamine was not discovered until 1979. Subsequent research in the early 1980s estab-

lished that the "PCP receptor" was, in fact, a binding site located within the ion channel belonging to the newly described NMDA-type GLU receptor. At that time, the role of GLU as a neurotransmitter within the mammalian nervous system had only recently been established. This confluence of findings, in the late 1980s, led to the first proposals that dysfunction of NMDA receptors, or of NMDA's modulatory circuitry, might underlie key symptoms in schizophrenia (reviewed in Javitt and Zukin 1991). As opposed to DA agents such as amphetamine, NMDA antagonists induce a syndrome that includes negative and positive symptoms and reproduce many of the neuropsychological deficits associated with schizophrenia.

The basic hypotheses underlying glutamatergic models have not changed since they were first proposed in the late 1980s. However, research since then has provided a fuller understanding of the roles of GLU and NMDA receptors in normal cognition and of the mechanisms whereby NMDA dysfunction may occur in schizophrenia.

GLUTAMATERGIC TRANSMISSION

Glutamate as a Neurotransmitter

GLU is the primary excitatory neurotransmitter in mammalian brain; aspartate and GLU make up the class of excitatory amino acid neurotransmitters. Approximately 60% of the neurons in the brain, including all cortical pyramidal neurons and thalamic relay neurons, use GLU as their primary neurotransmitter. Furthermore, glutamatergic terminals account for approximately 40% of all brain synapses (reviewed in Javitt 2004). GLU concentrations in the brain are more than 1,000-fold higher than concentrations of DA, serotonin, or any other monoaminergic neurotransmitters.

The high concentration of GLU in the brain and its participation in multiple metabolic pathways formed the initial basis of an argument against its potential role as a physiologically relevant neurotransmitter. This argument was resolved by the subsequent demonstration that the neurotransmitter pool of GLU is segregated from the metabolic pool and regulated independently. GLU is released from presynaptic terminals in response to neuronal depolarization and is recycled by excitatory amino acid transporters located on both neurons and glia. Within glia, GLU is converted to glutamine and released into extracellular fluid, where it is reabsorbed into presynaptic terminals and converted back to GLU via action of neuronal glutaminase.

Glutamate Receptors

The receptors for GLU are divided into two broad families: ionotropic and metabotropic. Ionotropic receptors are differentiated on the basis of sensitivity to the synthetic GLU derivatives NMDA, α-amino-3-hydroxy-5-methyl-4-isoxazolepropionic acid (AMPA), and kainate. Metabotropic receptors, which are G protein coupled and mediate longer-term neuromodulatory effects of GLU, are divided into groups on the basis of effector coupling and ligand sensitivity. Despite the differential sensitivity of these receptors to specific synthetic ligands, the endogenous neurotransmitter for all receptors is GLU and, to a lesser extent, the closely related amino acid aspartate.

NMDA receptors.   NMDA receptors are the most complex of the ionotropic receptors and a primary therapeutic target for psychiatric disorders. NMDA receptors contain not only the recognition site for GLU but also an allosteric modulatory site that binds the endogenous brain amino acids glycine and D-serine. This glycine binding site, like the benzodiazepine site of the GABA$_A$ receptor, regulates the channel open time and the desensitization rate in the presence of the agonist (GLU) but does not, in itself, induce channel opening. Like the benzodiazepine site, this site may be an ideal target for drug development.

Both glycine and D-serine are present in high concentration in the brain. However, NMDA receptors appear to be protected from high glycine and D-serine levels by the presence of amino acid transporters that are colocalized with NMDA receptors. Glycine type-1 transporters (GLYT1) may play a key role, although other small neutral amino acid transporters also may contribute (Javitt et al. 2005). As with the glycine site itself, these transporters have become a prominent target for drug development.

In addition, the NMDA receptor complex contains regulatory sites that are sensitive to polyamines, zinc (Zn^{2+}), protons, and oxidation-reduction agents such as glutathione. The multiple influences that converge on NMDA receptors speak to its critical role played in a multitude of brain processes.

NMDA receptors are blocked in a voltage-sensitive fashion by magnesium (Mg^{2+}), which binds to a site within the NMDA ion channel. As a result, NMDA receptors have a unique voltage, as well as being ligand (GLU) sensitive. This property permits NMDA receptors to play a unique role in the regulation of the connection strength between neurons through a process known as long-term potentiation. In addition, because NMDA receptors can be turned "on" or "off" simply by varying the membrane voltage, they serve as a key element in circuits related to attention, gating, and feedback regulation.

NMDA receptors are composed of multiple subunits, including at least one NR1 subunit and one or more modulatory subunits from the NR2 (NR2A–NR2D) and NR3 (NR3A, NR3B) families. These subunits significantly alter the functional properties of native NMDA receptors, including their voltage sensitivity and peak conductance and the degree to which they are influenced by the endogenous modulators glycine and D-serine. Interestingly, the modulatory agents glycine and D-serine have similar, excitatory effects on NMDA receptors containing NR2 subunits, but they have the opposite effects on receptors containing NR3 subunits, with glycine serving to activate NR3-containing receptors and D-serine serving to inhibit them (Chatterton et al. 2002).

PCP receptors.   PCP, ketamine, and other dissociative anesthetics bind to a site located within the ion channel formed by the NMDA complex. Note, however, that these agents also bind to a host of other receptors with varying affinities, leading to historical debate as to which receptors mediate the psychotomimetic effects of these agents. For example, PCP binds to a class of receptor termed the *sigma opiate* receptors, as well as to transporter

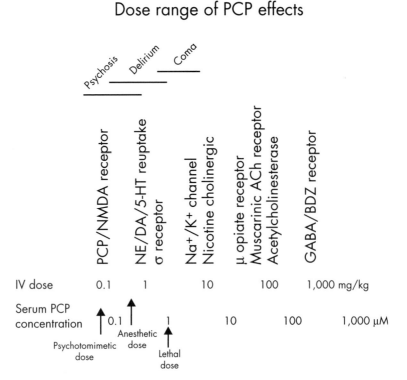

FIGURE 6–6.   Molecular targets of phencyclidine (PCP).

PCP induces symptoms that resemble those of schizophrenia when administered at doses of 0.1 mg/kg intravenously (IV). These doses produce plasma levels in the range of approximately 70 nM (0.07 μM). Although PCP has been reported to interact with a wide variety of molecular targets in brain, at doses associated with psychosis, PCP interacts primarily with the *N*-methyl-D-aspartate (NMDA)–associated "PCP receptor." Other psychotomimetic drugs, such as ketamine, also induce psychosis by blocking NMDA receptors. ACh=acetylcholine; BDZ=benzodiazepine; DA=dopamine; GABA=γ-aminobutyric acid; 5-HT=serotonin; K$^+$=potassium; Na$^+$=sodium; NE=norepinephrine.

sites for monoaminergic neurotransmitters such as DA and serotonin (Figure 6–6). Furthermore, these agents may interact at high concentration with D$_2$ or 5-HT$_{2A}$ receptors. These cross-reactivities have led, over the years, to suggestions that other receptors, besides the NMDA receptor, may mediate the psychotomimetic effects of PCP and ketamine.

A critical issue is not only the absolute potency with which PCP and ketamine induce their psychotomimetic effects but also the relative potency. In both animal models and clinical challenge studies, PCP is about 10-fold more potent than ketamine. Moreover, a variety of developed "designer drugs" (e.g., TCP [thienylcyclohexylpiperidine]) and pharmaceuticals (e.g., MK-801) show an even higher affinity for the PCP receptor than does PCP itself. These agents are similarly more effective than PCP in producing dissociative anesthetic-like symptoms in both animal models and clinical studies, strongly implicating NMDA receptors in the etiology of PCP-induced psychosis. Finally, the difference between the behavioral

profile induced by NMDA antagonists such as PCP and ketamine and the pattern induced by dopaminergic agents such as amphetamine and methylphenidate makes it difficult to attribute their effects to dopaminergic dysfunction alone.

AMPA receptors.   The other main class of the ionotropic neurotransmitters that may be involved in schizophrenia is the AMPA receptor. AMPA receptors are composed of the combinations of GluR1–4 subunits and work heavily in concert with NMDA receptors. Mature AMPA receptors containing the GluR2 subunit are calcium impermeant (Tanaka et al. 2000) and thus do not directly trigger long-term potentiation. Nevertheless, AMPA receptors provide the primary depolarization necessary to unblock NMDA receptors and to permit calcium entry into the cell.

Synergistically, calcium entry through unblocked NMDA receptors triggers AMPA insertion into the postsynaptic density and synaptic strengthening. AMPA receptors, however, are continuously recycled, leading to gradual synaptic weakening. If AMPA density falls below a critical threshold, levels of depolarization are insufficient to unblock NMDA channels, preventing subsequent AMPA activation. Such synapses, despite containing histologically identifiable NMDA, are functionally silent and cannot be recovered by electrical stimulation alone (Isaac et al. 1999). To the extent that silencing of synapses occurs in schizophrenia, it may limit the degree of recovery to be expected even if normal glutamatergic functioning could be restored.

At present, two main theories exist concerning the potential role of AMPA receptors in schizophrenia. One theory holds that cognitive dysfunction in schizophrenia is not directly related to NMDA dysfunction, but instead represents rebound glutamatergic hyperactivity operating through non-NMDA receptors. This theory predicts that blocking AMPA receptors should be therapeutically beneficial (Moghaddam et al. 1997). Other theories propose that schizophrenia may be associated with a global reduction in GLU release, which would affect AMPA and NMDA receptors. These theories predict that AMPA-stimulating agents should be beneficial (e.g., Tsai et al. 1998a). AMPA receptors desensitize quickly following direct stimulation. However, indirect modulators, termed *AMPAkines*, may be able to stimulate AMPA receptors without causing desensitization. Such compounds have been tested in schizophrenia only to a limited degree (Goff et al. 2001) and without conclusive evidence for or against efficacy.

Metabotropic receptors. Unlike ionotropic receptors, which are linked directly to ion channels, metabotropic receptors are linked to second-messenger systems. A particular role of glutamatergic metabotropic receptors is the regulation of presynaptic GLU release and postsynaptic sensitivity. Metabotropic receptors are divided into three groups according to functional activity. Group I receptors function predominantly to potentiate both presynaptic GLU release and postsynaptic NMDA neurotransmission. In contrast, group II and group III receptors serve to limit GLU release, particularly during conditions of GLU spillover from the synaptic cleft. Thus, group I agonists would be expected to stimulate neurotransmission mediated by ionotropic GLU receptors, whereas agonists for groups II and III receptors would be expected to have the opposite effect. At present, metabotropic agonists and antagonists are under development for clinical use by various pharmaceutical companies for treatment of schizophrenia. One agent in particular—LY354740, a group II agonist—has been found to reverse the acute effects of NMDA antagonists in both rodents and humans

(Krystal et al. 2005; Moghaddam and Adams 1998). Despite these intriguing results, clinical data with metabotropic agonists or antagonists have not yet been reported.

EVIDENCE SUPPORTING GLUTAMATERGIC MODELS OF SCHIZOPHRENIA

Pharmacological Evidence

Aversive pharmacological effects. The first studies detailing neurocognitive effects of PCP were performed in the 1960s before the development of modern rating scales and neuropsychological instruments. More recent studies with ketamine, however, have confirmed and extended the original findings.

One consistent finding was the close similarity of PCP- and ketamine-induced symptoms to those observed in schizophrenia. When formal rating scales are used, such as the Brief Psychiatric Rating Scale or the Positive and Negative Syndrome Scale for Schizophrenia, highly significant increases are observed not only in positive symptoms but also in negative symptoms and in disorganization (Krystal et al. 1994; Lahti et al. 2001; Malhotra et al. 1996). Auditory hallucinations are rare, whereas perceptual distortions are common. When patients with schizophrenia are exposed to ketamine, they also show increases in positive symptoms, as well as negative symptoms, and in particular show an increase in hallucinatory activity (Lahti et al. 2001; Malhotra et al. 1997). For most individuals with schizophrenia, the reactivated symptoms closely resemble their initial presenting symptoms, further validating glutamatergic theories of the disorder.

In addition to reproducing the severity and the type of symptoms observed in schizophrenia, ketamine induces a pattern of cognitive dysfunction strikingly similar to that observed in schizophrenia. The most disturbed function in schizophrenia is typically verbal declarative memory, a task that localizes strongly to the hippocampus (Bilder et al. 2000). This task is also strongly affected by PCP and ketamine, with amnesia being one of the hallmarks of dissociative anesthesia. The pattern of learning and memory deficits in schizophrenia, moreover, differs from that of Alzheimer's disease or other dementing illnesses in that patients have a delayed ability to learn new information but an intact ability to retain information once it is learned (Bilder et al. 2000). This type of deficit is not seen following structural lesions of hippocampus but is seen following selective NMDA receptor blockade (Newcomer et al. 1999). Thus, NMDA antagonists induce not only the domains of deficit similar to those seen in schizophrenia but also similar patterns within a domain.

Schizophrenia is also associated with disturbances in many prefrontal functions, such as executive functioning and working memory. These deficits are operationalized with tests such as the Wisconsin Card Sorting Test or "AX"-type Continuous Performance Test. In both of these tasks, ketamine is found to induce a pattern of deficit closely resembling that seen in schizophrenia (Krystal et al. 1994; Umbricht et al. 2000).

Ketamine infusion also reproduces both the severity and the type of thought disorder seen in schizophrenia; both types of thought disorder are associated with high levels of poverty of speech, circumstantiality, and loss of goal and relatively low levels of distractive, stilted speech or paraphasias (Adler et al. 1999). Conversely, processes that are relatively unimpaired in schizophrenia, such as implicit memory and priming, also appear unaffected by ketamine infusion. Furthermore, as observed in schizophrenia, specific neurocognitive changes are not accompanied by global impairments, as measured by instruments such as the Mini-Mental State Examination, so that the specificity of the effects is preserved.

Even the potent anesthetic abilities of ketamine are of interest given the well-documented but currently unexplained findings of increased sensation and pain thresholds in individuals with schizophrenia (Kudoh et al. 2000). Thereby, NMDA dysfunction may serve as a unifying model to explain the otherwise complex and idiosyncratic pattern of neurocognitive dysfunction in schizophrenia.

Therapeutic pharmacological effects.   A second line of evidence supporting the NMDA model comes from clinical studies of drugs that stimulate NMDA receptor–mediated neurotransmission. At present, the glycine binding site has proven most amenable to pharmacological intervention. The primary agents available for clinical study, to date, include the endogenous brain compounds glycine and D-serine, as well as the synthetic compound D-cycloserine, which fortuitously cross-reacts with the glycine binding site. As opposed to glycine and D-serine, which are full NMDA agonists, D-cycloserine functions as a partial agonist, leading to 40%–60% of the activation seen with glycine or D-serine.

Because of poor permeation into the brain and extensive peripheral metabolism, therapeutic dosages of glycine are in the range of 30–60 g/day. D-Serine, which is less extensively metabolized peripherally, appears to be effective at dosages as low as 2 g/day, although dose-response studies with this agent have not yet been conducted. D-Cycloserine appears most effective when given at a dosage of 50 mg/day. At higher doses, antagonist effects of D-cycloserine predominate, and clinical worsening of psychosis is observed.

When given at the previously mentioned dosages, results of clinical trials conducted with NMDA receptor agonists have been consistent across studies (Table 6–2). Studies with full agonists have reported highly significant, large effect size (0.9–2.1 SD units) improvements in negative and cognitive symptoms when these agents were added to typical antipsychotics or newer atypical antipsychotics, such as risperidone and olanzapine. The percentage of improvement in the negative symptoms ranged from 16% to 39% (weighted mean = 30%) for trials between 6 and 12 weeks. The level of cognitive and positive symptom improvement, across studies, was about 15%. Studies with D-cycloserine also had significant results, although the level of improvement was more modest. Because of the modest effects, some studies with D-cycloserine reported significant improvement, whereas others did not.

In some studies with glycine, D-serine, and D-cycloserine, the degree of negative symptom improvement correlates significantly with baseline glycine levels, suggesting that patients with the lowest pretreatment levels respond best to NMDA agonist treatment. In general, improvement has been less pronounced in patients receiving clozapine, raising the possibility that the atypical effects of clozapine may already reflect significant glutamatergic potentiation. The combination of D-cycloserine and clozapine has been found in some studies to worsen symptoms, suggesting that in such a combination, the NMDA antagonist effects of D-cycloserine may predominate (Goff et al. 1999a).

In addition to those studies with glycine site agonists, one recent clinical trial used the GLYT1 inhibitor *N*-methylglycine (sarcosine). This agent produced a highly significant, approximately 15% reduction in negative symptoms, along with a significant reduction in positive and cognitive symptoms and in the total Positive and Negative Syndrome Scale for Schizophrenia score (Tsai et al. 2004a), further supporting NMDA models.

Genetic Evidence

Genetic studies, over recent years, have begun to shed light on possible causes of NMDA dysfunction. As with postmortem studies, primary deficits may involve NMDA receptors themselves, including either the NR1 or the associated NR2 subunits, or proteins that regulate NMDA function indirectly.

To date, limited evidence implicates NMDA receptors directly in the genetics of schizophrenia. One positive study linking NMDA and genetics was reported in an African Bantu population but has not been replicated (Riley et al. 1997). More recent studies also have reported some linkages between NR2 subunits and schizophrenia itself

TABLE 6–2. Summary of clinical findings with the full *N*-methyl-D-aspartate receptor glycine-site agonists glycine (GLY) and D-serine (DSER) and the partial agonist D-cycloserine (DCS) in combination with typical, atypical, or mixed antipsychotics in schizophrenia

Study	Agonist	AP	N	Negative		Cognitive		Positive	
				% Change	P	% Change	P	% Change	P
Heresco-Levy et al. 1999	GLY	Mixed	22[a]	−39	<0.001	−24	0.01	−20	NS
Javitt et al. 2001	GLY	Mixed	12[a]	−34	<0.05	−12	0.1	−11	0.08
Heresco-Levy et al. 2004	GLY	OLZ/RISP	17[a]	−23	<0.0001	−9	0.02	−11	0.006
Evins et al. 2000	GLY	Clozapine	27	−4	NS	—	—	−7	NS
Tsai et al. 1998b	DSER	Mixed	29	−20	<0.001	−18	0.004	−22	0.004
Heresco-Levy et al. 2005	DSER	OLZ/RISP	39[a]	−16	<0.001	−12	0.001	−13	0.001
Tsai et al. 1999	DSER	Clozapine	20	−3	NS	−1	NS	−4	NS
Goff et al. 1999b	DCS	Conventional	47	−23	<0.022[b]	—	—	—	NS
Heresco-Levy et al. 2002	DCS	Mixed	21[a]	−14	<0.05	—	—	—	NS
Goff et al. 1999a	DCS	Clozapine	17[a]	+133[c]	<0.005	—	—	—	NS

Note. AP=antipsychotic; NS=not significant; —=not determined; OLZ=olanzapine; RISP=risperidone.
[a]Crossover study.
[b]Significant difference with Scale for the Assessment of Negative Symptoms only; Positive and Negative Syndrome Scale for Schizophrenia difference was not significant.
[c]Positive value represents significant worsening of symptoms.

(Di Maria et al. 2004) or clinical features of the disorder (Chiu et al. 2003; Itokawa et al. 2003). Nevertheless, this remains an area of active investigation.

Confirmed results have been reported for genes that regulate NMDA functioning indirectly. For example, D-amino acid oxidase (DAAO) is the primary enzyme responsible for degrading D-serine in the brain. D-Serine, in turn, is a primary regulator of NMDA functioning. Links have been reported between schizophrenia and both DAAO and G72, a novel protein that regulates DAAO functioning in primates (Chumakov et al. 2002; Korostishevsky et al. 2004), with the most active combinations of DAAO and G72 leading to the greatest susceptibility to schizophrenia.

Other confirmed links to schizophrenia, such as neuregulin, dysbindin, RGS4, or GRM3, also affect glutamatergic function and converge on NMDA receptors (Moghaddam 2003), primarily to produce a hypoglutamatergic state.

We should add that environmental factors that contribute to the development of schizophrenia also may converge on NMDA receptors. For example, it has been hypothesized that perinatal hypoxia, an important risk factor for schizophrenia, leads to neurotoxic degeneration of NMDA-bearing cells, an effect that may produce only behavioral symptoms later in development (Olney et al. 1999). Similarly, schizophrenia recently has been associated with decreased plasma levels of the NMDA agonists glycine (Sumiyoshi et al. 2004) and D-serine (Hashimoto et al. 2003) and increased levels of homocysteine (J. Levine et al. 2002; Susser et al. 1998), an agent that may act as a functional NMDA antagonist. Kynurenic acid levels also may be high in schizophrenia, whereas glutathione levels are low (Erhardt et al. 2001; Schwarcz et al. 2001), potentially affecting NMDA receptor neurotransmission. To the extent that these abnormalities are confirmed, they suggest that normalization of metabolic deficits may be a critical first step in the treatment and prevention of schizophrenia.

Preclinical Evidence

A final line of evidence supporting glutamatergic theories of schizophrenia comes from effects of NMDA alterations in animals. For example, mice with "knockdown" of the

NR1 subunit (knockouts are lethal) show several behaviors reminiscent of schizophrenia, including hyperactivity and decreased social affiliation (Miyamoto et al. 2001; Mohn et al. 1999; Tang et al. 1999). Similar findings are observed in animals with knockout of only the mice equivalent of the NR2A subunit (Ballard et al. 2002). In contrast, mice with increased NMDA expression or reduced GLYT1 expression (which presumably increases brain glycine levels) show increased learning ability, which may be viewed as a protective characteristic against the development of schizophrenia (Tsai et al. 2004b).

Postmortem Evidence

Although postmortem studies cannot, in themselves, provide an etiological basis for glutamatergic dysfunction in schizophrenia, they can help evaluate potential mechanisms whereby glutamatergic functioning might be impaired. First, it is easy to suspect that NMDA receptors themselves might be reduced in schizophrenia. Some evidence certainly supports this theory. Decreased expression of NMDA receptors has been reported in both the hippocampus (Gao et al. 2000), a region implicated in the memory disturbances associated with schizophrenia, and the thalamus, particularly in the nuclei with reciprocal connections to the limbic cortex (Ibrahim et al. 2000). AMPA receptors also have been reported to be decreased in these same regions (Eastwood et al. 1997; Meador-Woodruff and Healy 2000), suggesting that both deficits may operate in parallel.

An intriguing study evaluated patients antemortem until demise. The findings of the study showed that NMDA receptors in the temporal cortex were reduced only in patients who were found to have antemortem cognitive deficits (Humphries et al. 1996), suggesting a direct link between NMDA dysfunction and cognition. Nevertheless, findings of reduced NMDA expression have not been completely consistent across studies, and it remains unclear whether receptor expression alone is enough to account for the severity of deficit seen in schizophrenia.

An alternative possibility is that the receptors themselves function relatively normally but are dysregulated because of other factors. For example, in microarray studies of schizophrenia, many of the genes implicated code for presynaptic proteins, such as RGS4, which would be expected to affect glutamatergic neurotransmission primarily (Mirnics et al. 2001).

NMDA receptors must "dock" to the protein scaffolding through proteins such as PSD95, which also may be downregulated in schizophrenia. Similarly, dysfunction of other systems, such as nicotinic, serotonergic, or dopaminergic, may lead to secondary alterations in NMDA

functioning that may in some patients produce or exacerbate a basic flaw in glutamatergic functioning (see below).

Conclusion

Of the three alleged alterations of neurotransmission associated with schizophrenia discussed in this chapter (increased subcortical DA activity at D_2 receptors, decreased cortical DA activity at D_1 receptors, decreased GLU transmission at NMDA receptors), the second and third theories still lack unambiguous direct evidence (Table 6–1). Direct proof of decreased NMDA function in schizophrenia is lacking because postmortem studies failed to generate a consistent picture, and no method is currently available to study NMDA receptors in vivo in the human brain. However, a considerable amount of clinical and preclinical evidence supports the heuristic value of this model because it potentially accounts for the full spectrum of the illness (positive, negative, and cognitive domains). The significant effects of treatment support this hypothesis, especially given the fact that current treatments are all natural substances that may potentiate NMDA responsivity in brain to only a limited extent.

GLUTAMATE–DOPAMINE INTERACTIONS

A growing body of preclinical and imaging evidence suggests that the DA endophenotype associated with schizophrenia might emerge as a consequence of disconnectivity of the PFC and its connection involving alterations in NMDA transmission.

NEURONAL CIRCUITRY MODEL OF GLUTAMATE–DOPAMINE INTERACTIONS

The activity of DA neurons is modulated by projections involving GLU transmission from the PFC and other areas, such as the amygdala and subthalamic nuclei. A general model for GLU modulation of DA neurons in the substantia nigra/ventral tegmental area (VTA) is presented in Figure 6–7 (Carlsson et al. 1999; Kegeles et al. 2000; Laruelle et al. 2003). This model provides an anatomical framework relating the three fundamental putative neurochemical dysregulations involved in schizophrenia: 1) a deficit in GLU transmission, 2) a deficit in cortical DA transmission, and 3) a dysregulation of striatal DA transmission.

According to this model, the PFC modulates activity of midbrain DA neurons via an activating pathway (the "accelerator") and an inhibitory pathway (the "brake"),

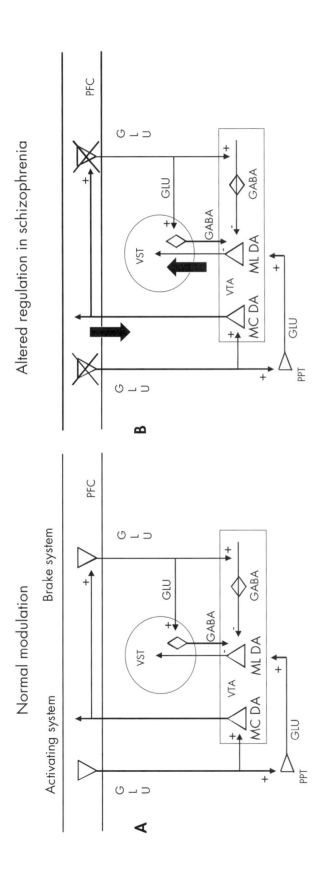

FIGURE 6–7. Neuronal circuitry models of glutamate–dopamine Interactions.

(**A**) Model of modulation of dopamine (DA) cell activity by cortical projections. This model, adapted from Carlsson et al. (1999), proposes a bimodal modulation of DA activity in the ventral tegmental area (VTA) by glutamatergic (GLU) projections originating in the frontal cortex. Stimulation of VTA DA neurons by GLU projections is represented on the left ("activating system"). These neurons exert a tonic excitatory influence on DA activity. Evidence in rodents suggests that direct stimulation of DA neurons by GLU afferents from the prefrontal cortex (PFC) is restricted to DA neurons that project back to the cortex (mesocortical DA system [MC DA]). Stimulation of mesolimbic (ML) DA neurons by GLU afferents from the cortex is polysynaptic, involving relays in the pedunculopontine tegmentum or other areas. The "brake system," represented on the right, exerts an inhibitory influence on DA activity via N-methyl-D-aspartate (NMDA) receptor–mediated stimulation of VTA γ-aminobutyric acid (GABA)ergic interneurons or striatotegmental GABA neurons and comes predominantly into play when DA activity is increased (such as from stress). In addition, the brake system regulating ML DA activity is activated by MC DA projections. (**B**) Model predicting that a deficiency in NMDA transmission in the cortex would result in decreased MC DA activity and would have unpredictable effects on ML DA activity under "baseline" conditions. Yet it would result in an increase in stress (or amphetamine)–induced ML DA release. See text for references. VST = ventral striatum.

which enables the PFC to fine tune dopaminergic activity. The activating pathway is composed of direct and indirect GLU projections onto the DA cells and acts preferentially on mesocortical DA neurons (see discussion and references in Carr and Sesack 2000). The inhibitory pathway is provided by PFC glutamatergic efferents to midbrain GABAergic interneurons and to striatomesencephalic GABA neurons and acts preferentially on subcortical DA neurons (Jackson et al. 2001). For example, blockade of GLU transmission in the VTA increases DA release in the accumbens and decreases DA release in the PFC (Takahata and Moghaddam 2000). This observation illustrates a GLU-mediated tonic inhibitory regulation of subcortical DA neurons and a tonic excitatory regulation of mesocortical DA neurons.

In schizophrenia, a reduced prefrontal activity, possibly secondary to an NMDA transmission deficiency, could result in a decrease in mesocortical DA activity (further worsening prefrontal-related cognitive impairment) and, under conditions of stress (such as stimulation of the DA system by the amygdala), a failure of the PFC to regulate DA activity properly in subcortical regions (Figure 6–7). If sustained, this dysregulation of subcortical DA might precipitate positive symptoms.

The scheme presented in Figure 6–7 encompasses only a limited aspect of GLU–DA interaction, leaving out interactions at the level of terminals and at the intracellular level. Nonetheless, it provides a general organizing principle and generates testable hypotheses. Because this model is derived mainly from rodent studies, its relevance to humans remains to be ascertained. For example, evidence of glutamatergic projections from the PFC to midbrain DA cell bodies is still lacking in primates.

IMAGING STUDIES OF GLUTAMATE–DOPAMINE INTERACTIONS

Imaging Studies of the Effect of GLU on DA Striatal Transmission

Imaging studies reviewed earlier showed that enhanced amphetamine-induced DA release is a salient endophenotype of schizophrenia. In microdialysis studies that used rodents (Miller and Abercrombie 1996), acute NMDA receptor blockade resulted in enhanced amphetamine-stimulated striatal DA release. We recently confirmed this mechanism in humans (Kegeles et al. 2000). Amphetamine-induced decrease in [^{123}I]-IBZM binding changed from $5.5 \pm 3.5\%$ under control conditions (amphetamine alone = 0.25 mg/kg) to $12.8 \pm 8.8\%$ under conditions of NMDA blockade, induced by ketamine ($P = 0.023$) (see Figure 6–8). The increase in amphetamine-induced DA

release induced by ketamine in healthy control subjects was comparable in magnitude to the exaggerated response seen in patients with schizophrenia to amphetamine administration (Abi-Dargham et al. 1998; Breier et al. 1997; Laruelle et al. 1996). These data are consistent with the hypothesis that the dysregulation of DA function after the amphetamine challenge in schizophrenia might be a result of a disruption of GLU neuronal systems regulating DA cell activity.

However, the net effect of acute ketamine administration on GLU transmission is complex. Ketamine blocks NMDA receptors but also induces GLU release, resulting in stimulation of other GLU receptors (Moghaddam and Adams 1998; Moghaddam et al. 1997). Therefore, acute effects of ketamine might result from either a deficit in NMDA transmission or an excess of GLU transmission at non-NMDA receptors. To resolve this issue, Van Berckel et al. (2001), using PET, examined the effects of the metabotropic glutamate receptor (mGlu) 2/3 agonist LY354740 on amphetamine-induced DA release in baboons. Amphetamine-induced DA release measured by the reduction of [^{11}C]raclopride binding potential was elevated following pretreatment with LY354740. Because activation of mGlu 2/3 receptors reduces GLU release (Battaglia et al. 1997; East et al. 1995), this study clarified the role that the inhibition of GLU transmission plays on the increase in amphetamine-induced DA release and provided additional support to the hypothesis that dysregulation of DA function, as shown by the amphetamine challenge in schizophrenia, might stem from a deficit in GLU transmission.

A limitation of these studies is that they involved acute NMDA disruption rather than mimicking or mirroring what might be a chronic disruption in schizophrenia. Therefore, studying the effect of sustained NMDA dysfunction on amphetamine-induced DA release will be important in further validating this model.

Importantly, altered amphetamine-induced DA release might be the result of a more general alteration in cortical development. For example, studies in rodents found that exposure to the DNA methylating agent methylazoxymethanol (MAM) at embryonic day 17 resulted in the emergence of behavioral and histological alterations reminiscent of schizophrenia in the adult rat (Flagstad et al. 2004, 2005; Grace 2000). After puberty, the MAM rat shows increased locomotor response to amphetamine. Microdialysis studies in the MAM rat reported elevated amphetamine-induced DA release in the nucleus accumbens (Flagstad et al. 2004). This observation suggests that in patients with schizophrenia, this altered response might emerge after puberty as a long-term consequence of the abnormal embryonic neurodevelop-

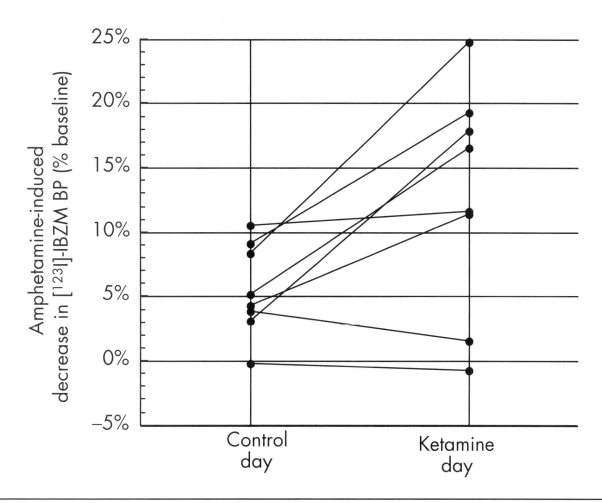

FIGURE 6–8.   Ketamine modulation of striatal amphetamine-induced dopamine release in healthy volunteers, showing a significantly larger release in eight healthy volunteers pretreated with intravenous ketamine compared with control conditions (repeated-measures analysis of variance, *P*=0.023).

These data indicate that, in humans, amphetamine-induced dopamine release in the striatum is modulated by glutamatergic circuits involving *N*-methyl-D-aspartate transmission. BP=binding potential.

mental processes. The contribution of abnormal GLU-mediated cortical regulation of DA function to this altered response to amphetamine in the MAM rat remains to be elucidated.

Imaging Studies of the Effect of GLU Transmission on DA Prefrontal Transmission

The model presented in Figure 6–7 also suggests that a sustained dysfunction of NMDA transmission would result in decreased prefrontal DA function. This hypothesis has been supported by studies in rodents and primates showing that chronic exposure to the NMDA receptor antagonists PCP and MK-801 (dizocilpine maleate) results in decreased DA levels in the PFC (Jentsch and Roth 1999; Jentsch et al. 1997, 1998; Tsukada et al. 2005). In monkeys,

chronic exposure to the NMDA antagonist MK-801 gradually lowered DA levels in the PFC and gradually upregulated [^{11}C]-NNC-112 in vivo binding in this region but not in other cortical regions. This finding was highly reminiscent of the increased [^{11}C]-NNC-112 binding observed in patients with schizophrenia in the dorsolateral PFC but not in other cortical regions (Abi-Dargham et al. 2002). Furthermore, in the Tsukada et al. monkey study, upregulated prefrontal [^{11}C]-NNC-112 binding potential was associated with impaired working memory performance, a relation observed in patients with schizophrenia as well (Abi-Dargham et al. 2002). These data supported the hypothesis that in schizophrenia, increased [^{11}C]-NNC-112 binding potential is a compensatory response to a sustained deficit in prefrontal DA function stemming from a sustained deficit in NMDA transmission.

To further validate this model in humans, D_1 receptor availability was evaluated in a group of subjects who regularly use ketamine for recreational purposes (chronic ketamine users). This study detected an increase in $[^{11}C]$-NNC-112 binding potential in chronic ketamine users that reached significance only in the dorsolateral PFC (Narendran et al., in press). This result indicates that DA transmission in the human dorsolateral PFC is particularly vulnerable to the detrimental effects of repeated NMDA antagonists and generally supports the hypothesis that altered DA transmission in the dorsolateral PFC of patients with schizophrenia might be a long-term consequence of deficient NMDA function.

DOPAMINE–GLUTAMATE INTERACTIONS

The data reviewed earlier in this chapter are consistent with the general hypothesis that the DA endophenotype of schizophrenia might be secondary to sustained NMDA hypofunction; however, it is also important to examine how such a DA endophenotype might contribute to or worsen NMDA transmission.

DOPAMINE–GLUTAMATE INTERACTIONS IN THE STRIATUM

Cortical glutamatergic afferents and DA projections converge on GABAergic medium spiny neurons in the striatum (Figure 6–9) usually on dendritic shafts and spines (for review, see Kotter 1994; Smith and Bolam 1990; Starr 1995). At this convergence point, DA has potent modulatory effects on GLU transmission (for review, see Cepeda and Levine 1998; Konradi and Heckers 2003; Nicola et al. 2000). Overall, D_2 receptor stimulation inhibits NMDA-mediated GLU transmission and long-term potentiation, and D_1 receptor stimulation facilitates GLU transmission and long-term potentiation (Centonze et al. 2001; M.S. Levine et al. 1996). The effect of D_2 receptor stimulation on GLU transmission involves both pre- and postsynaptic effects (Figure 6–9): D_2 stimulation inhibits GLU release and reduces the excitability of medium spiny neurons (Cepeda and Levine 1998; Cepeda et al. 2001; Leveque et al. 2000; Nicola et al. 2000; Onn et al. 2000; Peris et al. 1988; West and Grace 2002). In contrast, D_1 receptor stimulation generally promotes NMDA function and medium spiny neuron excitability (Figure 6–9), specifically when the cells are in a depolarized "up-state" as a result of the convergence of excitatory inputs (Dunah and Standaert 2001; Flores-Hernandez et al. 2002; Hernan-

dez-Lopez et al. 1997; Marti et al. 2002; Morari et al. 1994; West and Grace 2002; Wilson and Kawaguchi 1996).

These opposite effects of D_1 and D_2 receptor stimulation on NMDA transmission in the striatum might be relevant to both the pathophysiology and the treatment of schizophrenia. From a pathophysiology standpoint, excess D_2 receptor stimulation in schizophrenia, as documented by the imaging studies reviewed earlier, would inhibit GLU-mediated information flow into cortico-striato-thalamic-cortical loops and might worsen an already deficient NMDA transmission. As a result, the ability of the cortex to send information successfully to be processed in these loops would be impaired. Impairment of NMDA transmission also would inhibit plasticity in these loops.

By blocking D_2 receptors, antipsychotic drugs restore GLU transmission in the striatum, the ability of the striatum to receive and process cortical information, and the plasticity required for the shaping of cognitive processes by experience. This model also accounts for the fact that D_1 receptor antagonists are not antipsychotic drugs (de Beaurepaire et al. 1995; Den Boer et al. 1995; Karle et al. 1995; Karlsson et al. 1995).

DOPAMINE–GLUTAMATE INTERACTIONS IN THE CORTEX

In the PFC, DA modulates pyramidal cell excitability, both directly and indirectly, via modulation of GABAergic interneurons (Mrzljak et al. 1996; Smiley et al. 1994; Yang et al. 1999). Stimulation of DA receptors located on GABAergic interneurons is generally viewed as promoting a GABA-mediated inhibition of pyramidal cells (Del Arco and Mora 2000; Gorelova et al. 2002; Grobin and Deutch 1998; Seamans et al. 2001b). The effect of D_1 receptor stimulation on prefrontal pyramidal neurons is more complex. Stimulation of D_1 receptors enhances excitability of activated neurons and further stabilizes inactivated neurons (Fienberg et al. 1998; Seamans et al. 2001a; Yang et al. 1999). These "activity-dependent" actions of DA, especially at D_1 receptors, would allow the maintenance of firing in circuits activated during the processing of task-relevant information, while reducing the excitability of neurons that are not receiving sufficient excitatory input and are not relevant to the task at hand.

Thus, DA acts, via D_1 receptors, as a "reinforcer" in prefrontal cellular circuits. First, DA causes direct stimulation of D_1 receptors on pyramidal cells, leading to potentiation of the response of stimulated pyramidal neurons and silencing unstimulated neurons. Second, DA

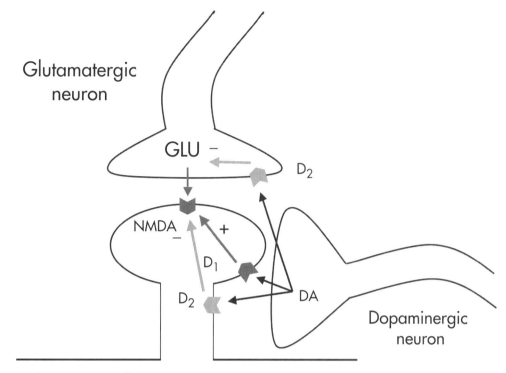

Glutamatergic neuron

GLU −

D_2

NMDA −

D_1 +

D_2

DA

Dopaminergic neuron

Dendritic spine of GABAergic medium spiny neuron

FIGURE 6–9. Opposite modulations of *N*-methyl-D-aspartate (NMDA) transmission by dopamine (DA) D_2 and D_1 receptors in γ-aminobutyric acid (GABA)–ergic medium spiny neurons in the striatum.

D_2 and D_1 receptors inhibit and facilitate, respectively, glutamate (GLU) transmission. Thus, an excess of D_2 receptor stimulation in schizophrenia would further impair NMDA-mediated information flow from the cortex into the striatum. By blocking D_2 receptors, antipsychotic drugs promote NMDA transmission. Conversely, D_1 receptor antagonists weaken NMDA transmission and are not antipsychotic drugs. See text for references.

promotes activity of GABAergic interneurons, contributing to a generalized inhibitory tone or "background noise reduction" (only neurons subjected to high excitatory inputs escape from this inhibition). Via these mechanisms, DA enhances the signal to noise in prefrontal circuits (Gorelova et al. 2002; Seamans et al. 2001b). Thus, a deficit in D_1 receptor stimulation in the PFC in schizophrenia might deteriorate function in already compromised NMDA transmission in the dorsolateral PFC of patients with schizophrenia.

CONCLUSION

Over the last 40 years, the DA model has been the leading neurochemical hypothesis of schizophrenia. This model has proven heuristically valuable, with all current medica-

tions for schizophrenia functioning primarily through the mechanism of D_2 receptor blockade. Yet it is unlikely that dopaminergic dysfunction, on its own, can fully account for the wide range of symptoms and neurocognitive deficits seen in schizophrenia. Glutamatergic models provide an alternative approach for conceptualizing the brain abnormalities associated with schizophrenia. Whether glutamatergic deficits are driven by dopaminergic dysfunction or whether they are the drivers remains to be determined and may vary across patients and across illness subtypes. Furthermore, the two models produce complementary views of the disorder, with the DA model accounting primarily for positive symptoms and prefrontal dysfunction and the GLU model accounting for negative symptoms and more global neuropsychological deficits. At present, no approved medications are available for treatment of either negative symptoms or neurocognitive dysfunction. New treatment approaches aimed at stimulating prefrontal DA release and D_1 receptor stimulation, or potentiating glutamatergic neurotransmission, however, do offer hope for future clinical development.

REFERENCES

Abi-Dargham A, Gil R, Krystal J, et al: Increased striatal dopamine transmission in schizophrenia: confirmation in a second cohort. Am J Psychiatry 155:761–767, 1998

Abi-Dargham A, Simpson N, Kegeles L, et al: PET studies of binding competition between endogenous dopamine and the D1 radiotracer [11C]NNC 756. Synapse 32:93–109, 1999

Abi-Dargham A, Martinez D, Mawlawi O, et al: Measurement of striatal and extrastriatal dopamine D1 receptor binding potential with [11C]NNC 112 in humans: validation and reproducibility. J Cereb Blood Flow Metab 20:225–243, 2000a

Abi-Dargham A, Rodenhiser J, Printz D, et al: Increased baseline occupancy of D2 receptors by dopamine in schizophrenia. Proc Natl Acad Sci U S A 97:8104–8109, 2000b

Abi-Dargham A, Mawlawi O, Lombardo I, et al: Prefrontal dopamine D1 receptors and working memory in schizophrenia. J Neurosci 22:3708–3719, 2002

Abi-Dargham A, Laruelle M: Mechanisms of action of second generation antipsychotic drugs in schizophrenia: insights from brain imaging studies. Eur Psychiatry 20:15–27, 2005

Adler CM, Malhotra AK, Elman I, et al: Comparison of ketamine-induced thought disorder in healthy volunteers and thought disorder in schizophrenia. Am J Psychiatry 156:1646–1649, 1999

Akil M, Pierri JN, Whitehead RE, et al: Lamina-specific alterations in the dopamine innervation of the prefrontal cortex in schizophrenic subjects. Am J Psychiatry 156:1580–1589, 1999

Akil M, Edgar CL, Pierri JN, et al: Decreased density of tyrosine hydroxylase-immunoreactive axons in the entorhinal cortex of schizophrenic subjects. Biol Psychiatry 47:361–370, 2000

Andersen PH, Gronvald FC, Hohlweg R, et al: NNC-112, NNC-687 and NNC-756, new selective and highly potent dopamine D1 receptor antagonists. Eur J Pharmacol 219:45–52, 1992

Angrist BM, Gershon S: The phenomenology of experimentally induced amphetamine psychosis—preliminary observation. Biol Psychiatry 2:95–107, 1970

Angrist B, van Kammen DP: CNS stimulants as a tool in the study of schizophrenia. Trends Neurosci 7:388–390, 1984

Arnsten AF, Cai JX, Murphy BL, et al: Dopamine D1 receptor mechanisms in the cognitive performance of young adult and aged monkeys. Psychopharmacology 116:143–151, 1994

Ballard TM, Pauly-Evers M, Higgins GA, et al: Severe impairment of NMDA receptor function in mice carrying targeted point mutations in the glycine binding site results in drug-resistant nonhabituating hyperactivity. J Neurosci 22:6713–6723, 2002

Battaglia G, Monn JA, Schoepp DD: In vivo inhibition of veratridine-evoked release of striatal excitatory amino acids by the group II metabotropic glutamate receptor agonist LY354740 in rats. Neurosci Lett 229:161–164, 1997

Bell DS: The experimental reproduction of amphetamine psychosis. Arch Gen Psychiatry 29:35–40, 1973

Benes FM, Todtenkopf MS, Taylor JB: Differential distribution of tyrosine hydroxylase fibers on small and large neurons in layer II of anterior cingulate cortex of schizophrenic brain. Synapse 25:80–92, 1997

Bilder RM, Goldman RS, Robinson D, et al: Neuropsychology of first-episode schizophrenia: initial characterization and clinical correlates. Am J Psychiatry 157:549–559, 2000

Boileau I, Dagher A, Leyton M, et al: Sensitization to psychostimulants: a PET/ [11C]-raclopride study in healthy volunteers. ACNP Annual Meeting Abstracts 2003

Bowen F, Kamienny R, Burn M, et al: Parkinsonism: effect of levodopa treatment on concept formation. Neurology 25:701–704, 1975

Breier A, Su TP, Saunders R, et al: Schizophrenia is associated with elevated amphetamine-induced synaptic dopamine concentrations: evidence from a novel positron emission tomography method. Proc Natl Acad Sci U S A 94:2569–2574, 1997

Brozowski TJ, Brown RM, Rosvold HE, et al: Cognitive deficit caused by regional depletion of dopamine in prefrontal cortex of rhesus monkey. Science 205:929–932, 1979

Bunzow JR, Van Tol HH, Grandy DK, et al: Cloning and expression of a rat D2 dopamine receptor cDNA. Nature 336:783–787, 1988

Burt DR, Creese I, Snyder SS: Antischizophrenic drugs: chronic treatment elevates dopamine receptors binding in brain. Science 196:326–328, 1977

Cai JX, Arnsten AFT: Dose-dependent effects of the dopamine D1 receptor agonists A77636 or SKF81297 on spatial working memory in aged monkeys. J Pharmacol Exp Ther 283:183–189, 1997

Carlsson A, Lindqvist M: Effect of chlorpromazine or haloperidol on formation of 3-methoxytyramine and normetanephrine in mouse brain. Acta Pharmacol Toxicol 20:140–144, 1963

Carlsson A, Waters N, Carlsson ML: Neurotransmitter interactions in schizophrenia—therapeutic implications. Biol Psychiatry 46:1388–1395, 1999

Carr DB, Sesack SR: Projections from the rat prefrontal cortex to the ventral tegmental area: target specificity in the synaptic associations with mesoaccumbens and mesocortical neurons. J Neurosci 20:3864–3873, 2000

Castner SA, Williams GV, Goldman-Rakic PS: Reversal of antipsychotic-induced working memory deficits by short-term dopamine D1 receptor stimulation [see comments]. Science 287:2020–2022, 2000

Centonze D, Picconi B, Gubellini P, et al: Dopaminergic control of synaptic plasticity in the dorsal striatum. Eur J Neurosci 13:1071–1077, 2001

Cepeda C, Levine MS: Dopamine and N-methyl-D-aspartate receptor interactions in the neostriatum. Dev Neurosci 20:1–18, 1998

Cepeda C, Hurst RS, Altemus KL, et al: Facilitated glutamatergic transmission in the striatum of D2 dopamine receptor-deficient mice. J Neurophysiol 85:659–670, 2001

Chatterton JE, Awobuluyi M, Premkumar LS, et al: Excitatory glycine receptors containing the NR3 family of NMDA receptor subunits. Nature 415:793–798, 2002

Chen GM, Weston JK: The analgesic and anesthetic effects of 1-(1-phenylcyclohexyl)-piperidine HCl on the monkey. Anesth Analg 39:132–137, 1960

Chinaglia G, Alvarez FJ, Probst A, et al: Mesostriatal and mesolimbic dopamine uptake binding sites are reduced in Parkinson's disease and progressive supranuclear palsy: a quantitative autoradiographic study using [3H]mazindol. Neuroscience 49:317–327, 1992

Chiu HJ, Wang YC, Liou YJ, et al: Association analysis of the genetic variants of the N-methyl-D-aspartate receptor subunit 2b (NR2b) and treatment-refractory schizophrenia in the Chinese. Neuropsychobiology 47:178–181, 2003

Chumakov I, Blumenfeld M, Guerassimenko O, et al: Genetic and physiological data implicating the new human gene G72 and the gene for D-amino acid oxidase in schizophrenia. Proc Natl Acad Sci U S A 99:13675–13680, 2002

Connell PH: Amphetamine Psychosis. London, England, Chapman & Hill, 1958

Creese I, Burt DR, Snyder SH: Dopamine receptor binding predicts clinical and pharmacological potencies of antischizophrenic drugs. Science 19:481–483, 1976

Cross AJ, Crow TJ, Owen F: 3H-Flupenthixol binding in post-mortem brains of schizophrenics: evidence for a selective increase in dopamine D2 receptors. Psychopharmacology (Berl) 74:122–124, 1981

Cross AJ, Crow TJ, Ferrier IN, et al: Dopamine receptor changes in schizophrenia in relation to the disease process and movement disorder. J Neural Transm Suppl 18:265–272, 1983

Crow TJ: Molecular pathology of schizophrenia: more than one disease process? BMJ 280:66–68, 1980

Czudek C, Reynolds GP: [3H] GBR 12935 binding to the dopamine uptake site in post-mortem brain tissue in schizophrenia. J Neural Transm 77:227–230, 1989

Dao-Castellana MH, Paillere-Martinot ML, Hantraye P, et al: Presynaptic dopaminergic function in the striatum of schizophrenic patients. Schizophr Res 23:167–174, 1997

Davis KL, Kahn RS, Ko G, et al: Dopamine in schizophrenia: a review and reconceptualization. Am J Psychiatry 148:1474–1486, 1991

de Beaurepaire R, Labelle A, Naber D, et al: An open trial of the D1 antagonist SCH 39166 in six cases of acute psychotic states. Psychopharmacology (Berl) 121:323–327, 1995

Dearry A, Gingrich JA, Falardeau P, et al: Molecular cloning and expression of the gene for a human D1 dopamine receptor. Nature 347:72–76, 1990

Del Arco A, Mora F: Endogenous dopamine potentiates the effects of glutamate on extracellular GABA in the prefrontal cortex of the freely moving rat. Brain Res Bull 53:339–345, 2000

Delay J, Deniker P, Harl JM: Therapeutic use in psychiatry of phenothiazine of central elective action (4560 RP). Ann Med Psychol (Paris) 110:112–117, 1952

Den Boer JA, van Megen HJ, Fleischhacker WW, et al: Differential effects of the D1-DA receptor antagonist SCH39166 on positive and negative symptoms of schizophrenia. Psychopharmacology (Berl) 121:317–322, 1995

Di Maria E, Gulli R, Begni S, et al: Variations in the NMDA receptor subunit 2B gene (GRIN2B) and schizophrenia: a case-control study. Am J Med Genet 128B:27–29, 2004

Dunah AW, Standaert DG: Dopamine D1 receptor-dependent trafficking of striatal NMDA glutamate receptors to the postsynaptic membrane. J Neurosci 21:5546–5558, 2001

East SJ, Hill MP, Brotchie JM: Metabotropic glutamate receptor agonists inhibit endogenous glutamate release from rat striatal synaptosomes. Eur J Pharmacol 277:117–121, 1995

Eastwood SL, Kerwin RW, Harrison PJ: Immunoautoradiographic evidence for a loss of alpha-amino-3-hydroxy-5-methyl-4-isoxazole propionate-preferring non-N-methyl-D-aspartate glutamate receptors within the medial temporal lobe in schizophrenia. Biol Psychiatry 41:636–643, 1997

Egan MF, Goldberg TE, Kolachana BS, et al: Effect of COMT Val108/158 Met genotype on frontal lobe function and risk for schizophrenia. Proc Natl Acad Sci U S A 98:6917–6922, 2001

Ellinwood EH Jr: Amphetamine psychosis, I: description of the individuals and process. J Nerv Ment Dis 144:273–283, 1967

Ellinwood EH, Sudilovsky A, Nelson LM: Evolving behavior in the clinical and experimental amphetamine model psychosis. Am J Psychiatry 130:1088–1093, 1973

Erhardt S, Blennow K, Nordin C, et al: Kynurenic acid levels are elevated in the cerebrospinal fluid of patients with schizophrenia. Neurosci Lett 313:96–98, 2001

Evins AE, Fitzgerald SM, Wine L, et al: Placebo-controlled trial of glycine added to clozapine in schizophrenia. Am J Psychiatry 157:826–828, 2000

Farde L, Nordström AL, Wiesel FA, et al: Positron emission tomography analysis of central D_1 and D_2 dopamine receptor occupancy in patients treated with classical neuroleptics and clozapine. Arch Gen Psychiatry 49:538–544, 1992

Fienberg AA, Hiroi N, Mermelstein PG, et al: DARPP-32: regulator of the efficacy of dopaminergic neurotransmission. Science 281:838–842, 1998

Flagstad P, Mork A, Glenthoj BY, et al: Disruption of neurogenesis on gestational day 17 in the rat causes behavioral changes relevant to positive and negative schizophrenia symptoms and alters amphetamine-induced dopamine release in nucleus accumbens. Neuropsychopharmacology 29:2052–2064, 2004

Flagstad P, Glenthoj BY, Didriksen M: Cognitive deficits caused by late gestational disruption of neurogenesis in rats: a preclinical model of schizophrenia. Neuropsychopharmacology 30:250–260, 2005

Flores-Hernandez J, Cepeda C, Hernandez-Echeagaray E, et al: Dopamine enhancement of NMDA currents in dissociated medium-sized striatal neurons: role of D1 receptors and DARPP-32. J Neurophysiol 88:3010–3020, 2002

Frankle WG, Gil R, Hackett E, et al: Occupancy of dopamine D2 receptors by the atypical antipsychotic drugs risperidone and olanzapine: theoretical implications. Psychopharmacology (Berl) 175:473–480, 2004

Fujita M, Verhoeff NP, Varrone A, et al: Imaging extrastriatal dopamine D(2) receptor occupancy by endogenous dopamine in healthy humans. Eur J Pharmacol 387:179–188, 2000

Gao XM, Sakai K, Roberts RC, et al: Ionotropic glutamate receptors and expression of N-methyl-D-aspartate receptor subunits in subregions of human hippocampus: effects of schizophrenia. Am J Psychiatry 157:1141–1149, 2000

Gessa GL, Devoto P, Diana M, et al: Dissociation of haloperidol, clozapine, and olanzapine effects on electrical activity of mesocortical dopamine neurons and dopamine release in the prefrontal cortex. Neuropsychopharmacology 22:642–649, 2000

Glenthoj BY, Hemmingsen R: Dopaminergic sensitization: implications for the pathogenesis of schizophrenia. Prog Neuropsychopharmacol Biol Psychiatry 21:23–46, 1997

Goff DC, Coyle JT: The emerging role of glutamate in the pathophysiology and treatment of schizophrenia. Am J Psychiatry 158:1367–1377, 2001

Goff DC, Henderson DC, Evins AE, et al: A placebo-controlled crossover trial of D-cycloserine added to clozapine in patients with schizophrenia. Biol Psychiatry 45:512–514, 1999a

Goff DC, Tsai G, Levitt J, et al: A placebo-controlled trial of D-cycloserine added to conventional neuroleptics in patients with schizophrenia. Arch Gen Psychiatry 56:21–27, 1999b

Goff DC, Leahy L, Berman I, et al: A placebo-controlled pilot study of the ampakine CX516 added to clozapine in schizophrenia. J Clin Psychopharmacol 21:484–487, 2001

Goldman-Rakic PS, Muly EC 3rd, Williams GV: D(1) receptors in prefrontal cells and circuits. Brain Res Brain Res Rev 31:295–301, 2000

Gorelova N, Seamans JK, Yang CR: Mechanisms of dopamine activation of fast-spiking interneurons that exert inhibition in rat prefrontal cortex. J Neurophysiol 88:3150–3166, 2002

Grace AA: Gating of information flow within the limbic system and the pathophysiology of schizophrenia. Brain Res Brain Res Rev 31:330–341, 2000

Griffith JJ, Oates J, Cavanaugh J: Paranoid episodes induced by drugs. JAMA 205:39, 1968

Grobin AC, Deutch AY: Dopaminergic regulation of extracellular gamma-aminobutyric acid levels in the prefrontal cortex of the rat. J Pharmacol Exp Ther 285:350–357, 1998

Guo N, Hwang D, Abdellhadi S, et al: The effect of chronic DA depletion on D1 ligand binding in rodent brain. Abstr Soc Neurosci 27, 2001

Gurevich EV, Bordelon Y, Shapiro RM, et al: Mesolimbic dopamine D-3 receptors and use of antipsychotics in patients with schizophrenia—a postmortem study. Arch Gen Psychiatry 54:225–232, 1997

Hall H, Sedvall G, Magnusson O, et al: Distribution of D1- and D2-dopamine receptors, and dopamine and its metabolites in the human brain. Neuropsychopharmacology 11:245–256, 1994

Halldin C, Stone-Elander S, Farde L, et al: Preparation of ^{11}C-labelled SCH 23390 for the in vivo study of dopamine D1 receptors using positron emission tomography. Appl Radiat Isot 37:1039–1043, 1986

Halldin C, Foged C, Chou YH, et al: Carbon-11-NNC 112: a radioligand for PET examination of striatal and neocortical D1-dopamine receptors. J Nucl Med 39:2061–2068, 1998

Hashimoto K, Fukushima T, Shimizu E, et al: Decreased serum levels of D-serine in patients with schizophrenia: evidence in support of the N-methyl-D-aspartate receptor hypofunction hypothesis of schizophrenia. Arch Gen Psychiatry 60:572–576, 2003

Heresco-Levy U, Javitt DC, Ermilov M, et al: Efficacy of high-dose glycine in the treatment of enduring negative symptoms of schizophrenia. Arch Gen Psychiatry 56:29–36, 1999

Heresco-Levy U, Ermilov M, Shimoni J, et al: Placebo-controlled trial of D-cycloserine added to conventional neuroleptics, olanzapine, or risperidone in schizophrenia. Am J Psychiatry 159:480–482, 2002

Heresco-Levy U, Ermilov M, Lichtenberg P, et al: High-dose glycine added to olanzapine and risperidone for the treatment of schizophrenia. Biol Psychiatry 55:165–171, 2004

Heresco-Levy U, Javitt DC, Ebstein R, et al: D-serine efficacy as add-on pharmacotherapy to risperidone and olanzapine for treatment-refractory schizophrenia. Biol Psychiatry 57:577–585, 2005

Hernandez-Lopez S, Bargas J, Surmeier DJ, et al: D1 receptor activation enhances evoked discharge in neostriatal medium spiny neurons by modulating an L-type Ca2+ conductance. J Neurosci 17:3334–3342, 1997

Hess EJ, Bracha HS, Kleinman JE, et al: Dopamine receptor subtype imbalance in schizophrenia. Life Sci 40:1487–1497, 1987

Hietala J, Syvalahti E, Vuorio K, et al: Presynaptic dopamine function in striatum of neuroleptic-naive schizophrenic patients. Lancet 346:1130–1131, 1995

Hietala J, Syvalahti E, Vilkman H, et al: Depressive symptoms and presynaptic dopamine function in neuroleptic-naive schizophrenia. Schizophr Res 35:41–50, 1999

Hirai M, Kitamura N, Hashimoto T, et al: [3H]GBR-12935 binding sites in human striatal membranes: binding characteristics and changes in parkinsonians and schizophrenics. Jpn J Pharmacol 47:237–243, 1988

Hirvonen J, Nagren K, Kajander J, et al: Measurement of cortical dopamine D1 receptor binding with 11C[SCH23390]: a test-retest analysis. J Cereb Blood Flow Metab 21:1133–1145, 2001

Humphries C, Mortimer A, Hirsch S, et al: NMDA receptor mRNA correlation with antemortem cognitive impairment in schizophrenia. Neuroreport 7:2051–2055, 1996

Hwang DR, Kegeles LS, Laruelle M: (–)-N-[(11)C]propyl-norapomorphine: a positron-labeled dopamine agonist for PET imaging of D(2) receptors. Nucl Med Biol 27:533–539, 2000

Ibrahim HM, Hogg AJ Jr, Healy DJ, et al: Ionotropic glutamate receptor binding and subunit mRNA expression in thalamic nuclei in schizophrenia. Am J Psychiatry 157:1811–1823, 2000

Ichikawa J, Ishii H, Bonaccorso S, et al: 5-HT(2A) and D(2) receptor blockade increases cortical DA release via 5-HT(1A) receptor activation: a possible mechanism of atypical antipsychotic-induced cortical dopamine release. J Neurochem 76:1521–1531, 2001

Isaac JT, Nicoll RA, Malenka RC: Silent glutamatergic synapses in the mammalian brain. Can J Physiol Pharmacol 77:735–737, 1999

Itokawa M, Yamada K, Yoshitsugu K, et al: A microsatellite repeat in the promoter of the N-methyl-D-aspartate receptor 2A subunit (GRIN2A) gene suppresses transcriptional activity and correlates with chronic outcome in schizophrenia. Pharmacogenetics 13:271–278, 2003

Jackson ME, Frost AS, Moghaddam B: Stimulation of prefrontal cortex at physiologically relevant frequencies inhibits dopamine release in the nucleus accumbens. J Neurochem 78:920–923, 2001

Javitt DC: Glutamate as a therapeutic target in psychiatric disorders. Mol Psychiatry 9:984–997, 2004

Javitt DC, Zukin SR: Recent advances in the phencyclidine model of schizophrenia. Am J Psychiatry 148:1301–1308, 1991

Javitt DC, Silipo G, Cienfuegos A, et al: Adjunctive high-dose glycine in the treatment of schizophrenia. Int J Neuropsychopharmacol 4:385–392, 2001

Javitt DC, Duncan L, Balla A, et al: Inhibition of System A–mediated glycine transport in cortical synaptosomes by therapeutic concentrations of clozapine: implications for mechanisms of action. Mol Psychiatry 10:275–287, 2005

Jentsch JD, Redmond DE Jr, Elsworth JD, et al: Enduring cognitive deficits and cortical dopamine dysfunction in monkeys after long-term administration of phencyclidine. Science 277:953–955, 1997

Jentsch JD, Elsworth JD, Taylor JR, et al: Dysregulation of mesoprefrontal dopamine neurons induced by acute and repeated phencyclidine administration in the nonhuman primate: implications for schizophrenia. Adv Pharmacol 42:810–814, 1998

Jentsch JD, Roth RH: The neuropsychopharmacology of phencyclidine: from NMDA receptor hypofunction to the dopamine hypothesis of schizophrenia. Neuropsychopharmacology 20:201–225, 1999

Joyce JN, Meador-Woodruff JH: Linking the family of D2 receptors to neuronal circuits in human brain: insights into schizophrenia. Neuropsychopharmacology 16:375–384, 1997

Joyce JN, Lexow N, Bird E, et al: Organization of dopamine D1 and D2 receptors in human striatum: receptor autoradiographic studies in Huntington's disease and schizophrenia. Synapse 2:546–557, 1988

Kalivas PW, Sorg BA, Hooks MS: The pharmacology and neural circuitry of sensitization to psychostimulants. Behav Pharmacol 4:315–334, 1993

Kapur S: Psychosis as a state of aberrant salience: a framework linking biology, phenomenology, and pharmacology in schizophrenia. Am J Psychiatry 160:13–23, 2003

Kapur S, Zipursky R, Jones C, et al: Relationship between dopamine D(2) occupancy, clinical response, and side effects: a double-blind PET study of first-episode schizophrenia. Am J Psychiatry 157:514–520, 2000

Karle J, Clemmesen L, Hansen L, et al: NNC 01–0687, a selective dopamine D1 receptor antagonist, in the treatment of schizophrenia. Psychopharmacology (Berl) 121:328–329, 1995

Karlsson P, Smith L, Farde L, et al: Lack of apparent antipsychotic effect of the D1-dopamine receptor antagonist SCH39166 in acutely ill schizophrenic patients. Psychopharmacology (Berl) 121:309–316, 1995

Karlsson P, Farde L, Halldin C, et al: PET study of D(1) dopamine receptor binding in neuroleptic-naive patients with schizophrenia. Am J Psychiatry 159:761–767, 2002

Kebabian JW, Calne DB: Multiple receptors for dopamine. Nature 277:93–96, 1979

Keefe RS, Silva SG, Perkins DO, et al: The effects of atypical antipsychotic drugs on neurocognitive impairment in schizophrenia: a review and meta-analysis. Schizophr Bull 25:201–222, 1999

Kegeles LS, Abi-Dargham A, Zea-Ponce Y, et al: Modulation of amphetamine-induced striatal dopamine release by ketamine in humans: implications for schizophrenia. Biol Psychiatry 48:627–640, 2000

Knable MB, Weinberger DR: Dopamine, the prefrontal cortex and schizophrenia. J Psychopharmacol 11:123–131, 1997

Knable MB, Hyde TM, Herman MM, et al: Quantitative autoradiography of dopamine-D1 receptors, D2 receptors, and dopamine uptake sites in postmortem striatal specimens from schizophrenic patients. Biol Psychiatry 36:827–835, 1994

Knable MB, Hyde TM, Murray AM, et al: A postmortem study of frontal cortical dopamine D1 receptors in schizophrenics, psychiatric controls, and normal controls. Biol Psychiatry 40:1191–1199, 1996

Konradi C, Heckers S: Molecular aspects of glutamate dysregulation: implications for schizophrenia and its treatment. Pharmacol Ther 97:153–179, 2003

Korostishevsky M, Kaganovich M, Cholostoy A, et al: Is the G72/G30 locus associated with schizophrenia? Single nucleotide polymorphisms, haplotypes, and gene expression analysis. Biol Psychiatry 56:169–176, 2004

Kotter R: Postsynaptic integration of glutamatergic and dopaminergic signals in the striatum. Prog Neurobiol 44:163–196, 1994

Krystal JH, Karper LP, Seibyl JP, et al: Subanesthetic effects of the noncompetitive NMDA antagonist, ketamine, in humans: psychotomimetic, perceptual, cognitive, and neuroendocrine responses. Arch Gen Psychiatry 51:199–214, 1994

Krystal JH, Abi-Saab W, Perry E, et al: Preliminary evidence of attenuation of the disruptive effects of the NMDA glutamate receptor antagonist, ketamine, on working memory by pretreatment with the group II metabotropic glutamate receptor agonist, LY354740, in healthy human subjects. Psychopharmacology (Berl) 179:303–309, 2005

Kudoh A, Ishihara H, Matsuki A: Current perception thresholds and postoperative pain in schizophrenic patients. Reg Anesth Pain Med 25:475–479, 2000

Laakso A, Vilkman H, Alakare B, et al: Striatal dopamine transporter binding in neuroleptic-naive patients with schizophrenia studied with positron emission tomography. Am J Psychiatry 157:269–271, 2000

Laakso A, Bergman J, Haaparanta M, et al: Decreased striatal dopamine transporter binding in vivo in chronic schizophrenia. Schizophr Res 52:115–120, 2001

Lahti RA, Roberts RC, Conley RR, et al: Dopamine D2, D3 and D4 receptors in human postmortem brain sections: comparison between normals and schizophrenics. Schizophr Res 18:173, 1996a

Lahti RA, Roberts RC, Conley RR, et al: D2-type dopamine receptors in postmortem human brain sections from normal and schizophrenic subjects. Neuroreport 7:1945–1948, 1996b

Lahti AC, Weiler MA, Tamara Michaelidis BA, et al: Effects of ketamine in normal and schizophrenic volunteers. Neuropsychopharmacology 25:455–467, 2001

Laruelle M: Imaging dopamine transmission in schizophrenia: a review and meta-analysis. Q J Nucl Med 42:211–221, 1998

Laruelle M: Imaging synaptic neurotransmission with in vivo binding competition techniques: a critical review. J Cereb Blood Flow Metab 20:423–451, 2000a

Laruelle M: The role of endogenous sensitization in the pathophysiology of schizophrenia: implications from recent brain imaging studies. Brain Res Rev 31:371–384, 2000b

Laruelle M: Dopamine transmission in the schizophrenic brain, in Schizophrenia, 2nd Edition. Edited by Weinberger DR, Hirsch S. Oxford, UK, Blackwell, 2003, pp 365–387

Laruelle M, Casanova M, Weinberger D, et al: Postmortem study of the dopaminergic D1 receptors in the dorsolateral prefrontal cortex of schizophrenics and controls. Schizophr Res 3:30–31, 1990

Laruelle M, Abi-Dargham A, van Dyck CH, et al: Single photon emission computerized tomography imaging of amphetamine-induced dopamine release in drug free schizophrenic subjects. Proc Natl Acad Sci U S A 93:9235–9240, 1996

Laruelle M, D'Souza CD, Baldwin RM, et al: Imaging D2 receptor occupancy by endogenous dopamine in humans. Neuropsychopharmacology 17:162–174, 1997a

Laruelle M, Iycr RN, Al-Tikriti MS, et al: Microdialysis and SPECT measurements of amphetamine-induced dopamine release in nonhuman primates. Synapse 25:1–14, 1997b

Laruelle M, Abi-Dargham A, Gil R, et al: Increased dopamine transmission in schizophrenia: relationship to illness phases. Biol Psychiatry 46:56–72, 1999

Laruelle M, Abi-Dargham A, van Dyck C, et al: Dopamine and serotonin transporters in patients with schizophrenia: an imaging study with [^{123}I]beta-CIT. Biol Psychiatry 47:371–379, 2000

Laruelle M, Kegeles LS, Abi-Dargham A: Glutamate, dopamine, and schizophrenia: from pathophysiology to treatment. Ann N Y Acad Sci 1003:138–158, 2003

Lavalaye J, Linszen DH, Booij J, et al: Dopamine transporter density in young patients with schizophrenia assessed with [123]FP-CIT SPECT. Schizophr Res 47:59–67, 2001

Lee T, Seeman P, Tourtelotte WW, et al: Binding of ^{3}H-neuroleptics and ^{3}H-apomorphine in schizophrenic brains. Nature 274:897–900, 1978

Leveque JC, Macias W, Rajadhyaksha A, et al: Intracellular modulation of NMDA receptor function by antipsychotic drugs. J Neurosci 20:4011–4020, 2000

Levine J, Stahl Z, Sela BA, et al: Elevated homocysteine levels in young male patients with schizophrenia. Am J Psychiatry 159:1790–1792, 2002

Levine MS, Li Z, Cepeda C, et al: Neuromodulatory actions of dopamine on synaptically evoked neostriatal responses in slices. Synapse 24:65–78, 1996

Lieberman JA, Kane JM, Alvir J: Provocative tests with psychostimulant drugs in schizophrenia. Psychopharmacology (Berl) 91:415–433, 1987a

Lieberman JA, Kane JM, Sarantakos S, et al: Prediction of relapse in schizophrenia. Arch Gen Psychiatry 44:597–603, 1987b

Lieberman JA, Kinon BL, Loebel AD: Dopaminergic mechanisms in idiopathic and drug-induced psychoses. Schizophr Bull 16:97–110, 1990

Lieberman JA, Sheitman BB, Kinon BJ: Neurochemical sensitization in the pathophysiology of schizophrenia: deficits and dysfunction in neuronal regulation and plasticity. Neuropsychopharmacology 17:205–229, 1997

Lindstrom LH, Gefvert O, Hagberg G, et al: Increased dopamine synthesis rate in medial prefrontal cortex and striatum in schizophrenia indicated by L-(beta-11C) DOPA and PET. Biol Psychiatry 46:681–688, 1999

Lindvall O, Björklund A: Dopamine- and norepinephrine-containing neuron systems: their anatomy in the rat brain, in Chemical Neuroanatomy. Edited by Emson P. New York, Raven, 1983, pp 229–255

Mackay AV, Iversen LL, Rossor M, et al: Increased brain dopamine and dopamine receptors in schizophrenia. Arch Gen Psychiatry 39:991–997, 1982

Malhotra AK, Pinals DA, Weingartner H, et al: NMDA receptor function and human cognition: the effects of ketamine in healthy volunteers. Neuropsychopharmacology 14:301–307, 1996

Malhotra AK, Pinals DA, Adler CM, et al: Ketamine-induced exacerbation of psychotic symptoms and cognitive impairment in neuroleptic-free schizophrenics. Neuropsychopharmacology 17:141–150, 1997

Marti M, Mela F, Bianchi C, et al: Striatal dopamine-NMDA receptor interactions in the modulation of glutamate release in the substantia nigra pars reticulata in vivo: opposite role for D1 and D2 receptors. J Neurochem 83:635–644, 2002

Marzella PL, Hill C, Keks N, et al: The binding of both [H-3] nemonapride and [H-3]raclopride is increased in schizophrenia. Biol Psychiatry 42:648–654, 1997

Matthysse S: Dopamine and the pharmacology of schizophrenia: the state of the evidence. J Psychiatr Res 11:107–113, 1974

McGowan S, Lawrence AD, Sales T, et al: Presynaptic dopaminergic dysfunction in schizophrenia: a positron emission tomographic [18F]fluorodopa study. Arch Gen Psychiatry 61:134–142, 2004

Meador-Woodruff JH, Healy DJ: Glutamate receptor expression in schizophrenic brain. Brain Res Brain Res Rev 31:288–294, 2000

Meador-Woodruff JH, Damask SP, Wang J, et al: Dopamine receptors mRNA expression in human striatum and neocortex. Neuropsychopharmacology 15:17–29, 1996

Meador-Woodruff JH, Haroutunian V, Powchik P, et al: Dopamine receptor transcript expression in striatum and prefrontal and occipital cortex: focal abnormalities in orbitofrontal cortex in schizophrenia. Arch Gen Psychiatry 54:1089–1095, 1997

Melis M, Diana M, Gessa GL: Clozapine potently stimulates mesocortical dopamine neurons. Eur J Pharmacol 366:R11–R13, 1999

Meyer-Lindenberg A, Miletich RS, Kohn PD, et al: Reduced prefrontal activity predicts exaggerated striatal dopaminergic function in schizophrenia. Nat Neurosci 5:267–271, 2002

Miller DW, Abercrombie ED: Effects of MK-801 on spontaneous and amphetamine-stimulated dopamine release in striatum measured with in vivo microdialysis in awake rats. Brain Res Bull 40:57–62, 1996

Mirnics K, Middleton FA, Lewis DA, et al: Analysis of complex brain disorders with gene expression microarrays: schizophrenia as a disease of the synapse. Trends Neurosci 24:479–486, 2001

Missale C, Nash SR, Robinson SW, et al: Dopamine receptors: from structure to function. Physiol Rev 78:189–225, 1998

Mita T, Hanada S, Nishino N, et al: Decreased serotonin S2 and increased dopamine D2 receptors in chronic schizophrenics. Biol Psychiatry 21:1407–1414, 1986

Miyamoto Y, Yamada K, Noda Y, et al: Hyperfunction of dopaminergic and serotonergic neuronal systems in mice lacking the NMDA receptor epsilon1 subunit. J Neurosci 21:750–757, 2001

Mogenson GJ, Jones DL, Yim CY: From motivation to action: functional interface between the limbic system and the motor system. Prog Neurobiol 14:69–97, 1980

Moghaddam B: Bringing order to the glutamate chaos in schizophrenia. Neuron 40:881–884, 2003

Moghaddam B, Adams BW: Reversal of phencyclidine effects by a group II metabotropic glutamate receptor agonist in rats. Science 281:1349–1352, 1998

Moghaddam B, Adams B, Verma A, et al: Activation of glutamatergic neurotransmission by ketamine: a novel step in the pathway from NMDA receptor blockade to dopaminergic and cognitive disruptions associated with the prefrontal cortex. J Neurosci 17:2921–2927, 1997

Mohn AR, Gainetdinov RR, Caron MG, et al: Mice with reduced NMDA receptor expression display behaviors related to schizophrenia. Cell 98:427–436, 1999

Monsma F Jr, Mahan LC, McVittie LD, et al: Molecular cloning and expression of a D1 dopamine receptor linked to adenylyl cyclase activation. Proc Natl Acad Sci U S A 87:6723–6727, 1990

Morari M, O'Connor WT, Ungerstedt U, et al: Dopamine D1 and D2 receptor antagonism differentially modulates stimulation of striatal neurotransmitter levels by N-methyl-D-aspartic acid. Eur J Pharmacol 256:23–30, 1994

Mrzljak L, Bergson C, Pappy M, et al: Localization of dopamine D4 receptors in GABAergic neurons of the primate brain. Nature 381:245–248, 1996

Murray AM, Hyde TM, Knable MB, et al: Distribution of putative D4 dopamine receptors in postmortem striatum from patients with schizophrenia. J Neurosci 15:2186–2191, 1995

Narendran R, Hwang DR, Slifstein M, et al: In vivo vulnerability to competition by endogenous dopamine: comparison of the D2 receptor agonist radiotracer (-)-N-[11C]propyl-norapomorphine ([11C]NPA) with the D2 receptor antagonist radiotracer [11C]-raclopride. Synapse 52:188–208, 2004

Narendran R, Frankle G, Keefe RS, et al: Altered prefrontal dopaminergic function in chronic recreational ketamine users. Am J Psychiatry (in press)

Newcomer JW, Farber NB, Jevtovic-Todorovic V, et al: Ketamine-induced NMDA receptor hypofunction as a model of memory impairment and psychosis. Neuropsychopharmacology 20:106–118, 1999

Nicola SM, Surmeier J, Malenka RC: Dopaminergic modulation of neuronal excitability in the striatum and nucleus accumbens. Annu Rev Neurosci 23:185–215, 2000

Nordstrom AL, Farde L, Wiesel FA, et al: Central D2-dopamine receptor occupancy in relation to antipsychotic drug effects: a double-blind PET study of schizophrenic patients. Biol Psychiatry 33:227–235, 1993

Okubo Y, Suhara T, Suzuki K, et al: Decreased prefrontal dopamine D1 receptors in schizophrenia revealed by PET. Nature 385:634–636, 1997

Olney JW, Farber NB: Glutamate receptor dysfunction and schizophrenia. Arch Gen Psychiatry 52:998–1007, 1995

Olney JW, Newcomer JW, Farber NB: NMDA receptor hypofunction model of schizophrenia. J Psychiatr Res 33:523–533, 1999

Onn SP, West AR, Grace AA: Dopamine-mediated regulation of striatal neuronal and network interactions. Trends Neurosci 23:S48–S56, 2000

Owen F, Cross AJ, Crow TJ, et al: Increased dopamine-receptor sensitivity in schizophrenia. Lancet 2:223–226, 1978

Palermo-Neto J: Dopaminergic systems: dopamine receptors. Psychiatr Clin North Am 20:705–721, 1997

Parsey RV, Oquendo MA, Zea-Ponce Y, et al: Dopamine D(2) receptor availability and amphetamine-induced dopamine release in unipolar depression. Biol Psychiatry 50:313–322, 2001

Pearce RK, Seeman P, Jellinger K, et al: Dopamine uptake sites and dopamine receptors in Parkinson's disease and schizophrenia. Eur Neurol 30 (suppl 1):9–14, 1990

Pehek EA, Yamamoto BK: Differential effects of locally administered clozapine and haloperidol on dopamine efflux in the rat prefrontal cortex and caudate-putamen. J Neurochem 63:2118–2124, 1994

Peris J, Dwoskin LP, Zahniser NR: Biphasic modulation of evoked [3H]D-aspartate release by D-2 dopamine receptors in rat striatal slices. Synapse 2:450–456, 1988

Piccini P, Pavese N, Brooks DJ: Endogenous dopamine release after pharmacological challenges in Parkinson's disease. Ann Neurol 53:647–653, 2003

Pimoule C, Schoemaker H, Reynolds GP, et al: [3H]SCH 23390 labelled D1 dopamine receptors are unchanged in schizophrenia and Parkinson's disease. Eur J Pharmacol 114:235–237, 1985

Reith J, Benkelfat C, Sherwin A, et al: Elevated dopa decarboxylase activity in living brain of patients with psychosis. Proc Natl Acad Sci U S A 91:11651–11654, 1994

Reynolds GP: Increased concentrations and lateral asymmetry of amygdala dopamine in schizophrenia. Nature 305:527–529, 1983

Reynolds GP: Beyond the dopamine hypothesis: the neurochemical pathology of schizophrenia. Br J Psychiatry 155:305–316, 1989

Reynolds GP, Czudek C: Status of the dopaminergic system in postmortem brain in schizophrenia. Psychopharmacol Bull 24:345–347, 1988

Reynolds GP, Mason SL: Are striatal dopamine D-4 receptors increased in schizophrenia? J Neurochem 63:1576–1577, 1994

Reynolds GP, Czudek C, Bzowej N, et al: Dopamine receptor asymmetry in schizophrenia. Lancet 1:979, 1987

Riley BP, Tahir E, Rajagopalan S, et al: A linkage study of the N-methyl-D-aspartate receptor subunit gene loci and schizophrenia in southern African Bantu-speaking families. Psychiatr Genet 7:57–74, 1997

Robinson TE, Becker JB: Enduring changes in brain and behavior produced by chronic amphetamine administration: a review and evaluation of animal models of amphetamine psychosis. Brain Res Rev 11:157–198, 1986

Rollema H, Lu Y, Schmidt AW, et al: 5-HT(1A) receptor activation contributes to ziprasidone-induced dopamine release in the rat prefrontal cortex. Biol Psychiatry 48:229–237, 2000

Sato M, Chen CC, Akiyama K, et al: Acute exacerbation of paranoid psychotic state after long-term abstinence in patients with previous methamphetamine psychosis. Biol Psychiatry 18:429–440, 1983

Sawaguchi T, Goldman-Rakic PS: D1 dopamine receptors in prefrontal cortex: involvement in working memory. Science 251:947–950, 1991

Sawaguchi T, Goldman-Rakic PS: The role of D1-dopamine receptor in working memory: local injections of dopamine antagonists into the prefrontal cortex of rhesus monkeys performing an oculomotor delayed-response task. J Neurophysiol 71:515–528, 1994

Schneider JS, Sun ZQ, Roeltgen DP: Effects of dopamine agonists on delayed response performance in chronic low-dose MPTP-treated monkeys. Pharmacol Biochem Behav 48:235–240, 1994

Schwarcz R, Rassoulpour A, Wu HQ, et al: Increased cortical kynurenate content in schizophrenia. Biol Psychiatry 50:521–530, 2001

Seamans JK, Floresco SB, Phillips AG: D-1 receptor modulation of hippocampal-prefrontal cortical circuits integrating spatial memory with executive functions in the rat. J Neurosci 18:1613–1621, 1998

Seamans JK, Durstewitz D, Christie BR, et al: Dopamine D1/D5 receptor modulation of excitatory synaptic inputs to layer V prefrontal cortex neurons. Proc Natl Acad Sci U S A 98:301–306, 2001a

Seamans JK, Gorelova N, Durstewitz D, et al: Bidirectional dopamine modulation of GABAergic inhibition in prefrontal cortical pyramidal neurons. J Neurosci 21:3628–3638, 2001b

Seeman P: Brain dopamine receptors in schizophrenia: PET problems [published erratum appears in Arch Gen Psychiatry 46:99, 1989]. Arch Gen Psychiatry 45:598–600, 1988

Seeman P: Dopamine receptor sequences: therapeutic levels of neuroleptics occupy D2 receptors, clozapine occupies D4. Neuropsychopharmacology 7:261–284, 1992

Seeman P, Lee T: Antipsychotic drugs: direct correlation between clinical potency and presynaptic action on dopamine neurons. Science 188:1217–1219, 1975

Seeman P, Ulpian C, Bergeron C, et al: Bimodal distribution of dopamine receptor densities in brains of schizophrenics. Science 225:728–731, 1984

Seeman P, Bzowej NH, Guan HC, et al: Human brain D1 and D2 dopamine receptors in schizophrenia, Alzheimer's, Parkinson's, and Huntington's diseases. Neuropsychopharmacology 1:5–15, 1987

Seeman P, Guan H-C, Niznik HB: Endogenous dopamine lowers the dopamine D$_2$ receptor density as measured by [^{3}H]raclopride: implications for positron emission tomography of the human brain. Synapse 3:96–97, 1989

Seeman P, Guan HC, Van Tol HHM: Dopamine D4 receptors elevated in schizophrenia. Nature 365:411–445, 1993

Seeman P, Guan HC, Van Tol HH: Schizophrenia: elevation of dopamine D4-like sites, using [3H]nemonapride and [125I]-epidepride. Eur J Pharmacol 286:R3–5, 1995

Smiley JF, Levey AI, Ciliax BJ, et al: D1 dopamine receptor immunoreactivity in human and monkey cerebral cortex: predominant and extrasynaptic localization in dendritic spines. Proc Natl Acad Sci U S A 91:5720–5724, 1994

Smith AD, Bolam JP: The neural network of the basal ganglia as revealed by the study of synaptic connections of identified neurones. Trends Neurosci 13:259–265, 1990

Snyder SH: Amphetamine psychosis: a "model" schizophrenia mediated by catecholamines. Am J Psychiatry 130:61–67, 1973

Sokoloff P, Giros B, Martres M-P, et al: Molecular cloning and characterization of a novel dopamine receptor D3 as a target for neuroleptics. Nature 347:146–151, 1990

Starr MS: Glutamate/dopamine D1/D2 balance in the basal ganglia and its relevance to Parkinson's disease. Synapse 19:264–293, 1995

Stern Y, Langston JW: Intellectual changes in patients with MPTP-induced parkinsonism. Neurology 35:1506–1509, 1985

Stevens J: An anatomy of schizophrenia? Arch Gen Psychiatry 29:177–189, 1973

Sumiyoshi T, Stockmeier CA, Overholser JC, et al: Dopamine D4 receptors and effects of guanine nucleotides on [3H]raclopride binding in postmortem caudate nucleus of subjects with schizophrenia or major depression. Brain Res 681:109–116, 1995

Sumiyoshi T, Anil AE, Jin D, et al: Plasma glycine and serine levels in schizophrenia compared to normal controls and major depression: relation to negative symptoms. Int J Neuropsychopharmacol 7:1–8, 2004

Sunahara RK, Guan H-C, O'Dowd BF, et al: Cloning of the gene for a human dopamine D5 receptor with higher affinity for dopamine than D1. Nature 350:614–619, 1991

Susser E, Brown AS, Klonowski E, et al: Schizophrenia and impaired homocysteine metabolism: a possible association. Biol Psychiatry 44:141–143, 1998

Takahata R, Moghaddam B: Target-specific glutamatergic regulation of dopamine neurons in the ventral tegmental area. J Neurochem 75:1775–1778, 2000

Talbot PS, Laruelle M: The role of in vivo molecular imaging with PET and SPECT in the elucidation of psychiatric drug action and new drug development. Eur Neuropsychopharmacol 12:503–511, 2002

Tamminga CA, Holcomb HH, Gao XM, et al: Glutamate pharmacology and the treatment of schizophrenia: current status and future directions. Int Clin Psychopharmacol 3:29–37, 1995

Tanaka H, Grooms SY, Bennett MV, et al: The AMPAR subunit GluR2: still front and center-stage. Brain Res 886:190–207, 2000

Tang YP, Shimizu E, Dube GR, et al: Genetic enhancement of learning and memory in mice. Nature 401:63–69, 1999

Taylor SF, Koeppe RA, Tandon R, et al: In vivo measurement of the vesicular monoamine transporter in schizophrenia. Neuropsychopharmacology 23:667–675, 2000

Tiberi M, Jarvie KR, Silvia C, et al: Cloning, molecular characterization, and chromosomal assignment of a gene encoding a second D1 dopamine receptor subtype: differential expression pattern in rat brain compared with the D1A receptor. Proc Natl Acad Sci U S A 88:7491–7495, 1991

Tsai G, van Kammen DP, Chen S, et al: Glutamatergic neurotransmission involves structural and clinical deficits of schizophrenia. Biol Psychiatry 44:667–674, 1998a

Tsai G, Yang P, Chung LC, et al: D-serine added to antipsychotics for the treatment of schizophrenia. Biol Psychiatry 44:1081–1089, 1998b

Tsai GE, Yang P, Chung LC, et al: D-serine added to clozapine for the treatment of schizophrenia. Am J Psychiatry 156:1822–1825, 1999

Tsai G, Lane HY, Yang P, et al: Glycine transporter I inhibitor, N-methylglycine (sarcosine), added to antipsychotics for the treatment of schizophrenia. Biol Psychiatry 55:452–456, 2004a

Tsai G, Ralph-Williams RJ, Martina M, et al: Gene knockout of glycine transporter 1: characterization of the behavioral phenotype. Proc Natl Acad Sci U S A 101:8485–8490, 2004b

Tsukada H, Nishiyama S, Fukumoto D, et al: Chronic NMDA antagonism impairs working memory, decreases extracellular dopamine, and increases D1 receptor binding in prefrontal cortex of conscious monkeys. Neuropsychopharmacology 30:1861–1869, 2005

Umbricht D, Schmid L, Koller R, et al: Ketamine-induced deficits in auditory and visual context-dependent processing in healthy volunteers: implications for models of cognitive deficits in schizophrenia. Arch Gen Psychiatry 57:1139–1147, 2000

Van Berckel BNM, Waterhouse RN, Hwang DR, et al: Enhanced amphetamine-induced striatal [11C]raclopride displacement by the group II metabotropic glutamate receptor agonist L354740 in baboons. Abstr Soc Neurosci 454.3, 2001

van Rossum JM: The significance of dopamine receptor blockade for the mechanism of action of neuroleptic drugs. Arch Int Pharmacodyn Ther 160:492–494, 1966

Van Tol HHM, Bunzow JR, Guan H-C, et al: Cloning of the gene for a human dopamine D4 receptor with high affinity for the antipsychotic clozapine. Nature 350:610–614, 1991

Verhoeff NP, Kapur S, Hussey D, et al: A simple method to measure baseline occupancy of neostriatal dopamine D2 receptors by dopamine in vivo in healthy subjects. Neuropsychopharmacology 25:213–223, 2001

Verhoeff NP, Hussey D, Lee M, et al: Dopamine depletion results in increased neostriatal D(2), but not D(1), receptor binding in humans. Mol Psychiatry 7:233, 322–328, 2002

Villemagne VL, Wong DF, Yokoi F, et al: GBR12909 attenuates amphetamine-induced striatal dopamine release as measured by [(11)C]raclopride continuous infusion PET scans. Synapse 33:268–273, 1999

Weinberger DR: Implications of the normal brain development for the pathogenesis of schizophrenia. Arch Gen Psychiatry 44:660–669, 1987

West AR, Grace AA: Opposite influences of endogenous dopamine D1 and D2 receptor activation on activity states and electrophysiological properties of striatal neurons: studies combining in vivo intracellular recordings and reverse microdialysis. J Neurosci 22:294–304, 2002

Wickens JR: Dopamine regulation of synaptic plasticity in the neostriatum: a cellular model of reinforcement, in Brain Dynamics and the Striatal Complex. Edited by Miller R, Wickens JR. London, England, Harwood Academic Publishers, 2000, pp 65–76

Wilson CJ, Kawaguchi Y: The origins of two-state spontaneous membrane potential fluctuations of neostriatal spiny neurons. J Neurosci 16:2397–2410, 1996

Yang CR, Seamans JK, Gorelova N: Developing a neuronal model for the pathophysiology of schizophrenia based on the nature of electrophysiological actions of dopamine in the prefrontal cortex. Neuropsychopharmacology 21:161–194, 1999

Young D, Scoville WB: Paranoid psychosis in narcolepsy and the possible dangers of benzedrine treatment. Med Clin North Am 22:637, 1938

Youngren KD, Inglis FM, Pivirotto PJ, et al: Clozapine preferentially increases dopamine release in the rhesus monkey prefrontal cortex compared with the caudate nucleus. Neuropsychopharmacology 20:403–412, 1999

Zhou QY, Grandy DK, Thambi L, et al: Cloning and expression of human and rat D1 dopamine receptors. Nature 347:76–80, 1990

PHOSPHOLIPIDS IN SCHIZOPHRENIA

Sahebarao P. Mahadik, Ph.D.

Jeffrey K. Yao, Ph.D., F.A.C.B.

Schizophrenia is a devastating neuropsychiatric disorder that has no clearly identified pathophysiology. The disorder has a similar incidence (0.6%–1.1%) around the world, but it progresses at varying degrees of severity (Craig et al. 1997; Eaton 1986; Jablensky et al. 1991). Many hypotheses about the etiology of schizophrenia based on varying degrees of pathophysiology, psychopathology, and response to pharmacological agents have been proposed, primarily focusing on neurotransmitter systems. Current long-term treatment of schizophrenia includes administering antipsychotic (predominantly antidopaminergic) medication, enlisting family and community support, providing patient education, and facilitating rehabilitation. Whereas 50%–68% of treated patients have long-term favorable outcomes (Hegarty et al. 1994), many obtain less than optimal results from current medications. The current antipsychotics typically prescribed reduce the most disturbing symptoms of the disease, such as anxiety, hallucinations, delusions, and rage, but leave unchanged the most disabling symptoms of the disorder, such as negative symp-

toms and cognitive deficits, and introduce side effects (Carpenter and Buchanan 1994; Kane and Marder 1993).

Among several pathophysiological hypotheses about schizophrenia, neuronal maldevelopment and consequent abnormal neurotransmission—resulting from defective genes, malnutrition, viral infections, and autoimmune dysfunction—is one that has attracted general interest. Although several etiopathogenetic mechanisms have shown promise for explaining the disorder, most do not account for the multitude of dissimilar clinical and biological characteristics demonstrated in schizophrenic individuals (Lieberman and Koreen 1993). Moreover, recent studies have shown that the average reduction in baseline symptoms has been in the range of 12%–18% after administration of either first- or second-generation antipsychotic medications to normalize the neurotransmitter defects (Khan et al. 2001). These limitations and the emergent morbidities, such as weight gain, insulin resistance, cardiovascular problems, and abnormal lipid metabolism, lead to a decline in the patient's quality of life and even to increased mortality (McIntyre et al. 2001; Wirshing 2003). When these facts are considered together with the earlier observations by Hegarty and colleagues (1994), one realizes that the long-term outcomes for today's patients with schizophrenia are not significantly different from the outcomes for patients 100 years ago in terms of ability to maintain employment and reintegrate into the community. This disturbing realization reflects the limitations of current antipsychotic treatment.

On the other hand, the neuronal membrane pathology can serve as a point of convergence for the previously mentioned hypothesis of schizophrenia. The neuronal membrane is the structural and functional site of neurotransmitter receptors, ion channels, signal transduction, and drug effects. The membrane also is a point where there is a natural intersection between genetic and environmental factors. Alternative ideas postulated over the years led to the phospholipid/fatty acid hypothesis for schizophrenia (Horrobin 1996, 1998; Horrobin et al. 1994; Rotrosen and Wolkin 1987). Numerous studies have shown that in both central and peripheral tissue, patients with schizophrenia have increased phospholipid breakdown and decreased levels of various essential polyunsaturated fatty acids (EPUFAs), particularly arachidonic acid (AA) and docosahexaenoic acid (DHA) (Peet et al. 2003; Yao 2003). Phospholipids represent a major class of lipids that are exclusively localized in the cellular membranes of all subcellular organelles, such as plasma membrane, microsomes, mitochondria, and nuclei. The dynamic state of all membranes, particularly neuronal, is solely dependent on their phospholipid composition.

The functions and levels of membrane phospholipids may be altered in response to environmental factors such as nutrition, physical and emotional stress, temperature, and infections. Furthermore, membrane damage, specifically free radical–mediated phospholipid peroxidation, can significantly alter a broad range of membrane functions. A putative role for free radicals in some domains of schizophrenia pathophysiology has thus been proposed (Cadet and Kahler 1994; Mahadik and Mukherjee 1996; Reddy and Yao 1996; Yao et al. 2001). Therefore, membrane dysfunction can be partly secondary to free radical–mediated pathology. Given the diverse physiological functions of membrane phospholipids and EPUFAs in neural growth, differentiation, and survival under a variety of pathophysiological conditions, an elucidation of their role in schizophrenia pathophysiology may provide novel strategies for the treatment of this disorder.

In this chapter, we provide a brief introduction on structural diversity and mechanisms of phospholipid metabolism and then summarize the evidence for phospholipid pathology, possible underlying mechanisms, neuro-

pathological and clinical implications, and therapeutic potential in schizophrenia.

PHOSPHOLIPIDS AND CELLULAR MEMBRANES

STRUCTURE AND METABOLISM

The parent compound of phospholipids is glycerol, with the primary glycerol group esterified to phosphoric acid at carbon sn-3, and other hydroxyl groups at carbon positions sn-1 and sn-2 are esterified to fatty acids F1 and F2, respectively (see Figure 7–1). In the brain, four main polar head groups—choline, ethanolamine, inositol, and serine—are attached to phosphoric acid at sn-3, and the resulting phosphoglycerolipids are referred to as phosphatidylcholines, phosphatidylethanolamines, phosphatidylinositols, and phosphatidylserines, respectively. Fatty acids attached to carbons sn-1 and sn-2 may be of many types depending on the length of the carbon (C14 to C26) chains, the number of double bonds in the chain, the precise position of the double bonds, and whether each double bond is in cis or $trans$ configuration. F1 fatty acids are generally nonessential saturated or monosaturated, whereas F2 fatty acids are almost entirely essential polyunsaturated fatty acids. These differences in substructure (e.g., head groups, type and position of fatty acids) contribute to the molecular diversity of phospholipids.

The phospholipid composition differs significantly among the subcellular membranes (plasma membrane, microsomes, Golgi complex, mitochondria, peroxisomes, lysosomes, endosomes, vesicles, and nuclei) of every cell type (Findley and Evans 1990). Phospholipids are organized in a lipid bilayer in which glycerol with fatty acids is embedded inside and polar head groups align at the surface. Phospholipids are highly enriched in neural membranes (65%) compared with nonneural tissues (15%–35%) (Horrocks et al. 1982; Suzuki 1981). There are mainly four types of phospholipids: phosphatidylcholines (45%), phosphatidylethanolamines (25%), phosphatidylinositols (10%), and phosphatidylserines (7%). These phospholipids are highly enriched (over 45% of the total fatty acid) in essential polyunsaturated fatty acids, predominantly AA and DHA (O'Brien et al. 1965). Phosphatidylcholine is predominantly localized in the outer layer.

FUNCTIONAL ROLE

The unique phospholipid composition and organization of neural plasma membrane regulate its wide range of functions such as cell-cell recognition and contact inhibi-

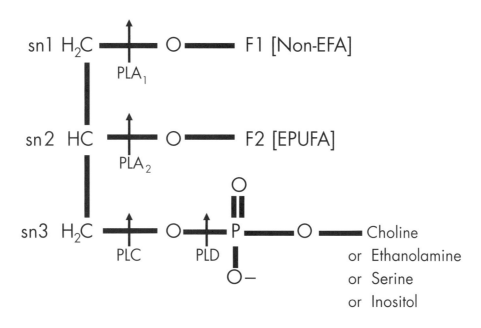

FIGURE 7–1. General structures and sites of enzymatic breakdown of typical membrane phosphoglycerides. The three carbons of primary structure (glycerol) are designated *sn1*, *sn2*, and *sn3*. The carbons sn1 and sn2 are esterified with fatty acids F1 (nonessential fatty acids) and F2 (essential polyunsaturated fatty acids, predominantly arachidonic acid and docosahexaenoic acid in the brain), respectively. The carbon sn3 is esterified with phosphoric acid, which is esterified by choline, ethanolamine, inositol, or serine, generating corresponding phosphoglycerides, phosphatidylcholine, phosphatidylethanolamine, phosphatidylinositol, or phosphatidylserine.

Arrows indicate the sites of the phospholipid breakdown by enzymes—phospholipase A_1 (PLA_1), phospholipase A_2 (PLA_2), phospholipase C (PLC), and phospholipase D (PLD)—which are specifically and differentially activated during membrane receptor signal transduction. EPUFA=essential polyunsaturated fatty acid; non-EFA=nonessential fatty acid.

tion through complex glycoconjugates, ion and nutritional transport, membrane receptor–mediated signal transduction, and response to a wide range of environmental factors (Figure 7–2). These processes lead to activation of specific phospholipases that cause generation of a whole range of phospholipid-derived second messengers such as AA, DHA, diacylglycerol, inositol polyphosphate, phosphoserine, and prostaglandins and endocannabinoids that are synthesized from AA and DHA. Particularly, AA plays a predominant role as a second messenger in signal transduction of several neurotransmitters (e.g., dopamine, serotonin, acetylcholine, norepinephrine, glutamate) and of some trophic factors such as basic fibroblast growth factor, nerve growth factor, and brain-derived neurotrophic factor (Axelrod 1990; Piomelli et al. 1991; Rana and Hokin 1990). These second messengers alter the cellular physiological response to environment, including by way of gene activation, and trigger further generation and propagation of action potential. Furthermore, these physiological responses can also alter the phospholipid metabolism, which may cause adaptive and maladaptive membrane structural changes and thereby alter function. All these processes are critical to neuronal growth, mainte-

nance, survival, and repair throughout the life span, because all these cellular processes have been found to be altered in patients with schizophrenia.

MEMBRANE PHOSPHOLIPIDS AND SCHIZOPHRENIA

ALTERED MEMBRANE PHOSPHOLIPIDS AND POLYUNSATURATED FATTY ACIDS

Peripheral Tissues: Red Blood Cells, Platelets, Plasma, and Skin Fibroblasts

The rationale for using peripheral tissues to determine phospholipid pathology in the brain has been that phospholipid metabolism is systemically regulated. That is, parallel changes in levels of phospholipid EPUFA occur in brain and peripheral tissues under a variety of pathophysiological situations (Carlson et al. 1986; Connor et al. 1990; Neuringer et al. 1986). Rotrosen and Wolkin (1987) summarized the earlier studies done on red blood cell (RBC) and platelet phospholipids from chronically medi-

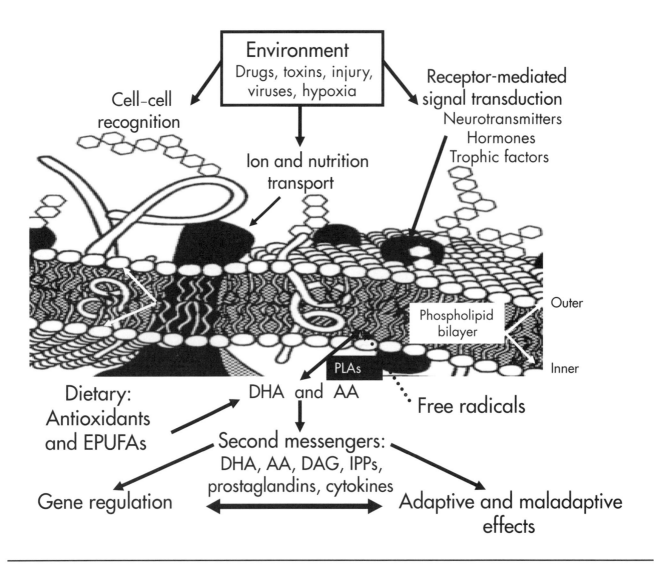

FIGURE 7–2.   Plasma membrane model depicting the key structural constituents and their functional roles in cell–cell interaction, interaction with environmental factors, and receptor-mediated signal transduction.

The membrane model shows the phospholipid bilayer, in which are embedded the receptors for neurotransmitters, physiological mediators and growth factors, transporters for ions and nutritional ingredients, and signal transduction machinery. The phospholipid bilayer is made up of four major phospholipids (phosphatidylcholine [PC], phosphatidylethanolamine [PE], phosphatidylinositol [PI], phosphatidylserine [PS]), which are asymmetrically localized (i.e., PC predominantly on outer lipid layer and PE, PI, PS on inner lipid layer). PE, PI, and PS are highly enriched in arachidonic acid (AA) and docosahexaenoic acid (DHA), which are released by receptor-mediated phospholipases (PLAs). AA and DHA and their metabolic products, diacylglycerol (DAG), inositol polyphosphates (IPPs), and prostaglandins, work as second messengers and physiological mediators, including gene modulation, and thus lead to adaptive and maladaptive cellular changes. EPUFA=essential polyunsaturated fatty acid.

cated schizophrenic patients. The majority of those studies found reduced levels of phosphatidylethanolamine, a phospholipid rich in AA and DHA. Reduced levels of phosphatidylethanolamine were also reported in the RBCs of drug-naive first-episode patients (Keshavan et al. 1993). Subsequently, however, more systematic analyses of phospholipid and fatty acid levels of RBCs were published from well clinically characterized patients with chronic schizophrenia (both those taking and those not

taking medication) (Yao et al. 1994) and in patients with predominantly positive and predominantly negative symptoms (Glen et al. 1994). These studies clearly demonstrated that reduced level of EPUFAs, particularly lower levels of AA and DHA, were present in patients with predominantly negative symptoms and a higher severity of symptoms. It was also demonstrated that the levels of phospholipids and their bound EPUFAs had been altered in the cultured skin fibroblasts of drug-naive first-episode patients (Mahadik et al. 1994, 1996a). Recent studies of drug-naive first-episode patients have also reported reduced levels of predominantly AA and DHA (Arvindakshan et al. 2003b; Khan et al. 2002; Reddy et al. 2004). These studies have indicated that the reduced levels of phospholipid EPUFA pathology may be associated with the onset of psychopathology and are not related to medication administered to the patient or to the number of years of illness.

Brain: Postmortem and De Novo ^{31}P-Magnetic Resonance Spectroscopy

If altered membrane dynamics plays a role in modulating the diverse cognitive and perception aberrations found in schizophrenia, then phospholipid and polyunsaturated fatty acid (PUFA) abnormalities likely are present in the brain. Altered levels of phospholipids and their EPUFAs in postmortem brain tissues from patients with schizophrenia have been reported (Horrobin et al. 1991; Yao et al. 2000). Specifically, there are decreased levels of phosphatidylethanolamine and phosphatidylcholine with concomitant reductions in total PUFA levels, which were largely attributable to decreases in AA and, to a lesser extent, its precursors, linoleic and eicosadienoic acid.

De novo magnetic resonance spectroscopy (MRS) studies have also demonstrated altered phospholipid metabolism, reduced phospholipid synthesis (reduced phosphomonoesters), and increased phospholipid breakdown (increased phosphodiesters) in both drug-naive first-episode patients with schizophrenia and medicated patients with chronic schizophrenia (Pettegrew et al. 1991; Stanley et al. 1995; Williamson et al. 1996). Levels of phosphomonoesters and phosphodiesters were found to be associated with the severity of psychopathology, particularly negative symptoms (Fukuzako et al. 1996). Recently, multiple lines of evidence have also converged to implicate oligodendroglial dysfunction, with subsequent abnormalities in myelin (70%–85% of its mass is lipid) maintenance and repair underlying the pathogenetic mechanism of schizophrenia, particularly in more severely ill patients (for reviews, see Bartzokis et al. 2003; Davis et al. 2003).

Correlation Between Peripheral and Central Findings

Myriad evidence has accumulated that reveals altered phospholipid and PUFA levels in both the peripheral and central tissue of patients with schizophrenia. However, it is necessary to confirm that the peripheral biochemical findings obtained in schizophrenia correlate with phospholipid/PUFA metabolism in the brain (Smesny et al. 2000). In nonhuman primates, RBC PUFA concentrations have been shown to reflect levels in the frontal cortex (Connor et al. 1990). Also, initial work in healthy human subjects has revealed that brain levels of the phospholipid breakdown product phosphodiesters (assessed with ^{31}P-MRS) correlate with reduced RBC concentrations of DHA and eicosapentaenoic acid (EPA) (Richardson et al. 2001). More recently, Yao and colleagues (2002) demonstrated that such correlations also occur in the peripheral and central phospholipids and PUFAs of schizophrenic patients. This line of evidence adds validity to using changes in peripheral lipid levels as a measure in schizophrenia and further supports the proposed hypothesis that schizophrenia may be a systemic phospholipid disorder (Horrobin 1998).

POSSIBLE MECHANISMS OF ALTERED PHOSPHOLIPID METABOLISM

Several mechanisms can lead to the type of membrane fatty acid defects identified in schizophrenia (Figure 7–3). Some of these mechanisms, such as increased phospholipid degradation, low dietary intake of essential fatty acids (EFAs) and their decreased incorporation into phospholipids, and free radical–mediated peroxidation, are examined later in this chapter.

Increased Phospholipid Turnover

Increased degradation by phospholipases. Increased levels of phospholipases (PLAs), particularly PLA$_2$, have been reported in patients with schizophrenia (Gattaz et al. 1990; Ross et al. 1997). However, the increase in plasma PLA$_2$ is inconsistent (Katila et al. 1997) and is considered a generalized "stressor" response (Noponen et al. 1993). The increased oxidative stress–mediated lipid peroxidation (see later in this section) has also been found to be associated with parallel increase in the PLA2 levels in several organs in animals (Burgess and Kuo 1996).

The discrepancies in previous data could be explained by the differential changes in the subtypes of the PLA$_2$ enzyme (Nigam and Scheve 2000). The superfamily of PLA$_2$ is divided into three types of enzymes: calcium (Ca^{2+})–dependent cytosolic PLA$_2$ (cPLA$_2$), Ca^{2+}-dependent secretory PLA$_2$ (sPLA$_2$), and Ca^{2+}-independent PLA$_2$ (iPLA$_2$) (Chakraborti 2003). Ross and colleagues (1997) showed that increased iPLA$_2$, not Ca^{2+}-dependent PLA$_2$, was found in serum of patients with schizophrenia. The PLA$_2$ levels correlated with general psychopathology scores and positive symptoms but not with negative symptoms. Recently, Gattaz's laboratory has replicated their earlier find-

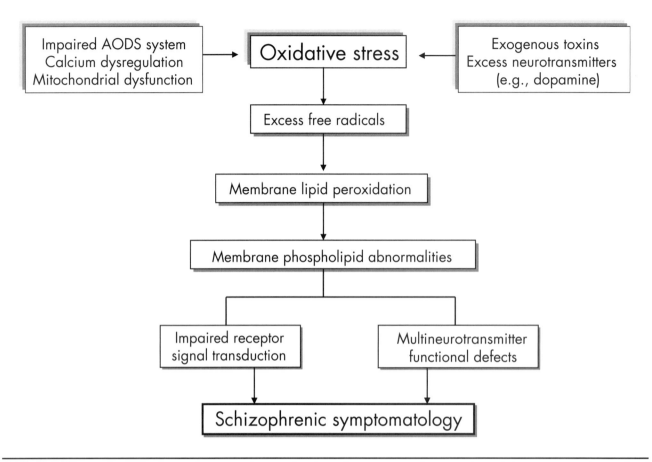

FIGURE 7–3.   Flow diagram depicting the mechanisms (e.g., impaired antioxidant defense system [AODS]) of oxidative stress that may lead to membrane phospholipid peroxidative breakdown and its pathophysiological consequences that may contribute to the development of schizophrenia symptomatology.
Source.   Adapted from Yao et al. 2001.

ings of increased PLA_2 activities in drug-free schizophrenia patients, and the increased levels were found in patients without a response to niacin (Tavares et al. 2003).

In addition to PLA_2, phospholipase C (PLC) and phospholipase D (PLD) are also involved in phospholipid degradation (Figure 7–1). The receptor-stimulated hydrolysis of inositol phospholipids, particularly phosphatidylinositol 4,5-bisphosphate (PI-4,5-P_2), is initiated by a specific PLC (Berridge and Irvine 1984). The resulting diacylglycerol and inositol 1,4,5-trisphosphate (1,4,5-IP_3) lead to activation of protein kinase C (PKC) and elevation of cytosolic Ca^{2+}, which provides molecular links between extracellular signals and intracellular events (Nishizuka 1992). Increased PLC activity may be involved in reported hyperactivity of the phosphatidylinositol pathway in schizophrenia (discussed later in this section).

Low dietary intake of essential polyunsaturated fatty acids.   Unlike saturated/monounsaturated fatty acids, EPUFAs cannot be synthesized de novo by the mam-

malian body. Therefore, the EPUFA precursors linoleic (n-6, 18:2n-6) and alpha-linolenic (n-3, 18:3n-3) acid (ALA) must be ingested through dietary sources. Increased intake of n-6 fatty acids or reduced intake of both n-6 and n-3 fatty acids can cause deficits in brain and behavioral development (Simopoulos 1991; Wainwright 1992). A large degree of variability exists in the quantity of EFAs, particularly n-3 EFA consumption among different cultures, primarily because of the local availability of these substances in the diet, in addition to the effects of lifestyle and consumption of antioxidants (Mahadik et al. 1999b; Peet et al. 1995). Christensen and Christensen (1988) found that differences in the clinical outcome of patients with schizophrenia in different countries studied by the World Health Organization were related to differences in the patients' dietary intake of oils from fish and vegetables, which are rich in n-3 EFAs, ALA, and DHA. In addition, the increased incidence of schizophrenia seen in children born during the Dutch famine (Hoek et al. 1998; Hulshoff Pol et al. 2000) suggests that this may have been related to a reduced consumption of fresh fruits and vegetables, which are a primary source of antioxidants and precursor EFAs.

Decreased EPUFA incorporation in phospholipids. In the brain, in addition to the dietary intake of the EPUFA precursors n-6 (linoleic acid) and n-3 (ALA) enzymatic regulation of phospholipid synthesis is significantly influenced by precursor levels and utilization by conversion into predominantly AA and DHA, respectively (Thompson 1992).

The utilization of precursor n-6 and n-3 EFAs may involve their conversion into AA and DHA, respectively; transport to the brain; and incorporation into phospholipids. Demisch and colleagues (1992) have shown that incorporation of ^{14}C-labeled AA into platelet phospholipids was significantly lower in untreated patients (>6 months) with a schizophreniform or schizoaffective disorder but not greater than in patients with chronic schizophrenia compared with normal control subjects. Subsequently, Yao and colleagues (1996) demonstrated that the total incorporation of ^{3}H-labeled AA in both relapsed and non-relapsed drug-free patients was significantly lower than in the same individuals receiving haloperidol treatment or in normal control subjects. A defective conversion of ALA to DHA was also found in skin fibroblasts from drug-naive first-episode patients (Mahadik et al. 1996b). The clinical significance of possible altered AA incorporation needs to be investigated systematically.

Antipsychotic treatments. The effects of antipsychotics on the dietary availability of EPUFAs and their incorporation into membrane phospholipids and hydrolysis by phospholipases are still unclear, except that haloperidol reduces EPUFA incorporation in vitro (Horrobin et al. 1994). A variety of antipsychotic drugs also inhibit PLA_2 activity (Taniguchi et al. 1988). However, no association was reported between RBC levels of EPUFAs and the type and dose of medication in individuals with schizophrenia (Glen et al. 1994; Yao et al. 1994). Treatment with some newer antipsychotics has been found to increase the levels of phospholipid AA and DHA in the RBC membranes of schizophrenic patients (Arvindakshan et al. 2003b; Evans et al. 2003; Horrobin 1999; Khan et al. 2002). It has been suggested that this increase may be partly related to the increased expression of apolipoprotein D, a protein that binds AA. Apolipoprotein D has been found in rat brain (Khan et al. 2003; Thomas et al. 2001b) and in the plasma of schizophrenic patients (Mahadik et al. 2002; Thomas et al. 2001a). Recently, its plasma levels have been found to correlate with the levels of RBC AA (Yao et al. 2005).

Increased Free Radical–Mediated Membrane Phospholipid Degradation

Free radicals. Free radicals are also commonly referred to as the reactive oxygen species, such as superoxides, hydroxyl radicals, and nitric oxides. These are generated in vivo during many normal biochemical reactions, such as the mitochondrial electron transfer chain, NADPH-dependent oxidase, auto-oxidation of EPUFAs, and catecholamines involving oxygen and nitric oxide.

Antioxidant defense systems. Under physiological conditions, the potential for free radical–mediated damage is kept in check by the antioxidant defense system, which is composed of a series of enzymatic and nonenzymatic components. The critical antioxidant enzymes include superoxide dismutase, catalase, and glutathione peroxidase. These enzymes act cooperatively at different sites in the metabolic pathway of free radicals. Superoxide dismutase converts free radicals into hydrogen peroxide, which is then decomposed into water and oxygen by catalase, thereby preventing the formation of hydroxy radicals that initiate lipid peroxidation. Selenium-dependent glutathione peroxidase protects against lipid peroxidation by converting hydrogen peroxide to water or more critically by converting toxic hydroperoxides to less toxic alcohols. The nonenzymatic antioxidants that are also equally important in the overall antioxidant defense systems (AODSs) are albumin, uric acid, bilirubin, glutathione, α-tocopherol (vitamin E), ascorbic acid (vitamin C), and β-carotene. These antioxidants inactivate free radicals by scavenging.

Oxidative stress and membrane phospholipid peroxidation. Oxidative stress is a state in which there is an increased free radical production and/or inefficient AODS, which can lead to membrane lipid peroxidation and thus may contribute to pathophysiology and thereby psychopathology (Figure 7–3). Phospholipid EPUFAs are highly susceptible to free radical interaction and auto-oxidation to form peroxyradicals and lipid peroxide intermediates. The existence of such peroxides within cell membranes results in altered membrane stability, fluidity, and permeability, and in impaired signal transduction (Ernster 1993). The brain, which is rich in EPUFAs, is particularly vulnerable to free radical–mediated damage (Halliwell 1992).

OXIDATIVE STRESS AND FREE RADICAL PATHOLOGY IN SCHIZOPHRENIA

Hoffer and colleagues (1954) first proposed a role for free radicals in the etiology of schizophrenia. Most of the studies have generally examined indirect measures of free radical activity because direct measures of free radicals in vivo are cumbersome. Initial studies done in medicated patients with chronic schizophrenia suggest that free radical pathology in schizophrenia may be a consequence of first-generation antipsychotic treatment, because treatment with these antipsychotics was found to cause oxidative injury in animals (Cadet and Lohr 1987; Mahadik and Mukherjee 1996). However, studies in drug-naive first-episode psychotic patients, as well as those in chronic patients both taking or not taking antipsychotic treatment, suggest that defects in AODS may play an important role in the pathophysiological mechanisms of schizophrenia (see later in this chapter). These studies have found altered levels of antioxidant enzymes in RBCs and skin fibroblasts, altered levels of antioxidants in plasma, and increased lipid peroxides in both plasma and cerebrospinal fluid (Mahadik and Mukherjee 1996; Mahadik et al. 1998; Mukherjee et al. 1996; Reddy and Yao 1996, 2003; Reddy et al. 1991; Yao et al. 2001). The plasma levels of vitamin E (Liday et al. 1995; McCreadie et al. 1995), vitamin C (Suboticanec et al. 1990), albumin (Yao et al. 2000), and uric acid (Yao et al. 1998) are lower in patients with schizophrenia.

In addition to membrane lipid peroxidation, researchers have found that free radicals in protein oxidation, gene modification, mitochondrial dysfunction, and neuronal dendritic and synaptic apoptosis may play a role (Mahadik et al. 2001; Simonian and Coyle 1996).

Factors That Influence Oxidative Stress

Cigarette smoking.   It is well documented that the majority of patients with schizophrenia are heavy smokers (Leon 1996; Scottish Schizophrenia Research Group 2000). In addition to numerous other chemicals, cigarette smoke contains reactive oxygen species, hydrogen peroxide, peroxynitrate, and peroxynitrite (Pryor and Stone 1993). Increased plasma lipid peroxidation products have been reported in heavy smokers compared with nonsmokers. Plasma levels of lipid peroxidation products return to levels similar to those in nonsmokers after 2 weeks of abstinence (Morrow et al. 1995). These oxidants not only put the lungs at risk but also seriously affect the central nervous system. Also, a report that heavy smoking by mothers during pregnancy increases the risk for behavioral problems in children in late adolescence (Fergusson et al. 1998) is compatible with the view that free radicals in the cigarette smoke may contribute to the abnormal neurodevelopment in some patients with schizophrenia.

Recent study by Hibbeln and colleagues (2003) found reductions in DHA and EPA but not AA in patients with chronic schizophrenia who smoked compared with nonsmokers. However, it is not clear whether patients with schizophrenia had reduced RBC PUFA levels (a most replicated fact) independent of smoking status because there was no normal control group. Carefully designed studies indicate that the altered antioxidant defense, as well as levels of EPUFAs, is not associated with the degree of smoking in schizophrenia patients (Yao et al. 2001).

Other factors.   Among other factors, such as the lifestyle of individuals with schizophrenia, particularly little or no exercise, high levels of alcohol consumption, and high-fat and high-calorie diets are unhealthy and pro-oxidant (Brown et al. 1999). A recent study of patients with chronic schizophrenia ($N=81$) found that they had a higher total calorie intake and high fat intake than the normal intake for the U.S. population (Strassnig et al. 2003). High caloric intake has been suggested to cause peroxidative brain damage and cognitive deficits in animals (Sohal et al. 1994). Mechanisms of the effects of other factors, such as season of birth, prenatal and postnatal birth complications, viral infections, drug use, and the mother's alcohol consumption during pregnancy, on fetal phospholipid metabolism can be very complex and are discussed in depth (Mahadik et al. 1999a, 1999b, 2001; McCreadie 1997; Mednick et al. 1988; Reddy and Yao 2003).

Antipsychotic treatments.   Antipsychotics can alter oxidative stress by altering antioxidant defense enzymes and generating reactive oxygen species (Mahadik et al. 2003a). Generally, typical antipsychotics such as haloperidol can increase oxidative stress by impairing antioxidant defense and increasing monoamine metabolism, and via its conversion to a free radical (Jedding et al. 1995; Mahadik and Mukherjee 1996; Mahadik et al. 1999b, 2003b). The increased oxidative stress then will contribute to free radical–mediated EPUFA loss, whereas atypical antipsychotics do not increase oxidative stress in rat brain because these agents do not reduce the expression of antioxidant enzymes and do not increase lipid peroxides similar to haloperidol (Parikh et al. 2002). Rather, atypical antipsychotics such as clozapine, olanzapine, and risperidone can improve the levels of RBC antioxidant enzymes, reduce plasma lipid peroxides, and increase levels of RBC EPUFAs in patients (Evans et al. 2003; Horrobin 1999; Mahadik et al. 2003a). However, altered blood antioxidant enzymes and related trace elements have been reported in patients with clozapine-induced agranulocytosis (Liday et al. 1995). In addition, the contribution of a very high caloric (food) intake (known to increase oxidative stress) by clozapine and olanzapine is still unknown.

PATHOPHYSIOLOGICAL SIGNIFICANCE

As discussed earlier, the phospholipids that are particularly enriched in AA and DHA are critical for normal brain and behavioral development and for their maintenance and functional performance throughout life (Bourre et al. 1992; Simopoulos 1991; Wainwright 1992). Therefore, altered phospholipid metabolism in schizophrenia may contribute to abnormal neurodevelopment and altered membrane receptor–mediated signal transduction by growth factors and neurotransmitters. It is also important to point out that the richness of the molecular diversity of these phospholipids in almost every tissue in the body may affect, in addition to brain function, other sensory functions, immunity, and serious medical morbidities such as cardiovascular disorders and type II diabetes.

Abnormal Neurodevelopment and Membrane EPUFA Deficits

There is overwhelming evidence that abnormal neurodevelopment is associated with schizophrenia (Weinberger 1996). This includes the following findings: impaired psychomotor and neuropsychological development ("neurointegrative defect") in children genetically at risk for schizophrenia (Fish et al. 1992), premorbid dysfunction (Cannon et al. 1997), and minor physical anomalies (Gupta et al. 1995; Lane et al. 1997). Brain structural studies have reported altered in vivo morphology (Degreef et al. 1992; DeLisi et al. 1992; Lawrie and Abukmeil 1998; Lieberman et al. 1992; Suddath et al. 1990) and postmortem neuropathology (Arnold et al. 1998; Glantz and Lewis 2000; Heckers 1997; Selemon et al. 1995). These studies have indicated, in particular, the differential reductions in volumes of certain brain regions, disorganized neuronal networks, and increased ventricular size. All of these changes likely predate (i.e., begin during neurogenesis) the onset of illness, and these areas progressively deteriorate by way of proposed increased "pruning" (excessive removal of nerve endings and processes) but not by classical degeneration (Keshavan et al. 1994).

Although such a neurodevelopmental hypothesis seems highly tenable, there must be a biochemical substrate through which the gene–environment interactions are expressed. Phospholipids, specifically AA and DHA, are highly involved in the developmental process. Reduced AA may explain reduced dendrites and synapses because it activates phosphorylation of growth-associated protein-43 (GAP-43), a key protein that contributes to dendrite growth and synaptogenesis (Benowitz and Routtenberg 1997). Furthermore, the proposed apoptosis may occur in schizophrenia (Catts and Catts 2000; Margolis et al. 1994) under increased oxidative stress (which is known to trigger apoptosis) (Wood and Youle 1994) and under reduced levels of growth factors (Bersani et al. 1999; Parikh et al. 2003). Apoptotic neuronal, dendritic, and synaptic loss could explain, at least in part, excessive pruning loss of dendritic and synaptic processes contributing to progressive deteriorating course of illness in some patients (Davis et al. 1998; Jaskiw et al. 1994; Nair et al. 1997). It is also important to indicate that the cultured skin fibroblasts from drug-naive first-episode patients had increased oxidative stress, altered levels of phospholipids and EPUFAs, reduced rate of growth and adhesion, increased senescence, and reduced response to growth factors (Mahadik and Mukherjee 1996).

Membrane Receptor–Mediated Signal Transduction

Phospholipid pathology may be the most important factor in the suggested abnormal receptor-mediated signal transduction of several neurotransmitters (e.g., dopamine, serotonin, glutamate, acetylcholine, γ-aminobutyric acid, and norepinephrine) and growth factors in schizophrenia (Hudson et al. 1993; Mahadik et al. 2001). This may happen by two ways: by way of altered phospholipid-dependent fluidity (Yao and van Kammen 1994) and by altered phospholipid-derived second messengers such as AA, DHA, diacylglycerol, inositol polyphosphates, prostaglandins, cytokines, and endocannabinoids that are generated by these neurotransmitters and growth factors (Yao and van Kammen 2004). Therefore, depleted levels of second messengers including AA may be one of the key factors in possible altered membrane signal transduction and neuronal deficits in schizophrenia (Skosnik and Yao 2003; Yao and Reddy 2003).

Hyperactivity of phosphoinositide pathways. Increased turnover of platelet phosphatidylinositol was found in both drug-treated and drug-free patients (Das et al. 1992; Yao et al. 1992) but was not found in drug-naive patients (Essali et al. 1990). The increased production of IP_3 may be because of an increase in the precursor $PI\text{-}4,5\text{-}P_2$, associated with a desensitization of the intracellular IP_3 receptor by neuroleptics (Das et al. 1992). On the other hand, Zilberman-Kaufman and colleagues (1992) reported an increased inositol-1-phosphatase in RBC of patients with chronic schizophrenia. Similarly, an increased formation of diacylglycerol has also been reported in patients with schizophrenia (Kaiya et al. 1989; Yao et al. 1996). Further, the hyperactivity of the G-protein–coupled phosphatidylinositol signaling system in schizophrenia has also been demonstrated in the postmortem brain to differ from that of major depression and bipolar mood disorder (Jope et al. 1998).

Eicosanoids. A variety of biologically active metabolites, which are derived from the newly released AA through the concerted reactions of cyclooxygenase and lipoxygenases, are collectively referred to as *eicosanoids* or *prostaglandins*, which modulate neural cell function as well as play a role in pathophysiological processes (Bazan 1999). A deficiency of prostaglandins has previously been related to schizophrenia (Horrobin 1977). One of the AA metabolites, prostaglandin D_2 (PGD_2), mediates vasodilatation during the inflammatory response. Therefore, reduced AA availability may explain in part a variety of clinical observations such as absence of arthritis and some inflammatory diseases, greater resistance to pain, and remission of psychosis during fever that are usually ignored by the receptor-based etiological hypotheses (Horrobin 1998).

Endocannabinoid system. Use of cannabis, Δ-9-tetrahydrocannabinol, induces psychosis that has been suggested to resemble schizophrenia psychopathology (Halikas et al. 1972; Thacore and Shukla 1976). The brain contains two endogenous cannabinoid receptor (CB_1) ligands, anandamide and 2-arachidonoylglycerol. Localization of CB_1 system in cortical and limbic brain areas suggests its possible role in neurocognitive deficits and behavior functions in schizophrenia (Emrich et al. 1997). Moreover, CB1 closely interacts with the dopaminergic system, which is implicated in schizophrenia pathology.

CLINICAL IMPLICATIONS

Clinical implications of the type of phospholipid pathology may also represent a very broad range of symptoms, with varying degree of severity and course, which are general characteristics of schizophrenia. Each patient may represent a unique phenotype based on the molecular diversity of phospholipid pathology combined with pathophysiological heterogeneity and their susceptibility to further change with the influence of environmental factors. Further support for these studies will be based on the reduced clinical severity by dietary supplementation of antioxidants and EPUFAs (see subsection "Therapeutic Implications" later in this chapter).

Psychopathology/Outcome

Christinsen and Christinsen (1988) first reported an association between clinical outcome (severity of symptomatology and course) and the intake of dietary fat (discussed previously). Patients with dietary intake of fat from fish and vegetables (rich in n-3 EPUFAs and antioxidants) had better outcomes compared with those of patients with dietary intake of fat from farmed animals (poor in n-3 EPUFAs and antioxidants and higher in calories). Subsequently, Glen and colleagues (1994) reported that the reduced RBC AA and DHA were present in patients with predominant negative symptoms (typical of poor outcome) but not in patients with positive symptoms. Peet and colleagues (1995) also showed that the dietary intake of EPUFAs was correlated with levels of RBC EPUFAs and the severity of psychopathology. One study has reported a significant relationship between AA or DHA and degree of symptom severity in early psychotic never-medicated and medicated-chronic patients with schizophrenia (Arvindakshan et al. 2003b). Further investigations are needed to clarify whether AA has a role in the development, illness presentation, and treatment of schizophrenia and related disorders.

Abnormal Involuntary Movements: Tardive Dyskinesia

There is evidence that movement disorders are part of the psychotic disorders and that older (atypical) antipsychotics exacerbate these, particularly tardive dyskinesia (TD) (American Psychiatric Association 1980; McCreadie et al. 1995). This finding suggested the role for reduced EPUFAs in TD. Decreased platelet membrane fluidity in TD patients (Zubenko and Cohen 1986) was an initial indirect piece of evidence. Vaddadi and colleagues (1989) subsequently found that psychiatric patients with TD (mostly schizophrenia) had lower n-6 and n-3 fatty acid levels in RBCs than patients without TD. Additionally, the magnitude of the decrease in PUFAs increased as TD severity increased. Peet and colleagues (1993) found that TD patients had higher levels of plasma lipid peroxides and lower RBC EPUFAs than non-TD patients did. A more recent finding indicates that newer (atypical) antipsychotics that do not induce oxidative stress and increase lipid peroxides in rat brain also do not induce extrapyramidal symptoms (Parikh et al. 2002).

It was hypothesized that these differences in EPUFA levels in the TD subpopulation were caused by dietary factors, drug therapy, and hospitalization status (Vaddadi et al. 1989). Although it is unclear as to the mechanism or connection between these findings and schizophrenia, there is now evidence that low plasma AA levels are associated with increased risk for dyskinesias in the general elderly population (Nilsson et al. 1996).

Pediatric Behavioral, Neurological, and Language Disorders

Several pediatric behavioral, neurological, and language disorders, such as dyslexia (Richardson et al. 2003), autism, and Asperger's syndrome (Bell et al. 2003), and attention-deficit/hyperactivity disorders (Arnold et al. 1994; Burgess and Stevens 2003) have been found to be associated with altered levels of phospholipids EPUFAs. Some of these disorders are associated with increased risk for subsequent development of adult psychotic disorders (Keshavan et al. 2003b). Dyslexia is a developmental disorder that is marked by visual dysfunction and difficulties in learning to read and write. It has been noted that dyslexia is associated with increased schizotypal personality features and shares many of the neuropsychological features of schizophrenia, including language, attentional, and working memory deficits (Maher 1991; Richardson 1994). Initial studies in a small group of schizophrenic patients have shown impaired electroretinogram in patients with reduced levels of RBC DHA (Peet et al. 2003). Likewise, receptive language difficulties have been observed repeatedly in both schizophrenic patients and in the siblings of individuals with schizophrenia spectrum disorder (Condray et al. 2002). It is possible that because these disorders are also found to be associated with increased risk for subsequent development of adult psychotic disorders (Keshavan et al. 2003a), these illnesses are related, albeit qualitatively different, and represent a continuum of membrane/phospholipid spectrum disorders.

Decreased Niacin-Induced Flushing

It is well known that the B vitamin niacin (nicotinic acid) induces a flushing response on the skin when orally administered at high doses. The molecular mechanism involves the niacin receptor–mediated release of AA, which is subsequently converted into prostaglandin D_2 (PGD_2) by cyclooxygenase. PGD_2 induces vasodilation and increased blood flow (Morrow et al. 1989). Therefore, schizophrenia patients with reduced levels of AA will have decreased niacin-induced flushing. It has been known for several decades that the majority of schizophrenia patients with predominantly negative symptoms, who have consistent reduced levels of AA and DHA, fail to flush when given oral doses of niacin, particularly those who exhibit low levels of AA (Horrobin 1980; Waldo 2003).

THERAPEUTIC IMPLICATIONS

Investigating PUFAs metabolism has proved fruitful for generating and testing novel etiological hypotheses and

new therapeutic agents for schizophrenia (Fenton et al. 2000). Oxidative stress–mediated peroxidation and availability and use of EFAs (linoleic acid and ALA, precursors of AA and DHA, respectively) can influence the phospholipids-EPUFA metabolism. It is conceivable that such membrane perturbations occur at early stages of illness and continue and perhaps worsen during the course of schizophrenia. Supplementation of antioxidants and EPUFAs may thus provide an alternative approach to examining the clinical relevance of PUFA deficits in schizophrenia.

Evidence indicates that the dysregulation of phospholipid metabolism may be related primarily to availability and/or metabolism of EPUFAs in patients with schizophrenia. Studies for the past 50 years have shown that disorders associated with EPUFA deficits can be prevented, and some of the cellular pathophysiologies can be corrected, by proper supplementation in the diet. Supplementation with antioxidants such as vitamins A and C and beta-carotene alone can prevent the loss of membrane EPUFAs and restore part of the EPUFAs. However, supplementation with a combination of antioxidants and EPUFAs may be preferred for more effective correction of EPUFA deficits. Also, because neuroleptics are still the drugs of choice for the effective control of psychosis, the most serious symptom of schizophrenia, adjunctive treatment with antioxidants and EPUFAs may prove important in the early course and outcome of schizophrenia and in the reduction of serious comorbidities.

Factors Influencing the Efficacy of Dietary PUFA Supplementation

Previous studies in EPUFA or antioxidant supplementation were carried out mainly in patients with chronic schizophrenia who had been treated with a variety of typical and/or atypical antipsychotic drugs. Several important issues concerning clinical design should be addressed.

Age and duration of illness.   It is generally accepted that antioxidant defense declines and EPUFA degradation increases in subjects with age over 55 years, and the duration of illness and antipsychotic treatment may also contribute to increased membrane pathology. Fenton and colleagues (2001), who did not find any therapeutic improvement in patients with chronic schizophrenia after EPA supplementation, have suggested that such treatment may be beneficial in younger patients at their early stages of illness (Fenton et al. 2000).

Source of EPUFA and antioxidants.   Recently, dietary supplementation with EPA, a precursor of DHA, has shown promising results in decreasing some of the clinical symptoms of schizophrenia (Peet et al. 2001; Puri et al. 2000; Richardson et al. 2000) and improving cognitive performance in patients with dyslexia and attention-deficit/hyperactivity disorder (Richardson et al. 2003). Alternatively, a mixture of EPA and DHA supplements may also be used to correct PUFA deficits (Arvindakshan et al. 2003a). On the other hand, both vitamins E and C are needed to provide antioxidant defense in membrane and cytosol, respectively.

Dosage. It is known that high doses of EPUFAs, if not balanced with dietary antioxidants, may increase levels of toxic peroxides (Rafalowska et al. 1989). Recent data indicate that the dose of 2 g of EPA alone or 180:120 mg EPA:DHA three times per day may be adequate. The dosage for vitamins E and C may be 400 IU and 500 mg, respectively, twice per day.

Caloric intake. The dose of both EPUFAs and antioxidants depends very much on the patient's dietary intake and total caloric intake, because caloric intake of greater than 2,600 calories is known to increase the EPUFA peroxidative breakdown.

Duration of treatment. Earlier studies suggested that supplementation for at least 4 months is required to restore RBC as well as brain membrane EPUFAs to steady-state levels (Mahadik and Evans 1997). However, one study demonstrated that supplementation with EPA had therapeutic effects within a few weeks, indicating a possible indirect role for EPA or for its metabolites (Peet et al. 2001).

Adjunctive medication. Typical antipsychotics such as haloperidol have pro-oxidant properties (Jedding et al. 1995), whereas some atypical antipsychotics may have neuroprotective effects against oxidative cell injury by way of increased AODS (Parikh et al. 2002). These medications can also affect EPUFA metabolism (Horrobin et al. 1994). Thus newer atypical antipsychotics not only have antioxidant effects but also improve membrane EPUFA levels (Horrobin 1999; Khan et al. 2002; Mahadik et al. 2003a).

Placebo control. Because all psychiatric disorders show a significant placebo effect on symptom reduction, well-designed placebo-controlled, dose-ranging studies would be critical for determining the therapeutic effects (Peet and Horrobin 2002).

Supplementation of Antioxidants

A total of 14 studies have been done using primarily vitamin E (800–1,600 IU daily) supplement in chronic schizophrenic patients with TD (Adler et al. 1999; Mahadik

and Gowda 1996; Reddy and Yao 1996). All but two studies (Adler et al. 1999; Shriqui et al. 1992) have found vitamin E to be beneficial in controlling some symptoms of TD and psychopathology. These studies have clearly indicated that vitamin E (800–1,600 IU daily) is efficacious if given to patients younger than 45 years and within 5 years of onset of TD. This observation has been interpreted as indicating that the use of antioxidant supplements may prevent the deteriorating course at early stages of illness (Mahadik and Gowda 1996; Mahadik and Scheffer 1996; Peet et al. 1993; Reddy and Yao 2003).

Supplementation of Essential Fatty Acids

Specific findings from the most recent studies with supplementation of only EPA and/or DHA are described here. Findings from a dose-ranging study using ethyl-EPA (placebo, 1, 2, or 4 g/day for 12 weeks) in patients with persistent schizophrenia symptoms taking clozapine or another atypical antipsychotic (olanzapine, risperidone, or quetiapine) or one of the typical psychotics have been published (Peet and Horrobin 2002). Placebo consisted of 4 g/day of liquid paraffin and had no complications, since liquid paraffin has been used up to 15–30 g/day as a laxative. No serious adverse effects were reported. It was concluded that 2 g/day had the maximum therapeutic effect. However, patients taking typical antipsychotics and new atypical drugs did not show improvement over that seen with the patients receiving placebo, who showed very significant improvements from baseline. The clozapine group had very little placebo effect, and therefore responses to the 2-g dose of ethyl-EPA were substantially better than placebo. The elevated levels of membrane EPA or DHA did not show correlation with clinical improvements, but levels of AA did show strong correlation. The authors explained this finding as an inhibition of AA incorporation by ethyl-EPA in membranes. However, ethyl-EPA is a potent inhibitor of PLA_2 that may upset some of the effects on AA. Because these studies found a therapeutic effect of 2 g ethyl-EPA in a small group of patients, further work is needed to explore the full therapeutically potential EPUFAs.

Finally, because most of the published studies that have reported therapeutic effects of EPUFA supplementation in schizophrenia have been done by a small group of investigators, it will be important to have replication studies done by many other investigators. It may even be preferable to do multinational studies, in which patients differ significantly in their racial background, lifestyle, socioeconomic status, and dietary patterns because all of these factors have a significant influence on membrane phospholipid EPUFA metabolism.

Supplementation of a Combination of Antioxidants and EPUFAs

As was discussed previously, increased oxidative stress–mediated EPUA peroxidative degradation, as well as defective phospholipid EPUFA metabolism, exists in schizophrenia, so the use of a combination of EPUFAs and antioxidants (e.g., vitamins E and C) for supplementation may be preferable (Mahadik et al. 2001). Antioxidants have been found to be very effective in protecting membrane EPUFAs in addition to preventing oxidative damage of vital cellular proteins, mitochondria, and DNA. Earlier studies also used only vitamin E, and supplementation with vitamin C, an effective intracellular antioxidant, has not yet been tried.

One study reported the effects of 4-month supplementation of a combination of EPA:DHA (360:240) and vitamins E:C (800 IU:1 g) per day in two equal doses in 34 chronic schizophrenic patients whose medication (both typical and atypical antipsychotics) had been stabilized (Arvindakshan et al. 2003a). All the patients showed over 25% reductions in most of the psychopathological scores, and these effects were significantly sustained up to 4 months after termination of supplementation. This study, though, did not have a placebo group. However, the membrane EPA and DHA levels were elevated from baseline to equal or even slightly higher than those in matched control subjects without any change in the plasma lipid peroxides. This outcome indicated that low-dose EPUFA treatment is adequate to correct the preexisting membrane EPUFA deficits and probably antioxidants prevented the degradation. Pretreatment AA levels were similar to those in control subjects, being significantly reduced at posttreatment and returning to pretreatment levels after 4 months of termination of supplementation. This finding suggests that supplementation of omega-3 EPUFAs such as EPA alone (Peet and Horrobin 2002), or a mixture of EPA and DHA as in this study, probably reduces AA incorporation in membranes by competition.

Further placebo-controlled supplementation studies with a combination of EPUFAs (EPA+DHA) and a mixture of vitamins E and C should be preferably considered. Although EPA is found to be effective in reducing some symptoms, it is not a major membrane fatty acid. Levels of its metabolites such as eicosanoids may increase at high doses. These metabolites have not been found to be therapeutic and may have some unwanted effects. Also, the reduction of membrane AA levels either by competition for incorporation or by inhibition of PLA_2 is not good idea. Normal levels of membrane AA and PLA_2 are critical for membrane receptor–mediated signal transduction of several neurotransmitters and growth factors in schizophrenia.

CONCLUSION

We do not wish to detract from the importance of developing safer and more efficient antipsychotics. However, it is tempting to suggest that the dietary supplementation of antioxidants and n-3 fatty acids with current conventional pharmacotherapy may be timely. The current therapy is very limited in reducing the negative symptoms and improving cognitive performance and in slowing down the deteriorating course of illness to improve clinical outcome with acceptable quality of life of patients. Nevertheless, for effective augmentation with these supplements, the knowledge of the molecular nature of abnormal phospholipid-EPUFA metabolism and its relationship to the degree of psychopathology within subjects is still missing. This lack of knowledge about the relationship between abnormal phospholipid-EPUFA metabolism and psychopathology is partly a result of the large number of factors involved in phospholipid metabolism, some of which are very difficult to control for, and partly due to the molecular diversity of phospholipids.

There is also need for a study involving a large number of drug-naive first-episode patients and well-matched control subjects that controls for dietary and socioeconomic status in addition to usual age, gender, and ethnic origin—a very difficult undertaking in a community setup. This may be partly possible in cohorts from U.S. Army personnel or better yet in cohorts in countries, such as India and China, in which the population is racially homogeneous, reasonably stable, and has similar lifestyles. Furthermore, it is important to establish the relationship between biochemical indices of oxidative stress and oxidative phospholipid-EPUFA degradation, and psychopathology at baseline and intermittently over a 2-year follow-up period. It is also necessary to investigate the effects of current medications on these indices. Regarding the molecular nature of pathology, although evidence points to the involvement of endogenous antioxidant enzyme genes, phospholipases, fatty acid carrier proteins, and desaturases, systematic studies are warranted.

Another important issue is the time of initiation of pathology. If it has prenatal origin, it may be important to have dietary supplementation during this period. The benefits of supplementation in adults may be limited because the adult brain may be difficult to remodel.

REFERENCES

Adler LA, Rotrosen J, Edson R, et al: Vitamin E treatment for tardive dyskinesia: Veterans Affairs Cooperative Study #394 Study Group. Arch Gen Psychiatry 56:836–841, 1999

American Psychiatric Association: Tardive Dyskinesia: A Task Force Report of the American Psychiatric Association. Washington, DC, American Psychiatric Association, 1980

Arnold LE, Kleykamp D, Votolato N, et al: Potential link between dietary intake of fatty acids and behavior: pilot exploration of serum lipids in attention-deficit hyperactivity disorder. J Child Adolesc Psychopharmacol 4:171–182, 1994

Arnold SE, Trojanowski JQ, Gur RE, et al: Absence of neurodegenerative and neural injury in the cerebral cortex in a sample of elderly patients with schizophrenia. Arch Gen Psychiatry 55:225–232, 1998

Arvindakshan M, Ghate M, Ranjekar PK, et al: Supplementation with a combination of omega-3 fatty acids and antioxidants (vitamins E and C) improves the outcome of schizophrenia. Schizophr Res 62:195–204, 2003a

Arvindakshan M, Sitasawad S, Debsikdar V, et al: Membrane essential polyunsaturated fatty acids (EPUFA) and schizophrenia outcome: EPUFA and lipid peroxide levels in never-medicated and medicated schizophrenics. Biol Psychiatry 53:56–64, 2003b

Axelrod J: Receptor-mediated activation of phospholipase A2 and arachidonic acid release in signal transduction. Biochem Soc Trans 18:503–507, 1990

Bazan NG: Eicosanoids, platelet-activating factor and inflammation, in Basic Neurochemistry: Molecular, Cellular, and Medical Aspects. Edited by Siegel GJ, Agranoff BW, Albers WR, et al. New York, Lippincott-Raven, 1999, pp 731–741

Bartzokis G, Nuechterlein KH, Lu PH, et al: Dysregulated brain development in adult men with schizophrenia: a magnetic resonance imaging study. Biol Psychiatry 53:412–421, 2003

Bell JG, Dick JR, MacKinlay EE, et al: Abnormal fatty acid metabolism in autism and Asperger's syndrome, in Phospholipid Spectrum Disorders in Psychiatry and Neurology. Edited by Peet M, Glen I, Horrobin D. Carnforth, UK, Marius Press, 2003, pp 521–528

Benowitz LI, Routtenberg A: GAP-43: an intrinsic determinant of neuronal development and plasticity. Trends Neurosci 20:84–91, 1997

Berridge MJ, Irvine RF: Inositol triphosphate, a novel second messenger in cellular signal transduction. Nature 312:315–321, 1984

Bersani G, Iannitelli A, Maselli P, et al: Low nerve growth factor plasma levels in schizophrenic patients: a preliminary study. Schizophr Res 37:197–203, 1999.

Bourre JM, Bonneil M, Chaudiere J, et al: Structural and functional importance of dietary polyunsaturated fatty acids in the nervous system. Adv Exp Med Biol 318:211–229, 1992

Brown S, Birtwistle J, Roi L, et al: The unhealthy lifestyle of people with schizophrenia. Psychol Med 29:697–701, 1999

Burgess JR, Kuo CF: Increased calcium-dependent phospholipase A2 activity in vitamin E, and selenium-deficient rat lung, liver and spleen cytosol is time-dependent and reversible. J Nutr Biochem 7:366–374, 1996

Burgess JR, Stevens LJ: Essential fatty acids in relation to attention deficit hyperactivity disorder: an update, in Phospholipid Spectrum Disorders in Psychiatry and Neurology. Edited by Peet M, Glen I, Horrobin D. Carnforth, UK, Marius Press, 2003, pp 511–520

Cadet JL, Kahler LA: Free radical mechanisms in schizophrenia and tardive dyskinesia. Neurosci Biobehav Rev 18:457–467, 1994

Cadet JL, Lohr JB: Free radicals and the developmental pathology of schizophrenic burnout. Integrative Psychiatry 5:40–48, 1987

Cannon M, Jones P, Gilvarry C, et al: Premorbid social functioning in schizophrenia and bipolar disorder: similarities and differences. Am J Psychiatry 154:1544–1550, 1997

Carlson SE, Rhodes PG, Ferguson MG, et al: Docosahexaenoic acid status of preterm infants at birth and following feeding with human milk or formula. Am J Clin Nutr 44:798–804, 1986

Carpenter WT Jr, Buchanan RW: Schizophrenia. N Engl J Med 330:681–690, 1994

Catts VS, Catts SV: Review: Apoptosis and schizophrenia: is the tumor suppressor gene, p53, a candidate susceptibility gene? Schizophr Res 41:405–415, 2000

Chakraborti S: Phospholipase A_2 isoforms: a perspective. Cell Signaling 15:637–665, 2003

Christinsen O, Christinsen E: Fat consumption and schizophrenia. Acta Psychiat Scand 78:587–591, 1988

Condray R, Steinhauer SR, van Kammen DP, et al: The language system in schizophrenia: effects of capacity and linguistic structure. Schizophr Bull 28:475–490, 2002

Connor WE, Neuringer M, Lin DS: Dietary effects on brain fatty acid composition: the reversibility of n-3 fatty acid deficiency and turnover of docosahexaenoic acid in the brain, erythrocytes, and plasma of rhesus monkeys. J Lipid Res 31:237–247, 1990

Craig TJ, Siegel C, Hopper K, et al: Outcome in schizophrenia and related disorders compared between developing and developed countries. Br J Psychiatry 170:229–233, 1997

Das I, Essali MA, deBelleroche J, et al: Inositol phospholipid turnover in platelet of schizophrenic patients. Prostaglandins Leukot Essent Fatty Acids 46:65–66, 1992

Davis KL, Buchsbaum MS, Shihabuddin L, et al: Ventricular enlargement in poor-outcome schizophrenia. Biol Psychiatry 43:783–793, 1998

Davis KL, Stewart DG, Friedman JI, et al: White matter changes in schizophrenia: evidence for myelin-related dysfunction. Arch Gen Psychiatry 60:443–456, 2003

Degreef G, Ashtari M, Bogerts B, et al: Volumes of ventricular system subdivisions measured from magnetic resonance images in first-episode schizophrenic patients. Arch Gen Psychiatry 49:531–537, 1992

DeLisi LE, Hoff A, Kushner M, et al: Ventricular enlargement at the onset of psychosis is associated with diagnostic outcome. Biol Psychiatry 32:199–201, 1992

Demisch L, Heinz K, Gerbaldo H, et al: Increased concentrations of phosphatidylinositol and decreased esterification of arachidonic acid into phospholipids in platelets from patients with schizoaffective disorders or atypic phasic psychoses. Prostaglandins Leukot Essent Fatty Acids 46:47–52, 1992

Eaton WW: The epidemiology of schizophrenia, in Handbook of Studies on Schizophrenia, Part 1: Epidemiology, Etiology, and Clinical Features. Edited by Burrows GD, Norman TC, Rubinstein G. Amsterdam, Elsevier, 1986, pp 11–33

Emrich HM, Leweke FM, Schneider U: Towards a cannabinoid hypothesis of schizophrenia: cognitive impairments due to dysregulation of the endogenous cannabinoid system. Pharmacol Biochem Behav 56:803–807, 1997

Ernster I: Lipid peroxidation in biological membranes: mechanisms and implications, in Active Oxygen Species, Lipid Peroxides, and Antioxidants. Edited by Yagi K. Tokyo, CRC Press, 1993, pp 11–38

Essali MA, Das R, de Belleroche J, et al: The platelet polyphosphoinositide system in schizophrenia: the effects of neuroleptic treatment. Biol Psychiatry 28:478–487, 1990

Evans DR, Parikh VV, Khan MM, et al: Red blood cell membrane essential fatty acid metabolism in early psychotic patients following antipsychotic drug treatment. Prostaglandins Leukot Essent Fatty Acids 69:393–399, 2003

Fenton WS, Hibbeln J, Knable M, et al: Essential fatty acids, lipid membrane abnormalities, and the diagnosis and treatment of schizophrenia. Biol Psychiatry 47:8–21, 2000

Fenton WS, Dickerson F, Boronow J, et al: A placebo controlled trial of omega-3 fatty acids (ethyl eicosapentaenoic acid) supplementation for residual symptoms and cognitive impairment in schizophrenia. Am J Psychiatry 158:2071–2074, 2001

Fergusson DM, Woodward LJ, Horwood LJ: Maternal smoking during pregnancy and psychiatric adjustment in late adolescence. Arch Gen Psychiatry 55:721–727, 1998

Findley JBG, Evans WH (eds): Biological Membranes: A Practical Approach. Ithaca, NY, IRL Press, 1990

Fish B, Marcus J, Hans S, et al: Infants at risk for schizophrenia: sequelae of a genetic neurointegrative defect. Arch Gen Psychiatry 49:221–235, 1992

Fukuzako H, Fukuzako T, Takeuchi K, et al: Phosphorus magnetic resonance spectroscopy in schizophrenia: correlation between membrane PL metabolism in the temporal lobe and positive symptoms. Prog Neuropsychopharmacol Biol Psychiatry 20:629–640, 1996

Gattaz WF, Hubner CK, Nevalainen TJ, et al: Increased serum phospholipase A2 activity in schizophrenia: a replication study. Biol Psychiatry 28:495–501, 1990

Glantz LA, Lewis DA: Decreased dendritic spine density on prefrontal cortical pyramidal neurons in schizophrenia. Arch Gen Psychiatry 57:65–73, 2000

Glen AIM, Glen EMT, Horrobin DF, et al: A red cell membrane abnormality in a subgroup of schizophrenic patients: evidence for two diseases. Schizophr Res 12:53–61, 1994

Gupta S, Andreasen NC, Arndt S, et al: Neurological soft signs in neuroleptic-naive and neuroleptic treated schizophrenic patients and normal comparison subjects. Am J Psychiatry 152:191–196, 1995

Halikas JA, Goodwin DW, Guze SB: Marijuana use and psychiatric illness. Arch Gen Psychiatry 27:162–165, 1972

Halliwell B: Reactive oxygen species and the central nervous system. J Neurochem 59:1609–1623, 1992

Heckers S: Neuropathology of schizophrenia: cortex, thalamus, basal ganglia, and neurotransmitter-specific projection system. Schizophr Bull 23:403–421, 1997

Hegarty JD, Baldessarini RJ, Tohen M, et al: One hundred years of schizophrenia: a meta-analysis of the outcome literature. Am J Psychiatry 151:1409–1416, 1994

Hibbeln JR, Makino KK, Martin CE, et al: Smoking, gender, and dietary influences on erythrocyte essential fatty acid composition among patients with schizophrenia or schizoaffective disorder. Biol Psychiatry 53:431–441, 2003

Hoek HW, Brown AS, Susser E, et al: The Dutch famine and schizophrenia spectrum disorders. Soc Psychiatry Psychiatr Epidemiol 33:373–379, 1998

Hoffer A, Osmond H, Smythies J: Schizophrenia: a new approach. J Ment Sci 100:29–52, 1954

Horrobin DF: Schizophrenia as a prostaglandin deficiency disease. Lancet 1:936–937, 1977

Horrobin DF: Niacin flushing, prostaglandin E and evening primrose oil: a possible objective test for monitoring therapy in schizophrenia. J Orthomolec Psychiatry 9:33–34, 1980

Horrobin DF: Schizophrenia as a membrane lipid disorder, which is expressed throughout the body. Prostaglandins Leukot Essent Fatty Acids 55:3–8, 1996

Horrobin DF: The membrane phospholipid hypothesis as a biochemical basis for the neurodevelopmental concept of schizophrenia. Schizophr Res 30:193–208, 1998

Horrobin DF: The effects of antipsychotic drugs on membrane phospholipids: a possible novel mechanism of action of clozapine, in Phospholipid Spectrum Disorders in Psychiatry. Edited by Horrobin D, Glen AL, Peet M. Carnforth, UK, Marius Press, 1999, pp 113–117

Horrobin DF, Manku MS, Hillman S, et al: Fatty acid levels in brains of schizophrenics and normal controls. Biol Psychiatry 30:795–805, 1991

Horrobin DF, Glen AIM, Vaddadi KS, et al: The membrane hypothesis of schizophrenia. Schizophr Res 13:195–208, 1994

Horrocks LA, Ansell GB, Porcellati G (eds): Phospholipids in the Nervous System, Vol 1: Metabolism. New York, Raven, 1982

Hudson CJ, Young LT, Li PP, et al: CNS signal transduction in the pathophysiology and pharmacology of affective disorders and schizophrenia. Synapse 13:278–293, 1993

Hulshoff Pol HE, Hoek HW, Susser E, et al: Prenatal exposure to famine and brain morphology in schizophrenia. Am J Psychiatry 157:1170–1172, 2000

Jablensky A, Sartorius N, Ernberg G, et al: Schizophrenia: manifestations, incidence and course in different cultures. Psychol Med Monogr Suppl 20:1–97, 1991

Jaskiw GE, Juliano DM, Goldberg TE, et al: Cerebral ventricular enlargement in schizophreniform disorder does not progress: a seven year follow-up study. Schizophr Res 14:23–28, 1994

Jedding I, Evans PJ, Akanmu D, et al: Characterization of the potential antioxidant and pro-oxidant actions of some neuroleptic drugs. Biochem Pharmacol 49:359–365, 1995

Jope RS, Song L, Grimes CA, et al: Selective increases in phosphoinositide signaling activity and G protein levels in postmortem brain from subjects with schizophrenia or alcohol dependence. J Neurochem 70:763–771, 1998

Kaiya H, Nishida A, Imai A, et al: Accumulation of diacylglycerol in platelet phosphoinositides turnover in schizophrenia: a biological marker of good prognosis? Biol Psychiatry 26:669–676, 1989

Kane JM, Marder SR: Psychopharmacologic treatment of schizophrenia. Schizophr Bull 19:287–302, 1993

Katila H, Appleberg B, Rimon R: No differences in phospholipase-A2 activity between acute psychiatric patients and controls. Schizophr Res 26:103–105, 1997

Keshavan MS, Mallinger AG, Pettegrew JW, et al: Erythrocyte membrane phospholipids in psychotic patients. Psychiatry Res 49:9–95, 1993

Keshavan MS, Anderson S, Pettegrew JW: Is schizophrenia due to excessive synaptic pruning in the prefrontal cortex? The Feinberg hypothesis revisited. J Psychiatric Res 28:239–265, 1994

Keshavan MS, Stanley JA, Montrose DM, et al: Prefrontal membrane phospholipid metabolism of child and adolescent offspring at risk for schizophrenia or schizoaffective disorder: an in vivo ^{31}P MRS study. Mol Psychiatry 8:316–323, 2003a

Keshavan MS, Sujata A, Mehra M, et al: Psychosis proneness and ADHD in young relatives of schizophrenia patients. Schizophr Res 59:85–92, 2003b

Khan A, Khan SR, Leventhal RM: Symptom reduction and suicide risk among treated with placebo in antipsychotic clinical trials: an analysis of the Food and Drug Administration database. Am J Psychiatry 158:1449–1454, 2001

Khan MM, Evans DR, Gunna V, et al: Reduced erythrocyte membrane essential fatty acids and increased lipid peroxides in schizophrenia at the never-medicated first-episode of psychosis and after years of treatment with antipsychotics. Schizophr Res 58:1–10, 2002

Khan MM, Parikh V, Mahadik SP: Antipsychotic drugs differentially modulate apolipoprotein D in rat brain. J Neurochemistry 86:1089–1100, 2003

Lane A, Kinsella A, Murphy P, et al: The anthropometric assessment of dysmorphic features in schizophrenia as an index of its developmental origins. Psychol Med 27:1155–1172, 1997

Lawrie SM, Abukmeil SS: Brain abnormality in schizophrenia: a systematic and quantitative review of volumetric magnetic resonance imaging studies. Br J Psychiatry 172:119–120, 1998

Leon JD: Smoking and vulnerability for schizophrenia. Schizophr Bull 22:405–409, 1996

Lieberman JA, Koreen AR: Neurochemistry and neuroendocrinology of schizophrenia: a selective review. Schizophr Bull 19:371–429, 1993

Lieberman J, Bogerts B, Degreef G, et al: Qualitative assessment of brain morphology in acute and chronic schizophrenia. Am J Psychiatry 149:784–794, 1992

Liday LA, Pippenger CE, Howard AA, et al: Free radical scavenging enzyme activity and related trace metals in clozapine-induced agranulocytosis: a pilot study. J Clin Psychopharmacology 15:353–360, 1995

Mahadik SP, Evans D: Essential fatty acids in the treatment of schizophrenia. Drugs Today 33:5–17, 1997

Mahadik SP, Gowda S: Antioxidants in the treatment of schizophrenia. Drugs Today 32:1–13, 1996

Mahadik SP, Mukherjee S: Free radical pathology and the antioxidant defense in schizophrenia. Schizophr Res 19:1–18, 1996

Mahadik SP, Scheffer RE: Oxidative injury and potential use of antioxidants in schizophrenia. Prostaglandins Leukot Essent Fatty Acids 55:45–54, 1996

Mahadik SP, Mukherjee S, Correnti E, et al: Distribution of plasma membrane phospholipids and cholesterol in skin fibroblasts from drug-naive patients at the onset of psychosis. Schizophr Res 13:239–247, 1994

Mahadik SP, Mukherjee S, Horrobin D, et al: Plasma membrane phospholipid fatty acid composition of cultured skin fibroblasts from schizophrenic patients: comparison with bipolar and normal controls. Psychiatry Res 63:133–142, 1996a

Mahadik SP, Shendarkar NS, Scheffer R, et al: Utilization of precursor essential fatty acids in culture by skin fibroblasts from schizophrenic patients and normal controls. Prostaglandins Leukot Essent Fatty Acids 55:65–70, 1996b

Mahadik SP, Mukherjee S, Correnti E, et al: Elevated plasma lipid peroxides at the onset of nonaffective psychosis. Biol Psychiatry 43:674–679, 1998

Mahadik SP, Mulchandani M, Hegde MV, et al: Cultural and socioeconomic differences in dietary intake of essential fatty acids and antioxidants-effects on the outcome, in Phospholipid Spectrum Disorders in Psychiatry. Edited by Horrobin D, Glen AL, Peet M. Carnforth, UK, Marius Press, 1999a, pp 167–179

Mahadik SP, Sitasawad V, Mulchandani M: Membrane peroxidation and the neuropathology of Schizophrenia, in Phospholipid Spectrum Disorders in Psychiatry. Edited by Horrobin D, Glen AL, Peet M. Carnforth, UK, Marius Press, 1999b, pp 99–111

Mahadik SP, Evans D, Lal H: Oxidative stress and the role of antioxidant and omega-3 essential fatty acid supplementation in schizophrenia. Prog Neuropsychopharmacol Biol Psychiatry 25:463–493, 2001

Mahadik SP, Khan MM, Evans DR, et al: Elevated plasma level of apolipoprotein D in schizophrenia and its treatment and outcome. Schizophr Res 58:55–62, 2002

Mahadik SP, Khan MM, Parikh V: Effects of antipsychotic drugs on rat brain, and on essential fatty acids in the erythrocytes of schizophrenic patients: implications of outcome, in Phospholipid Spectrum Disorders in Psychiatry and Neurology. Edited by Peet M, Glen I, Horrobin D. Carnforth, UK, Marius Press, 2003a, pp 289–298

Mahadik SP, Parikh V, Khan MM: The role of oxidative stress in modulating membrane and phospholipid function in schizophrenia, in Phospholipid Spectrum Disorders in Psychiatry and Neurology. Edited by Peet M, Glen I, Horrobin D. Carnforth, UK, Marius Press, 2003b, pp 277–288

Maher BA: Language and schizophrenia, in Handbook of Schizophrenia: Neuropsychology, Psychophysiology, and Information Processing, Vol 5. Edited by Steinhauer SR, Gruzelier JH, Zubin J. Amsterdam, Elsevier, 1991, pp 437–464

Margolis RL, Chung D-M, Post RM: Programmed cell death: implications for neuropsychiatric disorders. Biol Psychiatry 35:946–956, 1994

McCreadie RG: The Nithsdale Schizophrenia Surveys 16: breast-feeding and schizophrenia: preliminary results and hypothesis. Br J Psychiatry 170:234–237, 1997

McCreadie RG, MacDonald E, Wiles D, et al: The Nithsdale Schizophrenia Surveys 14: plasma lipid peroxide and serum vitamin E levels in patients with and without tardive dyskinesia and in normal subjects. Br J Psychiatry 167:1–8, 1995

McIntyre RS, McCann SM, Kennedy SH: Antipsychotic metabolic effects: weight gain, diabetes mellitus and lipid abnormalities. Can J Psychiatry 46:272–281, 2001

Mednick SA, Machon RA, Huttunen MO: Adult schizophrenia following prenatal exposure to an influenza epidemic. Arch Gen Psychiatry 45:189–192, 1988

Morrow J, Parsons W, Roberts L: Release of markedly increased quantities of prostaglandin D2 in vivo in humans following the administration of nicotinic acid. Prostaglandins 38:263–274, 1989

Morrow JD, Frei B, Longmire AW, et al: Increase in circulating products of lipid peroxidation (F2-isoprostanes) in smokers: smoking as a cause of oxidative damage. N Engl J Med 332:1198–1203, 1995

Mukherjee S, Mahadik SP, Correnti EE, et al: The antioxidant defense system at the onset of psychosis. Schizophr Res 19:19–26, 1996

Nair TR, Christensen JD, Kingsbury SJ, ct al: Progression of cerebroventricular enlargement and the subtyping of schizophrenia. Psychiatry Res 74:141–150, 1997

Neuringer M, Connor WE, Lin DS, et al: Biochemical and functional effect of prenatal and postnatal omega-3 fatty acid deficiency on retina and brain in rhesus monkeys. Proc Natl Acad Sci U S A 83:4021–4025, 1986

Nigam S, Scheve T: Phospholipase A2s and lipid peroxidation. Biochim Biophys Acta 1488:167–181, 2000

Nilsson A, Horrobin DF, Rosengren A, et al: Essential fatty acids and abnormal involuntary movements in the general male population: a study of men born in 1933. Prostaglandins Leukot Essent Fatty Acids 55:83–87, 1996

Nishizuka Y: Intracellular signaling by hydrolysis of phospholipids and activation of protein kinase C. Science 258:607–614, 1992

Noponen M, Sanfilipo M, Samanich K, et al: Elevated PLA2 activity in schizophrenics and other psychiatric patients. Biol Psychiatry 34:641–649, 1993

O'Brien JS, Samson EL: Lipid composition of the normal human brain: gray matter, white matter, and myelin. J Lipid Res 6:537–544, 1965

Parikh V, Khan MM, Mahadik SP: Differential effects of antipsychotics on expression of antioxidant enzymes and membrane lipid peroxidation in rat brain. J Psychiatr Res 37:43–51, 2002

Parikh V, Evans DR, Khan MM, et al: Nerve growth factor levels in never medicated first episode psychotic patients and medicated chronic schizophrenic patients. Schizophr Res 60:117–123, 2003

Peet M, Horrobin DF: In association with the E-E Multicenter Study Group: a dose-ranging exploratory study of the effects of ethyl-eicosapentaenoate in patients with persistent schizophrenic symptoms. J Psychiatric Res 36:7–18, 2002

Peet M, Laugharne J, Rangarajan N, et al: Tardive dyskinesia, lipid peroxidation, and sustained amelioration with vitamin E treatment. Int Clin Psychopharmacol 8:151–153, 1993

Peet M, Laugharne J, Rangarajan N, et al: Depleted red cell membrane essential fatty acid in drug treated schizophrenic patients. J Psychiatr Res 29:227–232, 1995

Peet M, Brind J, Ramchand CN, et al: Two double blind placebo-controlled pilot studies of eicosapentaenoic acid in the treatment of schizophrenia. Schizophr Res 49:243–251, 2001

Peet M, Glen I, Horrobin D (eds): Phospholipid Spectrum Disorders in Psychiatry and Neurology. Carnforth, Lancashire, UK, Marius Press, 2003

Pettegrew JW, Keshavan MS, Minshew NJ: Alterations in brain high-energy phosphate and membrane phospholipid metabolism in first-episode, drug-naive schizophrenics: a pilot study of the dorsal prefrontal cortex using in vivo phosphorus 31 nuclear magnetic resonance spectroscopy. Arch Gen Psychiatry 48:563–568, 1991

Piomelli D, Pilon C, Giros B, et al: Dopamine activation of the arachidonic acid cascade as a basis for D1/D2 receptor synergism. Nature 353:164–167, 1991

Pryor WA, Stone K: Oxidants in cigarette smoke: radicals hydrogen peroxide, peroxynitrate, and peroxynitrate. Ann N Y Acad Sci 686:12–27, 1993

Puri BK, Richardson AJ, Horrobin DF, et al: Eicosapentaenoic acid treatment in schizophrenia associated with symptom remission, normalization of blood fatty acids, reduced neuronal membrane phospholipid turnover and structural brain changes. Int J Clin Pract 54:57–63, 2000

Rafalowska U, Liu G -J, Floyd RA: Peroxidation induced changes in synaptosomal transport of dopamine and gamma-aminobutyric acid. Free Rad Biol Med 6:485–492, 1989

Rana RS, Hokin LE: Role of phosphoinositols in transmembrane signaling. Physiol Rev 70:115–164, 1990

Reddy R, Yao J: Free radical pathology in schizophrenia: a review. Prostaglandins Leukot Essent Fatty Acids 55:33–43, 1996

Reddy R, Yao J: Membrane protection in schizophrenia: concepts and therapeutic opportunities, in Phospholipid Spectrum Disorders in Psychiatry and Neurology. Edited by Peet M, Glen I, Horrobin D. Carnforth, UK, Marius Press, 2003, pp 299–314

Reddy RD, Mahadik SP, Mukherjee S, et al: Enzymes of the antioxidant defense system in chronic schizophrenic patients. Biol Psychiatry 30:409–412, 1991

Reddy RD, Keshavan MS, Yao JK: Reduced red blood cell membrane polyunsaturated fatty acids in first-episode schizophrenia at neuroleptic-naïve baseline. Schizophr Bull 30:901–911, 2004

Richardson AJ: Dyslexia, handedness and syndromes of psychosis proneness. Int J Psychophysiol 18:251–263, 1994

Richardson AJ, Easton T, Puri BK: Red cell and plasma fatty acid changes accompanying symptom remission in a patient with schizophrenia treated with eicosapentaenoic acid. Eur Neuropsychopharmacol 10:189–193, 2000

Richardson AJ, Allen SJ, Hajnal JV, et al: Association between central and peripheral measures of phospholipid breakdown revealed by cerebral 31-phosphorus magnetic resonance spectroscopy and fatty acid composition of erythrocyte membranes. Prog Neuropsychopharmacol Biol Psychiatry 25:1513–1521, 2001

Richardson AJ, Cyhlarova E, Puri EK: Clinical and biochemical fatty acid abnormalities in dyslexia, dyspraxia and schizotypy: an overview, in Phospholipid Spectrum Disorders in Psychiatry and Neurology. Edited by Peet M, Glen I, Horrobin D. Carnforth, UK, Marius Press, 2003, pp 477–490

Ross BM, Hudson C, Erlich J, et al: Increased phospholipid breakdown in schizophrenia: evidence for the involvement of a calcium-dependent phospholipase A2. Arch Gen Psychiatry 54:487–494, 1997

Rotrosen J, Wolkin A: Phospholipid and prostaglandin hypotheses of schizophrenia, in Psychopharmacology: The Third Generation of Progress. Edited by Meltzer HY. New York, Raven, 1987, pp 759–764

Scottish Schizophrenia Research Group: Smoking habits and plasma lipid peroxides and vitamin E in never medicated first-episode schizophrenic patients with schizophrenia. Br J Psychiatry 176:290–293, 2000

Selemon LD, Rajkowska G, Goldman-Rakic PS: Abnormally high neuronal density in the schizophrenic cortex. Arch Gen Psychiatry 52:805–818, 1995

Shriqui CL, Bradjewejn J, Annable I, et al: Vitamin E in the treatment of tardive dyskinesia: a double-blind placebo-controlled study. Am J Psychiatry 149:391–393, 1992

Simonian NA, Coyle JT: Oxidative stress in neurodegenerative diseases. Annu Rev Pharmacol Toxicol 36:82–106, 1996

Simopoulos AP: Omega-3 fatty acids in health and disease, and in growth and development. Am J Clin Nutr 54:438–463, 1991

Skosnik PD, Yao JK: From membrane phospholipids to neurotransmission: is arachidonic acid a nexus in the pathophysiology of schizophrenia? Prostaglandins Leukot Essent Fatty Acids 69:367–384, 2003

Smesny S, Volz HP, Riehemann S, et al: Diseases of phospholipid metabolism as possible pathogenetic factors in schizophrenia: current findings and critical evaluation. Fortschr Neurol Psychiatr 68:301–312, 2000

Sohal RS, Ku HH. Agarwal S, et al: Oxidative damage, mitochondrial oxidant generation and antioxidant defenses during ageing and in response to food restriction in the mouse. Mech Ageing Dev 74(1–2):121–133, 1994

Stanley JA, Williamson PC, Drost DJ, et al: An in vivo study of the prefrontal cortex of schizophrenic patients at different age of illness via phosphorous magnetic resonance spectroscopy. Arch Gen Psychiatry 52:399–406, 1995

Strassnig M, Brar JS, Ganguli R: Nutritional assessment of patients with schizophrenia. Schizophr Bull 29:393–397, 2003

Suboticanec K, Folnegovic V, Korbar M, et al: Vitamin C status in chronic schizophrenia. Biol Psychiatry 28:959–966, 1990

Suddath RL, Christison GW, Torrey EF, et al: Anatomical abnormalities in the brains of monozygotic twins discordant for schizophrenia. N Engl J Med 322:789–794, 1990

Suzuki K: Chemistry and metabolism of brain lipids, in Basic Neurochemistry, 3rd Edition. Edited by Seigel DJ, Albers RW, Agranoff BW. Boston, MA, Little, Brown, 1981, pp 355–370

Taniguchi K, Urakami M, Takanaka K: Effects of various drugs on superoxide generation, arachidonic acid release and phospholipase A2 in polymorphonuclear leukocytes. Jpn J Pharmacol 46:275–284, 1988

Tavares H, Yacubian J, Talib LL, et al: Increased phospholipase A2 activity in schizophrenia with absent response to niacin. Schizophr Res 61:1–6, 2003

Thacore VR, Shukla SR: Cannabis psychosis and paranoid schizophrenia. Arch Gen Psychiatry 33:383–386, 1976

Thomas EA, Danielson PE, Nelson PA, et al: Clozapine increases apolipoprotein D expression in rodent brain: towards a mechanism for neuroleptic pharmacotherapy. J Neurochem 76:789–796, 2001a

Thomas EA, Dean B, Pavey G, et al: Increased CNS levels of apolipoprotein D in schizophrenic and bipolar subjects: implications for the pathophysiology of psychiatric disorder. Proc Natl Acad Sci U S A 98:4066–4071, 2001b

Thompson GA (ed): The Regulation of Membrane Lipid Metabolism, 2nd Edition. Boca Raton, FL, CRC Press, 1992

Vaddadi KS, Courtney P, Gilleard CS, et al: A double-blind trial of essential fatty acid supplementation in patients with tardive dyskinesia. Psychiatry Res 27:313–323, 1989

Wainwright PE: Do essential fatty acids play a role in brain and behavioral development? Neurosci Biobehav Rev 16:193–205, 1992

Waldo MC: Niacin flush response in families of schizophrenic patients, in Phospholipid Spectrum Disorders in Psychiatry and Neurology. Edited by Peet M, Glen I, Horrobin D. Carnforth, UK, Marius Press, 2003, pp 346–352

Weinberger DR: On the plausibility of the neurodevelopmental hypothesis of schizophrenia. Neuropsychopharmacology 14: 1S–11S, 1996

Williamson PC, Brauer M, Leonard S, et al: 31P magnetic resonance spectroscopy studies in schizophrenia. Prostaglandins Leukot Essent Fatty Acids 55:115–118, 1996

Wirshing DA: Adverse effects of second-generation antipsychotics. J Clin Psychiatry 62 (suppl 21):7–10, 2003

Wood KA, Youle RJ: Apoptosis and free radicals. Ann N Y Acad Sci 738:400–407, 1994

Yao JK: Abnormalities of fatty acid metabolism in red cells, platelets and brain in schizophrenia, in Phospholipid Spectrum Disorders in Psychiatry and Neurology. Edited by Peet M, Glen I, Horrobin D. Carnforth, UK, Marius Press, 2003, pp 193–212

Yao JK, Reddy RD: Membrane pathology in schizophrenia: Implication for arachidonic acid signaling. Current Medicinal Chemistry-Central Nervous System Agents 3:57–65, 2003

Yao JK, van Kammen DP: Red blood cell membrane dynamics in schizophrenia, I: membrane fluidity. Schizophr Res 11: 209–216, 1994

Yao JK, van Kammen DP: Membrane phospholipids and cytokine interaction in schizophrenia. Int Rev Neurobiol 59: 297–326, 2004

Yao JK, Yasaei P, van Kammen DP: Increased turnover of platelet phosphatidylinositol in schizophrenia. Prostaglandins Leukot Essent Fatty Acids 46:39–46, 1992

Yao JK, van Kammen DP, Welker JA: Red cell membrane dynamics in schizophrenia, II: fatty acid composition. Schizophr Res 13:217–226, 1994

Yao JK, van Kammen DP, Gurklis J: Abnormal incorporation of arachidonic acid into platelets of drug-free patients with schizophrenia. Psychiatry Res 60:11–21, 1996

Yao JK, Reddy R, van Kammen DP: Reduced level of plasma antioxidant uric acid in schizophrenia. Psychiatry Res 80:29–39, 1998

Yao JK, Leonard S, Reddy RD: Membrane phospholipid abnormalities in postmortem brain from schizophrenic patients. Schizophr Res 42:7–17, 2000

Yao JK, Reddy RD, van Kammen DP: Oxidative damage and schizophrenia: an overview of its evidence and therapeutic implications. CNS Drugs 15:287–310, 2001

Yao JK, Stanley JA, Reddy RD, et al: Correlations between peripheral polyunsaturated fatty acid content and in vivo membrane phospholipid metabolites. Biol Psychiatry 52:823–830, 2002

Yao JK, Thomas EA, Reddy RD, et al: Association of apolipoprotein D with membrane arachidonic acid levels in schizophrenia. Schizophr Res 72:259–266, 2005

Zilberman-Kaufman M, Agam G, Moscowits L, et al: Raised monophosphate activity in schizophrenic patients. Clin Chim Acta 209(1–2):89–93, 1992

Zubenko GS, Cohen BM: A cell membrane correlate of tardive dyskinesia in patients treated with phenothiazines. Psychopharmacology (Berl) 88(2):230–236, 1986

CHAPTER

8

NEUROPROGRESSIVE THEORIES

L. FREDRIK JARSKOG, M.D.

JOHN H. GILMORE, M.D.

Neurodegenerative features of schizophrenia were noted by Kraepelin, who described "dementia praecox" as a progressive illness with a deteriorating clinical course (Kraepelin 1919). Originally, the hypothesis of schizophrenia as a progressive neurodegenerative disorder was supported both by Alzheimer and by Southard, who in the early twentieth century reported loss of cortical neurons and cerebral atrophy in postmortem tissue (Bogerts 1999). However, most subsequent studies were unable to replicate these early findings, and the concept of schizophrenia as a neurodegenerative disorder largely faded. The articulation of schizophrenia as a neurodevelopmental disorder in the 1980s found broad support, given the absence of classic neurodegenerative features and the epidemiological studies that found associations between early life insults and a higher incidence of schizophrenia (Murray and Lewis 1987; Weinberger 1987).

The neurodevelopmental hypothesis states that early life environmental insults (e.g., infection, trauma) can alter the course of neurodevelopment to yield static brain deficits that later manifest as psychosis. This hypothesis has clearly advanced our understanding of schizophrenia

with regard to the influence of developmental factors in the etiology of the disorder. However, this perspective is unable to account for several cardinal features of schizophrenia, including the long period of symptomatic dormancy between the early life insults and the eventual manifestation of clinical symptoms, the progressive loss of function that affects a substantial proportion of patients, evidence for progressive structural changes in multiple brain regions, and evidence that antipsychotic medications can modify the course of illness.

By definition a neurodegenerative disorder is a progressive disease of the nervous system that is initiated by specific biochemical changes—often with an underlying genetic basis—that ultimately lead to a distinct histopathology with associated clinical manifestations (Hardy and Gwinn-Hardy 1998). The onset of clinical symptoms depends on interactions of the underlying pathophysiology with normal maturational processes as well as the individual's capacity for adaptive neuroplastic responses and their cognitive reserve. Neurodegenerative disorders may remain clinically dormant until a threshold level of pathophysiological damage has occurred. The absence of a

This work was supported in part by National Institute of Mental Health (NIMH) grants MH01752 and MH60352 and the UNC Schizophrenia Research Center and by a grant from the NIMH Silvio O. Conte Center for the Neuroscience of Mental Disorders (MH64065).

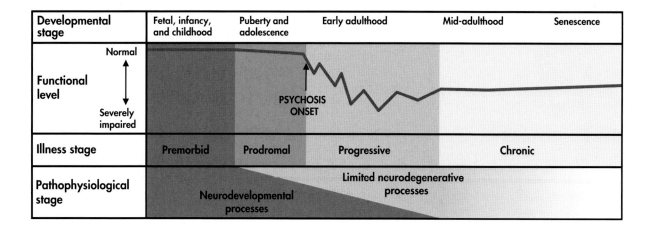

FIGURE 8–1.   Proposed neuroprogressive model of schizophrenia.

The model incorporates a limited neurodegenerative process within a neurodevelopmental framework. The solid line in upper portion of figure represents the average functional level over the lifetime of patients with schizophrenia superimposed on the intersection of neurodevelopmental *(darkly shaded area to left)* and neurodegenerative *(lightly shaded area to right)* processes. It is hypothesized that the mechanism(s) that underlie the progressive events are most active around the onset of psychosis and diminish with time.

pathognomonic cellular phenotype in schizophrenia has been cited as evidence against a neurodegenerative hypothesis (Weinberger and McClure 2002). However, a set of subtle yet increasingly reproducible histopathological, neurochemical, and neurostructural deficits is emerging. Although these deficits appear nonspecific and are not found in all patients with schizophrenia, the pathology may reveal more distinct biochemical and histological characteristics as novel and more sensitive cellular and molecular techniques are brought to bear on the illness. Further, recent evidence suggests that certain clinical and neurostructural features are progressive—a feature that is consistent with a neurodegenerative component.

In this chapter, we advance the hypothesis that schizophrenia represents a limited neurodegenerative disorder with neurodevelopmental antecedents (see Figure 8–1). We review clinical, neurocognitive, neuroimaging, and neuropathological studies in a critical analysis of this hypothesis. We then review specific mechanisms that could contribute to the progressive features of schizophrenia, including the potential roles of apoptosis, excitotoxicity, oxidative stress, and neurochemical sensitization.

PSYCHOPATHOLOGY AND NEUROCOGNITIVE DEFICITS

Given the genetic and early life events that have been linked to schizophrenia, the pathophysiological onset of schizophrenia clearly predates the onset of psychosis. The

presymptomatic period is generally known as the *premorbid phase*, whereas the period that encompasses nonspecific psychiatric symptoms without psychosis is termed the *prodromal phase*. Not surprisingly, substantial data indicate that the premorbid phase of schizophrenia is characterized by subtle cognitive, social, and motor deficits. From this baseline of mild impairment, most patients with schizophrenia begin to experience deterioration in their overall level of function during the prodromal phase of illness, and this deterioration typically accelerates following the formal onset of psychosis (Huber et al. 1980; Lieberman et al. 2001b; Pfohl and Winokur 1982). Interestingly, the functional deterioration is not inexorable; it is generally limited to the first 5 years after the onset of psychosis after which a plateau is reached (McGlashan 1988). A longitudinal study measuring social adjustment found that deterioration was generally limited to the first year of illness after which it remained stable for over a decade (Mason et al. 1996).

Although most would agree that the functional level of patients with schizophrenia declines after the onset of psychosis, the basis for this decline remains uncertain. One possibility is that the psychopathological dimension of schizophrenia—positive, negative, and cognitive symptoms—contributes to the functional decline. Although it might seem that positive symptoms ought to be associated with a decline in function, most studies have found that positive symptoms correlate poorly with functional outcome (Green 1996). Further, several studies report that positive symptoms do not tend to progress or worsen after the first year of illness (Eaton et al. 1995; Mason et al.

1996). On the other hand, it appears that negative symptoms are at least somewhat correlated with overall level of function and long-term outcome (Buchanan and Gold 1996). One study found that primary negative symptoms progressed in severity over the first 5 years after the onset of psychosis and that development of the deficit syndrome was associated with poor outcome and long-term disability (Fenton and McGlashan 1994). However, first-episode patients had lower rates of the deficit syndrome than patients with chronic schizophrenia (Mayerhoff et al. 1994), and Eaton and colleagues (1995) found that negative symptoms were stable after the first 2 years of illness. Thus it appears that progression of negative symptoms may occur in a subset of patients following the onset of psychosis, and, for these patients, negative symptoms may be associated with worsening functional status.

Mounting data indicate that the strongest predictor of overall functional outcome in schizophrenia is neurocognitive function (Green et al. 2000). Therefore, deteriorating neurocognitive function could represent a cause of functional decline. Whereas early studies described the presence of progressive cognitive impairment in individuals with schizophrenia (Abrahamson 1983; Bilder et al. 1992; Smith 1964), a number of subsequent studies have not found such evidence (Rund 1998). Studies have found cognitive decline in chronically institutionalized geriatric patients (Friedman et al. 2002; Harvey et al. 1999). However, a study of older outpatients found no differences in age-related cognitive decline (Eyler Zorrilla et al. 2000), and a longitudinal study of neuropsychological deficits in a cohort with a mean age of approximately 50 years found cognitive function to be stable (Heaton et al. 2001). Cross-sectional comparisons of cognitive functioning in first-episode and chronic schizophrenia have found similar degrees of impairment, further suggesting that cognitive deficits do not generally progress (Addington and Addington 2002; Moritz et al. 2002; Saykin et al. 1994). Longitudinal studies in first-episode patients have found either no progression (Hoff et al. 1999) or even improvement of cognitive impairments (Nopoulos et al. 1994). Taken together, these studies suggest that progressive cognitive deterioration in schizophrenia is generally limited to a subset of geriatric and chronically institutionalized patients.

Although neurocognitive deficits may not progress appreciably after the onset of psychosis except in certain cases involving older patients with poor outcome, it has also been considered that neurocognitive function may deteriorate earlier, during the premorbid and prodromal phases of schizophrenia. An increasing number of studies provide support for this hypothesis. A variety of cognitive, motor, and social abnormalities have been identified in individuals in the premorbid phase of illness (Cannon et al. 2002; Caspi et al. 2003; Done et al. 1994; Jones et al. 1994; Kremen et al. 1994), but impairment in these domains tends to be significantly more severe after the formal onset of psychosis, suggesting that some deterioration has occurred. In a longitudinal study of 51 subjects with prodromal symptoms, neurocognitive function generally was at an intermediate level between matched control subjects and individuals with schizophrenia (Hambrecht et al. 2002; see also Figure 8–2). In the 15-month follow-up period, worsening self-perceived neuropsychological function (e.g., concentration, visual and auditory perception) was predictive of transition to psychosis in the small number of subjects ($n=5$) who developed a first episode of psychosis. A retrospective study of patients with schizophrenia found that their performance on a standardized scholastic test had worsened significantly from grade 8 to grade 11 before the onset of psychosis (Fuller et al. 2002). Deterioration in the premorbid/prodromal phase was also suggested in another retrospective study which found that individuals who eventually developed schizophrenia often did not complete high school despite having normal academic performance in elementary school (Cannon et al. 1999).

Although still preliminary, these data increasingly suggest that progressive deterioration of cognitive function does occur during the late premorbid and prodromal phases of schizophrenia. After the first episode of psychosis, neurocognitive functioning appears to remain relatively stable except in geriatric, chronically institutionalized patients. Negative symptoms can progress for several years after the onset of psychosis before reaching a plateau. Similarly, overall functional level in patients with schizophrenia worsens for at least several years after the onset of psychosis and then reaches a plateau. Thus evidence of progressive changes in psychopathology could represent the clinical phenotype of a limited neurodegenerative process that is temporally restricted to the late premorbid and prodromal phases as well as several years after the onset of psychosis (see Figure 8–1).

POSTMORTEM NEUROPATHOLOGY

Despite intensive study, investigators have been unable to identify a specific phenotype that defines the neuropathology of schizophrenia (Harrison 1999). Almost all studies report no increase in gliosis or glial fibrillary acidic protein staining (Arnold et al. 1998; Benes et al. 1991; Purohit et al. 1998; Roberts et al. 1986, 1987; Stevens 1982). The absence of gliosis clearly distinguishes the neuropathology of schizophrenia from that of Alzheimer's disease and other classic neurodegenerative disorders in which gliosis is present. In fact, increasing numbers of

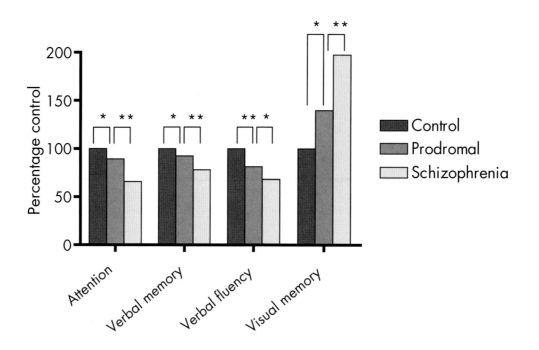

FIGURE 8–2.   Comparison of selected neurocognitive measures in healthy control subjects, prodromal patients, and patients with schizophrenia (n=29 in each group).

This graph was derived from data reported by Hambrecht and colleagues (2002) on neurocognitive function assessed at entry in a longitudinal study of psychosis prodrome. For each measure, the data from each group were normalized to the mean of the control group. A Mann-Whitney U test was used to perform two statistical comparisons: 1) prodromal patients versus normal control subjects and 2) prodromal patients versus patients with schizophrenia (*P<0.05; **P<0.01). On measures of attention (Continuous Performance Test), verbal memory (Auditory Verbal Learning Test), and verbal fluency (word generation in 1 minute), lower scores represent poorer performance, whereas for visual memory (Rey-Osterrieth Complex Figure Test), higher scores represent poorer performance. The data demonstrate that patients with prodromal symptoms of psychosis have neurocognitive deficits that fall between the function of healthy control subjects and patients with schizophrenia.

studies have found reduced numbers of cortical glia in schizophrenia, including in prefrontal, motor, and anterior cingulate cortices (Benes et al. 1986; Cotter et al. 2001; Stark et al. 2004).

Another prominent feature of classic neurodegenerative disorders is large-scale neuronal loss. However, most studies of schizophrenia have not identified fewer cortical neurons (Akbarian et al. 1995b; Pakkenberg 1993; Selemon et al. 1995, 1998; Thune et al. 2001). Several studies in anterior cingulate cortex have identified layer-specific reductions in density of pyramidal and nonpyramidal neurons (Benes et al. 1991, 2001). Also, lower neuron counts have been found in mediodorsal thalamus (Byne et al. 2002; Cullen et al. 2003; Pakkenberg 1990; Popken et al. 2000; Young et al. 2000). Thus certain subpopulations of cortical neurons and glia as well as discrete subcortical neuron populations may be reduced in schizophrenia, but overall these reductions are modest.

Increasing evidence suggests that the cortical neuropathology of schizophrenia is characterized by limited

neuronal atrophy. Selemon and colleagues (1995, 1998) found that neuron density was increased in areas 9 and 46 and that gray matter thickness was somewhat thinner, indicating that cortical neuropil was reduced. This finding gave rise to the reduced neuropil hypothesis of schizophrenia (Selemon et al. 1995). Supporting this hypothesis are studies that show fewer dendritic spines and dendrite length in the prefrontal cortex (Black et al. 2004; Garey et al. 1998; Glantz and Lewis 2000) and reduced synaptic marker proteins in schizophrenia (Eastwood and Harrison 1995; Glantz and Lewis 1997; Karson et al. 1999; Thompson et al. 1998). Smaller somal volume of neurons also has been reported in the prefrontal cortex of patients with schizophrenia (Pierri et al. 2001; Rajkowska et al. 1998). Neuron somal size is known to correlate with the degree of axonal and dendritic arborization (Harrison and Eastwood 2001); therefore, the presence of smaller neuronal soma is consistent with the aforementioned evidence of shorter dendrites and reduced synaptic markers in schizophrenia.

Thus although pathognomonic neuropathological lesions are absent in schizophrenia, a number of subtle synaptic and dendritic deficits appear to characterize the disorder. Because the postmortem findings do not provide a longitudinal perspective, they do not offer much insight into when the deficits might have emerged. Further, a number of potential confounding variables must be considered when interpreting human postmortem studies including postmortem interval, medications, and diagnostic uncertainty. However, when the postmortem deficits are considered in context with neuroimaging data indicating that progressive brain morphologic changes occur in schizophrenia (discussed in the next section), it raises the possibility that limited progressive neuronal atrophy may occur after the onset of clinical symptoms.

NEUROIMAGING PATHOLOGY

STRUCTURAL STUDIES

Numerous magnetic resonance imaging (MRI) studies have demonstrated structural brain abnormalities in schizophrenia, including ventricular enlargement and reduced cortical gray matter volume (Harrison 1999; Shenton et al. 2001). Because most of these studies were cross-sectional in design, it was unknown whether the volume changes were progressive. More recently, investigators have applied longitudinal designs to structural MRI studies, and the issue of progression has been addressed in various patient groups including patients with prodromal symptoms, those with childhood-onset schizophrenia, those with first-episode schizophrenia, and chronic patient populations. In prodromal patients considered to be at "ultra-high risk" for the development of psychosis, progressive gray matter loss was identified in inferior frontal, medial temporal, and cingulate cortices only in those patients who transitioned to psychosis (Pantelis et al. 2003). Studies of subjects with childhood-onset schizophrenia have identified progressive brain volume changes in several regions including enlargement of lateral ventricles (Rapoport et al. 1997) and loss of frontal, temporal, and parietal cortical gray matter (Gogtay et al. 2004; Jacobsen et al. 1998; Rapoport et al. 1999; Thompson et al. 2001) compared with normal healthy control subjects (see Figure 8–3).

In first-episode schizophrenia, several groups (Cahn et al. 2002; DeLisi et al. 1997, 2004; Lieberman et al. 2001a), but not all (Gur et al. 1998), have identified progressive ventricular enlargement. Progressive cortical volume loss in first-episode schizophrenia compared with matched control subjects has also been reported in cerebral hemispheres (DeLisi et al. 1997), total cerebral gray matter (Cahn et al. 2002), whole frontal cortex (Gur et al. 1998), and superior temporal gyrus gray matter (Kasai et al. 2003). In adults with chronic schizophrenia, progressive ventricular enlargement has been reported in male patients (Mathalon et al. 2001) including those with poor outcome (Davis et al. 1998). In another study, patients found to have progressive ventricular enlargement were thought to have a distinct pathophysiological subtype of schizophrenia (Nair et al. 1997). Progressive loss of fronto-temporal cortical gray matter has also been associated with males with chronic schizophrenia (Mathalon et al. 2001).

The longitudinal structural MRI studies provide increasing evidence that the pathophysiology of schizophrenia represents, in part, a progressive process, especially around the onset of illness. Although the MRI studies do not indicate the nature of the progressive structural changes, the postmortem results indicate that neural atrophy and neuropil loss may represent a cellular basis for progression (see Figure 8–4).

The hypothesis that schizophrenia represents a neuroprogressive disorder has been challenged based on grounds that the reported gray matter loss is too pervasive and rapid to be physiologically plausible (Weinberger and McClure 2002). Although it is true that evidence for progressive gray matter loss has emerged at different stages of schizophrenia and that the loci of progressive loss have differed across some of the studies, it is likely that future longitudinal studies that use larger cohorts and employ higher resolution neuroimaging techniques will help to define the process more precisely. Further, as proposed here and previously (Lieberman 1999), the nature of a limited degenerative process does not predicate a classic gliotic neurodegeneration, nor does it discount the substantial impact of late neuromaturational processes such as synaptic pruning and cortical myelination. Potential mechanisms underlying limited neuroprogression in schizophrenia are discussed in the last section.

FUNCTIONAL AND SPECTROSCOPIC STUDIES

Reduced metabolic activity has been demonstrated in the prefrontal cortex in schizophrenia with positron emission tomography (PET) and functional MRI (fMRI) (Andreasen et al. 1997; Weinberger et al. 1986). Although these findings are consistent with postmortem evidence of reduced neuropil and structural MRI findings that show reduced gray matter in frontal cortex, the PET and fMRI studies were not longitudinal, and it is not known whether the reduction in metabolic activity is also progressive. Magnetic resonance spectroscopy (MRS) studies may shed more light on this issue. In subjects with first-episode schizo-

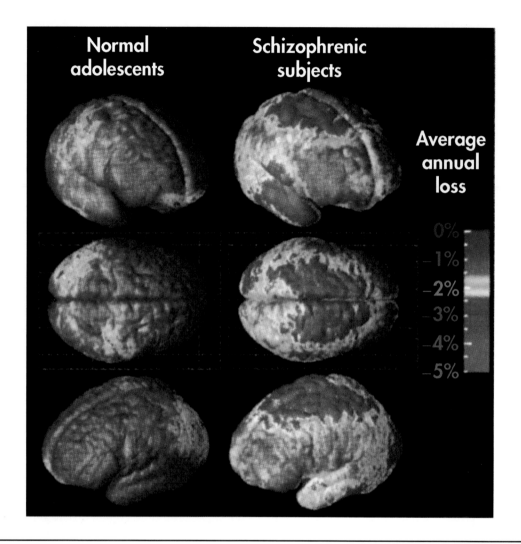

FIGURE 8–3.   Average rates of gray matter loss in adolescents with childhood-onset schizophrenia and in matched healthy control subjects.

These three-dimensional maps, derived from MRI images acquired sequentially from the same subjects over a 5-year interval, demonstrate substantial gray matter loss in schizophrenia. Average rates of gray matter loss from 13 to 18 years of age are displayed on average cortical models for the group. Severe loss (red and pink colors; up to 5% annually) occurs in parietal, superior frontal, and temporal cortices, whereas inferior frontal cortex remains stable (blue; 0–1% loss).

Source.   Reprinted from Thompson PM, Vidal C, Giedd JN, et al.: "Mapping Adolescent Brain Change Reveals Dynamic Wave of Accelerated Gray Matter Loss in Very Early Onset Schizophrenia." *Proceedings of the National Academy of Sciences U S A* 98:11650–11655, 2001. Copyright 2001, National Academy of Sciences. Used with permission.

phrenia, phosphorus-31 (^{31}P) MRS in the prefrontal cortex has demonstrated decreased phosphomonoesters and increased phosphodiesters (Hinsberger et al. 1997; Pettegrew et al. 1991; Stanley et al. 1995). The combination of lower phosphomonoester and higher phosphodiester levels is thought to reflect an increased rate of membrane phospholipid breakdown (Pettegrew et al. 1993), which could represent evidence of active neuronal and/or glial breakdown. Lower levels of *N*-acetylaspartate (NAA) have also been reported in the temporal and frontal cortex using proton (^{1}H) MRS in subjects with schizophrenia (Ber-

tolino et al. 1998; Cecil et al. 1999). NAA is considered a nonspecific marker of neuronal metabolism, and lower NAA levels may indicate reduced neuronal viability.

As with fMRI and PET studies, ^{1}H- and ^{31}P-MRS findings appear consistent with the postmortem and structural MRI literature, but the absence of longitudinal studies using these methodologies limits the extent to which the findings support a progressive process in the pathophysiology of schizophrenia. The use of longitudinal fMRI, PET, and MRS study designs could provide important insights in this regard.

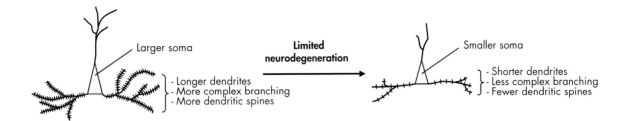

FIGURE 8–4. Proposed progression of neuronal cytopathology associated with a limited neurodegenerative model of schizophrenia.

This model proposes that progressive neuronal atrophy accompanies progressive cortical gray matter loss that has been demonstrated in longitudinal neuroimaging studies. Depicted is a cortical pyramidal neuron that is decreasing in somal size, dendrite length and number, and dendritic spine number.

CORRELATION OF NEUROPATHOLOGY WITH PSYCHOPATHOLOGY

In a meta-analysis, investigators found that a long duration of untreated psychosis in first-episode schizophrenia is correlated with poorer treatment response and lower overall level of functioning (Perkins et al. 2005). These data provide support for the hypothesis that untreated psychosis is neurotoxic (Wyatt 1991). To explore the potential neurostructural consequences of this hypothesis, several groups have examined whether longer periods of untreated psychosis are associated with greater structural brain abnormalities. To date, no such relationship has emerged (Fannon et al. 2000; Ho et al. 2003; Hoff et al. 2000), but these analyses are somewhat limited by their retrospective designs.

More insight into this issue is provided by longitudinal studies in which clinical symptoms and neurostructural measures have been assessed concurrently over time. In patients with new-onset schizophrenia, worse functional outcome correlated with the rate of cortical gray matter loss and ventricular enlargement (Cahn et al. 2002; Lieberman et al. 2001a), and loss of frontal cortical volume correlated with less negative symptom improvement but greater positive symptom improvement (Gur et al. 1998); however, no relationship was found between progressive superior temporal gyrus loss and clinical measures (Kasai et al. 2003). In previously treated patients, reduction in cortical volume was associated with greater neurocognitive decline (Gur et al. 1998), and in male patients with chronic schizophrenia, greater cortical gray matter loss and ventricular enlargement correlated with clinical symptom severity (Mathalon et al. 2001). Similarly, Davis and colleagues (1998) found progressive ventricular enlargement in patients with poor outcome. In childhood-onset schizophrenia, progressive loss of superior temporal gyrus has correlated with worse clinical outcome (Jacobsen et al. 1998), and progressive frontal and temporal cortical loss was associated with worse positive and negative symptoms and worse neurocognitive function (Thompson et al. 2001).

Accumulating evidence suggests a general link between progressive neurostructural deficits and less favorable clinical and cognitive outcomes. However, this association has not been found in all studies and is not consistent across brain regions or outcome domains. This inconsistency could stem from considerable variability among individuals in their capacity to maintain normal cognitive function in the face of neurostructural progression. A number of potential confounds must also be considered, including the influence of antipsychotic medications, drug abuse, and cigarette smoking, as well as the effects of overall environmental stimulation experienced by different patients. At this time, it remains uncertain how to reconcile those studies reporting structural progression with other studies that have found generally stable clinical and cognitive functioning. Further studies using longitudinal designs and larger cohorts, correlating structural, clinical, and cognitive variables in carefully defined patient subgroups, must be conducted to clarify this important issue.

POTENTIAL MECHANISMS UNDERLYING NEUROPROGRESSION

A number of potential mechanisms have been proposed to underlie neuroprogressive changes in schizophrenia. These include glutamate excitotoxicity, oxidative stress, neurochemical sensitization, and altered activation of apoptosis. Evidence supporting these will be discussed in the following sections. Because a role for apoptosis has been proposed in several of the other mechanisms, we first review apoptosis to provide a context for the remainder of the discussion.

APOPTOSIS

Apoptosis has increasingly been considered as a potential contributing mechanism to the pathophysiology of schizophrenia (Benes 2004; Jarskog et al. 2000). Apoptosis is a cell death mechanism that is crucial to normal neurodevelopment and is also implicated in a number of neuropathological conditions. Given that the pathology of schizophrenia primarily involves neuropil loss and synaptic disconnectivity without large-scale cortical neuron loss (Lewis and Lieberman 2000), a role for apoptosis would need to be able to account for this neuropathological profile. In fact, emerging data have demonstrated that apoptotic mechanisms can lead to reductions in neuronal viability (Ona et al. 1999) as well as contribute to pathological elimination of synapses (Gylys et al. 2004; Mattson et al. 1998) and terminal neurites (Garden et al. 2002; Ivins et al. 1998) without causing cell death, so-called synaptic apoptosis.

Altered levels of apoptotic regulatory proteins have been identified in postmortem temporal cortex in schizophrenia, including a reduction in Bcl-2, a potent antiapoptotic protein (Jarskog et al. 2000), as well as an increase of the Bax/Bcl-2 ratio (Jarskog et al. 2004). Bax is a pro-apoptotic protein, and higher Bax/Bcl-2 ratios are associated with greater apoptotic susceptibility (Oltvai et al. 1993). However, caspase-3—a downstream apoptosis-effector protein and a useful marker of apoptotic activity—was not increased in temporal cortex (Jarskog et al. 2004), indicating that neuronal apoptosis may not be active in chronic schizophrenia, the stage of illness represented by most postmortem brain samples. This conclusion is also consistent with evidence that the rate of single-stranded DNA breaks is reduced in postmortem anterior cingulate cortex in schizophrenia (Benes et al. 2003). The absence of increased apoptosis in chronic schizophrenia is perhaps not surprising given that structural neuroimaging studies have generally found progressive brain volume changes limited to early phases of the disorder. Therefore, if gray matter loss is mediated by apoptotic activity, it may be episodic rather than continuous and may be generally limited to the first onset of schizophrenia. Given the evidence for increased pro-apoptotic vulnerability in schizophrenia cortex and the evidence that nonlethal apoptotic activity can lead to synaptic and/or dendritic loss, we propose that such a mechanism could represent the primary pathological consequence of apoptotic dysfunction in schizophrenia.

GLUTAMATE EXCITOTOXICITY

The glutamate hypothesis of schizophrenia posits a role for abnormal glutamate neurotransmission in the pathophysiology of schizophrenia. This hypothesis is supported in part by the observation that antagonism of the glutamatergic N-methyl-D-aspartate (NMDA) receptor by phencyclidine (PCP) can produce transient expression of many of the clinical dimensions of schizophrenia in normal healthy individuals and exacerbate psychosis in patients with schizophrenia (Goff and Coyle 2001). Further, it has been proposed that NMDA receptor hypofunction causes reduced activation of inhibitory γ-aminobutyric acid (GABA) neurons, leading to glutamatergic disinhibition and excitotoxicity (Coyle 1996; Olney and Farber 1995).

Despite the theoretical appeal of this hypothesis and increasing evidence of glutamatergic system abnormalities in schizophrenia, little neuropathological evidence specifically supports glutamatergic excitotoxicity (Goff and Coyle 2001). Nevertheless, because excitotoxicity can produce neuronal degeneration by acute necrosis or delayed apoptosis, excitotoxic damage may be difficult to detect in postmortem specimens if it occurred via apoptotic mechanisms (which can proceed without gliosis), especially if the excitotoxicity was limited to earlier stages of the disorder (e.g., around the first episode of psychosis). Further, because schizophrenia is characterized more by neuronal atrophy and neuropil loss rather than actual neuron loss, it is of interest that brief focal application of glutamate to distal dendrites in vitro has been shown to produce a local activation of apoptotic mechanisms without inducing neuronal death (Mattson et al. 1998). Another study found increased levels of the unedited $GluR_2$ subunit of the glutamatergic AMPA receptor in frontal cortex in schizophrenia, which has been associated with increased calcium permeability of the receptor channel (Akbarian et al. 1995a). High calcium flux in synapses and dendritic spines can produce dendrite retraction and neurotoxicity via apoptotic mechanisms (Mattson et al. 1998).

OXIDATIVE STRESS

Oxidative stress occurs when the levels of oxygen radicals exceed the antioxidant capacity of a given system. Persistent oxidative stress is known to produce cumulative damage that is thought to contribute to several classic neurodegenerative disorders (Barnham et al. 2004). Given the evidence for progressive pathology, an oxidative stress hypothesis has been considered in schizophrenia. One potential source of oxidative stress is excess glutamate, as described in the previous section (Coyle and Puttfarcken

1993). Further, altered peripheral levels of antioxidant enzymes have been documented in new-onset psychosis (Mukerjee et al. 1996), as have abnormalities in the phospholipase A_2 system (Hudson et al. 1996; Ross et al. 1997). Thus, several lines of evidence implicate oxidative stress as a mechanism that could contribute to the progressive changes seen in schizophrenia.

Glucocorticoid-induced stress represents another potential stress-related mechanism underlying neurostructural changes observed in certain psychiatric disorders, including affective, anxiety, and psychotic disorders (Arango et al. 2001; Church et al. 2002). For example, it has been proposed that glucocorticoid toxicity could underlie reduced hippocampal volumes in schizophrenia (Benes 1997). Supporting evidence includes increased plasma levels of cortisol and related stress markers in schizophrenia (Breier and Buchanan 1992; Risch et al. 1992).

NEUROCHEMICAL SENSITIZATION

The neurochemical sensitization hypothesis proposes that the symptoms of schizophrenia could be caused by deficits in neural regulation during neurodevelopment that result in a pathological form of neurochemical sensitization (Lieberman et al. 1997). This is analogous to preclinical models of pharmacologically induced behavioral sensitization, a phenomenon in which intermittent pharmacological stimulation can lead to enduring enhancement of a behavioral response (Wolf et al. 1993). This condition, if sustained, could in turn lead to neurotoxic effects and account for progressive and persistent morbidity paralleling the functional decline often associated with schizophrenia. Several lines of evidence are consistent with the neurochemical sensitization hypothesis, including the ability of amphetamine and other psychotomimetic drugs to induce psychotic symptoms in healthy subjects, the increased susceptibility of patients with schizophrenia to the psychotogenic effects of dopamine agonists, and the development of sensitization to psychosis-inducing effects of stimulants in chronic stimulant abusers (Lieberman et al. 1997). Interactions between dopaminergic and glutamatergic systems have also been demonstrated in animal models of chronic PCP use that have been found to promote subcortical dopamine release and induce sensitization to the behavioral effects of subsequent NMDA antagonist exposure (Goff and Coyle 2001). In schizophrenia, the development of neurochemical sensitization is proposed to occur in response to environmental stimulation (e.g., stressful life events, drug abuse) during late adolescence and early adulthood in individuals who already have specific genetic and/or epi-

genetic vulnerability to the disorder. Ultimately, self-limiting neurotoxicity has been proposed to occur as a consequence of elevated excitatory amino acid activity, potentially via apoptosis (Coyle 1996).

CONCLUSION

This chapter represents an overview of the clinical and neuropathological evidence that schizophrenia has neuroprogressive features. When first articulated, the neurodevelopmental hypothesis represented a paradigm shift in our understanding of schizophrenia. It provided a mechanistic framework for evidence that early life neurobiological insults were associated with higher rates of schizophrenia in adulthood. However, the neurodevelopmental hypothesis does not account for the long dormancy of psychotic symptoms after the early life insult(s) or the evidence for limited progressive loss of function and progressive neurostructural changes.

In this chapter, we have advanced the argument that schizophrenia represents a neurodevelopmental disorder that also encompasses limited neurodegenerative features. This conclusion is supported by recent neuroimaging studies that have reported progressive loss of cortical gray matter and progressive ventricular enlargement as well as studies that indicate a limited progression of clinical psychopathology and neurocognitive function.

It is important to recognize that neither the pathophysiology nor the clinical course of schizophrenia resembles those of a classic neurodegenerative disorder such as Alzheimer's disease. Any evidence of degeneration is subtle and confined primarily to the loss of dendritic processes and synaptic elements rather than loss of neurons. Further, the progressive process appears generally limited to the early stages of clinical symptoms including the prodromal period and several years following the onset of psychosis. Nevertheless, the possibility that a limited, but as yet uncharacterized, neurodegenerative mechanism is involved remains plausible and merits further investigation. The importance of this issue is most clearly related to the treatment of schizophrenia because a progressive process is potentially modifiable. If the functional decline in schizophrenia can be slowed early in the course of the disorder, then improved long-term outcomes may be achieved.

REFERENCES

Abrahamson D: Schizophrenic deterioration, 4. Br J Psychiatry 143:82–83, 1983

Addington J, Addington D: Cognitive functioning in first-episode schizophrenia. J Psychiatry Neurosci 27:188–192, 2002

Akbarian S, Smith MA, Jones EG: Editing for an AMPA receptor subunit RNA in prefrontal cortex and striatum in Alzheimer's disease, Huntington's disease and schizophrenia. Brain Res 699:297–304, 1995a

Akbarian S, Kim JJ, Potkin SG, et al: Gene expression for glutamic acid decarboxylase is reduced without loss of neurons in prefrontal cortex of schizophrenics. Arch Gen Psychiatry 52:258–266, 1995b

Andreasen NC, O'Leary DS, Flaum M, et al: Hypofrontality in schizophrenia: distributed dysfunctional circuits in neuroleptic-naive patients. Lancet 349:1730–1734, 1997

Arango C, Kirkpatrick B, Koenig J: At issue: stress, hippocampal neuronal turnover, and neuropsychiatric disorders. Schizophr Bull 27:477–480, 2001

Arnold SE, Trojanowski JQ, Gur RE, et al: Absence of neurodegeneration and neural injury in the cerebral cortex in a sample of elderly patients with schizophrenia. Arch Gen Psychiatry 55:225–232, 1998

Barnham KJ, Masters CL, Bush AI: Neurodegenerative diseases and oxidative stress. Nat Rev Drug Discov 3:205–214, 2004

Benes FM: The role of stress and dopamine-GABA interactions in the vulnerability for schizophrenia. J Psychiatr Res 31:257–275, 1997

Benes FM: The role of apoptosis in neuronal pathology in schizophrenia and bipolar disorder. Curr Opin Psychiatry 17:189–190, 2004

Benes FM, Davidson J, Bird ED: Quantitative cytoarchitectural studies of the cerebral cortex of schizophrenics. Arch Gen Psychiatry 43:31–35, 1986

Benes FM, McSparren J, Bird ED, et al: Deficits in small interneurons in prefrontal and cingulate cortices of schizophrenic and schizoaffective patients. Arch Gen Psychiatry 48:996–1001, 1991

Benes FM, Vincent SL, Todtenkopf M: The density of pyramidal and nonpyramidal neurons in anterior cingulate cortex of schizophrenic and bipolar subjects. Biol Psychiatry 50:395–406, 2001

Benes FM, Walsh J, Bhattacharyya S, et al: DNA fragmentation decreased in schizophrenia but not bipolar disorder. Arch Gen Psychiatry 60:359–364, 2003

Bertolino A, Callicott JH, Nawroz S, et al: Reproducibility of proton magnetic resonance spectroscopic imaging in patients with schizophrenia. Neuropsychopharmacology 18:1–9, 1998

Bilder RM, Lipschutz-Broch L, Reiter G, et al: Intellectual deficits in first-episode schizophrenia: evidence for progressive deterioration. Schizophr Bull 18:437–448, 1992

Black JE, Kodish IM, Grossman AW, et al: Pathology of layer V pyramidal neurons in the prefrontal cortex of patients with schizophrenia. Am J Psychiatry 161:742–724, 2004

Bogerts B: The neuropathology of schizophrenic diseases: historical aspects and present knowledge. Eur Arch Psychiatry Clin Neurosci 249 (suppl 4):2–13, 1999

Breier A, Buchanan RW: The effects of metabolic stress on plasma progesterone in healthy volunteers and schizophrenic patients. Life Sci 51:1527–1534, 1992

Buchanan RW, Gold JM: Negative symptoms: diagnosis, treatment and prognosis. Int Clin Psychopharmacol 11 (suppl 2):3–11, 1996

Byne W, Buchsbaum MS, Mattiace LA, et al: Postmortem assessment of thalamic nuclear volumes in subjects with schizophrenia. Am J Psychiatry 159:59–65, 2002

Cahn W, Pol HE, Lems EB, et al: Brain volume changes in first-episode schizophrenia: a 1-year follow-up study. Arch Gen Psychiatry 59:1002–1010, 2002

Cannon M, Jones P, Huttunen MO, et al: School performance in Finnish children and later development of schizophrenia: a population-based longitudinal study. Arch Gen Psychiatry 56:457–463, 1999

Cannon M, Caspi A, Moffitt TE, et al: Evidence for early childhood, pan-developmental impairment specific to schizophreniform disorder: results from a longitudinal birth cohort. Arch Gen Psychiatry 59:449–456, 2002

Caspi A, Reichenberg A, Weiser M, et al: Cognitive performance in schizophrenia patients assessed before and following the first psychotic episode. Schizophr Res 65:87–94, 2003

Cecil KM, Lenkinski RE, Gur RE, et al: Proton magnetic resonance spectroscopy in the frontal and temporal lobes of neuroleptic naive patients with schizophrenia. Neuropsychopharmacology 20:131–140, 1999

Church SM, Cotter D, Bramon E, et al: Does schizophrenia result from developmental or degenerative processes? J Neural Transm Suppl 63:129–147, 2002

Cotter DR, Pariante CM, Everall IP: Glial cell abnormalities in major psychiatric disorders: the evidence and implications. Brain Res Bull 55:585–595, 2001

Coyle JT: The glutamatergic dysfunction hypothesis for schizophrenia. Harv Rev Psychiatry 3:241–253, 1996

Coyle JT, Puttfarcken P: Oxidative stress, glutamate, and neurodegenerative disorders. Science 262:689–695, 1993

Cullen TJ, Walker MA, Parkinson N, et al: A postmortem study of the mediodorsal nucleus of the thalamus in schizophrenia. Schizophr Res 60:157–166, 2003

Davis KL, Buchsbaum MS, Shihabuddin L, et al: Ventricular enlargement in poor-outcome schizophrenia. Biol Psychiatry 43:783–793, 1998

DeLisi LE, Sakuma M, Tew W, et al: Schizophrenia as a chronic active brain process: a study of progressive brain structural change subsequent to the onset of schizophrenia. Psychiatry Res 74:129–140, 1997

DeLisi LE, Sakuma M, Maurizio AM, et al: Cerebral ventricular change over the first 10 years after the onset of schizophrenia. Psychiatry Res 130:57–70, 2004

Done DJ, Crow TJ, Johnstone EC, et al: Childhood antecedents of schizophrenia and affective illness: social adjustment at ages 7 and 11. BMJ 309:699–703, 1994

Eastwood SL, Harrison PJ: Decreased synaptophysin in the medial temporal lobe in schizophrenia demonstrated using immunoautoradiography. Neuroscience 69:339–343, 1995

Eaton WW, Thara R, Federman B, et al: Structure and course of positive and negative symptoms in schizophrenia. Arch Gen Psychiatry 52:127–134, 1995

Eyler Zorrilla LT, Heaton RK, McAdams LA, et al: Cross-sectional study of older outpatients with schizophrenia and healthy comparison subjects: no differences in age-related cognitive decline. Am J Psychiatry 157:1324–1326, 2000

Fannon D, Chitnis X, Doku V, et al: Features of structural brain abnormality detected in first-episode psychosis. Am J Psychiatry 157:1829–1834, 2000

Fenton WS, McGlashan TH: Antecedents, symptom progression, and long-term outcome of the deficit syndrome in schizophrenia. Am J Psychiatry 151:351–356, 1994

Friedman JI, Harvey PD, McGurk SR, et al: Correlates of change in functional status of institutionalized geriatric schizophrenic patients: focus on medical comorbidity. Am J Psychiatry 159:1388–1394, 2002

Fuller R, Nopoulos P, Arndt S, et al: Longitudinal assessment of premorbid cognitive functioning in patients with schizophrenia through examination of standardized scholastic test performance. Am J Psychiatry 159:1183–1189, 2002

Garden GA, Budd SL, Tsai E, et al: Caspase cascades in human immunodeficiency virus-associated neurodegeneration. J Neurosci 22:4015–4024, 2002

Garey LJ, Ong WY, Patel TS, et al: Reduced dendritic spine density on cerebral cortical pyramidal neurons in schizophrenia. J Neurol Neurosurg Psychiatry 65:446–453, 1998

Glantz LA, Lewis DA: Reduction of synaptophysin immunoreactivity in the prefrontal cortex of subjects with schizophrenia: regional and diagnostic specificity. Arch Gen Psychiatry 54:943–952, 1997

Glantz LA, Lewis DA: Decreased dendritic spine density on prefrontal cortical pyramidal neurons in schizophrenia. Arch Gen Psychiatry 57:65–73, 2000

Goff DC, Coyle JT: The emerging role of glutamate in the pathophysiology and treatment of schizophrenia. Am J Psychiatry 158:1367–1377, 2001

Gogtay N, Sporn A, Clasen LS, et al: Comparison of progressive cortical gray matter loss in childhood-onset schizophrenia with that in childhood-onset atypical psychoses. Arch Gen Psychiatry 61:17–22, 2004

Green MF: What are the functional consequences of neurocognitive deficits in schizophrenia? Am J Psychiatry 153:321–330, 1996

Green MF, Kern RS, Braff DL, et al: Neurocognitive deficits and functional outcome in schizophrenia: are we measuring the "right stuff"? Schizophr Bull 26:119–136, 2000

Gur RE, Cowell P, Turetsky BI, et al: A follow-up magnetic resonance imaging study of schizophrenia: relationship of neuroanatomical changes to clinical and neurobehavioral measures. Arch Gen Psychiatry 55:145–152, 1998

Gylys KH, Fein JA, Wiley DJ, et al: Rapid annexin-V labeling in synaptosomes. Neurochem Int 44:125–131, 2004

Hambrecht M, Lammertink M, Klosterkotter J, et al: Subjective and objective neuropsychological abnormalities in a psychosis prodrome clinic. Br J Psychiatry 43 (suppl):S30–S37, 2002

Hardy J, Gwinn-Hardy K: Genetic classification of primary neurodegenerative disease. Science 282:1075–1079, 1998

Harrison PJ: The neuropathology of schizophrenia: a critical review of the data and their interpretation. Brain 122 (part 4):593–624, 1999

Harrison PJ, Eastwood SL: Neuropathological studies of synaptic connectivity in the hippocampal formation in schizophrenia. Hippocampus 11:508–519, 2001

Harvey PD, Silverman JM, Mohs RC, et al: Cognitive decline in late-life schizophrenia: a longitudinal study of geriatric chronically hospitalized patients. Biol Psychiatry 45:32–40, 1999

Heaton RK, Gladsjo JA, Palmer BW, et al: Stability and course of neuropsychological deficits in schizophrenia. Arch Gen Psychiatry 58:24–32, 2001

Hinsberger AD, Williamson PC, Carr TJ, et al: Magnetic resonance imaging volumetric and phosphorus 31 magnetic resonance spectroscopy measurements in schizophrenia. J Psychiatry Neurosci 22:111–117, 1997

Ho BC, Alicata D, Ward J, et al: Untreated initial psychosis: relation to cognitive deficits and brain morphology in first-episode schizophrenia. Am J Psychiatry 160:142–148, 2003

Hoff AL, Sakuma M, Wieneke M, et al: Longitudinal neuropsychological follow-up study of patients with first-episode schizophrenia. Am J Psychiatry 156:1336–1341, 1999

Hoff AL, Sakuma M, Razi K, et al: Lack of association between duration of untreated illness and severity of cognitive and structural brain deficits at the first episode of schizophrenia. Am J Psychiatry 157:1824–1828, 2000

Huber G, Gross G, Schuttler R, et al: Longitudinal studies of schizophrenic patients. Schizophr Bull 6:592–605, 1980

Hudson CJ, Kennedy JL, Gotowiec A, et al: Genetic variant near cytosolic phospholipase A2 associated with schizophrenia. Schizophr Res 21:111–116, 1996

Ivins KJ, Bui ET, Cotman CW: Beta-amyloid induces local neurite degeneration in cultured hippocampal neurons: evidence for neuritic apoptosis. Neurobiol Dis 5:365–378, 1998

Jacobsen LK, Giedd JN, Castellanos FX, et al: Progressive reduction of temporal lobe structures in childhood-onset schizophrenia. Am J Psychiatry 155:678–685, 1998

Jarskog LF, Gilmore JH, Selinger ES, et al: Cortical bcl-2 protein expression and apoptotic regulation in schizophrenia. Biol Psychiatry 48:641–650, 2000

Jarskog LF, Selinger ES, Lieberman JA, et al: Apoptotic proteins in the temporal cortex in schizophrenia: high Bax/Bcl-2 ratio without caspase-3 activation. Am J Psychiatry 161:109–115, 2004

Jones P, Rodgers B, Murray R, et al: Child development risk factors for adult schizophrenia in the British 1946 birth cohort. Lancet 344:1398–1402, 1994

Karson CN, Mrak RE, Schluterman KO, et al: Alterations in synaptic proteins and their encoding mRNAs in prefrontal cortex in schizophrenia: a possible neurochemical basis for "hypofrontality." Mol Psychiatry 4:39–45, 1999

Kasai K, Shenton ME, Salisbury DF, et al: Progressive decrease of left superior temporal gyrus gray matter volume in patients with first-episode schizophrenia. Am J Psychiatry 160:156–164, 2003

Kraepelin E: Dementia Praecox and Paraphrenia. Translated by Barclay RM. New York, Robert E Krieger Publishing Company, 1919

Kremen WS, Seidman LJ, Pepple JR, et al: Neuropsychological risk indicators for schizophrenia: a review of family studies. Schizophr Bull 20:103–119, 1994

Lewis DA, Lieberman JA: Catching up on schizophrenia: natural history and neurobiology. Neuron 28:325–334, 2000

Lieberman JA: Is schizophrenia a neurodegenerative disorder? A clinical and neurobiological perspective. Biol Psychiatry 46:729–739, 1999

Lieberman JA, Sheitman BB, Kinon BJ: Neurochemical sensitization in the pathophysiology of schizophrenia: deficits and dysfunction in neuronal regulation and plasticity. Neuropsychopharmacology 17:205–229, 1997

Lieberman JA, Chakos M, Wu H, et al: Longitudinal study of brain morphology in first episode schizophrenia. Biol Psychiatry 49:487–499, 2001a

Lieberman JA, Perkins D, Belger A, et al: The early stages of schizophrenia: speculations on pathogenesis, pathophysiology, and therapeutic approaches. Biol Psychiatry 50:884–897, 2001b

Mason P, Harrison G, Glazebrook C, et al: The course of schizophrenia over 13 years. A report from the International Study on Schizophrenia (ISoS) coordinated by the World Health Organization. Br J Psychiatry 169:580–586, 1996

Mathalon DH, Sullivan EV, Lim KO, et al: Progressive brain volume changes and the clinical course of schizophrenia in men: a longitudinal magnetic resonance imaging study. Arch Gen Psychiatry 58:148–157, 2001

Mattson MP, Keller JN, Begley JG: Evidence for synaptic apoptosis. Exp Neurol 153:35–48, 1998

Mayerhoff DI, Loebel AD, Alvir JM, et al: The deficit state in first-episode schizophrenia. Am J Psychiatry 151:1417–1422, 1994

McGlashan TH: A selective review of recent North American long-term follow-up studies of schizophrenia. Schizophr Bull 14:515–542, 1988

Moritz S, Andresen B, Perro C, et al: Neurocognitive performance in first-episode and chronic schizophrenic patients. Eur Arch Psychiatry Clin Neurosci 252:33–37, 2002

Mukerjee S, Mahadik SP, Scheffer R, et al: Impaired antioxidant defense at the onset of psychosis. Schizophr Res 19:19–26, 1996

Murray RM, Lewis SW: Is schizophrenia a neurodevelopmental disorder? Br Med J (Clin Res Ed) 295:681–682, 1987

Nair TR, Christensen JD, Kingsbury SJ, et al: Progression of cerebroventricular enlargement and the subtyping of schizophrenia. Psychiatry Res 74:141–150, 1997

Nopoulos P, Flashman L, Flaum M, et al: Stability of cognitive functioning early in the course of schizophrenia. Schizophr Res 14:29–37, 1994

Olney JW, Farber NB: Glutamate receptor dysfunction and schizophrenia. Arch Gen Psychiatry 52:998–1007, 1995

Oltvai ZN, Milliman CL, Korsmeyer SJ: Bcl-2 heterodimerizes in vivo with a conserved homolog, Bax, that accelerates programmed cell death. Cell 74:609–619, 1993

Ona VO, Li M, Vonsattel JP, et al: Inhibition of caspase-1 slows disease progression in a mouse model of Huntington's disease. Nature 399:263–267, 1999

Pakkenberg B: Pronounced reduction of total neuron number in mediodorsal thalamic nucleus and nucleus accumbens in schizophrenics. Arch Gen Psychiatry 47:1023–1028, 1990

Pakkenberg B: Total nerve cell number in neocortex in chronic schizophrenics and controls estimated using optical disectors. Biol Psychiatry 34:768–772, 1993

Pantelis C, Velakoulis D, McGorry PD, et al: Neuroanatomical abnormalities before and after onset of psychosis: a cross-sectional and longitudinal MRI comparison. Lancet 361:281–288, 2003

Perkins DO, Gu H, Boteva K, et al: Relationship of duration of untreated psychosis and outcome in first episode schizophrenia: a critical review and meta-analysis. Am J Psychiatry 162:1795–1804, 2005

Pettegrew JW, Keshavan MS, Panchalingam K, et al: Alterations in brain high-energy phosphate and membrane phospholipid metabolism in first-episode, drug-naive schizophrenics: a pilot study of the dorsal prefrontal cortex by in vivo phosphorus 31 nuclear magnetic resonance spectroscopy. Arch Gen Psychiatry 48:563–568, 1991

Pettegrew JW, Keshavan MS, Minshew NJ: 31P nuclear magnetic resonance spectroscopy: neurodevelopment and schizophrenia. Schizophr Bull 19:35–53, 1993

Pfohl B, Winokur G: The evolution of symptoms in institutionalized hebephrenic/catatonic schizophrenics. Br J Psychiatry 141:567–572, 1982

Pierri JN, Volk CL, Auh S, et al: Decreased somal size of deep layer 3 pyramidal neurons in the prefrontal cortex of subjects with schizophrenia. Arch Gen Psychiatry 58:466–473, 2001

Popken GJ, Bunney WE Jr, Potkin SG, et al: Subnucleus-specific loss of neurons in medial thalamus of schizophrenics. Proc Natl Acad Sci U S A 97:9276–9280, 2000

Purohit DP, Perl DP, Haroutunian V, et al: Alzheimer disease and related neurodegenerative diseases in elderly patients with schizophrenia: a postmortem neuropathologic study of 100 cases. Arch Gen Psychiatry 55:205–211, 1998

Rajkowska G, Selemon LD, Goldman-Rakic PS: Neuronal and glial somal size in the prefrontal cortex: a postmortem morphometric study of schizophrenia and Huntington disease. Arch Gen Psychiatry 55:215–224, 1998

Rapoport JL, Giedd J, Kumra S, et al: Childhood-onset schizophrenia: progressive ventricular change during adolescence. Arch Gen Psychiatry 54:897–903, 1997

Rapoport JL, Giedd JN, Blumenthal J, et al: Progressive cortical change during adolescence in childhood-onset schizophrenia: a longitudinal magnetic resonance imaging study. Arch Gen Psychiatry 56:649–654, 1999

Risch SC, Lewine RJ, Kalin NH, et al: Limbic-hypothalamic-pituitary-adrenal axis activity and ventricular-to-brain ratio studies in affective illness and schizophrenia. Neuropsychopharmacology 6:95–100, 1992

Roberts GW, Colter N, Lofthouse R, et al: Gliosis in schizophrenia: a survey. Biol Psychiatry 21:1043–1050, 1986

Roberts GW, Colter N, Lofthouse R, et al: Is there gliosis in schizophrenia? Investigation of the temporal lobe. Biol Psychiatry 22:1459–1468, 1987

Ross BM, Hudson C, Erlich J, et al: Increased phospholipid breakdown in schizophrenia: evidence for the involvement of a calcium-independent phospholipase A2. Arch Gen Psychiatry 54:487–494, 1997

Rund BR: A review of longitudinal studies of cognitive functions in schizophrenia patients. Schizophr Bull 24:425–435, 1998

Saykin AJ, Shtasel DL, Gur RE, et al: Neuropsychological deficits in neuroleptic naive patients with first-episode schizophrenia. Arch Gen Psychiatry 51:124–131, 1994

Selemon LD, Rajkowska G, Goldman-Rakic PS: Abnormally high neuronal density in the schizophrenic cortex: a morphometric analysis of prefrontal area 9 and occipital area 17. Arch Gen Psychiatry 52:805–818; discussion 819–820, 1995

Selemon LD, Rajkowska G, Goldman-Rakic PS: Elevated neuronal density in prefrontal area 46 in brains from schizophrenic patients: application of a three-dimensional, stereologic counting method. J Comp Neurol 392:402–412, 1998

Shenton ME, Dickey CC, Frumin M, et al: A review of MRI findings in schizophrenia. Schizophr Res 49:1–52, 2001

Smith A: Mental deterioration in chronic schizophrenia. J Nerv Ment Dis 139:479–487, 1964

Stanley JA, Williamson PC, Drost DJ, et al: An in vivo study of the prefrontal cortex of schizophrenic patients at different stages of illness via phosphorus magnetic resonance spectroscopy. Arch Gen Psychiatry 52:399–406, 1995

Stark AK, Uylings HB, Sanz-Arigita E, et al: Glial cell loss in the anterior cingulate cortex, a subregion of the prefrontal cortex, in subjects with schizophrenia. Am J Psychiatry 161:882–888, 2004

Stevens JR: Neuropathology of schizophrenia. Arch Gen Psychiatry 39:1131–1139, 1982

Thompson PM, Sower AC, Perrone-Bizzozero NI: Altered levels of the synaptosomal associated protein SNAP-25 in schizophrenia. Biol Psychiatry 43:239–243, 1998

Thompson PM, Vidal C, Giedd JN, et al: Mapping adolescent brain change reveals dynamic wave of accelerated gray matter loss in very early onset schizophrenia. Proc Natl Acad Sci U S A 98:11650–11655, 2001

Thune JJ, Uylings HB, Pakkenberg B: No deficit in total number of neurons in the prefrontal cortex in schizophrenics. J Psychiatr Res 35:15–21, 2001

Weinberger DR: Implications of normal brain development for the pathogenesis of schizophrenia. Arch Gen Psychiatry 44:660–669, 1987

Weinberger DR, McClure RK: Neurotoxicity, neuroplasticity, and magnetic resonance imaging morphometry: what is happening in the schizophrenic brain? Arch Gen Psychiatry 59:553–558, 2002

Weinberger DR, Berman KF, Zec RF: Physiologic dysfunction of dorsolateral prefrontal cortex in schizophrenia, I: Regional cerebral blood flow evidence. Arch Gen Psychiatry 43:114–124, 1986

Wolf ME, White FJ, Nassar R, et al: Differential development of autoreceptor subsensitivity and enhanced dopamine release during amphetamine sensitization. J Pharmacol Exp Ther 264:249–255, 1993

Wyatt RJ: Neuroleptics and the natural course of schizophrenia. Schizophr Bull 17:325–351, 1991

Young KA, Manaye KF, Liang C, et al: Reduced number of mediodorsal and anterior thalamic neurons in schizophrenia. Biol Psychiatry 47:944–953, 2000

NEUROPATHOLOGY AND NEURAL CIRCUITS IMPLICATED IN SCHIZOPHRENIA

L. Fredrik Jarskog, M.D.

Trevor W. Robbins, Ph.D.

Despite the prominent clinical manifestations of schizophrenia, a clear cellular phenotype of this devastating disorder has not been defined. Early in the twentieth century, Kraeplin suggested that schizophrenia was characterized by a degenerative pathology, and early studies by Alzheimer and by Southard supported this view. Subsequent studies, however, did not find evidence of degeneration, and during the reign of psychoanalytic psychiatry, many questioned the neurobiological underpinnings of schizophrenia. Fortunately, the development of better study designs and more sophisticated immunohistochemical and molecular techniques provided a limited set of subtle yet relatively reproducible neuropathological findings (Harrison 1999).

In part, neuropathology in schizophrenia is characterized by deficits in cortical neuropil and synaptic connectivity as well as a notable absence of glial proliferation. These deficits may underlie evidence for abnormal brain circuitry. Our aim in this chapter is first to highlight pertinent positive and negative histopathological and neurochemical findings in brain regions that have been implicated consistently in schizophrenia and then to explore the effect of these deficits on relevant brain circuitry. We examine the involvement of frontostriatothalamic, frontocingulate, and frontotemporal circuits, given the current research interest in these circuits and the accumulated neuropathological and neuroimaging findings within the respective brain regions. We begin, though, by reviewing normal cortical cytoarchitecture.

This work was supported in part by National Institute of Mental Health (NIMH) grant MH01752 and the University of North Carolina Schizophrenia Research Center and by a grant from the NIMH Silvio O. Conte Center for the Neuroscience of Mental Disorders (MH064065).

NORMAL CORTICAL CYTOARCHITECTURE

PYRAMIDAL AND NONPYRAMIDAL NEURONS

Pyramidal neurons represent the primary source of glutamatergic neurotransmission and constitute about 70% of all cortical neurons. These excitatory neurons have a single apical dendrite that extends toward the pial surface and multiple basilar dendrites that extend laterally. Dendrites are covered by small protrusions called dendritic spines that receive most excitatory input. In addition, inhibitory terminals are found on dendrites, cell soma, and the axon initial segment. Most pyramidal neurons also have a principal axon that extends into the white matter. Intrinsic collaterals project from the principal axons before entering the white matter, extending horizontally and then vertically in the cortical gray matter.

Nonpyramidal neurons provide inhibitory neurotransmission in the cerebral cortex, and almost all use the neurotransmitter γ-aminobutyric acid (GABA). GABAergic neurons are classified according to morphological and neurochemical characteristics. Subtypes of GABA neurons exert specific roles in the circuitry of dorsal prefrontal cortex (DPFC). For example, axon terminals of chandelier neurons synapse with the axon initial segment of pyramidal neurons to provide localized inhibition. In contrast, axon terminals of basket neurons spread horizontally much farther than chandelier neurons and are thus able to exert inhibitory regulation over more distal pyramidal neuron populations (Levitt et al. 1993).

CORTICAL LAMINAE AND CORTICAL PROJECTIONS

Neurons in cortical association areas are generally arranged in six layers (Amaral 2000) (see Figure 9–1). Layer I is thin and contains relatively few cells, but most neurons in this layer are GABAergic. Layers II and IV consist primarily of tightly packed, small pyramidal neurons and are often referred to as the *external* and *internal granular layers*, respectively. Layers III and V are generally the thickest layers and contain larger pyramidal neurons. Layer VI, also known as the *pleomorphic layer*, contains pyramidal neurons with atypical morphology.

The following is a brief overview of efferent projection patterns from cortical layers (Jones 1984). Pyramidal neurons in layer II and superficial layer III generally project to nearby cortical areas, whereas those in deep layer III project to more distal cortical regions. Pyramidal neurons in layer V project to multiple subcortical regions (not including thalamus), whereas those in layer VI project to the thalamus. In addition to their primary extrinsic projections, pyramidal neurons also provide local axon collaterals that have layer-specific patterns of intrinsic connections. The broad distribution of targets of efferent intrinsic and extrinsic projections from pyramidal neurons in the different cortical layers illustrates the extent to which even subtle abnormalities in a neuronal subtype with restricted laminar distribution could have significant effects on cortical connectivity.

In contrast to the layer-specific organization of efferent projections, afferent projections from other cortical regions are more evenly distributed in their synaptic terminations. Similarly, afferent projections from several subcortical regions are distributed evenly, including cholinergic projections from the nucleus basalis of Meynert and serotoninergic inputs from the raphe nucleus. However, afferent thalamic, dopaminergic, and noradrenergic projections to the DPFC each form more topographically restricted synaptic connections. Specifically, afferents from the mediodorsal thalamus terminate predominantly in cortical layer IV and deep layer III, whereas noradrenergic and dopaminergic afferents have a bimodal distribution in superficial and deep cortical layers (Lewis and Lieberman 2000).

HISTOPATHOLOGY OF SCHIZOPHRENIA

GLIAL NUMBERS AND MARKERS

Although an early study found an increase in periventricular and subependymal gliosis in schizophrenia (Stevens 1982), a general consensus has emerged that schizophrenia is characterized by an absence of glial proliferation (Arnold et al. 1998; Benes et al. 1991a; Roberts et al. 1986), and several recent reports even suggested that cortical glial density is decreased (Cotter et al. 2001; Stark et al. 2004; Uranova et al. 2004). Most studies also report normal glial fibrillary acidic protein (GFAP) staining (Arnold et al. 1998; Damadzic et al. 2001; Perrone-Bizzozero et al. 1996; Purohit et al. 1998; Roberts et al. 1987). GFAP is a structural protein that increases markedly in response to astrocytic infiltration following neuronal damage and is often elevated in classic neurodegenerative disorders such as Alzheimer's disease. Interestingly, a proteomic analysis of frontal cortex identified four proteins that were differentially expressed in schizophrenia compared with control, two of which were reductions in isoforms of GFAP (Johnston-Wilson et al. 2000). The absence of gliosis strongly suggests the absence of a classic neurodegenerative process, providing general support for schizophrenia as a disorder of neurodevelopment. It has been argued,

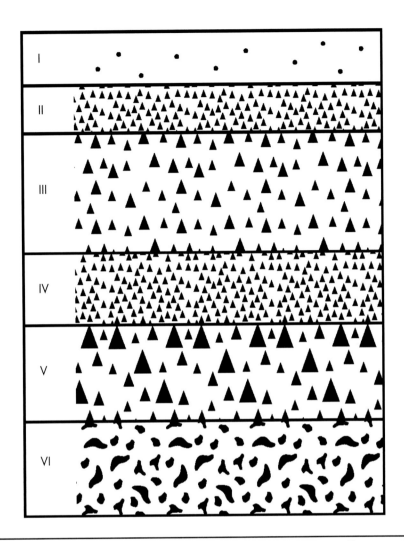

FIGURE 9–1.   Depiction of the six cortical layers, showing the lamina-specific differences in neuronal shape, size, and packing density.

Layer I is sparsely populated with small interneurons, layers II and IV are tightly packed with small pyramidal neurons, layers III and V are thickest and contain large pyramidal neurons, and layer VI contains pleomorphic cells.

however, that the absence of gliosis does not rule out a more limited degenerative process (Lieberman 1999; see Chapter 8, "Neuroprogressive Theories").

NEURONAL NUMBER AND DISTRIBUTION

Classic neurodegenerative disorders are generally characterized by large-scale neuronal loss, but little evidence suggests that schizophrenia is associated with substantial cortical neuronal loss. One study that used unbiased stereology found no change in total cortical neuronal number in schizophrenia compared with control subjects (Pakkenberg 1993). Likewise, several studies found no evidence of neuronal loss in DPFC in schizophrenia (Akbarian et al. 1995a; Selemon et al. 1995, 1998; Thune et al. 2001) but did find small but significant increases in

neuronal density in prefrontal and occipital cortex in schizophrenic compared with control subjects. The investigators interpreted these increases to reflect modest reductions in neuropil rather than absolute changes in neuronal counts (see Figure 9–2). However, several studies have found reductions in the densities of neuronal subpopulations, including interneurons in layer II of DPFC and in layers II–VI of the anterior cingulate cortex (ACC) (Benes et al. 1991a, 2001).

In contrast to cortex, reduced neuronal numbers have been found more consistently in subcortical areas in schizophrenia. An early stereological study reported about 30% fewer neurons in nucleus accumbens and mediodorsal thalamus in schizophrenia (Pakkenberg 1990). The mediodorsal thalamus findings have been replicated in many (Byne et al. 2002; Popken et al. 2000; K.A. Young et

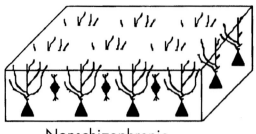

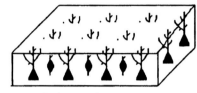

FIGURE 9–2.   Schematic depiction of the "reduced neuropil" hypothesis of schizophrenia.

The cortex of individuals with schizophrenia is thinner and the neurons are smaller and more densely packed as compared with the cortex of nonschizophrenic control subjects. However, the overall number of neurons is not different in schizophrenia compared with control subjects.

Source.   Reprinted from Selemon LD, Rajkowska G, Goldman-Rakic PS: "Abnormally High Neuronal Density in the Schizophrenic Cortex: A Morphometric Analysis of Prefrontal Area 9 and Occipital Area 17." *Archives of General Psychiatry* 52:805–818, 1995. Copyright 1995, American Medical Association. Used with permission.

al. 2000), but not all (Cullen et al. 2003; Dorph-Petersen et al. 2004), studies. In hippocampus, a meta-analysis of neuroimaging studies found consistent volume reductions (Nelson et al. 1998), but most postmortem studies have not reported an overall loss of neurons (Heckers et al. 1991; Walker et al. 2002). Notably, several studies have identified reductions in hippocampal neuronal subpopulations, specifically in GABAergic interneurons (Benes et al. 1998; Zhang and Reynolds 2002). Thus, although overall cortical neuronal numbers in schizophrenia appear mostly unchanged, discrete neuronal reductions may occur with laminar and regional specificity. Furthermore, several discrete subcortical nuclei appear to have more substantial neuronal reductions.

Investigators also have examined neuronal distribution and organization in schizophrenia. In entorhinal cortex, several studies have suggested abnormal lamination as well as neuronal disorganization, consistent with migrational deficits early in development (Arnold et al. 1991, 1997; Jakob and Beckmann 1986). In frontal and temporal cortices, abnormal distribution of nicotinamide-adenine dinucleotide phosphate-diaphorase (NADPH-D)–containing neurons in gray and white matter has been reported, thought to reflect deficits in migration or neuronal apoptosis (Akbarian et al. 1993a, 1993b, 1996a, 1996b).

Whereas evidence of neuronal maldistribution has been used to support the neurodevelopmental hypothesis of schizophrenia, other studies have failed to replicate these findings (Akil and Lewis 1997; Krimer et al. 1997). Taken together, these data are suggestive, but not conclusive, of neuronal disorganization in schizophrenia, and further studies are needed to clarify this important issue.

NEUROPIL AND SYNAPTIC MARKERS

As mentioned earlier, evidence suggests that the cortical neuropathology of schizophrenia involves a reduction in cortical neuropil (Selemon and Goldman-Rakic 1999) (see Figure 9–2). Neuropil is primarily composed of axons, dendrites, and synaptic terminals. Consistent with the "reduced neuropil" hypothesis is evidence of reduced dendritic spines and total dendritic length of pyramidal neurons in DPFC in schizophrenia (Black et al. 2004; Garey et al. 1998; Glantz and Lewis 2000), fewer parvalbumin (PV)– and GABA membrane transporter (GAT-1)–immunoreactive varicosities (Lewis et al. 2001; Pierri et al. 1999), and reduction in synaptophysin (a presynaptic marker) (Eastwood and Harrison 1995; Glantz and Lewis 1997; Karson et al. 1999; Perrone-Bizzozero et al. 1996) and SNAP-25 protein (Gabriel et al. 1997; Karson et

1999; Thompson et al. 1998). Synaptic pathology is also suggested in hippocampus, where investigators have found reduced synaptophysin (Eastwood and Harrison 1995; Vawter et al. 1999) and reduced SNAP-25 (C.E. Young et al. 1998). Two other recently described synaptic markers—complexin I and complexin II—are thought to be associated with inhibitory and excitatory neurons, respectively. Reductions of both complexins have been reported in medial temporal lobe in schizophrenia (Harrison and Eastwood 1998).

Neural cell adhesion molecule (NCAM), another protein increasingly appreciated for its diverse roles in neurodevelopment and synaptic stabilization, also has been implicated in schizophrenia. In schizophrenia, compared with controls, NCAM in the hippocampus has been reported as both reduced (Barbeau et al. 1995) and increased (Vawter et al. 1999), whereas in frontal cortex, NCAM appears unchanged (Barbeau et al. 1995).

The postmortem data implicating synaptic and neuropil changes in schizophrenia are also supported by a gene array study that identified reduced expression of multiple genes coding for synaptic gene products in DPFC (Mirnics et al. 2000). Taken together, the evidence implicating neuropil and synaptic abnormalities in the pathophysiology of schizophrenia is strong.

NEURONAL SOMA

Small but significant reductions in pyramidal neuronal size in DPFC have been reported in schizophrenia compared with controls (Pierri et al. 2001, 2003; Rajkowska et al. 1998). Other studies in DPFC and ACC did not find differences (Benes et al. 1986, 2000; Cotter et al. 2001). In hippocampus, several studies have reported smaller pyramidal neurons in schizophrenia (Arnold et al. 1995; Benes et al. 1991b, 1998; Zaidel et al. 1997). Because somal size is thought to be related in part to the extent of dendritic and axonal arborization (Elston and Rosa 1997; Jacobs et al. 1997), reduced somal size in schizophrenia is consistent with evidence for reduced dendritic spine density and dendritic length. Although the etiology remains unclear, smaller somal volumes could stem from early developmental agenesis or subtle atrophy at a later stage in a process not severe enough to induce gliosis (Rajkowska et al. 1998).

GABAERGIC SYSTEM

GABA represents the main inhibitory neurotransmitter of the cerebral cortex and is a critical modulator of cortical-subcortical connectivity. Deficits in the GABAergic system represent some of the most consistent neuropathological findings in schizophrenia. Glutamic acid decar-

boxylase (GAD), the enzyme that synthesizes GABA, exists as 65-kDa and 67-kDa isoforms. GAD_{67} mRNA, but not GAD_{65} mRNA, is reduced in DPFC in schizophrenia (Akbarian et al. 1995a; Guidotti et al. 2000; Volk et al. 2000). Consistent with these findings is increased $GABA_A$ receptor binding in ACC and DPFC in schizophrenia (Benes et al. 1992b; Dean et al. 1999), which may represent a compensatory upregulation in response to reduced GABA levels, and the increased receptor binding appears preferentially to affect pyramidal over nonpyramidal neurons (Benes et al. 1996). Furthermore, studies have found fewer GAT-1 cartridges in the GABAergic chandelier neurons of DPFC in schizophrenia (Pierri et al. 1999; Woo et al. 1998). GAT-1 cartridges reflect the vertical arrangement of axon terminals of chandelier cells that synapse at the axon initial segment of layer III pyramidal neurons and are thought to modulate excitatory output from pyramidal neurons.

Additional data come from studies of the calcium-binding proteins PV, calretinin, and calbindin, which are present in separate subpopulations of interneurons. One study found that PV-immunoreactive neurons were reduced in DPFC in schizophrenia (Beasley and Reynolds 1997; Lewis et al. 2001), but another study found no differences (Woo et al. 1997). This latter group did find fewer PV-immunoreactive varicosities in the middle layer of DPFC in schizophrenia (Lewis et al. 2001), but even though PV mRNA was also reduced, this reduction was on a per-neuron level rather than an overall reduction of PV mRNA-containing neurons (Hashimoto et al. 2003). Thus, it appears that GABAergic deficits occur in schizophrenia in several cortical regions, and although total interneuron numbers may not be altered, there is emerging evidence for changes in certain GABAergic neuron subpopulations as well as deficits of the GABAergic system.

GLUTAMATERGIC SYSTEM

The glutamatergic system is the principal excitatory neurotransmitter system of the human frontal cortex (Robinson and Coyle 1987). Four types of glutamate receptors have been identified, including the G protein–coupled metabotropic receptor family and the three ionotropic receptor families (N-methyl-D-aspartate [NMDA], AMPA, and kainate). The observation that the NMDA glutamate receptor antagonist phencyclidine (PCP) can reproduce positive, negative, and cognitive symptoms of schizophrenia in healthy control subjects (Krystal et al. 1994) and exacerbate psychosis in patients with schizophrenia (Lahti et al. 1995) has contributed significantly to the glutamate hypothesis of schizophrenia (Coyle 1996; Javitt and Zukin 1991; Olney and Farber 1995).

TABLE 9–1. Postmortem studies of glutamate receptor expression

Glutamate receptor subtype	Brain region	Increased subunit mRNA	Decreased subunit mRNA	Studies
N-methyl-D-aspartate (NMDA)	Prefrontal cortex	NR1, NR2A		Dracheva et al. 2001
		NR2D		Akbarian et al. 1996b
	Superior temporal cortex		NR1	Humphries et al. 1996
	Thalamus		NR1, NR2B, NR2C	Ibrahim et al. 2000b
		NR2B		Clinton and Meador-Woodruff 2004
	Hippocampus		NR1	Gao et al. 2000
AMPA	Prefrontal cortex	GluR2 (unedited form)		Akbarian et al. 1995b
	Thalamus		GluR1, GluR3	Ibrahim et al. 2000a
	Hippocampus		GluR1	Eastwood et al. 1997
Kainate	Prefrontal cortex	GluR7	KA2	Meador-Woodruff et al. 2001
	Thalamus		KA2	Ibrahim et al. 2000b
	Hippocampus		GluR6, KA2	Porter et al. 1997

The glutamatergic system has not been studied as extensively as the GABAergic system in schizophrenia, but emerging data are suggestive of glutamatergic dysfunction. Although ligand-binding studies of the NMDA receptor have been relatively unrevealing, real-time polymerase chain reaction and in situ hybridization techniques have identified significant alterations in each of the ionotropic glutamatergic receptor systems (see Table 9–1). Findings from ligand-binding studies of AMPA and kainate have been largely consistent with those of receptor expression (Meador-Woodruff and Healy 2000).

The complexity of glutamatergic neurotransmission makes the functional significance of postmortem changes in glutamate receptor levels uncertain. For instance, it is unknown whether changes found in NMDA receptor expression might lead to receptor hypofunction and the clinical picture of schizophrenia, as suggested by the link between PCP and schizophrenia-like symptoms. However, taken as a whole, the data are supportive of glutamatergic deficits at the neuropathological level in schizophrenia. Given the potential for new insights into the pathophysiology of schizophrenia and the potential therapeutic relevance of agents that modulate glutamate neurotransmission, research in this area is of considerable importance.

DOPAMINERGIC SYSTEM

The dopamine hypothesis has undergone significant revisions over the past 15 years. The current iteration suggests that subcortical hyperdopaminergia coexists with hypodopaminergia in frontal cortex and that the imbalance of subcortical-to-cortical dopamine levels may contribute to positive, negative, and cognitive symptoms of schizophrenia (Abi-Dargham and Moore 2003). Although a subcortical increase in dopamine transmission had long been hypothesized, direct evidence has emerged only recently. Several single photon emission computed tomography (SPECT) studies have reported increased striatal dopamine transmission in both first-episode neuroleptic-naive patients and previously treated chronically ill patients with acute psychosis (Abi-Dargham et al. 1998, 2000). These data have helped foster renewed interest in the dopamine hypothesis of schizophrenia (Laruelle et al. 2003). The hypothesis that the positive symptoms of schizophrenia are in part mediated (or exacerbated) by increased subcortical dopamine activity is consistent with the antipsychotic action of dopamine D_2 receptor antagonists, which are presumed to act mainly in the striatum (including the nucleus accumbens) because of the greater density of dopamine D_2 receptors in the striatum relative to the DPFC (Lidow and Goldman-Rakic 1994).

The most consistent postmortem finding has been that of increased dopamine D_2 receptor density in striatum in schizophrenia, confirmed by meta-analysis (Zakzanis and Hansen 1998). However, this finding is generally attributed to a compensatory upregulation in response to chronic neuroleptic treatment. Given that working memory relies in part on dopamine modulation in the DPFC and that working memory deficits have been extensively documented in schizophrenia (Park and Holzman 1992; Sawaguchi and Goldman-Rakic 1994), several groups have performed postmortem assessments of cortical dopamine tracts. Decreased lengths of tyrosine hydroxylase–immunoreactive axons and dopamine membrane transporter–positive axons in layer VI of DPFC and decreased density of tyrosine hydroxylase–immunoreactive axons in entorhinal cortex have been identified, and an analysis of these brain regions in haloperidol-treated monkeys did not indicate that these findings were relted to medication (Akil et al. 1999, 2000). Another study found no changes in tyrosine hydroxylase–immunoreactive varicosities in DPFC or ACC in schizophrenia compared with control subjects, although reductions in schizophrenia were found in several layers of ACC in medicated patients only (Benes et al. 1997). Changes also have been identified in dopamine receptor transcript expression in schizophrenia, including reduced levels of D_3 and D_4 receptor mRNA in DPFC (Mcador-Woodruff et al. 1997), whereas another study found increased D_4 receptor mRNA levels in DPFC but no change in caudate (Stefanis et al. 1998). Taken together, these postmortem data on the dopaminergic system suggest a pattern of dopaminergic dysregulation that is both cortical and subcortical; some findings appear related to antipsychotic treatment, but other changes are treatment independent.

NEURONAL CIRCUITS IMPLICATED IN SCHIZOPHRENIA

Accumulating postmortem and in vivo data make it abundantly clear that the pathophysiology of schizophrenia is not restricted to a single brain region or a single neuronal subtype. Indeed, studies have provided evidence of multiple brain region involvement, both within and between various cortical and subcortical areas, as well as deficits in multiple neuronal cell types with diverse functions. In this section, we review evidence for involvement of three key circuits that have been implicated in schizophrenia: 1) corticostriatothalamic, 2) prefrontal–anterior cingulate, and 3) frontotemporal. Furthermore, given our focus on postmortem neuropathology, in the last section, we examine the cellular basis of working memory impairment as an illustration of how postmortem neuropathological deficits could contribute to an important behavioral dimension of schizophrenia via circuit abnormalities. Deficits in working memory are well established in schizophrenia (Goldman-Rakic 1994), and their functional importance has clearly been established, given that working memory function has emerged as one of the

strongest predictors of long-term functional outcome in the disorder (Green et al. 2000).

CORTICOSTRIATOTHALAMIC CIRCUITRY

The corticostriatothalamic pathways represent at least five somewhat parallel cortical-subcortical circuits (Alexander et al. 1986). Specifically, these motor-cognitive-affective circuits link DPFC, orbitofrontal, anterior cingulate, oculomotor, and supplementary motor areas to the striatum, basal ganglia, and thalamus. Projections also link back from the thalamus to the frontal cortex to form closed loops, as well as project to other cortical and subcortical areas, forming open loop connections (Haber et al. 2000; Tekin and Cummings 2002).

In an effort to understand the symptomatology of schizophrenia in terms of brain function, particular attention has been paid to the connectivity between DPFC and striatum. Impairments in DPFC circuitry have been identified in a variety of paradigms, including in response to working memory challenges with functional magnetic resonance imaging (fMRI) (Callicott et al. 2003; Weinberger et al. 1986) and positron emission tomography (PET) (Schroeder et al. 1994). Numerous neuropsychological studies have linked executive function deficits to frontostriatal circuitry in schizophrenia (Pantelis et al. 1997; Robbins 1990). PET studies also have reported simultaneous changes in DPFC and basal ganglia, with evidence of reduced metabolic activity in basal ganglia and concomitant cortical hypofrontality (Buchsbaum et al. 1992; Siegel et al. 1993). Cortical hypofrontality also has been identified by magnetic resonance spectroscopy (MRS), showing reduced N-acetylaspartate (NAA) levels in DPFC (Bertolino et al. 1996); NAA is thought to be a measure of neuronal viability. Together, these data provide compelling evidence for deficits in frontostriatal circuitry in schizophrenia.

Interestingly, the evidence for metabolic hypofrontality in frontal cortex is also reflected in reduced level of cortical dopamine transmission, one of the key tenets of the updated dopamine hypothesis of schizophrenia. Use of ^{11}C-labeled NNC-112, a PET ligand for the dopamine D_1 receptor, showed increased availability of D_1 receptors in the frontal cortex of schizophrenic patients, and this was strongly associated with impaired working memory function (Abi-Dargham et al. 2002). This finding is thought to reflect evidence of compensatory D_1 receptor upregulation secondary to chronic hypodopaminergia in the frontal cortex. These data complement the data showing that schizophrenia is also associated with increased stimulation of striatal D_2 receptors (Abi-Dargham et al. 2000).

To examine the relation between cortical metabolism and striatal dopamine function, an elegant study measured both regional cerebral blood flow (rCBF) and presynaptic dopamine function with PET during a working memory task. Investigators found that reduced activation of DPFC was tightly linked and predictive of exaggerated striatal dopamine function (Meyer-Lindenberg et al. 2002). Thus, the balance of cortical and subcortical dopamine function appears to be a critical component of the pathophysiology of schizophrenia, and studies described here are beginning to provide direct evidence of the dopamine hypothesis via frontostriatal circuit abnormalities.

PREFRONTAL–ANTERIOR CINGULATE CIRCUITRY

Extensive reciprocal connectivity exists between ACC and DPFC (areas 9 and 46) as well as among other cortical (orbitofrontal, temporal) and subcortical (including amygdala, parahippocampus, and insula) regions (Mega et al. 1997). ACC has broad integrative functions that include affect regulation, motivation, and attention (Tamminga et al. 2000). In particular, recent studies have reported that ACC serves to signal the occurrence of conflicts in information processing, thereby triggering compensatory adjustments in cognitive control (reviewed by Botvinick et al. 2004). For example, investigators who used fMRI to examine brain activity in subjects performing a cognitive task designed to produce cognitive conflict (Stroop color-naming task) found that ACC conflict-related activity predicted both greater DPFC activity and adjustments in behavior, implicating ACC in conflict monitoring in the engagement of cognitive control (Kerns et al. 2004).

Several neuroimaging studies have shown abnormal activation of ACC in schizophrenia. For example, using PET, Tamminga et al. (1992) identified reduced glucose metabolism in ACC in medication-free schizophrenic patients compared with control subjects, without evidence of DPFC changes. PET also has been used to find hypometabolism in ACC during attentional tasks (e.g., Stroop task) (Carter et al. 1997; Yucel et al. 2002). Furthermore, in response to psychotomimetic ketamine, schizophrenic patients show significant activation of ACC, pointing to ACC involvement in ketamine-induced psychosis (Lahti et al. 1995).

Considerable neuropathological data corroborate the neuroimaging findings that implicate abnormalities in ACC in schizophrenia. Investigators have found reduced density of GABAergic interneurons in multiple layers of ACC in schizophrenia compared with healthy control subjects (Benes et al. 1986, 1991a, 2001). Evidence indicates increased $GABA_A$ receptor binding in ACC, prefer-

entially localized to pyramidal neurons in cortical layer II (Benes et al. 1992b). In addition, the number of vertical glutamatergic processes in layer II of ACC is increased (Benes et al. 1992a).

In summary, given the important role of ACC in regulating the activity of the DPFC during attentional tasks and evidence that attention and other high-order cognitive functions appear to be primary deficits in schizophrenia, the data reviewed suggest a prominent role for abnormal prefrontal–anterior cingulate circuitry in the disorder.

FRONTOTEMPORAL CIRCUITRY

The temporal lobe has mesial (hippocampus, amygdala, entorhinal, and perirhinal cortices) and nonmesial (inferior, middle, and superior temporal gyri and anterior temporal pole) subdivisions. The hippocampus and adjacent entorhinal and perirhinal cortices form the highly interconnected hippocampal complex, which connects with higher association areas including the cingulate cortex via Papez's circuit (Mega et al. 1997). As reviewed, considerable reciprocal connectivity exists between ACC and DPFC. Direct projections between the hippocampus and the PFC also have been described (Carr and Sesack 1996; Swanson 1981). Therefore, direct and indirect connectivity of mesolimbic structures can clearly influence DPFC function.

Considerable interest in frontotemporal connectivity in schizophrenia stems in part from the observation that neonatal hippocampal lesions in rats reproduce several behavioral, pharmacological, and molecular features that have been associated with schizophrenia. These include the delayed emergence of deficits starting in adolescence (postnatal days 40–60), behavioral abnormalities linked to increased striatal and mesolimbic dopamine transmission according to pharmacological challenge studies, impaired working memory function, and deficits in prepulse inhibition (Lipska and Weinberger 2003). However, it appears that altered development of the prefrontal cortex subsequent to neonatal hippocampal lesions contributes to several of the subsequent behavioral abnormalities (i.e., amphetamine-induced hyperlocomotion) (Lipska et al. 1998). Another study of adult nonhuman primates that had medial temporal lobe lesions either as neonates or as adults found that monkeys that were lesioned as adults had a reduction in striatal dopamine levels following amphetamine infusion into the DPFC, much as did unlesioned control animals. In contrast, monkeys that were lesioned as neonates had an increase in striatal dopamine levels following amphetamine infusion (Saunders et al.

1998). This crucial study highlights the importance of frontotemporal connectivity and its effect on distal brain regions (e.g., striatum and its interactions with the DPFC), especially when considered in the context of schizophrenia, which is widely accepted as a disorder of neurodevelopment.

Several studies have suggested frontotemporal dysconnectivity in schizophrenia. For example, when PET was used to measure brain activity during a cognitive task, control subjects showed reciprocal activation of prefrontal cortex with concomitant deactivation of superior temporal cortex, whereas subjects with schizophrenia had a failure of task-related deactivation of superior temporal cortex, suggesting significant frontotemporal dysconnectivity (Fletcher et al. 1996; Frith et al. 1995). Investigators have used electroencephalography to detect reduced coherence between frontal and temporal regions, suggesting impaired connectivity and potentially providing a basis for misattribution of inner thoughts to external voices in schizophrenia (Ford et al. 2002). Given that both DPFC and temporal cortex are extensively connected via ACC with considerably less direct connectivity, and given the extent to which cellular and functional pathology has been associated with ACC, an interesting consideration is the degree to which abnormalities in ACC might underlie frontotemporal deficits. Nevertheless, it is clear from both clinical and preclinical perspectives that frontotemporal circuit deficits contribute to the pathophysiology of schizophrenia.

CELLULAR BASIS OF WORKING MEMORY CIRCUITRY

In this section, we consider the neuropathological basis of the "working memory circuit." Working memory deficits were described earlier, especially in relation to frontostriatothalamic circuits and also hippocampal function. Considerable data on the cellular basis for working memory have emerged from studies in primates. In particular, the "delayed-response" task in monkeys is thought to be analogous to working memory tasks in humans. Studies have found that sustained neuronal firing in the DPFC of monkeys during the delay portion of the delayed-response task appears to be required for the animal to respond correctly (Funahashi et al. 1989). The phenomenon of active and sustained neuronal firing is thought to contribute to working memory function. Furthermore, studies of 2-deoxyglucose use suggest that layer III pyramidal neurons of the DPFC are involved (Friedman and Goldman-Rakic 1994; Goldman-Rakic 1995). Numerous postmortem studies implicate layer III pyramidal cells in DPFC in the neuropathology of schizophrenia, including evidence of re-

duced somal size (Pierri et al. 2001, 2003; Rajkowska et al. 1998), fewer dendritic spines (Garey et al. 1998; Glantz and Lewis 2000), and reduced total dendritic length. These data contribute to a potential cellular basis for impaired working memory function (Lewis and Akil 1997; Lewis and Lieberman 2000) (see Figure 9–3).

Specifically, layer III pyramidal neurons provide excitatory output in the DPFC, and the principal axons of these neurons also extend intrinsic collaterals prior to entering the white matter. These collaterals extend horizontally and organize into discrete clusters. Of these clustered axon collaterals, about half form excitatory synapses with dendritic spines of pyramidal neurons, and the other half synapse with dendritic shafts of GABAergic inhibitory neurons (Dorph-Petersen et al. 2004; Melchitzky et al. 2001), particularly those of the PV-containing class of interneurons (Melchitzky and Lewis 2003). In contrast, the axon collaterals that travel between clusters primarily form excitatory synapses with dendritic spines of layer III pyramidal neurons (Melchitzky et al. 1998). Together, these findings suggest an important role for layer III pyramidal neurons in the so-called reverberating excitatory circuit implicated in working memory (Pucak et al. 1996). Given that layer III pyramidal neurons interact both locally and distally within the DPFC, the neuropathological deficits described in schizophrenia have the potential to influence normal working memory function profoundly.

GABA INTERNEURONS

GABAergic chandelier cells form inhibitory synapses on layer III pyramidal neurons. These synapses arrange to form so-called cartridges on the axon initial segment of the pyramidal neurons. Because the excitatory output of layer III pyramidal cells is modulated by chandelier cell axon terminals, the chandelier neuron likely represents another important link in DPFC circuitry underlying working memory function.

Several studies have identified deficits in chandelier cells in schizophrenia (see Figure 9–3). Specifically, studies found a mean reduction of 40% of GAT-1 cartridges in DPFC (Woo et al. 1997), and these reductions were most apparent in deep layer III and layer IV (Pierri et al. 1999). Furthermore, the density of neurons containing GAT-1 mRNA was reduced by 21%–33% (Volk et al. 2001). Because the GAT-1 cartridges reflect the point at which the inhibitory chandelier cells synapse on the axon initial segment of layer III pyramidal neurons, it is hypothesized that the inhibitory modulation of excitatory output of pyramidal neurons is significantly altered in DPFC in schizophrenia, and this represents further evidence of disrupted DPFC circuitry in the disorder.

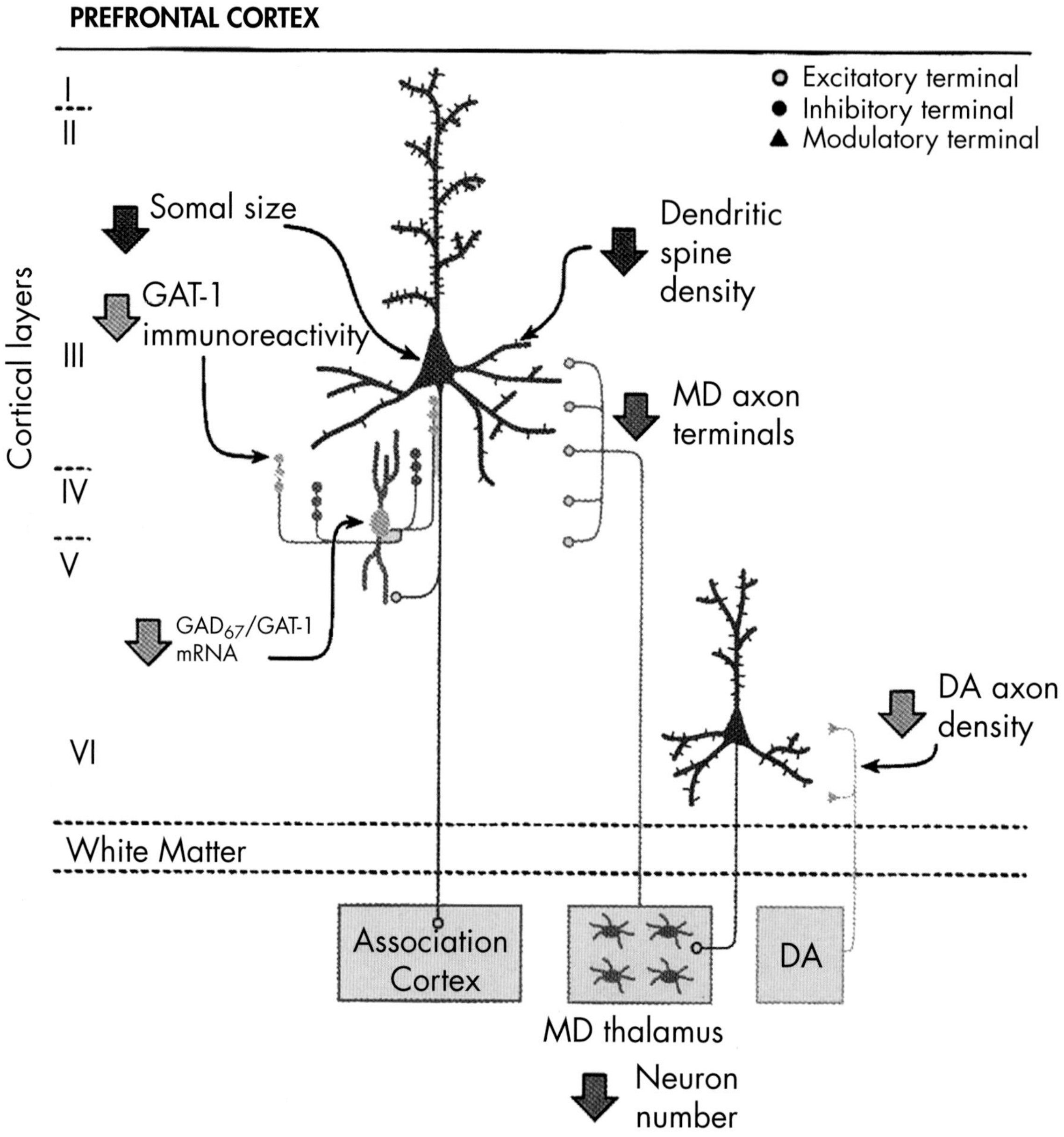

PREFRONTAL CORTEX

FIGURE 9–3. Cortical circuitry in schizophrenia.

Schematic diagram summarizing disturbances in the connectivity between the mediodorsal (MD) thalamic nucleus and the dorsal prefrontal cortex (PFC) in schizophrenia. Postmortem studies have reported that subjects with schizophrenia have 1) decreased number of neurons in the MD thalamic nucleus; 2) diminished density of parvalbumin-positive varicosities, a putative marker of thalamic axon terminals, selectively in deep layers III–IV, the termination zone of MD thalamic projections to the PFC; 3) reduced expression of the mRNA for glutamic acid decarboxylase (GAD_{67}), the synthesizing enzyme for γ-aminobutyric acid (GABA), in a subset of PFC GABA neurons; 4) decreased density of GABA transporter (GAT-1)–immunoreactive axon cartridges, the distinctive, vertically arrayed axon terminals of GABAergic chandelier neurons, which synapse exclusively on the axon initial segment of pyramidal neurons; and 5) decreased dopamine (DA) innervation of layer VI, the principal location of pyramidal neurons that provide corticothalamic feedback projections.

Source. Reprinted from Lewis DA, Lieberman JA: "Catching Up on Schizophrenia: Natural History and Neurobiology." *Neuron* 28:325–334, 2000. Used with permission of Elsevier.

THALAMIC PROJECTION NEURONS

Circuitry underlying working memory also has been shown to involve afferent projections from the mediodorsal thalamus (Isseroff et al. 1982). Thalamic afferents synapse on dendritic spines of pyramidal neurons in layers III and IV of DPFC (Giguere and Goldman-Rakic 1988; Melchitzky et al. 1999). In schizophrenia, several lines of histopathological evidence converge to indicate that thalamic afferent projections to the DPFC are reduced (Figure 9–3). First, as described earlier, fewer neurons in the mediodorsal thalamic nucleus in schizophrenia compared with control subjects have been found in many (Byne et al. 2002; Pakkenberg 1990; Popken et al. 2000; K.A. Young et al. 2000), but not all (Cullen et al. 2003; Dorph-Petersen et al. 2004), studies. This suggests that cortical projections from the thalamus are also reduced.

Second, evidence suggests that PV-immunoreactive varicosities are reduced in deep layer III and layer IV in area 9, whereas in the superficial cortical layers, the density of PV-immunoreactive varicosities is unchanged in schizophrenia (Lewis et al. 2001). Studies in monkey DPFC in deep layer III and layer IV have found that about 50% of PV-immunoreactive axon terminals are excitatory, but in layer II and superficial layer III, all PV-immunoreactive varicosities are inhibitory (Giguere and Goldman-Rakic 1988). This suggests that the reduction of PV-immunoreactive varicosities in middle cortical layers in DPFC in schizophrenia indeed reflects fewer afferent thalamic projections.

Finally, as reviewed earlier, the number of dendritic spines and the somal volume of layer III pyramidal neurons are reduced in schizophrenia, and both of these findings are consistent with a reduction in thalamic inputs. Together, these data are consistent with further disruption in DPFC circuitry that underlies working memory in schizophrenia.

DOPAMINERGIC AFFERENTS

A critical role for an intact DPFC dopaminergic system in maintaining normal working memory function was first identified in primates (Brozoski et al. 1979). Because dopaminergic afferents are known to synapse with both pyramidal neurons and GABAergic inhibitory neurons in DPFC (Sesack et al. 1998), the cortical dopamine projections can provide significant modulation of DPFC output. In schizophrenia, the total length of tyrosine hydroxylase–immunoreactive axons is reduced by approximately 30%, with a similar reduction in dopamine membrane transporter–positive axons in layer VI of DPFC (Akil et al. 1999) (Figure 9–3). Given that pyramidal neurons in layer

VI of DPFC project back to the thalamus, the observed deficits suggest another point of altered corticothalamic connectivity.

CONCLUSION

The neuropathology of schizophrenia is subtle and lacks pathognomonic lesions. Even for findings that are considered quite consistent, one or more studies often find opposite or negative results. Nevertheless, converging lines of investigation increasingly characterize and identify schizophrenia as a disorder of synaptic dysconnectivity involving multiple interconnected brain circuits.

Most studies find overall neuronal numbers in schizophrenia to be unchanged from those in healthy control subjects, although certain neuronal subpopulations appear to be reduced, including a marked reduction in mediodorsal thalamus, which may particularly influence corticothalamic connectivity. Several consistent neurochemical deficits have been identified, especially involving the GABAergic system in DPFC and ACC. Considerable neuropathological research has focused on DPFC, hippocampus, and ACC, but data also implicate other brain regions, including temporal, parietal, and occipital cortices as well as cerebellum, suggesting that the pathophysiology of schizophrenia is not narrowly restricted. One of the ongoing challenges is to identify etiopathogenic mechanism(s) that can account for the regional, cellular, and molecular diversity of findings that characterize schizophrenia.

REFERENCES

Abi-Dargham A, Moore H: Prefrontal DA transmission at D1 receptors and the pathology of schizophrenia. Neuroscientist 9:404–416, 2003

Abi-Dargham A, Gil R, Krystal J, et al: Increased striatal dopamine transmission in schizophrenia: confirmation in a second cohort. Am J Psychiatry 155:761–767, 1998

Abi-Dargham A, Rodenhiser J, Printz D, et al: Increased baseline occupancy of D_2 receptors by dopamine in schizophrenia. Proc Natl Acad Sci U S A 97:8104–8109, 2000

Abi-Dargham A, Mawlawi O, Lombardo I, et al: Prefrontal dopamine D1 receptors and working memory in schizophrenia. J Neurosci 22:3708–3719, 2002

Akbarian S, Bunney WE Jr, Potkin SG, et al: Altered distribution of nicotinamide-adenine dinucleotide phosphate-diaphorase cells in frontal lobe of schizophrenics implies disturbances of cortical development. Arch Gen Psychiatry 50:169–177, 1993a

Akbarian S, Vinuela A, Kim JJ, et al: Distorted distribution of nicotinamide-adenine dinucleotide phosphate-diaphorase neurons in temporal lobe of schizophrenics implies anomalous cortical development. Arch Gen Psychiatry 50:178–187, 1993b

Akbarian S, Kim JJ, Potkin SG, et al: Gene expression for glutamic acid decarboxylase is reduced without loss of neurons in prefrontal cortex of schizophrenics. Arch Gen Psychiatry 52:258–266, 1995a

Akbarian S, Smith MA, Jones EG: Editing for an AMPA receptor subunit RNA in prefrontal cortex and striatum in Alzheimer's disease, Huntington's disease and schizophrenia. Brain Res 699:297–304, 1995b

Akbarian S, Kim JJ, Potkin SG, et al: Maldistribution of interstitial neurons in prefrontal white matter of the brains of schizophrenic patients. Arch Gen Psychiatry 53:425–436, 1996a

Akbarian S, Sucher NJ, Bradley D, et al: Selective alterations in gene expression for NMDA receptor subunits in prefrontal cortex of schizophrenics. J Neurosci 16:19–30, 1996b

Akil M, Lewis DA: Cytoarchitecture of the entorhinal cortex in schizophrenia. Am J Psychiatry 154:1010–1012, 1997

Akil M, Pierri JN, Whitehead RE, et al: Lamina-specific alterations in the dopamine innervation of the prefrontal cortex in schizophrenic subjects. Am J Psychiatry 156:1580–1589, 1999

Akil M, Edgar CL, Pierri JN, et al: Decreased density of tyrosine hydroxylase-immunoreactive axons in the entorhinal cortex of schizophrenic subjects. Biol Psychiatry 47:361–370, 2000

Alexander GE, DeLong MR, Strick PL: Parallel organization of functionally segregated circuits linking basal ganglia and cortex. Annu Rev Neurosci 9:357–381, 1986

Amaral DG: The anatomical organization of the central nervous system, in Principles of Neural Science. Edited by Kandel ER, Schwartz JH, Jessell TM. New York, McGraw-Hill, 2000, pp 317–336

Arnold SE, Hyman BT, Van Hoesen GW, et al: Some cytoarchitectural abnormalities of the entorhinal cortex in schizophrenia. Arch Gen Psychiatry 48:625–632, 1991

Arnold SE, Franz BR, Gur RC, et al: Smaller neuron size in schizophrenia in hippocampal subfields that mediate cortical-hippocampal interactions. Am J Psychiatry 152:738–748, 1995

Arnold SE, Ruscheinsky DD, Han LY: Further evidence of abnormal cytoarchitecture of the entorhinal cortex in schizophrenia using spatial point pattern analyses. Biol Psychiatry 42:639–647, 1997

Arnold SE, Trojanowski JQ, Gur RE, et al: Absence of neurodegeneration and neural injury in the cerebral cortex in a sample of elderly patients with schizophrenia. Arch Gen Psychiatry 55:225–232, 1998

Barbeau D, Liang JJ, Robitalille Y, et al: Decreased expression of the embryonic form of the neural cell adhesion molecule in schizophrenic brains. Proc Natl Acad Sci U S A 92:2785–2789, 1995

Beasley CL, Reynolds GP: Parvalbumin-immunoreactive neurons are reduced in the prefrontal cortex of schizophrenics. Schizophr Res 24:349–355, 1997

Benes FM, Davidson J, Bird ED: Quantitative cytoarchitectural studies of the cerebral cortex of schizophrenics. Arch Gen Psychiatry 43:31–35, 1986

Benes FM, McSparren J, Bird ED, et al: Deficits in small interneurons in prefrontal and cingulate cortices of schizophrenic and schizoaffective patients. Arch Gen Psychiatry 48:996–1001, 1991a

Benes FM, Sorensen I, Bird ED: Reduced neuronal size in posterior hippocampus of schizophrenic patients. Schizophr Bull 17:597–608, 1991b

Benes FM, Sorensen I, Vincent SL, et al: Increased density of glutamate-immunoreactive vertical processes in superficial laminae in cingulate cortex of schizophrenic brain. Cereb Cortex 2:503–512, 1992a

Benes FM, Vincent SL, Alsterberg G, Bird ED, et al: Increased GABAA receptor binding in superficial layers of cingulate cortex in schizophrenics. J Neurosci 12:924–929, 1992b

Benes FM, Vincent SL, Marie A, et al: Up-regulation of GABAA receptor binding on neurons of the prefrontal cortex in schizophrenic subjects. Neuroscience 75:1021–1031, 1996

Benes FM, Todtenkopf MS, Taylor JB: Differential distribution of tyrosine hydroxylase fibers on small and large neurons in layer II of anterior cingulate cortex of schizophrenic brain. Synapse 25:80–92, 1997

Benes FM, Kwok EW, Vincent SL, et al: A reduction of nonpyramidal cells in sector CA2 of schizophrenics and manic depressives. Biol Psychiatry 44:88–97, 1998

Benes FM, Todtenkopf MS, Logiotatos P, et al: Glutamate decarboxylase(65)-immunoreactive terminals in cingulate and prefrontal cortices of schizophrenic and bipolar brain. J Chem Neuroanat 20:259–269, 2000

Benes FM, Vincent SL, Todtenkopf M: The density of pyramidal and nonpyramidal neurons in anterior cingulate cortex of schizophrenic and bipolar subjects. Biol Psychiatry 50:395–406, 2001

Bertolino A, Nawroz S, Mattay VS, et al: Regionally specific pattern of neurochemical pathology in schizophrenia as assessed by multislice proton magnetic resonance spectroscopic imaging. Am J Psychiatry 153:1554–1563, 1996

Black JE, Kodish IM, Grossman AW, et al: Pathology of layer V pyramidal neurons in the prefrontal cortex of patients with schizophrenia. Am J Psychiatry 161:742–744, 2004

Botvinick MM, Cohen JD, Carter CS: Conflict monitoring and anterior cingulate cortex: an update. Trends Cogn Sci 8:539–546, 2004

Brozoski TJ, Brown RM, Rosvold HE, et al: Cognitive deficit caused by regional depletion of dopamine in prefrontal cortex of rhesus monkey. Science 205:929–932, 1979

Buchsbaum MS, Haier RJ, Potkin SG, et al: Frontostriatal disorder of cerebral metabolism in never-medicated schizophrenics. Arch Gen Psychiatry 49:935–942, 1992

Byne W, Buchsbaum MS, Mattiace LA, et al: Postmortem assessment of thalamic nuclear volumes in subjects with schizophrenia. Am J Psychiatry 159:59–65, 2002

Callicott JH, Mattay VS, Verchinski BA, et al: Complexity of prefrontal cortical dysfunction in schizophrenia: more than up or down. Am J Psychiatry 160:2209–2215, 2003

Carr DB, Sesack SR: Hippocampal afferents to the rat prefrontal cortex: synaptic targets and relation to dopamine terminals. J Comp Neurol 369:1–15, 1996

Carter CS, Mintun M, Nichols T, et al: Anterior cingulate gyrus dysfunction and selective attention deficits in schizophrenia: [15O]H2O PET study during single-trial Stroop task performance. Am J Psychiatry 154:1670–1675, 1997

Clinton SM, Meador-Woodruff JH: Abnormalities of the NMDA receptor and associated intracellular molecules in the thalamus in schizophrenia and bipolar disorder. Neuropsychopharmacology 29:1353–1362, 2004

Cotter DR, Pariante CM, Everall IP: Glial cell abnormalities in major psychiatric disorders: the evidence and implications. Brain Res Bull 55:585–595, 2001

Coyle JT: The glutamatergic dysfunction hypothesis for schizophrenia. Harv Rev Psychiatry 3:241–253, 1996

Cullen TJ, Walker MA, Parkinson N, et al: A postmortem study of the mediodorsal nucleus of the thalamus in schizophrenia. Schizophr Res 60:157–166, 2003

Damadzic R, Bigelow LB, Krimer LS, et al: A quantitative immunohistochemical study of astrocytes in the entorhinal cortex in schizophrenia, bipolar disorder and major depression: absence of significant astrocytosis. Brain Res Bull 55:611–618, 2001

Dean B, Hussain T, Hayes W, et al: Changes in serotonin$_{2A}$ and GABA$_A$ receptors in schizophrenia: studies on the human dorsolateral prefrontal cortex. J Neurochem 72:1593–1599, 1999

Dorph-Petersen KA, Pierri JN, Sun Z, et al: Stereological analysis of the mediodorsal thalamic nucleus in schizophrenia: volume, neuron number, and cell types. J Comp Neurol 472:449–462, 2004

Dracheva S, Marras SA, Elhakem SL, et al: N-methyl-D-aspartic acid receptor expression in the dorsolateral prefrontal cortex of elderly patients with schizophrenia. Am J Psychiatry 158:1400–1410, 2001

Eastwood SL, Harrison PJ: Decreased synaptophysin in the medial temporal lobe in schizophrenia demonstrated using immunoautoradiography. Neuroscience 69:339–343, 1995

Eastwood SL, Kerwin RW, Harrison PJ: Immunoautoradiographic evidence for a loss of alpha-amino-3-hydroxy-5-methyl-4-isoxazole propionate-preferring non-N-methyl-D-aspartate glutamate receptors within the medial temporal lobe in schizophrenia. Biol Psychiatry 41:636–643, 1997

Elston GN, Rosa MG: The occipitoparietal pathway of the macaque monkey: comparison of pyramidal cell morphology in layer III of functionally related cortical visual areas. Cereb Cortex 7:432–452, 1997

Fletcher PC, Frith CD, Grasby PM, et al: Local and distributed effects of apomorphine on fronto-temporal function in acute unmedicated schizophrenia. J Neurosci 16:7055–7062, 1996

Ford JM, Mathalon DH, Whitfield S, et al: Reduced communication between frontal and temporal lobes during talking in schizophrenia. Biol Psychiatry 51:485–492, 2002

Friedman HR, Goldman-Rakic PS: Coactivation of prefrontal cortex and inferior parietal cortex in working memory tasks revealed by 2DG functional mapping in the rhesus monkey. J Neurosci 14:2775–2788, 1994

Frith CD, Friston KJ, Herold S, et al: Regional brain activity in chronic schizophrenic patients during the performance of a verbal fluency task. Br J Psychiatry 167:343–349, 1995

Funahashi S, Bruce CJ, Goldman-Rakic PS: Mnemonic coding of visual space in the monkey's dorsolateral prefrontal cortex. J Neurophysiol 61:331–349, 1989

Gabriel SM, Haroutunian V, Powchik P, et al: Increased concentrations of presynaptic proteins in the cingulate cortex of subjects with schizophrenia. Arch Gen Psychiatry 54:559–566, 1997

Gao XM, Sakai K, Roberts RC, et al: Ionotropic glutamate receptors and expression of N-methyl-D-aspartate receptor subunits in subregions of human hippocampus: effects of schizophrenia. Am J Psychiatry 157:1141–1149, 2000

Garey LJ, Ong WY, Patel TS, et al: Reduced dendritic spine density on cerebral cortical pyramidal neurons in schizophrenia. J Neurol Neurosurg Psychiatry 65:446–453, 1998

Giguere M, Goldman-Rakic PS: Mediodorsal nucleus: areal, laminar, and tangential distribution of afferents and efferents in the frontal lobe of rhesus monkeys. J Comp Neurol 277:195–213, 1988

Glantz LA, Lewis DA: Reduction of synaptophysin immunoreactivity in the prefrontal cortex of subjects with schizophrenia: regional and diagnostic specificity. Arch Gen Psychiatry 54:943–952, 1997

Glantz LA, Lewis DA: Decreased dendritic spine density on prefrontal cortical pyramidal neurons in schizophrenia. Arch Gen Psychiatry 57:65–73, 2000

Goldman-Rakic PS: Working memory dysfunction in schizophrenia. J Neuropsychiatry Clin Neurosci 6:348–357, 1994

Goldman-Rakic PS: Cellular basis of working memory. Neuron 14:477–485, 1995

Green MF, Kern RS, Braff DL, et al: Neurocognitive deficits and functional outcome in schizophrenia: are we measuring the "right stuff"? Schizophr Bull 26:119–136, 2000

Guidotti A, Auta J, Davis JM, et al: Decrease in reelin and glutamic acid decarboxylase$_{67}$ (GAD67) expression in schizophrenia and bipolar disorder: a postmortem brain study. Arch Gen Psychiatry 57:1061–1069, 2000

Haber SN, Fudge JL, McFarland NR: Striatonigrostriatal pathways in primates form an ascending spiral from the shell to the dorsolateral striatum. J Neurosci 20:2369–2382, 2000

Harrison PJ: The neuropathology of schizophrenia: a critical review of the data and their interpretation. Brain 122 (pt 4):593–624, 1999

Harrison PJ, Eastwood SL: Preferential involvement of excitatory neurons in medial temporal lobe in schizophrenia. Lancet 352:1669–1673, 1998

Hashimoto T, Volk DW, Eggan SM, et al: Gene expression deficits in a subclass of GABA neurons in the prefrontal cortex of subjects with schizophrenia. J Neurosci 23:6315–6326, 2003

Heckers S, Heinsen H, Geiger B, et al: Hippocampal neuron number in schizophrenia: a stereological study. Arch Gen Psychiatry 48:1002–1008, 1991

Humphries C, Mortimer A, Hirsch S, et al: NMDA receptor mRNA correlation with antemortem cognitive impairment in schizophrenia. Neuroreport 7:2051–2055, 1996

Ibrahim HM, Healy DJ, Hogg AJ Jr, et al: Nucleus-specific expression of ionotropic glutamate receptor subunit mRNAs and binding sites in primate thalamus. Brain Res Mol Brain Res 79:1–17, 2000a

Ibrahim HM, Hogg AJ Jr, Healy DJ, et al: Ionotropic glutamate receptor binding and subunit mRNA expression in thalamic nuclei in schizophrenia. Am J Psychiatry 157:1811–1823, 2000b

Isseroff A, Rosvold HE, Galkin TW, et al: Spatial memory impairments following damage to the mediodorsal nucleus of the thalamus in rhesus monkeys. Brain Res 232:97–113, 1982

Jacobs B, Driscoll L, Schall M: Life-span dendritic and spine changes in areas 10 and 18 of human cortex: a quantitative Golgi study. J Comp Neurol 386:661–680, 1997

Jakob H, Beckmann H: Prenatal developmental disturbances in the limbic allocortex in schizophrenics. J Neural Transm 65:303–326, 1986

Javitt DC, Zukin SR: Recent advances in the phencyclidine model of schizophrenia. Am J Psychiatry 148:1301–1308, 1991

Johnston-Wilson NL, Sims CD, Hofmann JP, et al: Disease-specific alterations in frontal cortex brain proteins in schizophrenia, bipolar disorder, and major depressive disorder. The Stanley Neuropathology Consortium. Mol Psychiatry 5:142–149, 2000

Jones EG: Laminar distribution of cortical efferent cells, in Cerebral Cortex. Edited by Peters AJEG. New York, Plenum, 1984, pp 521–553

Karson CN, Mrak RE, Schluterman KO, et al: Alterations in synaptic proteins and their encoding mRNAs in prefrontal cortex in schizophrenia: a possible neurochemical basis for "hypofrontality." Mol Psychiatry 4:39–45, 1999

Kerns JG, Cohen JD, MacDonald AW III, et al: Anterior cingulate conflict monitoring and adjustments in control. Science 303:1023–1026, 2004

Krimer LS, Jakab RL, Goldman-Rakic PS: Quantitative three-dimensional analysis of the catecholaminergic innervation of identified neurons in the macaque prefrontal cortex. J Neurosci 17:7450–7461, 1997

Krystal JH, Karper LP, Seibyl JP, et al: Subanesthetic effects of the noncompetitive NMDA antagonist, ketamine, in humans: psychotomimetic, perceptual, cognitive, and neuroendocrine responses. Arch Gen Psychiatry 51:199–214, 1994

Lahti AC, Holcomb HH, Medoff DR, et al: Ketamine activates psychosis and alters limbic blood flow in schizophrenia. Neuroreport 6:869–872, 1995

Laruelle M, Kegeles LS, Abi-Dargham A: Glutamate, dopamine, and schizophrenia: from pathophysiology to treatment. Ann N Y Acad Sci 1003:138–158, 2003

Levitt JB, Lewis DA, Yoshioka T, et al: Topography of pyramidal neuron intrinsic connections in macaque monkey prefrontal cortex (areas 9 and 46). J Comp Neurol 338:360–376, 1993

Lewis DA, Akil M: Cortical dopamine in schizophrenia: strategies for postmortem studies. J Psychiatr Res 31:175–195, 1997

Lewis DA, Lieberman JA: Catching up on schizophrenia: natural history and neurobiology. Neuron 28:325–334, 2000

Lewis DA, Cruz DA, Melchitzky DS, et al: Lamina-specific deficits in parvalbumin-immunoreactive varicosities in the prefrontal cortex of subjects with schizophrenia: evidence for fewer projections from the thalamus. Am J Psychiatry 158:1411–1422, 2001

Lidow MS, Goldman-Rakic PS: A common action of clozapine, haloperidol, and remoxipride on D1- and D2-dopaminergic receptors in the primate cerebral cortex. Proc Natl Acad Sci U S A 91:4353–4356, 1994

Lieberman JA: Is schizophrenia a neurodegenerative disorder? A clinical and neurobiological perspective. Biol Psychiatry 46:729–739, 1999

Lipska BK, Weinberger DR: Animal models of schizophrenia, in Schizophrenia. Edited by Hirsch SR, Weinberger DR. Malden, MA, Blackwell Science, 2003, pp 388–402

Lipska BK, Al-Amin HA, Weinberger DR: Excitotoxic lesions of the rat medial prefrontal cortex: effects on abnormal behaviors associated with neonatal hippocampal damage. Neuropsychopharmacology 19:451–464, 1998

Meador-Woodruff JH, Healy DJ: Glutamate receptor expression in schizophrenic brain. Brain Res Brain Res Rev 31:288–294, 2000

Meador-Woodruff JH, Haroutunian V, Powchik P, et al: Dopamine receptor transcript expression in striatum and prefrontal and occipital cortex: focal abnormalities in orbitofrontal cortex in schizophrenia. Arch Gen Psychiatry 54:1089–1095, 1997

Meador-Woodruff JH, Davis KL, Haroutunian V: Abnormal kainate receptor expression in prefrontal cortex in schizophrenia. Neuropsychopharmacology 24:545–552, 2001

Mega MS, Cummings JL, Salloway S, et al: The limbic system: an anatomic, phylogenetic, and clinical perspective, in The Neuropsychiatry of Limbic and Subcortical Disorders. Edited by Salloway S, Malloy P, Cummings JL. Washington, DC, American Psychiatric Press, 1997, pp 3–18

Melchitzky DS, Lewis DA: Pyramidal neuron local axon terminals in monkey prefrontal cortex: differential targeting of subclasses of GABA neurons. Cereb Cortex 13:452–460, 2003

Melchitzky DS, Sesack SR, Pucak ML, et al: Synaptic targets of pyramidal neurons providing intrinsic horizontal connections in monkey prefrontal cortex. J Comp Neurol 390: 211–224, 1998

Melchitzky DS, Sesack SR, Lewis DA: Parvalbumin-immunoreactive axon terminals in macaque monkey and human prefrontal cortex: laminar, regional, and target specificity of type I and type II synapses. J Comp Neurol 408:11–22, 1999

Melchitzky DS, Gonzalez-Burgos G, Barrionuevo G, et al: Synaptic targets of the intrinsic axon collaterals of supragranular pyramidal neurons in monkey prefrontal cortex. J Comp Neurol 430:209–221, 2001

Meyer-Lindenberg A, Miletich RS, Kohn PD, et al: Reduced prefrontal activity predicts exaggerated striatal dopaminergic function in schizophrenia. Nat Neurosci 5:267–271, 2002

Mirnics K, Middleton FA, Marquez A, et al: Molecular characterization of schizophrenia viewed by microarray analysis of gene expression in prefrontal cortex. Neuron 28:53–67, 2000

Nelson MD, Saykin AJ, Flashman LA, et al: Hippocampal volume reduction in schizophrenia as assessed by magnetic resonance imaging: a meta-analytic study. Arch Gen Psychiatry 55:433–440, 1998

Olney JW, Farber NB: Glutamate receptor dysfunction and schizophrenia. Arch Gen Psychiatry 52:998–1007, 1995

Pakkenberg B: Pronounced reduction of total neuron number in mediodorsal thalamic nucleus and nucleus accumbens in schizophrenics. Arch Gen Psychiatry 47:1023–1028, 1990

Pakkenberg B: Total nerve cell number in neocortex in chronic schizophrenics and controls estimated using optical disectors. Biol Psychiatry 34:768–772, 1993

Pantelis C, Barnes TR, Nelson HE, et al: Frontal-striatal cognitive deficits in patients with chronic schizophrenia. Brain 120 (pt 10):1823–1843, 1997

Park S, Holzman PS: Schizophrenics show spatial working memory deficits. Arch Gen Psychiatry 49:975–982, 1992

Perrone-Bizzozero NI, Sower AC, Bird ED, et al: Levels of the growth-associated protein GAP-43 are selectively increased in association cortices in schizophrenia. Proc Natl Acad Sci U S A 93:14182–14187, 1996

Pierri JN, Chaudry AS, Woo TU, et al: Alterations in chandelier neuron axon terminals in the prefrontal cortex of schizophrenic subjects. Am J Psychiatry 156:1709–1719, 1999

Pierri JN, Volk CL, Auh S, et al: Decreased somal size of deep layer 3 pyramidal neurons in the prefrontal cortex of subjects with schizophrenia. Arch Gen Psychiatry 58:466–473, 2001

Pierri JN, Volk CL, Auh S, et al: Somal size of prefrontal cortical pyramidal neurons in schizophrenia: differential effects across neuronal subpopulations. Biol Psychiatry 54:111–120, 2003

Popken GJ, Bunney WE Jr, Potkin SG, et al: Subnucleus-specific loss of neurons in medial thalamus of schizophrenics. Proc Natl Acad Sci U S A 97:9276–9280, 2000

Porter RH, Eastwood SL, Harrison PJ: Distribution of kainate receptor subunit mRNAs in human hippocampus, neocortex and cerebellum, and bilateral reduction of hippocampal GluR6 and KA2 transcripts in schizophrenia. Brain Res 751:217–231, 1997

Pucak ML, Levitt JB, Lund JS, et al: Patterns of intrinsic and associational circuitry in monkey prefrontal cortex. J Comp Neurol 376:614–630, 1996

Purohit DP, Perl DP, Haroutunian V, et al: Alzheimer disease and related neurodegenerative diseases in elderly patients with schizophrenia: a postmortem neuropathologic study of 100 cases. Arch Gen Psychiatry 55:205–211, 1998

Rajkowska G, Selemon LD, Goldman-Rakic PS: Neuronal and glial somal size in the prefrontal cortex: a postmortem morphometric study of schizophrenia and Huntington disease. Arch Gen Psychiatry 55:215–224, 1998

Robbins TW: The case of frontostriatal dysfunction in schizophrenia. Schizophr Bull 16:391–402, 1990

Roberts GW, Colter N, Lofthouse R, et al: Gliosis in schizophrenia: a survey. Biol Psychiatry 21:1043–1050, 1986

Roberts GW, Colter N, Lofthouse R, et al: Is there gliosis in schizophrenia? Investigation of the temporal lobe. Biol Psychiatry 22:1459–1468, 1987

Robinson MB, Coyle JT: Glutamate and related acidic excitatory neurotransmitters: from basic science to clinical application. FASEB J 1:446–455, 1987

Saunders RC, Kolachana BS, Bachevalier J, et al: Neonatal lesions of the medial temporal lobe disrupt prefrontal cortical regulation of striatal dopamine. Nature 393:169–171, 1998

Sawaguchi T, Goldman-Rakic PS: The role of D_1-dopamine receptor in working memory: local injections of dopamine antagonists into the prefrontal cortex of rhesus monkeys performing an oculomotor delayed-response task. J Neurophysiol 71:515–528, 1994

Schroeder J, Buchsbaum MS, Siegel BV, et al: Patterns of cortical activity in schizophrenia. Psychol Med 24:947–955, 1994

Selemon LD, Goldman-Rakic PS: The reduced neuropil hypothesis: a circuit based model of schizophrenia. Biol Psychiatry 45:17–25, 1999

Selemon LD, Rajkowska G, Goldman-Rakic PS: Abnormally high neuronal density in the schizophrenic cortex: a morphometric analysis of prefrontal area 9 and occipital area 17. Arch Gen Psychiatry 52:805–818, 1995

Selemon LD, Rajkowska G, Goldman-Rakic PS: Elevated neuronal density in prefrontal area 46 in brains from schizophrenic patients: application of a three-dimensional, stereologic counting method. J Comp Neurol 392:402–412, 1998

Sesack SR, Hawrylak VA, Melchitzky DS, et al: Dopamine innervation of a subclass of local circuit neurons in monkey prefrontal cortex: ultrastructural analysis of tyrosine hydroxylase and parvalbumin immunoreactive structures. Cereb Cortex 8:614–622, 1998

Siegel BV Jr, Buchsbaum MS, Bunney WE Jr, et al: Cortical-striatal-thalamic circuits and brain glucose metabolic activity in 70 unmedicated male schizophrenic patients. Am J Psychiatry 150:1325–1336, 1993

Stark AK, Uylings HB, Sanz-Arigita E, et al: Glial cell loss in the anterior cingulate cortex, a subregion of the prefrontal cortex, in subjects with schizophrenia. Am J Psychiatry 161: 882–888, 2004

Stefanis NC, Bresnick JN, Kerwin RW, et al: Elevation of D4 dopamine receptor mRNA in postmortem schizophrenic brain. Brain Res Mol Brain Res 53:112–119, 1998

Stevens JR: Neuropathology of schizophrenia. Arch Gen Psychiatry 39:1131–1139, 1982

Swanson LW: A direct projection from Ammon's horn to prefrontal cortex in the rat. Brain Res 217:150–154, 1981

Tamminga CA, Thaker GK, Buchanan R, et al: Limbic system abnormalities identified in schizophrenia using positron emission tomography with fluorodeoxyglucose and neocortical alterations with deficit syndrome. Arch Gen Psychiatry 49:522–530, 1992

Tamminga CA, Vogel M, Gao X, et al: The limbic cortex in schizophrenia: focus on the anterior cingulate. Brain Res Brain Res Rev 31:364–370, 2000

Tekin S, Cummings JL: Frontal-subcortical neuronal circuits and clinical neuropsychiatry: an update. J Psychosom Res 53:647–654, 2002

Thompson PM, Sower AC, Perrone-Bizzozero NI: Altered levels of the synaptosomal associated protein SNAP-25 in schizophrenia. Biol Psychiatry 43:239–243, 1998

Thune JJ, Uylings HB, Pakkenberg B: No deficit in total number of neurons in the prefrontal cortex in schizophrenics. J Psychiatr Res 35:15–21, 2001

Uranova NA, Vostrikov VM, Orlovskaya DD, et al: Oligodendroglial density in the prefrontal cortex in schizophrenia and mood disorders: a study from the Stanley Neuropathology Consortium. Schizophr Res 67:269–275, 2004

Vawter MP, Howard AL, Hyde TM, et al: Alterations of hippocampal secreted N-CAM in bipolar disorder and synaptophysin in schizophrenia. Mol Psychiatry 4:467–475, 1999

Volk DW, Austin MC, Pierri JN, et al: Decreased glutamic acid decarboxylase$_{67}$ messenger RNA expression in a subset of prefrontal cortical gamma-aminobutyric acid neurons in subjects with schizophrenia. Arch Gen Psychiatry 57:237–245, 2000

Volk D, Austin M, Pierri J, et al: GABA transporter-1 mRNA in the prefrontal cortex in schizophrenia: decreased expression in a subset of neurons. Am J Psychiatry 158:256–265, 2001

Walker MA, Highley JR, Esiri MM, et al: Estimated neuronal populations and volumes of the hippocampus and its subfields in schizophrenia. Am J Psychiatry 159:821–828, 2002

Weinberger DR, Berman KF, Zec RF: Physiologic dysfunction of dorsolateral prefrontal cortex in schizophrenia, I: regional cerebral blood flow evidence. Arch Gen Psychiatry 43: 114–124, 1986

Woo TU, Miller JL, Lewis DA: Schizophrenia and the parvalbumin-containing class of cortical local circuit neurons. Am J Psychiatry 154:1013–1015, 1997

Woo TU, Whitehead RE, Melchitzky DS, et al: A subclass of prefrontal gamma-aminobutyric acid axon terminals are selectively altered in schizophrenia. Proc Natl Acad Sci U S A 95:5341–5346, 1998

Young CE, Arima K, Xie J, et al: SNAP-25 deficit and hippocampal connectivity in schizophrenia. Cereb Cortex 8:261–268, 1998

Young KA, Manaye KF, Liang C, et al: Reduced number of mediodorsal and anterior thalamic neurons in schizophrenia. Biol Psychiatry 47:944–953, 2000

Yucel M, Pantelis C, Stuart GW, et al: Anterior cingulate activation during Stroop task performance: a PET to MRI coregistration study of individual patients with schizophrenia. Am J Psychiatry 159:251–254, 2002

Zaidel DW, Esiri MM, Harrison PJ: Size, shape, and orientation of neurons in the left and right hippocampus: investigation of normal asymmetries and alterations in schizophrenia. Am J Psychiatry 154:812–818, 1997

Zakzanis KK, Hansen KT: Dopamine D2 densities and the schizophrenic brain. Schizophr Res 32:201–206, 1998

Zhang ZJ, Reynolds GP: A selective decrease in the relative density of parvalbumin-immunoreactive neurons in the hippocampus in schizophrenia. Schizophr Res 55:1–10, 2002

STRUCTURAL AND FUNCTIONAL NEUROANATOMY

AYSENIL BELGER, PH.D.

GABRIEL DICHTER, PH.D.

Although schizophrenia was first identified and examined in the early studies by Emil Kraepelin (1856–1926) and Eugen Bleuler (1857–1939) nearly a century ago, the underlying etiology and pathophysiology of the disease remain unknown. Diagnosis requires the presence of hallucinations or delusions, and these positive symptoms generally improve with antipsychotic treatment. However, the subtler but perhaps more devastating aspects of schizophrenia, including negative symptoms (e.g., alogia, amotivation, affective flattening) and cognitive dysfunction (impairments in executive functioning, working memory, attention, social cognition), have proven much more difficult to combat and are becoming the primary targets of treatment-oriented research. As the clinical diagnosis of schizophrenia has become more refined, the hypothesis that it is a heterogeneous group of diseases rather than one clearly defined disorder has increased in popularity.

In the past quarter-century, increasingly advanced neuroimaging technologies have been used in research on the etiology and pathophysiology of schizophrenia. Beginning with the first computed tomography (CT) studies of schizophrenia by Johnstone and colleagues in 1976, imaging research has expanded to include the use of magnetic resonance imaging (MRI) technology in 1986, allowing for detailed visualization of brain anatomy. In 1996, the first functional MRI (fMRI) studies that led to an exciting and promising area of research by examining in vivo brain functioning were performed. fMRI has opened the door to analysis of the cortical dysfunction involved in the long underrecognized cognitive deficits of schizophrenia. Cross-sectional and longitudinal structural MRI studies have shown reductions in regional brain volumes and increases in cerebral spinal fluid spaces (including the lateral, third, and fourth ventricles), adding fuel to the debate about theories of developmental or degenerative etiology. Neuroimaging studies of schizophrenia—from very recent MRI studies of at-risk newborns, to prodromal or first-episode individuals, and to longitudinal analyses of chronically ill patients—continue to stimulate scientific inquiry into the etiology and pathophysiology of this complex disorder.

In this chapter, we provide an overview of the findings to date of morphological and functional neuropathology of schizophrenia as assessed through neuroimaging methodologies. In considering the findings of the studies of functional and structural neuroimaging, it is first useful to have an understanding of the methodologies used to acquire the evidence.

NEUROIMAGING METHODS

In this chapter, *neuroimaging* refers to a wide array of in vivo techniques that provide a window into the structural and functional properties of the human brain. These techniques include noninvasive ones, such as CT and nuclear magnetic resonance (NMR), as well as minimally invasive techniques, such as positron emission tomography (PET), requiring an intravenous injection of a radioactive material. Neuroimaging techniques provide a method to discover brain structure or function that is altered from normal and further enable the correlation of these differences with clinical signs and symptoms. In individuals with schizophrenia, the alterations in brain structure may be quite subtle, be difficult to detect, and appear as a variety of small planar, linear, volumetric, and, more recently, shape or geometric changes in brain morphology. Our purpose in this section is not only to describe the imaging techniques but also to discuss procedures that are used to analyze these images.

Nuclear Magnetic Resonance: Structural MRI, Functional MRI, and Diffusion Tensor Imaging

NMR or MRI provides a high-quality, three-dimensional image of organs and structures inside the body without X rays or other radiation. MRI uses a strong magnetic field to create images of biological tissue, enabling the visualization of anatomy in great detail. Longitudinal MRI studies can determine when the structural abnormalities first appeared in the course of a disease, how they will affect subsequent development, and precisely how their progression correlates with cognitive and emotional aspects of a disorder.

MRI technology is based on the principle that when the protons in the nucleus of a molecule are placed in an electromagnetic field, they absorb energy on the basis of the natural oscillation period (i.e., "spin") of the protons. After the protons absorb this energy, they quickly release the energy as they return to their initial energy state. The MRI signal detects this energy release. The strength of the MRI signal depends in part on the density of protons in the tissue; the greater the density, the greater the signal. The other factors that determine the signal strength are the time that it takes for protons to "relax"—that is, return to their initial energy state. Two parameters measure this relaxation time, T1 and T2, which vary according to the microenvironment of the protons. The MR signal can be manipulated by changing the way in which the nuclei are initially subjected to electromagnetic energy. This manipulation can change the dependence of the observed signal on these three signal parameters: proton density, T1, and T2.

Hence several different MRI techniques ("weightings") are available; some tissue properties are accentuated over others, which changes the ability to detect differences in tissue type. Magnetic coils in the MRI machine detect these signals, and a computer changes them into an image based on signal strength. For example, tissue that contains a lot of water and fat is proton dense and produces a strong signal and hence a bright image; tissue that contains little or no water, such as bone, produces a relatively weak signal and appears darker. MRI allows images to be constructed in any plane and thus is particularly valuable in studying the complex three-dimensional anatomy of the brain and spinal cord.

MRI enables not only the visualization of brain structures with a high spatial resolution but also the measurement of the metabolic correlates of localized neural activity in different brain regions. This technique, referred to as *functional MRI*, measures brain activity under resting and activated conditions. fMRI combines the high spatial resolution and noninvasive imaging of brain anatomy offered by standard MRI with a strategy for detecting changes in blood oxygenation levels driven by neuronal activity. It allows for more detailed maps of brain areas underlying human mental activities in health and disease.

Ample evidence suggests that signals detected by fMRI are valid measurements of local changes in neuronal activity (Boynton et al. 1996; Sereno et al. 1995). Nevertheless, it is important to note that fMRI creates images not of neural activity directly but of physiological activity that is correlated with neuronal activity. Neurons in the brain that are engaged during a cognitive task increase their metabolic demands and the associated energy requirements. Because the brain does not store energy, it must create adenosine triphosphate energy through the oxidation of glucose. Energy in the form of glucose and oxygen is delivered into cells through the vascular system; oxygen then binds to hemoglobin molecules. The increase of blood oxygen and oxygen delivery displaces deoxygenated hemoglobin from the capillaries, venules, and small veins in regions surrounding the active neurons. Because deoxygenated hemoglobin has magnetic field gradients that alter the spins of nearby diffusing hydrogen nuclei, its presence reduces the MR signal intensity in those regions. Thus, when deoxygenated hemoglobin is removed and replaced with oxygenated hemoglobin, the increases in blood flow aiming to replenish the energy demands of active neurons result in a local increase in MR signal. These changes can be mapped subsequently to localize the regions eliciting the neural activity.

To date, fMRI has been applied to the study of various functions of the brain ranging from studies of early sensory responses (Barch et al. 2003a; Druzgal and D'Esposito 2001) to higher-order, more complex, and abstract cognitive activities and decision-making processes (Ford et al. 2004; Kubicki et al. 2003; MacDonald and Carter 2003).

Most recently, MRI technology has been extended to the study of the microstructure and diffusion properties of white matter fibers connecting various brain regions. Diffusion tensor imaging combines MRI principles with those encoding molecular diffusion in the MRI signal to detect properties of white matter that are not accessible through standard structural MRI (for review, see Le Bihan et al. 2001). The random translational motion of molecules (Brownian movement) in tissue can be anisotropic (i.e., highly unidirectional), as in white matter. Such diffusion anisotropy measures can be characterized and can inform us about tissue microstructure. Various local properties of white matter tissue, such as apparent diffusion, fractional anisotropy (FA), and spatial orientation, will become new features for studying the integrity of connective fibers in neurodevelopmental or neurodegenerative brain changes. Global properties (i.e., the tracking of major fiber paths) may lead to a better understanding of brain connectivity or alterations thereof. In routine clinical MRI, most of the signal arises from water in tissue, and the visualization of changes in the diffusion properties of water in tissue with MRI has become a useful, multifaceted tool to characterize tissue structure and to identify and differentiate disease processes. Diffusion imaging also promises to further the understanding of brain disorders and abnormalities such as schizophrenia, in which evidence is growing for a more global, distributed pathology potentially affecting the development of major fiber networks in the brain leading to relative disconnection syndrome.

RADIOTRACER METHODOLOGIES: PET AND SPECT

The first series of neuroimaging studies describing functional changes in the brain of patients with schizophrenia examined regional cerebral blood flow and cerebral metabolism. Unlike MRI techniques, radiotracer methodologies such as PET and single photon emission computed tomography (SPECT) involve the administration of radioactively tagged pharmaceuticals that distribute in the brain according to specific and kinetic pharmacological properties. PET uses radioactively labeled biological probes, named *tracers*, to visualize blood flow changes related to neural activity (Raichle 1987). This method of measuring brain function is based on the detection of radioactivity emitted when positrons (positively charged particles) undergo radioactive decay in the brain. Depending on what brain function is under study, an appropriate compound is labeled with positron-emitting radionuclides to produce three-dimensional PET images. Depending on the labeled compound, the image may reflect blood flow or metabolic or other chemical activity in the brain. Numerous sources have shown that signals detected by PET are valid measurements of local changes in neuronal activity (DeYoe et al. 1996; Raichle 1987). Thus, PET studies can be used to map functional brain changes associated with cognitive functions such as learning, language, and attention and cognitive dysfunction in brain disorders such as schizophrenia. Localizing the neural sources of changes in these domains will promote a better understanding of the causes of schizophrenia and monitor the effectiveness of specific treatments.

In physiological studies of sensorimotor or cognitive systems, oxygen-15-labeled water can be used to identify all the brain structures that are involved in a particular task. Because oxygen-15 has a very short half-life, the injections can be repeated (every 15 minutes) to compare the regional values of blood flow at rest and during various cognitive tasks. This method can recognize the regions of the brain activated during hand movement, reading, listening, or the execution or imagination of a cognitive task. It also can be applied to identify the brain structures in which the metabolism is modified during drug treatment.

PET studies also can be used to determine the mode of action of various drugs. Most psychotropic substances and drugs act by binding to the recognition, transport, or degradation sites of neurotransmitters. When labeled with positron-emitting isotopes, they serve as remarkable tracers in visualizing these specific sites.

Although both PET and SPECT scanning methods use radiotracers, SPECT scanning relies on the detection of light signals (scintillation) associated with the emission of photons, rather than positrons, following nuclear transformation of the tracer agents penetrating the brain. These light signals are subsequently converted to electrical impulses, which are amplified and analyzed to determine the location and energy level of the photon. Both PET and SPECT scanning methods can be used for studying brain perfusion changes associated with increased neuronal metabolic activity, as well as the pharmacokinetic, brain uptake, and biodistribution of radioligands selective for brain receptor targets. Hence both methods can be used to evaluate the distribution and number of receptor sites that may be altered by schizophrenia or by antipsychotic drug treatments, further informing about the localization of the pathophysiology associated with schizophrenia.

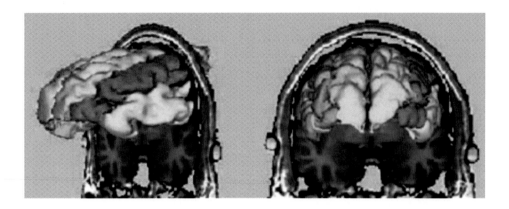

FIGURE 10–1. Surface rendering of the superior (*light beige/aqua*), middle (*blue/peach*), and inferior (*gold/yellow*) frontal lobe gyri with a coronal 1.5-mm slice that illustrates the relation of the gyri to the coronal slice.

Source. Reprinted from Shenton ME, Dickey CC, Frumin M, et al.: "A Review of MRI Findings in Schizophrenia." *Schizophrenia Research* 49:1–52, 2001. Used with permission.

STRUCTURAL NEUROANATOMY OF SCHIZOPHRENIA

Structural MRI studies of schizophrenia have yielded several promising results but also have been fraught with inconsistencies and contradictory findings. Difficulties in study recruitment with attendant small sample sizes, along with high dropout rates, have reduced the power of many studies. These problems are of concern enough for cross-sectional studies, and longitudinal designs have faced even more daunting challenges. However, since the first MRI studies in 1986, a body of evidence has accumulated that has produced some impressive results and will guide future research. With the increasing power and advancing precision of today's scanners, subsections of areas previously studied can be examined, perhaps producing more revealing and consistent findings. Advances in computer science, particularly those in the area of image processing, have made analysis of data more informative. This section serves to summarize most of the MRI findings in schizophrenia over the past 15 years. For detailed review, see Shenton et al. (2001) for an exhaustive analysis of work done in this area to the year 2000.

FRONTAL LOBE STRUCTURE

The frontal lobes are the "executive center" of the brain. Emotional, perceptual, cognitive, and volitional processes are integrated via the frontal lobes, and damage to the frontal lobes may cause diminished arousal and emotional functioning, difficulty planning and initiating activity, and decreased attention, concentration, and inhibition (Freed-

man et al. 1998). The frontal lobes are a highly complex region of the human brain (constituting about 30% of the neocortex in humans), having afferent and efferent connections to all other areas of the cortex as well as to limbic and basal ganglia structures (e.g., Fuster 1997). Prominent structures of the frontal lobes include 1) those areas governing motor movement, including the primary, premotor, and supplementary motor cortices, and the frontal eye fields; 2) Broca's speech production area; 3) the anterior cingulate gyrus, which maintains interconnections with the spinal cord, limbic system, and orbital frontal lobes that appear to exert hierarchical control over the limbic and autonomic system (Gray 1987); 4) the medial frontal lobes, which integrate volition, emotion, cognition, and motor function; and 5) the dorsolateral prefrontal cortex (DLPFC) , which governs executive decision making and planning of actions (for a review, see Devinsky et al. 1995; Joseph 1996). Figure 10–1 is a three-dimensional surface reconstruction of the prefrontal cortex and its subdivisions into superior, middle, and inferior gyri.

Research into frontal lobe anomalies in schizophrenia has been pursued because individuals with schizophrenia consistently show deficits on frontally mediated neuropsychological tasks (Bilder et al. 1992; de la Torre et al. 2005; Saykin et al. 1991, 1994). Additionally, frontal lobe lesions produce symptoms that are commonly observed in schizophrenia; for example, damage to the medial frontal lobes typically causes apathy, paratonic rigidity (gegenhalten), waxy flexibility, or uncontrollable movement of the extremities. Additionally, deep medial lesions of the frontal lobes may cause emotional blunting and catatonia (Luria 1980). Finally, orbital lesions in animals cause sensory disturbances, heightened general arousal, and decreased ability to shift attention appropriately (Fuster 1997) and produce perseveration in humans (Luria 1980).

Postmortem morphometric microscopy studies have documented increased neuronal density and decreased neuropil in frontal, temporal, and limbic areas (e.g., Arnold et al. 1991; Selemon et al. 1998), suggesting diminished connectivity between these regions and other brain structures. Several studies reported volume reductions in the frontal lobes of individuals with schizophrenia compared with healthy subjects. These include selective reductions in bilateral inferior prefrontal gray matter volume in subjects with schizophrenia relative to healthy subjects (Buchanan et al. 1998) and to individuals with alcohol dependence (Sullivan et al. 1998b). Wright et al. (1999) found significant reductions in dorsolateral prefrontal cortical gray matter volume in patients with schizophrenia relative to healthy control subjects. Finally, Gur and colleagues (1998) documented decreased frontal lobe volume in both first-episode and previously treated patients, relative to healthy control subjects, as well as a reduction in frontal lobe volume in patients 30 months later, suggesting that frontal lobe volumes progressively decline in schizophrenia (but see Vita et al. 1997).

Volume deficits are found to have functional consequences. For example, frontal lobe gray matter volumes have been associated with severity of negative symptoms, and Chua and colleagues (1997) found an inverse relation between psychomotor poverty and left ventromedial prefrontal gray matter volume in patients with schizophrenia.

Early structural neuroimaging studies of schizophrenia investigated volume differences in the frontal lobes as a whole: Wible and colleagues (1995) found no differences in frontal lobe volumes, although left prefrontal gray matter volume was significantly correlated with reductions in volume in several temporal lobe structures (see also Breier et al. 1992), as well as with negative symptom severity. Others have found reductions in prefrontal cortical thickness (Selemon et al. 1998) and relations between right prefrontal white matter volume and right amygdala–hippocampus volume (Breier et al. 1992).

More recent advances in imaging resolution have allowed for structural investigations of subregions of the frontal lobes. Such investigations have found decreased frontal volumes in the following areas: white matter (Buchanan et al. 1998); bilateral inferior gyri (Buchanan et al. 1998); middle frontal, middle, medial, and right fronto-orbital subregions (Goldstein et al. 1999); and dorsolateral prefrontal gray matter, which was associated with poor neurocognitive performance on executive function and attention tasks as well as with more severe negative symptom severity (Gur et al. 2000). Other recent high-resolution structural MRI studies have reported reduced

cortical gray matter volume and increased cerebrospinal fluid volume in the frontal and left temporal lobes in schizophrenia (Mitelman et al. 2003) and bilateral anterior cingulate gray matter volume reductions in patients with schizophrenia that were relatively greater than reductions in other prefrontal and temporolimbic regions (Yamasue et al. 2004). The latter result was confirmed by a diffusion tensor imaging study that found higher cingulate bundle white matter directionality in patients with auditory hallucinations, suggesting abnormal coactivation in regions related to the acoustical processing of external stimuli (Hubl et al. 2004).

An influential review of 193 MRI studies from 1988 to 2000 by Shenton and colleagues (2001) identified subtle but consistent structural abnormalities in schizophrenia across investigations, including ventricular enlargement (80% of studies reviewed), third ventricle enlargement (73%), and abnormalities of the medial (74%) and superior temporal lobes (100%). There was also evidence for frontal lobe abnormalities (59%), particularly in prefrontal gray matter and orbitofrontal regions; parietal lobe abnormalities (60%), particularly of the inferior parietal lobule; subcortical abnormalities (42%–92%, depending on the structure); and cerebellar abnormalities (31%).

Finally, a few research groups have examined individuals at high risk for developing schizophrenia but who do not meet current criteria for the disorder (e.g., individuals with a first-degree relative with schizophrenia). Harris and colleagues (2004) found increased right prefrontal lobe gyral folding in individuals who subsequently developed schizophrenia, and Molina and colleagues (2004) reported lower prefrontal gray matter volume in chronically ill (i.e., illness duration of more than 6 years) but not first-episode schizophrenic patients. Finally, Yucel and colleagues (2003) reported more poorly developed left paracingulate sulci in young men at ultrahigh risk for developing psychosis.

TEMPORAL LOBE STRUCTURE: SUPERIOR TEMPORAL GYRUS, HIPPOCAMPUS, AND AMYGDALA

The temporal lobes receive extensive projections from the somesthetic and visual projection areas and process a wide range of sensory information. The superior temporal lobes mediate auditory and linguistic functions, and the inferior temporal lobes, including the amygdala and hippocampus, subserve emotional, visual, and auditory memory and integration of other perceptual and visceral activity (Joseph 1996).

There are extensive reports of abnormal structural and neuroanatomical findings in temporal regions in schizophrenia, particularly in certain substructures of the temporal lobes, such as the hippocampus. Findings of temporal lobe pathology range from smaller temporal cortical volume (e.g., Anderson et al. 2002; Dickey et al. 2002a, 2003; Gur et al. 1998; Henn and Braus 1999; Hirayasu et al. 2000a, 2000b; Ho et al. 2003; Holinger et al. 1999; McCarley et al. 1999, 2002; Shenton et al. 2001; Sumich et al. 2002), to smaller Heschl's gyri (Dickey et al. 2002b; Kim et al. 2000; Kwon et al. 1999; Sumich et al. 2002), to smaller hippocampal formations (Deicken et al. 1998; Fannon et al. 2003; Kasai et al. 2003b; Nasrallah et al. 1997; Shenton et al. 2002; Sumich et al. 2002; Szeszko et al. 2003) detected as early as the first episode of the illness onset (Fannon et al. 2000; Hirayasu et al. 2000a; Kubicki et al. 2002a; Levitt et al. 2002; Sumich et al. 2002; Szeszko et al. 2003).

Recently, Narr et al. (2004) isolated regional volume deficits in patients experiencing their first episode of schizophrenia by using two novel and complementary comput-erized surface-based image analysis techniques (Figure 10–2). Specifically, the authors compared hippocampal radial distances and perihippocampal cerebrospinal fluid distributions between diagnostic groups at thousands of homologous hippocampal surface locations, allowing the identification of very local changes in hippocampal structure. Their findings indicated that volume reductions resulted from disturbed neurodevelopmental rather than neurodegenerative processes (Heckers 2001; Wood et al. 2001). Patients without any prior antipsychotic medication exposure also had smaller hippocampal volumes compared with the healthy group. Although these findings do not rule out the possibility that medications may affect hippocampal size, the results do show that substantial volume deficits are apparent before any treatment and that acute treatment does not appear to have a major effect.

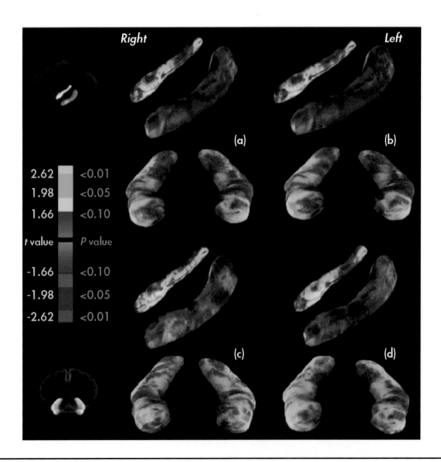

FIGURE 10–2.   Statistical maps showing significant differences in radial distances in color.

Color bar shows *t* values and the corresponding two-tailed probability values obtained at each hippocampal surface location. Positive *t* values indicate significant surface contractions in first-episode patients compared with control subjects in (a) the average atlas space of the entire sample and in (b) native scanner space. Significant differences in radial distances between diagnostic groups are also mapped within (c) female and (d) male groups in atlas space only.

Source.   Reprinted from Narr KL, Thompson PM, Szeszko P, et al.: "Regional Specificity of Hippocampal Volume Reductions in First-Episode Schizophrenia." *Neuroimage* 21:1563–1575, 2004. Used with permission.

Shenton and colleagues (2001) reported that of 51 MRI studies evaluating whole temporal lobe volume, 31 reported smaller volumes, whereas 20 reported no significant differences (an earlier review by the same researcher found that 17 of 31 studies indicated smaller temporal lobe volumes, and 16 of 31 found no difference). Shenton et al. attributed this disparity to methodological differences in MRI acquisition, including slice thickness and landmark and slice interpolation differences and the likelihood that diagnostic group differences would be more evident in structures within the temporal lobe than in the temporal lobe as a whole. For example, Shenton et al. (2001) reported that 74% of 49 MRI studies indicated decreased volume of medial temporal lobe structures (i.e., the amygdala-hippocampal complex and parahippocampal gyrus) relative to control subjects, although amygdala-hippocampal reductions also have been reported in patients with bipolar (Velakoulis et al. 1999), mood (Altshuler et al. 1998), posttraumatic stress (Bremner et al. 1995), and geriatric (Golomb et al. 1993) disorders. The nonspecificity of the amygdala-hippocampal volume reductions to schizophrenia indicates that this morphology may be related to a nonspecific risk factor for psychiatric illness and general cognitive decline, a conclusion strengthened by evidence that individuals at risk for Alzheimer's disease (Visser et al. 2002), unaffected siblings of patients with schizophrenia (Callicott et al. 1998), and prodromal individuals at ultra-high risk for developing psychosis (Lawrie et al. 2002; Seidman and Wencel 2003) show hippocampal volume reductions as well. More recent studies have reported correlations between hallucinations and smaller left middle and superior temporal gyrus volumes (Onitsuka et al. 2004), as well as progressive medial temporal volume decline over the course of illness (Velakoulis et al. 2002).

The superior temporal gyrus lies above the sylvian fissure and subsumes the primary auditory cortex and part of Wernicke's area on the left side. Electrical stimulation of anterior portions of this gyrus have produced auditory hallucinations in individuals without schizophrenia. Most structural studies have reported superior temporal gyrus volume reductions in schizophrenia, whether in just gray matter (see, e.g., Pearlson 1997) or in both gray and white matter (see Bryant et al. 1999), and relations between lateral ventricle size and left superior temporal gyral volumes have been reported (Chance et al. 2003; Gaser et al. 2004). Furthermore, brain scans at initial hospitalization and 18 months later showed progressive volume reduction of the left posterior superior temporal gyrus gray matter in patients with first-episode schizophrenia but not in patients with first-episode affective psychosis (Kasai et al. 2003a) and correlations between anterior su-

perior temporal gyrus volumes and psychotic and negative symptoms. Superior temporal gyrus volume reductions also have been documented in nonpsychotic offspring of patients with schizophrenia, suggesting that superior temporal gyrus volume reductions may be a marker of risk for schizophrenia (Rajarethinam et al. 2004). Note, however, that studies of subregions of the superior temporal gyrus (e.g., right posterior superior temporal gyrus; J.L. Taylor et al. 2005; see Figure 10–3) have detected volume *increases* in schizophrenia. In contrast to the medial temporal lobe volume reductions reported earlier, superior temporal gyrus volume reductions appear to be specific to schizophrenia spectrum disorders and apply to schizotypal outpatients as well (Dickey et al. 1999; Downhill et al. 2001).

Another temporal lobe structure reported to show abnormalities in schizophrenia is the planum temporale. The planum temporale is a critical brain structure for language processing, particularly in the left hemisphere. Structural findings generally indicate relatively less left-greater-than-right asymmetry in patients with schizophrenia relative to control subjects (for a review, see Shapleske et al. 1999), a difference generally attributed to a smaller left planum temporale in schizophrenic patients. In addition, reduced planum temporale volumes have been shown to be associated with positive symptoms (Crespo-Facorro et al. 2004). However, variations in the definitions of the planum temporale have led to some inconsistent findings (see Barta et al. 1995).

BASAL GANGLIA, THALAMUS, AND CAUDATE STRUCTURES

Basal Ganglia

As mentioned previously, in a review by Shenton and colleagues (2001), structural subcortical abnormalities were identified in 42%–92% of 193 studies. Because many antipsychotic medications act through dopaminergic receptors, and the basal ganglia (i.e., the caudate, putamen, globus pallidus, and nucleus accumbens) have extensive dopaminergic inputs, this subcortical structure has been the focus of recent research. Of the 25 MRI studies of basal ganglia volume reviewed by Shenton and colleagues (2001), 17 reported significant volumetric differences, with some indicating increases (Bryant et al. 1999; Shihabuddin et al. 1998) and others indicating decreases (Corey-Bloom et al. 1995; Lawrie et al. 1999) in basal ganglia volume.

Antipsychotic exposure seems to influence basal ganglia volume. Several research groups have reported increased volume over 18–24 months in first-episode pa-

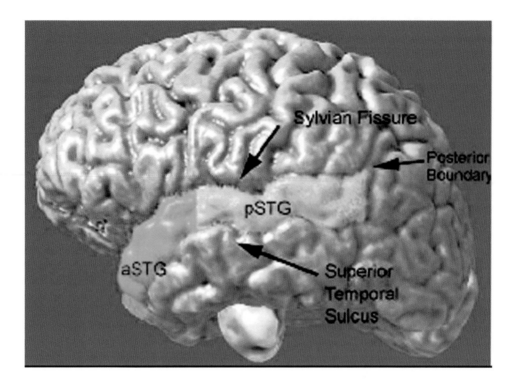

FIGURE 10–3. Three-dimensional view of the superior temporal gyrus (STG) and boundaries.

The STG was defined as the area between the superior temporal sulcus and the sylvian fissure, with the posterior boundary being the junction where the horizontal ramus of the sylvian fissure and the ascending ramus of the superior temporal sulcus meet (*green:* left anterior STG [aSTG]; *light blue:* left posterior STG [pSTG]).

Source. Reprinted from Taylor JL, Blanton RE, Levitt JG, et al.: "Superior Temporal Gyrus Differences in Childhood-Onset Schizophrenia." *Schizophrenia Research* 73:235–241, 2005. Used with permission.

tients and that antipsychotic dose predicted a larger caudate at the second assessment (Chakos et al. 1994; Keshavan et al. 1994). A few studies have reported increased basal ganglia volume in antipsychotic-naïve patients, indicating that increased basal ganglia volume is not simply an artifact of medication treatment (Keshavan et al. 1998).

Thalamus

The thalamus is a major relay station in the brain that receives input from many cortical and subcortical areas and that filters (e.g., "gates") relevant from irrelevant sensory input. Published literature is fairly evenly divided regarding whether structural thalamic differences are evident in schizophrenia. For example, Arciniegas and colleagues (1999) reported no significant differences in thalamic volumes between patients and control subjects. Deicken and colleagues (2002) also found no intergroup differences in total thalamic volume and thalamic asymmetry. However, Ettinger and colleagues (2001) found smaller thalamic volumes in first-episode patients, and Kemether et al. (2003) found that persons with schizo-

phrenia had significantly smaller thalamic subregion volumes (mediodorsal and pulvinar nuclei). Disagreement across studies with respect to thalamic volume differences may be due to the difficulty in identifying thalamic nuclei with structural fMRI (e.g., Deicken et al. 2002).

Caudate

The basal ganglia are a critical link in the corticostriatonigral-thalamocortical circuitry connecting subcortical to cortical regions (Braff and Swerdlow 1997), and dysfunction in the basal ganglia has been related to schizophrenia, Parkinson's disease, and Huntington's disease (Heimer et al. 1991). Similar to the basal ganglia, relations between caudate volume and schizophrenia appear to be moderated by antipsychotic effects: volumetric studies of the caudate in schizophrenia generally have found increases in caudate volume in patients taking typical neuroleptics (Chakos et al. 1994; Keshavan et al. 1994). However, follow-up studies noted volumetric decreases when these same patients were switched to atypical antipsychotics (Chakos et al. 1995; Frazier et al. 1996). Several studies of

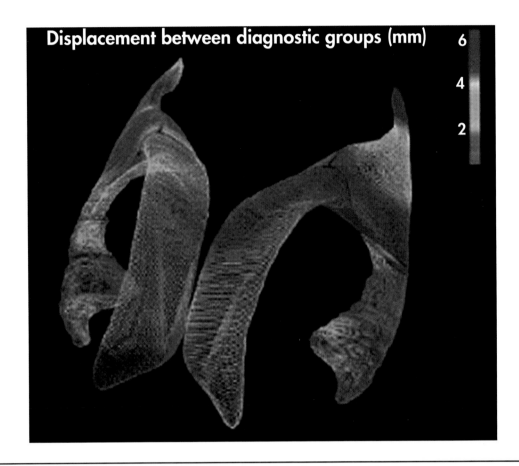

FIGURE 10–4.   Three-dimensional displacement maps of the lateral ventricles.

Top view of the lateral ventricles showing regional differences from average surface models between schizophrenic patients (*n*=25, SZ) and nonschizophrenic control subjects (*n*=28, NC) mapped across gender in both hemispheres. The color bar represents the root mean square magnitude of displacements in millimeters (mm). Diagnostic group displacements can be seen in the left posterior horn, on superior ventricular surfaces, and in the vicinity of the caudate nucleus (*highest displacement shown in red*).

Source.   Reprinted from Narr KL, Thompson PM, Sharma T, et al.: "Three-Dimensional Mapping of Temporo-Limbic Regions and the Lateral Ventricles in Schizophrenia: Gender Effects." *Biological Psychiatry* 50:84–97, 2001. Used with permission.

antipsychotic-naïve patients have documented smaller caudate volumes in persons with schizophrenia (e.g., Corson et al. 1999), suggesting that volumetric decreases are not just an artifact of medication treatment.

VENTRICULAR ENLARGEMENT

One of the most reproduced and consistent neuroimaging findings in persons with schizophrenia is lateral ventricular enlargement. Of particular interest is the apparent increase in ventricular size with progression of the disease (DeLisi et al. 1997; Lieberman et al. 2001).

Narr and colleagues (2001) found that persons with schizophrenia show displacements in the left posterior horn, on superior ventricular surfaces, and in the vicinity of the caudate nucleus (highest displacement shown in red; see Figure 10–4) relative to healthy individuals.

Chronically ill patients have shown marked ventricular enlargement, whereas first-episode patients generally show much less of an abnormality. Some studies also have found that the temporal horn of the left lateral ventricle is disproportionately enlarged in persons with schizophrenia (Chance et al. 2003; Gaser et al. 2004; Yotsutsuji et al. 2003). This evidence of lateralization and the proximity of this area to brain regions presumed dysfunctional in schizophrenia (hippocampus, amygdala, other temporal lobe structures) have fueled debate surrounding the etiology of the disease. Lateralization of defects has suggested a neurodevelopmental disease process, whereas ventricular enlargement as a whole has drawn comparisons to neurodegenerative processes such as Alzheimer's disease. This comparison also points out the lack of specificity of this finding. Patients with Alzheimer's disease, Parkinson's disease, Huntington's disease, and prolonged corticosteroid use all show evidence of ventricular enlargement, suggesting that lateral ventricular enlargement in and of itself is hardly pathognomonic for the disorder. Third ventricular enlargement has been noted in addition to increased lateral ventricular volume. Although relatively few studies have focused on the third ventricle, a substantial majority of the studies reviewed in Shenton et al. (2001) (24 of 33, or 73%) showed this region to be significantly enlarged in patients with schizophrenia. Because of the proximity of the thalamus to the third ventricle, this finding has been used in support of the theory of thalamic dysfunction in schizophrenia, posited by Andreasen (1997).

Many structural imaging studies have focused on regional changes in selected structures in schizophrenia, but other studies have focused on group differences in cortical gray matter concentration between patients with schizophrenia and healthy subjects. Narr and colleagues (2005), using such a method (Figure 10–5), reported significantly reduced intensity-based gray matter concentration in dorsolateral prefrontal cortex in first-episode patients compared with control subjects, most prominently in the middle frontal gyrus, and in the temporal lobe, particularly the superior temporal gyrus bilaterally. Further decreases are visible in inferior parietal regions and in occipital regions in the left hemisphere. No significant increases in intensity-based gray matter concentration were observed in patients with schizophrenia compared with control subjects.

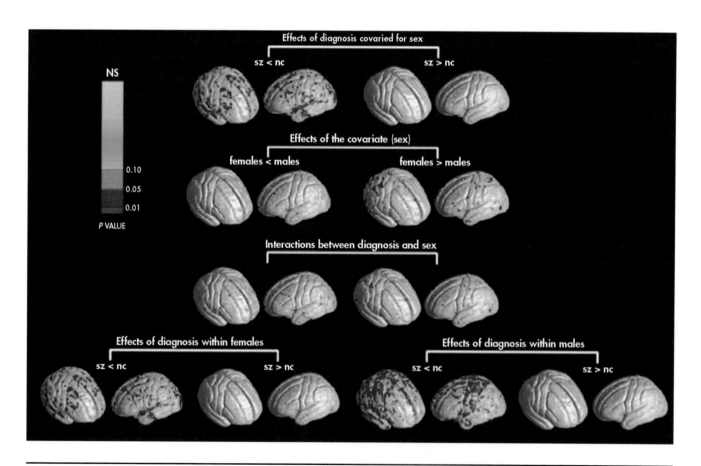

FIGURE 10–5. Statistical maps showing significant regional differences in cortical gray matter concentration in the comparison groups.

Top row: Patients with first-episode schizophrenia (sz) compared with healthy subjects (nc) after covarying for sex. **Second row:** Between male and female subjects across diagnostic groups. **Third row:** For interactions between diagnosis and sex. **Last row:** Between diagnostic groups within females (left) and males (right). Probability values, indexed in color, show positive and negative effects. NS=nonsignificant.

Source. Reprinted from Narr KL, Bilder RM, Toga AW, et al.: "Mapping Cortical Thickness and Gray Matter Concentration in First Episode Schizophrenia." *Cerebral Cortex* 15:708–719, 2005. Used with permission.

FUNCTIONAL NEUROANATOMY OF SCHIZOPHRENIA

Schizophrenia is a disorder characterized by multiple symptoms, with a varied course and outcome. The etiology is unknown, but multiple pathological processes or, equally likely, a unique pathophysiological process may be involved. The varied clinical and cognitive deficits observed across patients with schizophrenia suggest that different clusters of symptoms may reflect functional pathology coming from different cortical and subcortical neural circuits. Here, we review neuroimaging evidence of impaired functioning across a widely distributed cortical and subcortical network. We also discuss how these abnormalities might be related to specific signs and symptoms of schizophrenia.

The current diagnosis of schizophrenia is primarily phenomenological—that is, based on observation of the patient's behavior and subjective experiences. However, a growing body of evidence suggests that distinct neuropathological processes can be identified in postmortem brain tissues of individuals with schizophrenia, and novel neuroimaging methods enable in vivo studies of brain function and morphology both in individuals with schizophrenia and in their high-risk offspring. In particular, functional neuroimaging studies over the past decade have identified specific abnormalities in frontostriatal and frontolimbic regions in schizophrenia, identifiable as early as the first onset of the disorder, and have proposed that these neural dysfunctions may underlie the broad spectrum of cognitive deficits observed in this disorder.

PREFRONTAL CORTEX DYSFUNCTION

Although many classifications have been proposed to describe the complex array of deficits associated with schizophrenia (Grossberg 2000), all models have posited that many aspects of schizophrenia symptoms can be ascribed to a breakdown in various prefrontal cortical functions. For instance, poor performance on working memory and other executive function tasks has been associated with deficient dorsolateral prefrontal cortex function (Abi-Dargham et al. 2002; Barch et al. 2002, 2003b; Callicott et al. 2003a; Manoach 2003; Menon et al. 2001; Perlstein et al. 2003). Functional neuroimaging studies that used continuous performance tasks and working memory tasks repeatedly found reduced activation in dorsolateral prefrontal regions in schizophrenic patients (Braus et al. 2002; Ford et al. 2004; Fuentes 2001; Hazlett et al. 1998; Kiehl and Liddle 2001; MacDonald and Carter 2003; Perlstein et al. 2003; Volz et al. 1999). Prefrontal cortex dysfunction

becomes particularly pronounced under increased task complexity conditions (see Figure 10–6).

More recent studies have reported significantly greater activity in dorsolateral prefrontal cortex regions under certain task conditions in subjects with schizophrenia relative to healthy comparison subjects. Accordingly, some newer studies have proposed that the relation between task complexity and cortical activation in subjects with schizophrenia is characterized by a bell-shaped curve, so that greater effort is required to perform relatively simple tasks (corresponding to greater dorsolateral prefrontal cortex activation), and with greater task complexity, the person with schizophrenia begins to fail at the task (corresponding to lack of activation) (Callicott et al. 2003b; Manoach 2003).

Context-dependent response selection and execution deficits have been associated with dorsolateral prefrontal cortex activation deficits (Barch et al. 2002, 2003b; MacDonald and Carter 2003; Manoach et al. 1999, 2000), whereas deficits in the selection of responses according to their emotional valence and success in achieving rewards (Rushworth et al. 1997) have been closely associated with more ventral and orbitofrontal regions of the prefrontal cortex (Chemerinski et al. 2002; Crespo-Facorro and Arango 2000). Decreased prefrontal activity also has been associated with a reduction in incentive motivational signals from suppressed amygdala circuits that project to the prefrontal regions (Grady and Keightley 2002; Grossberg 2000; Paradiso et al. 2003; Shenton et al. 2001). By providing a motivational aspect to response selection, inferior or orbital prefrontal regions play an important role in the selection (Rubia et al. 2001; Spence 2000; S.F. Taylor et al. 1999) of task-inappropriate behaviors. Thus, in healthy individuals, the interaction between dorsolateral and more ventral prefrontal regions provides a balance between task-dependent rule-based response selection and motivational or incentive-based response inhibition, but in patients with schizophrenia, these prefrontal subregions appear to be imbalanced. In addition to the interaction between inferior and dorsal prefrontal regions, numerous studies have reported abnormal activation in anterior cingulate regions, more medial prefrontal areas involved in performance and response monitoring (Andreasen et al. 1995; Ardekani et al. 2002; Carter et al. 2001; Fletcher et al. 1999). Taken together, these findings suggest that the prefrontal cortical dysfunction in schizophrenia is rather widespread and distributed over the dorsolateral, ventral, and medial prefrontal regions, each contributing to specific aspects of the clinical and cognitive phenomenology.

Despite the overwhelming evidence of prefrontal cortex dysfunction, it remains unclear whether these deficits

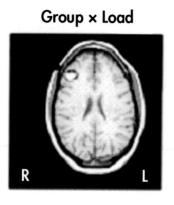

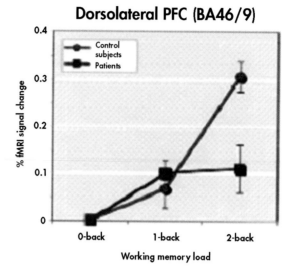

FIGURE 10–6.   Functional magnetic resonance imaging (fMRI) slices showing representative regions that had greater activation in control subjects relative to schizophrenic patients during a working memory task.

The plots on the right reflect signal intensity in the dorsolateral prefrontal cortex (DLPFC; BA 46/9) for healthy comparison subjects and subjects with schizophrenia as the percent change in signal intensity from the 0-back condition. Bars represent ±1 standard error.
Source.   Adapted from Perlstein WM, Dixit NK, Carter CS, et al.: "Prefrontal Cortex Dysfunction Mediates Deficits in Working Memory and Prepotent Responding in Schizophrenia." *Biological Psychiatry* 53:25–38, 2003. Used with permission.

are present early during the course of the disorder or whether they emerge following chronic psychotic episodes. Furthermore, it is also unclear whether selective regional functional abnormalities differentiate the various clinical manifestations of the disorder and show strong correlations with the severity of the expression of particular clusters of symptoms. Recent fMRI studies examining cortical functions in individuals at high risk for schizophrenia on the basis of subclinical (e.g., prodromal) symptoms (Morey et al. 2005) have reported significant deficits in the recruitment of prefrontal cortical regions, with further deterioration of prefrontal functions during the course of the illness (Figure 10–7). Furthermore, impairments were not found to be localized to selective prefrontal regions but rather reflected a distributed pathology involving frontal neocortex.

TEMPORAL CORTEX DYSFUNCTION

As significant as reports of prefrontal pathology, numerous neuroimaging and electrophysiological studies also have reported significant, early emerging, and neuroprogressive deficits in temporal cortical structure and function in schizophrenia (Dickey et al. 2003; Ho et al. 2003; Kasai et al. 2003a, 2003b; Kubicki et al. 2002a, 2002b; McCarley et al. 2002; Ngan et al. 2003; Sumich et al. 2002). Functional

imaging and electrophysiological studies also have shown abnormal cortical activation patterns during auditory selective attention tasks or auditory oddball tasks, which have been determined to rely on superior temporal cortical region processing (McCarley et al. 1993, 2002; O'Donnell et al. 1995, 1999; Shenton et al. 1989, 1993).

More recent studies have suggested specific deficits in frontotemporal connectivity, above and beyond potential localized frontal or temporal dysfunction, as measured by electroencephalogram coherence measures and measures of effective connectivity during auditory oddball tasks (Winterer et al. 2003).

FUNCTIONAL DEFICITS IN LIMBIC CORTEX AND MIDBRAIN PATHOLOGY

The limbic system consists of a band of cortical tissue on the medial sides of the cerebral hemispheres and includes the amygdala and the hippocampus. In addition to the cognitive functions described previously, the limbic system is believed to be associated with smell, eating, control of aggression, expression of emotion, and sexual response. Levels of dopamine have been shown to be elevated in the limbic system of individuals with schizophrenia, particularly in the left amygdala. Increased dopamine receptors also have been found in the thalamus (Gluck et al. 2002).

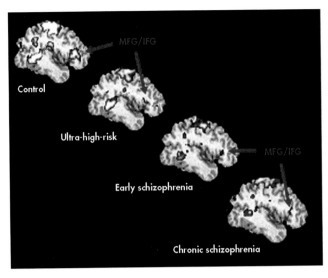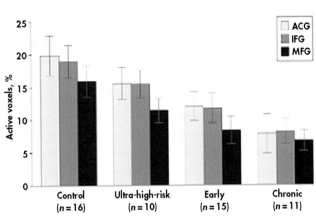

FIGURE 10–7. Group-averaged, target-related prefrontal activation in control, ultra-high-risk, early schizophrenia, and chronic schizophrenia groups.

Bar graph depicts the prefrontal target-related activation by group ($F_{3,48}$=4.6; $P<0.01$) and region ($F_{1,48}$=12.8; $P<0.001$), with greater activation in control subjects than in early and chronic groups. There was medial frontal activation for group ($F_{3,48}$=3.5; $P=0.02$), with greater activation in the control than in the chronically ill group. Bars=mean values; error bars=standard error. ACG=anterior cingulate gyrus; IFG=inferior frontal gyrus; MFG=middle frontal gyrus.

Source. Adapted from Morey RA, Inan S, Mitchell TV, et al.: "Imaging Frontostriatal Function in Ultra-High-Risk, Early, and Chronic Schizophrenia During Executive Processing." *Archives of General Psychiatry* 62:254–262, 2005. Used with permission.

Dopamine production is under the direct control of γ-aminobutyric acid (GABA)ergic neurons, such that an abnormally low GABA concentration promotes dopamine production. Although two GABA receptors have been identified, only $GABA_A$ has been consistently shown to be related to schizophrenia. Accumulating evidence suggests that $α_5$ GABA receptors play a prominent role in the abnormally high dopamine production that has been shown consistently to be related to schizophrenic symptomatology and can further be linked to abnormal thalamic regulation and gamma band synchrony in schizophrenia (Behrendt 2003). In particular, patients with schizophrenia show significant activation impairments during attention and vigilance tasks, especially lower bilateral activation in the thalamic nuclei and in the right head of the caudate nucleus (Salgado-Pineda et al. 2004). Similar findings were reported in the early PET studies by Siegel et al. (1993) that showed low metabolic activity rates in medial frontal cortical regions and in the basal ganglia, consistent with the importance of the cortical-striatal-thalamic pathways in schizophrenia.

Evidence of functional deficits in the midbrain area in patients with schizophrenia is abundant. These deficits are assessed with measures such as fMRI, PET, magnetoencephalography, and electrophysiological methods. The anatomical structures that have been found to be as-

sociated with activation deficits in schizophrenia include the basal ganglia, caudate, striate, thalamus, anterior cingulate cortex, and anterior cingulate gyrus. These deficits in brain activation are associated with neurocognitive deficits, particularly in the inability to select task-appropriate actions while inhibiting task-inappropriate ones.

Deficits in schizophrenia are apparent in a variety of domains, including impairments in affective and emotional processing (Kalus et al. 2005) and social and cognitive difficulties (Hempel et al. 2003). Consistent with such findings, activation deficits also have been found in patients with schizophrenia during tasks assessing emotional and affective competence. Despite behavioral results comparable to those of control subjects, patients showed less activation in several neural structures when completing a task viewing affective pictures. The researchers used evocative pictures to examine the automatic emotional response that requires no elaborate rating or categorization of stimuli. In patients, the right amygdala, bilateral hippocampal region, medial prefrontal cortex, basal ganglia, cerebellum, midbrain, and visual cortex were found to have less activation. In particular, decreased activation in the right amygdala appears to be an important finding related to dysfunctional emotional behavior in schizophrenia (Takahashi et al. 2004).

GLOBAL CHANGES: ABNORMAL CONNECTIVITY HYPOTHESIS

Although many of the studies reviewed in this chapter have focused on relatively circumscribed anatomical and functional deficits in schizophrenia, evidence is growing that schizophrenia is a disorder of cortical connectivity yielding more global, systemic alterations in cortical and subcortical structure and function. More specifically, recent diffusion tensor imaging studies have reported significant functional impairments in frontotemporal and frontoparietal connections (Burns et al. 2003), which suggest a structural disconnectivity in schizophrenia. In particular, reduced fractional anisotropy in the left uncinate fasciculus (Kubicki et al. 2002b) and left arcuate fasciculus in patients with schizophrenia compared with control subjects has been interpreted as reflecting frontotemporal and frontoparietal structural disconnectivity in schizophrenia.

More recent studies combining diffusion tensor imaging with magnetization transfer imaging (MTR), a technique sensitive to myelin and axonal alterations, have reported divergent findings from these two methods, suggesting that some of the diffusion abnormalities in schizophrenia are likely a result of abnormal coherence, or organization of the fiber tracts, but others may be attributed to or coincide with myelin or axonal disruption. Decreased diffusion anisotropy was reported in schizophrenia in multiple brain regions (Kubicki et al. 2005), including the fornix, bilaterally in the cingulum bundle, the superior occipitofrontal fasciculus, the internal capsule, the right inferior occipitofrontal fasciculus, and the left arcuate fasciculus. MTR maps, in contrast, showed changes in the corpus callosum, fornix, right internal capsule, and superior occipitofrontal fasciculus bilaterally; however, no changes were noted in the anterior cingulum bundle, the left internal capsule, the arcuate fasciculus, or the inferior occipitofrontal fasciculus. In addition, the right posterior cingulum bundle showed MTR but not FA changes in schizophrenia.

CONCLUSION

The implementation of complex cognitive and affective functions in the human brain not only depends on the proper functioning of individual regions but also necessitates the communication between brain regions that facilitates integration of cognitive, motor, and affective domains of function. As reviewed in this chapter, structural and functional impairments have been identified across multiple brain systems in schizophrenia, particularly along frontolimbic pathways and regions. Much of the current evidence from neuroimaging studies suggests dysfunctions to be prominently manifest in anterior components of the limbic circuitry, including the thalamus, basal ganglia, and hippocampus, as well as their target projection regions in frontal neocortex.

REFERENCES

Abi-Dargham A, Mawlawi O, Lombardo I, et al: Prefrontal dopamine D1 receptors and working memory in schizophrenia. J Neurosci 22:3708–3719, 2002

Altshuler LL, Bartzokis G, Grieder T, et al: Amygdala enlargement in bipolar disorder and hippocampal reduction in schizophrenia: an MRI study demonstrating neuroanatomic specificity. Arch Gen Psychiatry 55:663–664, 1998

Anderson JE, Wible CG, McCarley RW, et al: An MRI study of temporal lobe abnormalities and negative symptoms in chronic schizophrenia. Schizophr Res 58:123–134, 2002

Andreasen NC: Linking mind and brain in the study of mental illnesses: a project for a scientific psychopathology. Science 275:1586–1593, 1997

Andreasen NC, Swayze V, O'Leary DS, et al: Abnormalities in midline attentional circuitry in schizophrenia: evidence from magnetic resonance and positron emission tomography. Eur Neuropsychopharmacol 5(suppl):37–41, 1995

Arciniegas D, Rojas DC, Teale P, et al: The thalamus and the schizophrenia phenotype: failure to replicate reduced volume. Biol Psychiatry 45:1329–1335, 1999

Ardekani BA, Choi SJ, Hossein-Zadeh GA, et al: Functional magnetic resonance imaging of brain activity in the visual oddball task. Brain Res Cogn Brain Res 14:347–356, 2002

Arnold SE, Hyman BT, Van Hoesen GW, et al: Some cytoarchitectural abnormalities of the entorhinal cortex in schizophrenia. Arch Gen Psychiatry 48:625–632, 1991

Barch DM, Csernansky JG, Conturo T, et al: Working and long-term memory deficits in schizophrenia: is there a common prefrontal mechanism? J Abnorm Psychol 111:478–494, 2002

Barch DM, Mathews JR, Buckner RL, et al: Hemodynamic responses in visual, motor, and somatosensory cortices in schizophrenia. Neuroimage 20:1884–1893, 2003a

Barch DM, Sheline YI, Csernansky JG, et al: Working memory and prefrontal cortex dysfunction: specificity to schizophrenia compared with major depression. Biol Psychiatry 53:376–384, 2003b

Barta PE, Petty RG, McGilchrist I, et al: Asymmetry of the planum temporale: methodological considerations and clinical associations. Psychiatry Res 61:137–150, 1995

Behrendt RP: Hallucinations: synchronisation of thalamocortical gamma oscillations underconstrained by sensory input. Conscious Cogn 12:413–451, 2003

Bilder RM, Lipschutz-Broch L, Reiter G, et al: Intellectual deficits in first-episode schizophrenia: evidence for progressive deterioration. Schizophr Bull 18:437–448, 1992

Boynton GM, Engel SA, Glover GH, et al: Linear systems analysis of functional magnetic resonance imaging in human V1. J Neurosci 16:4207–4221, 1996

Braff DL, Swerdlow NR: Neuroanatomy of schizophrenia. Schizophr Bull 23:509–512, 1997

Braus DF, Weber-Fahr W, Tost H, et al: Sensory information processing in neuroleptic-naive first-episode schizophrenic patients: a functional magnetic resonance imaging study. Arch Gen Psychiatry 59:696–701, 2002

Breier A, Buchanan RW, Elkashef A, et al: Brain morphology and schizophrenia: a magnetic resonance imaging study of limbic, prefrontal cortex, and caudate structures. Arch Gen Psychiatry 49:921–926, 1992

Bremner JD, Krystal JH, Southwick SM, et al: Functional neuroanatomical correlates of the effects of stress on memory. J Trauma Stress 8:527–553, 1995

Bryant NL, Buchanan RW, Vladar K, et al: Gender differences in temporal lobe structures of patients with schizophrenia: a volumetric MRI study. Am J Psychiatry 156:603–609, 1999

Buchanan RW, Vladar K, Barta PE, et al: Structural evaluation of the prefrontal cortex in schizophrenia. Am J Psychiatry 155:1049–1055, 1998

Burns J, Job D, Bastin ME, et al: Structural disconnectivity in schizophrenia: a diffusion tensor magnetic resonance imaging study. Br J Psychiatry 182:439–443, 2003

Callicott JH, Egan MF, Bertolino A, et al: Hippocampal N-acetyl aspartate in unaffected siblings of patients with schizophrenia: a possible intermediate neurobiological phenotype. Biol Psychiatry 44:941–950, 1998

Callicott JH, Egan MF, Mattay VS, et al: Abnormal fMRI response of the dorsolateral prefrontal cortex in cognitively intact siblings of patients with schizophrenia. Am J Psychiatry 160:709–719, 2003a

Callicott JH, Mattay VS, Verchinski BA, et al: Complexity of prefrontal cortical dysfunction in schizophrenia: more than up or down. Am J Psychiatry 160:2209–2215, 2003b

Carter CS, MacDonald AW 3rd, Ross LL, et al: Anterior cingulate cortex activity and impaired self-monitoring of performance in patients with schizophrenia: an event-related fMRI study. Am J Psychiatry 158:1423–1428, 2001

Chakos MH, Lieberman JA, Bilder RM, et al: Increase in caudate nuclei volumes of first-episode schizophrenic patients taking antipsychotic drugs. Am J Psychiatry 151:1430–1436, 1994

Chakos MH, Lieberman JA, Alvir J, et al: Caudate nuclei volumes in schizophrenic patients treated with typical antipsychotics or clozapine. Lancet 345(8947):456–457, 1995

Chance SA, Esiri MM, Crow TJ: Ventricular enlargement in schizophrenia: a primary change in the temporal lobe? Schizophr Res 62:123–131, 2003

Chemerinski E, Nopoulos PC, Crespo-Facorro B, et al: Morphology of the ventral frontal cortex in schizophrenia: relationship with social dysfunction. Biol Psychiatry 52:1–8, 2002

Chua SE, Wright IC, Poline JB, et al: Grey matter correlates of syndromes in schizophrenia: a semi-automated analysis of structural magnetic resonance images. Br J Psychiatry 170:406–410, 1997

Corey-Bloom J, Jernigan T, Archibald S, et al: Quantitative magnetic resonance imaging of the brain in late-life schizophrenia. Am J Psychiatry 152:447–449, 1995

Corson PW, Nopoulos P, Andreasen NC, et al: Caudate size in first-episode neuroleptic-naive schizophrenic patients measured using an artificial neural network. Biol Psychiatry 46:712–720, 1999

Crespo-Facorro B, Arango C: [Schizophrenia: a brain disease, II: functional neuroimaging]. Actas Esp Psiquiatr 28:31–39, 2000

Crespo-Facorro B, Nopoulos PC, Chemerinski E, et al: Temporal pole morphology and psychopathology in males with schizophrenia. Psychiatry Res 132:107–115, 2004

de la Torre JC, Barrios M, Junque C: Frontal lobe alterations in schizophrenia: neuroimaging and neuropsychological findings. Eur Arch Psychiatry Clin Neurosci 255:236–244, 2005

Deicken RF, Zhou L, Schuff N, et al: Hippocampal neuronal dysfunction in schizophrenia as measured by proton magnetic resonance spectroscopy. Biol Psychiatry 43:483–488, 1998

Deicken RF, Eliaz Y, Chosiad L, et al: Magnetic resonance imaging of the thalamus in male patients with schizophrenia. Schizophr Res 58:135–144, 2002

DeLisi LE, Sakuma M, Tew W, et al: Schizophrenia as a chronic active brain process: a study of progressive brain structural change subsequent to the onset of schizophrenia. Psychiatry Res 74:129–140, 1997

Devinsky O, Morrell MJ, Vogt BA: Contributions of anterior cingulate cortex to behaviour. Brain 118(pt 1):279–306, 1995

DeYoe EA, Carman GJ, Bandettini P, et al: Mapping striate and extrastriate visual areas in human cerebral cortex. Proc Natl Acad Sci U S A 93:2382–2386, 1996

Dickey CC, McCarley RW, Voglmaier MM, et al: Schizotypal personality disorder and MRI abnormalities of temporal lobe gray matter. Biol Psychiatry 45:1393–1402, 1999

Dickey CC, McCarley RW, Shenton ME: The brain in schizotypal personality disorder: a review of structural MRI and CT findings. Harv Rev Psychiatry 10:1–15, 2002a

Dickey CC, McCarley RW, Voglmaier MM, et al: Smaller left Heschl's gyrus volume in patients with schizotypal personality disorder. Am J Psychiatry 159:1521–1527, 2002b

Dickey CC, McCarley RW, Voglmaier MM, et al: An MRI study of superior temporal gyrus volume in women with schizotypal personality disorder. Am J Psychiatry 160:2198–2201, 2003

Downhill JE Jr, Buchsbaum MS, Hazlett EA, et al: Temporal lobe volume determined by magnetic resonance imaging in schizotypal personality disorder and schizophrenia. Schizophr Res 48:187–199, 2001

Druzgal TJ, D'Esposito M: Activity in fusiform face area modulated as a function of working memory load. Brain Res Cogn Brain Res 10:355–364, 2001

Ettinger U, Chitnis XA, Kumari V, et al: Magnetic resonance imaging of the thalamus in first-episode psychosis. Am J Psychiatry 158:116–118, 2001

Fannon D, Chitnis X, Doku V, et al: Features of structural brain abnormality detected in first-episode psychosis. Am J Psychiatry 157:1829–1834, 2000

Fannon D, Simmons A, Tennakoon L, et al: Selective deficit of hippocampal N-acetylaspartate in antipsychotic-naive patients with schizophrenia. Biol Psychiatry 54:587–598, 2003

Fletcher P, McKenna PJ, Friston KJ, et al: Abnormal cingulate modulation of fronto-temporal connectivity in schizophrenia. Neuroimage 9:337–342, 1999

Ford JM, Gray M, Whitfield SL, et al: Acquiring and inhibiting prepotent responses in schizophrenia: event-related brain potentials and functional magnetic resonance imaging. Arch Gen Psychiatry 61:119–129, 2004

Frazier JA, Giedd JN, Kaysen D, et al: Childhood-onset schizophrenia: brain MRI rescan after 2 years of clozapine maintenance treatment. Am J Psychiatry 153:564–566, 1996

Freedman M, Black S, Ebert P, et al: Orbitofrontal function, object alternation and perseveration. Cereb Cortex 8:18–27, 1998

Fuentes LJ: [Selective attention deficit in schizophrenia]. Rev Neurol 32:387–391, 2001

Fuster JM: The Prefrontal Cortex: Anatomy, Physiology, and Neuropsychology of the Frontal Lobe. Philadelphia, PA, Lippincott-Raven, 1997

Gaser C, Nenadic I, Buchsbaum BR, et al: Ventricular enlargement in schizophrenia related to volume reduction of the thalamus, striatum, and superior temporal cortex. Am J Psychiatry 161:154–156, 2004

Gluck MR, Thomas RG, Davis KL, et al: Implications for altered glutamate and GABA metabolism in the dorsolateral prefrontal cortex of aged schizophrenic patients. Am J Psychiatry 159:1165–1173, 2002

Goldstein JM, Goodman JM, Seidman LJ, et al: Cortical abnormalities in schizophrenia identified by structural magnetic resonance imaging. Arch Gen Psychiatry 56:537–547, 1999

Golomb J, de Leon MJ, Kluger A, et al: Hippocampal atrophy in normal aging: an association with recent memory impairment. Arch Neurol 50:967–973, 1993

Grady CL, Keightley ML: Studies of altered social cognition in neuropsychiatric disorders using functional neuroimaging. Can J Psychiatry 47:327–336, 2002

Gray JA: The Psychology of Fear and Stress. New York, Oxford University Press, 1987

Grossberg S: The imbalanced brain: from normal behavior to schizophrenia. Biol Psychiatry 48:81–98, 2000

Gur RE, Cowell P, Turetsky BI, et al: A follow-up magnetic resonance imaging study of schizophrenia: relationship of neuroanatomical changes to clinical and neurobehavioral measures. Arch Gen Psychiatry 55:145–152, 1998

Gur RE, Cowell PE, Latshaw A, et al: Reduced dorsal and orbital prefrontal gray matter volumes in schizophrenia. Arch Gen Psychiatry 57:761–768, 2000

Harris JM, Whalley H, Yates S, et al: Abnormal cortical folding in high-risk individuals: a predictor of the development of schizophrenia? Biol Psychiatry 56:182–189, 2004

Hazlett EA, Buchsbaum MS, Haznedar MM, et al: Prefrontal cortex glucose metabolism and startle eyeblink modification abnormalities in unmedicated schizophrenia patients. Psychophysiology 35:186–198, 1998

Heckers S: Neuroimaging studies of the hippocampus in schizophrenia. Hippocampus 11:520–528, 2001

Heimer L, de Olmos J, Alheid GF, et al: "Perestroika" in the basal forebrain: opening the border between neurology and psychiatry. Prog Brain Res 87:109–165, 1991

Hempel A, Hempel E, Schonknecht P, et al: Impairment in basal limbic function in schizophrenia during affect recognition. Psychiatry Res 122:115–124, 2003

Henn FA, Braus DF: Structural neuroimaging in schizophrenia: an integrative view of neuromorphology. Eur Arch Psychiatry Clin Neurosci 249 (suppl 4):48–56, 1999

Hirayasu Y, McCarley RW, Salisbury DF, et al: Planum temporale and Heschl gyrus volume reduction in schizophrenia: a magnetic resonance imaging study of first-episode patients. Arch Gen Psychiatry 57:692–699, 2000a

Hirayasu Y, Shenton ME, Salisbury DF, et al: Hippocampal and superior temporal gyrus volume in first-episode schizophrenia. Arch Gen Psychiatry 57:618–619, 2000b

Ho BC, Andreasen NC, Nopoulos P, et al: Progressive structural brain abnormalities and their relationship to clinical outcome: a longitudinal magnetic resonance imaging study early in schizophrenia. Arch Gen Psychiatry 60:585–594, 2003

Holinger DP, Shenton ME, Wible CG, et al: Superior temporal gyrus volume abnormalities and thought disorder in left-handed schizophrenic men. Am J Psychiatry 156:1730–1735, 1999

Hubl D, Koenig T, Strik W, et al: Pathways that make voices: white matter changes in auditory hallucinations. Arch Gen Psychiatry 61:658–668, 2004

Johnstone EC, Crow TJ, Frith CD, et al: Cerebral ventricular size and cognitive impairment in chronic schizophrenia. Lancet 2(7992):924–926, 1976

Joseph R: Neuropsychiatry, Neuropsychology, and Clinical Neuroscience: Emotion, Evolution, Cognition, Language, Memory, Brain Damage, and Abnormal Behavior. Baltimore, MD, Williams & Wilkins, 1996

Kalus P, Slotboom J, Gallinat J, et al: The amygdala in schizophrenia: a trimodal magnetic resonance imaging study. Neurosci Lett 375:151–156, 2005

Kasai K, Shenton ME, Salisbury DF, et al: Progressive decrease of left Heschl gyrus and planum temporale gray matter volume in first-episode schizophrenia: a longitudinal magnetic resonance imaging study. Arch Gen Psychiatry 60:766–775, 2003a

Kasai K, Shenton ME, Salisbury DF, et al: Progressive decrease of left superior temporal gyrus gray matter volume in patients with first-episode schizophrenia. Am J Psychiatry 160:156–164, 2003b

Kemether EM, Buchsbaum MS, Byne W, et al: Magnetic resonance imaging of mediodorsal, pulvinar, and centromedian nuclei of the thalamus in patients with schizophrenia. Arch Gen Psychiatry 60:983–991, 2003

Keshavan MS, Bagwell WW, Haas GL, et al: Changes in caudate volume with neuroleptic treatment (letter). Lancet 344 (8934):1434, 1994

Keshavan MS, Rosenberg D, Sweeney JA, et al: Decreased caudate volume in neuroleptic-naive psychotic patients. Am J Psychiatry 155:774–778, 1998

Kiehl KA, Liddle PF: An event-related functional magnetic resonance imaging study of an auditory oddball task in schizophrenia. Schizophr Res 48:159–171, 2001

Kim JJ, Crespo-Facorro B, Andreasen NC, et al: An MRI-based parcellation method for the temporal lobe. Neuroimage 11:271–288, 2000

Kubicki M, Shenton ME, Salisbury DF, et al: Voxel-based morphometric analysis of gray matter in first episode schizophrenia. Neuroimage 17:1711–1719, 2002a

Kubicki M, Westin CF, Maier SE, et al: Uncinate fasciculus findings in schizophrenia: a magnetic resonance diffusion tensor imaging study. Am J Psychiatry 159:813–820, 2002b

Kubicki M, McCarley RW, Nestor PG, et al: An fMRI study of semantic processing in men with schizophrenia. Neuroimage 20:1923–1933, 2003

Kubicki M, McCarley R, Westin CF, et al: A review of diffusion tensor imaging studies in schizophrenia. J Psychiatr Res July 13, 2005 (Epub ahead of print)

Kwon JS, McCarley RW, Hirayasu Y, et al: Left planum temporale volume reduction in schizophrenia. Arch Gen Psychiatry 56:142–148, 1999

Lawrie SM, Whalley H, Kestelman JN, et al: Magnetic resonance imaging of brain in people at high risk of developing schizophrenia. Lancet 353:30–33, 1999

Lawrie SM, Whalley HC, Abukmeil SS, et al: Temporal lobe volume changes in people at high risk of schizophrenia with psychotic symptoms. Br J Psychiatry 181:138–143, 2002

Le Bihan D, Mangin JF, Poupon C, et al: Diffusion tensor imaging: concepts and applications. J Magn Reson Imaging 13:534–546, 2001

Levitt JJ, McCarley RW, Dickey CC, et al: MRI study of caudate nucleus volume and its cognitive correlates in neuroleptic-naive patients with schizotypal personality disorder. Am J Psychiatry 159:1190–1197, 2002

Lieberman J, Chakos M, Wu H, et al: Longitudinal study of brain morphology in first episode schizophrenia. Biol Psychiatry 49:487–499, 2001

Luria A: Higher Cognitive Functions in Man. New York, Basic Books, 1980

MacDonald AW 3rd, Carter CS: Event-related FMRI study of context processing in dorsolateral prefrontal cortex of patients with schizophrenia. J Abnorm Psychol 112:689–697, 2003

Manoach DS: Prefrontal cortex dysfunction during working memory performance in schizophrenia: reconciling discrepant findings. Schizophr Res 60:285–298, 2003

Manoach DS, Press DZ, Thangaraj V, et al: Schizophrenic subjects activate dorsolateral prefrontal cortex during a working memory task, as measured by fMRI. Biol Psychiatry 45:1128–1137, 1999

Manoach DS, Gollub RL, Benson ES, et al: Schizophrenic subjects show aberrant fMRI activation of dorsolateral prefrontal cortex and basal ganglia during working memory performance. Biol Psychiatry 48:99–109, 2000

McCarley RW, Shenton ME, O'Donnell BF, et al: Auditory P300 abnormalities and left posterior superior temporal gyrus volume reduction in schizophrenia. Arch Gen Psychiatry 50:190–197, 1993

McCarley RW, Wible CG, Frumin M, et al: MRI anatomy of schizophrenia. Biol Psychiatry 45:1099–1119, 1999

McCarley RW, Salisbury DF, Hirayasu Y, et al: Association between smaller left posterior superior temporal gyrus volume on magnetic resonance imaging and smaller left temporal P300 amplitude in first-episode schizophrenia. Arch Gen Psychiatry 59:321–331, 2002

Menon V, Anagnoson RT, Mathalon DH, et al: Functional neuroanatomy of auditory working memory in schizophrenia: relation to positive and negative symptoms. Neuroimage 13:433–446, 2001

Mitelman SA, Shihabuddin L, Brickman AM, et al: MRI assessment of gray and white matter distribution in Brodmann's areas of the cortex in patients with schizophrenia with good and poor outcomes. Am J Psychiatry 160:2154–2168, 2003

Molina V, Sanz J, Sarramea F, et al: Lower prefrontal gray matter volume in schizophrenia in chronic but not in first episode schizophrenia patients. Psychiatry Res 131:45–56, 2004

Morey RA, Inan S, Mitchell TV, et al: Imaging frontostriatal function in ultra-high-risk, early, and chronic schizophrenia during executive processing. Arch Gen Psychiatry 62:254–262, 2005

Narr KL, Thompson PM, Sharma T, et al: Three-dimensional mapping of temporo-limbic regions and the lateral ventricles in schizophrenia: gender effects. Biol Psychiatry 50:84–97, 2001

Narr KL, Thompson PM, Szeszko P, et al: Regional specificity of hippocampal volume reductions in first-episode schizophrenia. Neuroimage 21:1563–1575, 2004

Narr KL, Bilder RM, Toga AW, et al: Mapping cortical thickness and gray matter concentration in first episode schizophrenia. Cereb Cortex 15:708–719, 2005

Nasrallah HA, Sharma S, Olson SC: The volume of the entorhinal cortex in schizophrenia: a controlled MRI study. Prog Neuropsychopharmacol Biol Psychiatry 21:1317–1322, 1997

Ngan ET, Vouloumanos A, Cairo TA, et al: Abnormal processing of speech during oddball target detection in schizophrenia. Neuroimage 20:889–897, 2003

O'Donnell BF, Shenton ME, McCarley RW, et al: Conjoint left asymmetry of auditory P300 voltage and MRI volume of posterior superior temporal gyrus in schizophrenia: a quantitative evaluation. Electroencephalogr Clin Neurophysiol Suppl 44:387–394, 1995

O'Donnell BF, McCarley RW, Potts GF, et al: Identification of neural circuits underlying P300 abnormalities in schizophrenia. Psychophysiology 36:388–398, 1999

Onitsuka T, Shenton ME, Salisbury DF, et al: Middle and inferior temporal gyrus gray matter volume abnormalities in chronic schizophrenia: an MRI study. Am J Psychiatry 161:1603–1611, 2004

Paradiso S, Andreasen NC, Crespo-Facorro B, et al: Emotions in unmedicated patients with schizophrenia during evaluation with positron emission tomography. Am J Psychiatry 160:1775–1783, 2003

Pearlson GD: Superior temporal gyrus and planum temporale in schizophrenia: a selective review. Prog Neuropsychopharmacol Biol Psychiatry 21:1203–1229, 1997

Perlstein WM, Dixit NK, Carter CS, et al: Prefrontal cortex dysfunction mediates deficits in working memory and prepotent responding in schizophrenia. Biol Psychiatry 53:25–38, 2003

Raichle M: Circulatory and metabolic correlates of brain function in normal humans, in Handbook of Physiology: The Nervous System, Vol 5. Edited by Plum F, Mountcastle V. Bethesda, MD, American Physiological Association, 1987, pp 643–674

Rajarethinam R, Sahni S, Rosenberg DR, et al: Reduced superior temporal gyrus volume in young offspring of patients with schizophrenia. Am J Psychiatry 161:1121–1124, 2004

Rubia K, Russell T, Bullmore ET, et al: An fMRI study of reduced left prefrontal activation in schizophrenia during normal inhibitory function. Schizophr Res 52:47–55, 2001

Rushworth MF, Nixon PD, Eacott MJ, et al: Ventral prefrontal cortex is not essential for working memory. J Neurosci 17:4829–4838, 1997

Salgado-Pineda P, Junque C, Vendrell P, et al: Decreased cerebral activation during CPT performance: structural and functional deficits in schizophrenic patients. Neuroimage 21:840–847, 2004

Saykin AJ, Gur RC, Gur RE, et al: Neuropsychological function in schizophrenia: selective impairment in memory and learning. Arch Gen Psychiatry 48:618–624, 1991

Saykin AJ, Shtasel DL, Gur RE, et al: Neuropsychological deficits in neuroleptic naive patients with first-episode schizophrenia. Arch Gen Psychiatry 51:124–131, 1994

Seidman LJ, Wencel HE: Genetically mediated brain abnormalities in schizophrenia. Curr Psychiatry Rep 5:135–144, 2003

Selemon LD, Rajkowska G, Goldman-Rakic PS: Elevated neuronal density in prefrontal area 46 in brains from schizophrenic patients: application of a three-dimensional, stereologic counting method. J Comp Neurol 392:402–412, 1998

Sereno MI, Dale AM, Reppas JB, et al: Borders of multiple visual areas in humans revealed by functional magnetic resonance imaging. Science 268:889–893, 1995

Shapleske J, Rossell SL, Woodruff PW, et al: The planum temporale: a systematic, quantitative review of its structural, functional and clinical significance. Brain Res Brain Res Rev 29:26–49, 1999

Shenton ME, Faux SF, McCarley RW, et al: Correlations between abnormal auditory P300 topography and positive symptoms in schizophrenia: a preliminary report. Biol Psychiatry 25:710–716, 1989

Shenton ME, O'Donnell BF, Nestor PG, et al: Temporal lobe abnormalities in a patient with schizophrenia who has word-finding difficulty: use of high-resolution magnetic resonance imaging and auditory P300 event-related potentials. Harv Rev Psychiatry 1:110–117, 1993

Shenton ME, Dickey CC, Frumin M, et al: A review of MRI findings in schizophrenia. Schizophr Res 49:1–52, 2001

Shenton ME, Gerig G, McCarley RW, et al: Amygdala-hippocampal shape differences in schizophrenia: the application of 3D shape models to volumetric MR data. Psychiatry Res 115:15–35, 2002

Shihabuddin L, Buchsbaum MS, Hazlett EA, et al: Dorsal striatal size, shape, and metabolic rate in never-medicated and previously medicated schizophrenics performing a verbal learning task. Arch Gen Psychiatry 55:235–243, 1998

Siegel BV Jr, Buchsbaum MS, Bunney WE Jr, et al: Cortical-striatal-thalamic circuits and brain glucose metabolic activity in 70 unmedicated male schizophrenic patients. Am J Psychiatry 150:1325–1336, 1993

Spence SA: Commenting on neuroimaging (comment) [published erratum appears in Br J Psychiatry 177:471, 2000]. Br J Psychiatry 176:594, 2000

Stefanis N, Frangou S, Yakeley J, et al: Hippocampal volume reduction in schizophrenia: effects of genetic risk and pregnancy and birth complications. Biol Psychiatry 46:697–702, 1999

Sullivan EV, Mathalon DH, Lim KO, et al: Patterns of regional cortical dysmorphology distinguishing schizophrenia and chronic alcoholism. Biol Psychiatry 43:118–131, 1998b

Sumich A, Chitnis XA, Fannon DG, et al: Temporal lobe abnormalities in first-episode psychosis. Am J Psychiatry 159:1232–1235, 2002

Szeszko PR, Goldberg E, Gunduz-Bruce H, et al: Smaller anterior hippocampal formation volume in antipsychotic-naive patients with first-episode schizophrenia. Am J Psychiatry 160:2190–2197, 2003

Takahashi H, Koeda M, Oda K, et al: An fMRI study of differential neural response to affective pictures in schizophrenia. Neuroimage 22:1247–1254, 2004

Taylor JL, Blanton RE, Levitt JG, et al: Superior temporal gyrus differences in childhood-onset schizophrenia. Schizophr Res 73:235–241, 2005

Taylor SF, Tandon R, Koeppe RA: Global cerebral blood flow increase reveals focal hypoperfusion in schizophrenia. Neuropsychopharmacology 21:368–371, 1999

Velakoulis D, Pantelis C, McGorry PD, et al: Hippocampal volume in first-episode psychoses and chronic schizophrenia: a high-resolution magnetic resonance imaging study. Arch Gen Psychiatry 56:133–141, 1999

Velakoulis D, Wood SJ, Smith DJ, et al: Increased duration of illness is associated with reduced volume in right medial temporal/anterior cingulate grey matter in patients with chronic schizophrenia. Schizophr Res 57:43–49, 2002

Visser PJ, Verhey FR, Hofman PA, et al: Medial temporal lobe atrophy predicts Alzheimer's disease in patients with minor cognitive impairment. J Neurol Neurosurg Psychiatry 72: 491–497, 2002

Vita A, Dieci M, Giobbio GM, et al: Time course of cerebral ventricular enlargement in schizophrenia supports the hypothesis of its neurodevelopmental nature. Schizophr Res 23:25–30, 1997

Volz H, Gaser C, Hager F, et al: Decreased frontal activation in schizophrenics during stimulation with the continuous performance test—a functional magnetic resonance imaging study. Eur Psychiatry 14:17–24, 1999

Wible CG, Shenton ME, Hokama H, et al: Prefrontal cortex and schizophrenia: a quantitative magnetic resonance imaging study. Arch Gen Psychiatry 52(4):279–288, 1995

Winterer G, Coppola R, Egan MF, et al: Functional and effective frontotemporal connectivity and genetic risk for schizophrenia. Biol Psychiatry 54:1181–1192, 2003

Wood SJ, Velakoulis D, Smith DJ, et al: A longitudinal study of hippocampal volume in first episode psychosis and chronic schizophrenia. Schizophr Res 52:37–46, 2001

Wright IC, Sharma T, Ellison ZR, et al: Supra-regional brain systems and the neuropathology of schizophrenia. Cereb Cortex 9:366–378, 1999

Yamasue H, Iwanami A, Hirayasu Y, et al: Localized volume reduction in prefrontal, temporolimbic, and paralimbic regions in schizophrenia: an MRI parcellation study. Psychiatry Res 131:195–207, 2004

Yotsutsuji T, Saitoh O, Suzuki M, et al: Quantification of lateral ventricular subdivisions in schizophrenia by high-resolution three-dimensional magnetic resonance imaging. Psychiatry Res 122:1–12, 2003

Yucel M, Wood SJ, Phillips LJ, et al: Morphology of the anterior cingulate cortex in young men at ultra-high risk of developing a psychotic illness. Br J Psychiatry 182:518–524, 2003

CHAPTER

11

PSYCHOPATHOLOGY

J. P. LINDENMAYER, M.D.

ANZALEE KHAN, M.S.

Schizophrenia is a serious mental illness characterized by positive, negative, and cognitive symptoms that affect almost all aspects of mental activity, including perception, attention, memory, and emotion. Symptoms are associated with various degrees of more persistent social and functional impairments. Schizophrenia affects about 1% of the U.S. population. It is estimated that people with schizophrenia occupy 10% of hospital beds in the United States, and approximately 30% of people with the disease are hospitalized at one point in their lives.

The disorder begins usually in late adolescence and early adulthood. The median age at onset is about 23 years in men and 28 years in women. Onset is rare before 16 years and uncommon after 50 years. The disorder can have a relatively acute onset, over the course of 2–3 weeks, or an insidious one. Most individuals experience a prodromal phase before the first episode during which certain signs and symptoms will be present, yet the person does not fulfill all the criteria of the disorder (McGorry et al. 1996).

DIAGNOSIS OF SCHIZOPHRENIA

The definitions and criteria used to establish the diagnosis of schizophrenia have undergone important and wide changes over the years despite the fact that the definition and descriptions of the symptoms themselves have remained rather stable. The different diagnostic concepts used over time have been influenced by various factors outside the specific symptoms of the disorder and have introduced a significant amount of variability in the way schizophrenia has been diagnosed. Some of these factors are 1) the number and type of symptoms included in the diagnosis (narrow vs. broad definition), 2) short versus extended duration of symptoms, 3) inclusion of cross-sectional versus longitudinal course aspects of the disorder, and 4) inclusion versus exclusion of negative symptoms. Some of these changes in definition can be best understood in reviewing the historical perspective of the development of the diagnostic concept of schizophrenia.

Traditionally, American nosology was based on Bleuler's four "A's": disturbance in **A**ffect, **A**ssociation, **A**utism, and **A**mbivalence. These criteria tended to result in a relatively broad concept of schizophrenia, which was elaborated in DSM-II (American Psychiatric Association 1968). Other examples of this extended boundary of schizophrenia were Kasanin's (1933) schizoaffective schizophrenia, Hoch and Polatin's (1949) pseudoneurotic schizophrenia and Vaillant's (1964) good prognosis schizophrenia. DSM-III (American Psychiatric Association 1980) and DSM-III-R (American Psychiatric Association 1987) brought about a radical departure from this approach and introduced a much narrower concept with 1) a clear limitation of the number and type of symptoms, 2) a requirement

TABLE 11–1.   Schneider's first-rank symptoms

Symptoms	Description
Three special forms of auditory hallucinations	1. Hearing one's thoughts spoken aloud 2. Hearing voices referring to himself/herself, made in the third person 3. Auditory hallucinations in the form of a running commentary on one's activity
Thought withdrawal, insertion, and interruption	
Thought broadcasting	One's thoughts are broadcast to others
Somatic hallucinations	Somatic passivity, in which the patient is the passive and reluctant recipient of externally imposed bodily sensations
Delusional perception	A normal perception followed by delusional and highly personalized interpretation
Ideas of passivity	Feelings, impulses, or motor activity are experienced, influenced, or controlled by external agents

Note.   Schneider's diagnostic concept of schizophrenia has had considerable influence on almost all diagnostic systems subsequently developed. However, later studies have shown that Schneiderian first-rank symptoms are not entirely pathognomonic and that they can be found in other psychotic disorders as well, such as depression and mania (Carpenter et al. 1973; Wing and Nixon 1975).

for a specific duration of symptoms, and 3) the inclusion of a course criterion. This development was the result of critiques of the lack of reliability and validity of diagnosis (Beck et al. 1962; Spitzer and Fleiss 1974) and the important influence of the German phenomenological school with the introduction of Schneider's "first-rank symptoms" (Schneider 1959, 1974) (Table 11–1), which focused on specific allegedly pathognomonic symptoms of schizophrenia. In addition, the work of the Washington University School (Feighner et al. 1972) (Table 11–2) introduced the requirement of duration of at least 6 months before the diagnosis could be established. The symptoms included in the definition of schizophrenia in DSM-III were largely based on Schneiderian first-rank symptoms, with the requirement of 6 months' duration, which included prodromal and residual periods of illness. This definition resulted in a much narrower concept of schizophrenia, somewhat closer to the British and European concept of the disorder.

There was a further narrowing with the introduction of DSM-IV (American Psychiatric Association 1994) and DSM-IV-TR (American Psychiatric Association 2000), which include specific negative symptoms (Table 11–3). Criterion A in DSM-IV includes four positive symptoms and one negative symptom; at least two of these have to be present for this criterion to be fulfilled. The criterion for duration of acute phase symptoms was extended from 1 week to 1 month. If delusions (criterion A) are judged to be bizarre, only this single symptom is required to satisfy criterion A for schizophrenia. Similarly, the diagnosis of schizophrenia can be made with only hallucinations

within criterion A, if these consist of voices keeping up a running commentary on the person's behavior or thoughts or if two or three voices are conversing with each other. DSM-IV-TR uses the term *disorganized speech* instead of *incoherence* or *marked loosening of associations* for the schizophrenic thought disorder. Negative symptoms, such as affective flattening, alogia, and avolition, are now included in criterion A. For criterion B, the requirement for a decrease in social/occupational functioning is broadened. Criterion C requires continuous signs of the disorder for at least 6 months, whereas criterion D delineates schizophrenia from schizoaffective and mood disorders.

The definition of schizophrenia remains somewhat different in the International Classification of Diseases, 10th Revision (ICD-10; World Health Organization 1992) (Table 11–4). ICD-10 takes a more cross-sectional approach without including the decline in social/occupational functions as required by DSM-IV-TR. The requirement for duration of symptoms is reduced to only 1 month, in contrast to 6 months in DSM-IV-TR. Among the positive symptoms, Schneiderian symptoms are well represented, and only one is required for the diagnosis of schizophrenia, reflecting the pathognomonic importance ICD-10 continues to give to the Schneiderian first-rank symptoms. Negative symptoms such as marked apathy, paucity of speech, and blunting or incongruity of emotional responses are given more prominence as well. The ICD-10 definition is narrower than the DSM-IV-TR definition regarding positive symptoms in that it requires predominantly Schneiderian first-rank symptoms.

TABLE 11–2.   The Washington University criteria (Feighner criteria) for schizophrenia

For a diagnosis of schizophrenia, A through C are required:

A. Both of the following are necessary:

1. A chronic illness with at least 6 months of symptoms prior to the index evaluation without return to the premorbid level of psychosocial adjustment.

2. Absence of a period of depressive or manic symptoms sufficient to qualify for affective disorder or probable affective disorder.

B. The patient must have at least one of the following:

1. Delusions or hallucinations without significant perplexity or disorientation associated with them.

2. Verbal production that makes communication difficult because of a lack of logical or understandable organization. (In the presence of muteness the diagnostic decision must be deferred.)

C. At least three of the following manifestations must be present for a diagnosis of "definite" schizophrenia, and two for a diagnosis of "probable" schizophrenia.

1. Single

2. Poor premorbid social adjustment or work history

3. Family history of schizophrenia

4. Absence of alcoholism or drug abuse within 1 year of onset of psychosis

5. Onset of illness prior to age 40

Note.   The Washington University or St. Louis or Feighner criteria, published in 1972, represented the first diagnostic classification validated primarily by follow-up and family studies rather than by clinical judgment and experience (Feighner et al. 1972). Feighner criteria were also the first of the commonly used diagnostic criteria for schizophrenia to assign operational diagnostic criteria to each disorder included.
Source.   Reprinted from Feighner JP, Robbins E, Guze SB, et al.: "Diagnostic Criteria for Psychiatric Research." *Archives of General Psychiatry* 26:57–63, 1972. Used with permission.

Although ICD-10 includes a prodromal phase in schizophrenia, the criterion of greater than 1 month's duration of symptoms does not include the prodromal phase. Conversely, DSM-IV-TR acknowledges the prodromal phase, which may be prevalent during the 6-month diagnostic period and is part of the evolving disorder.

In terms of affective symptoms, DSM-IV-TR criteria for schizophrenia allow for the presence of affective symptoms if the symptoms are relatively brief, whereas ICD-10 specifies that they must follow the psychotic symptoms. The subtypes of ICD-10 and DSM-IV-TR are undifferentiated, residual, disorganized (hebephrenic in ICD-10), catatonic, and paranoid schizophrenia (Table 11–5). In addition, ICD-10 contains simple and postschizophrenic depression as subtypes. Table 11–6 provides a comparison between ICD-10 and DSM-IV-TR diagnostic systems.

DIAGNOSTIC ASSESSMENT TOOLS

The diagnostic classifications most often used in clinical practice are DSM-IV-TR and ICD-10. The Research Diagnostic Criteria (RDC; Spitzer et al. 1978) are mostly used in research. (The RDC, introduced in 1975, were modified and expanded from the Feighner criteria. The requirement of illness duration shortened from 6 months to 2 weeks [see Table 11–7].) The reliability of diagnostic assessments and of the characteristic symptoms of schizophrenia can be improved by the use of structured interview instruments. Among these are the Present State Examination (PSE; Wing 1970), Schedule for Affective Disorders and Schizophrenia (SADS; Endicott and Spitzer 1978), Diagnostic Interview Schedule (DIS; Robbins et al. 1981), Structured Clinical Interview for DSM-IV (SCID; First et al. 1997), and Comprehensive Assessment of Symptoms and History (CASH; Andreasen 1985).

In the following sections, we discuss the characteristic symptoms of schizophrenia, their differential diagnosis, their assessment, and some of their neurocognitive correlates. The symptoms are grouped into five syndromal domains—1) positive symptoms, 2) negative symptoms, 3) cognitive symptoms, 4) excitement symptoms, and 5) anxiety/depression symptoms—based on our own analyses of extensive psychometric data (Lindenmayer et al. 1994, 1995).

TABLE 11–3.   DSM-IV-TR diagnostic criteria for schizophrenia

A. Characteristic symptoms: Two (or more) of the following, each present for a significant portion of time during a 1-month period (or less if successfully treated):

1. Delusions
2. Hallucinations
3. Disorganized speech (e.g., frequent derailment or incoherence)
4. Grossly disorganized or catatonic behavior
5. Negative symptoms (i.e., affective flattening, alogia, or avolition)

Note.   Only one criterion A symptom is required if delusions are bizarre or hallucinations consist of a voice keeping up a running commentary on the person's behavior or thoughts, or two or more voices are conversing with each other.

B. Social/occupational dysfunction: For a significant portion of the time since the onset of the disturbance, one or more major areas of functioning such as work, interpersonal relations, or self-care are markedly below the level achieved prior to the onset (or when the onset is in childhood or adolescence, failure to achieve the expected level of interpersonal, academic, or occupational achievement).

C. Duration: Continuous signs of the disturbance persist for at least 6 months. This 6-month period must include least 1 month of symptoms (or less if successfully treated) that meet Criterion A (i.e., active-phase symptoms) and may include periods of prodromal and residual symptoms. During these prodromal or residual periods, the signs of the disturbance may be manifested by only negative symptoms or two or more symptoms listed in criterion A present in an attenuated form (e.g., odd beliefs, unusual perceptual experiences).

D. Schizoaffective and mood disorder exclusion: Schizoaffective disorder and mood disorder with psychotic features have been ruled out because either 1) no major depressive, manic, or mixed episodes have occurred concurrently with the active-phase symptoms; or 2) if mood episodes have occurred during active-phase symptoms, their total duration has been brief relative to the active and residual periods.

E. Substance/general medical condition exclusion: The disturbance is not due to the direct physiological effects of a substance (e.g., a drug of abuse, a medication) or a general medical condition.

F. Relationship to a pervasive developmental disorder: If there is a history of autistic disorder or another pervasive developmental disorder, the additional diagnosis of schizophrenia is made only if prominent delusions or hallucinations are also present for at least a month (or less if successfully treated).

Note.   The 4th edition of the DSM-IV was published in 1994 and the text revision in 2000. The greatest difference between the DSM-III-R (American Psychiatric Association 1987) and DSM-IV-TR (American Psychiatric Association 2000) criteria for schizophrenia is in the description of characteristic symptomatology. The criterion for duration of acute-phase symptoms is extended from 1 week to 1 month. Hallucinations are no longer required to be prominent. DSM-IV-TR uses the term *disorganized speech* instead of *incoherence or marked loosening of associations* for schizophrenic thought disorder. Negative symptoms were included in the criteria for the first time in the DSM system in the 4th edition.
Source.   Reprinted from American Psychiatric Association: *Diagnostic and Statistical Manual of Mental Disorders*, 4th Edition, Text Revision. Arlington, VA, American Psychiatric Association, 2000. Copyright 2000, American Psychiatric Association. Used with permission.

DEVELOPMENT OF THE SYNDROMAL CONCEPT OF SCHIZOPHRENIA

Schizophrenia is a disorder with a significant heterogeneous presentation of symptoms both in individual patients and over the course of the illness. Observations by more recent cross-sectional and longitudinal analysis of schizophrenic symptoms have led to the conceptualization of two replicable psychopathological domains of symptoms, the positive and negative symptom domains. The terms *positive* and *negative symptoms* were first used by the neurologist Hughlings Jackson (1887–1888), in his conceptualization of neurological organic brain disease. Positive symptoms include hallucinations, delusions, dis-

organized speech, behavior, and catatonic symptoms, whereas negative symptoms include affective blunting, poverty of speech, anhedonia, and avolition (Andreasen et al. 1995).

Crow (1980, 1985), in a seminal contribution, applied this concept to schizophrenia and described type I and type II schizophrenia, which he considered as dichotomous syndromes with relatively independent underlying pathophysiological processes. Crow postulated that the negative syndrome (type II schizophrenia) would be stable because it was hypothesized to reflect structural brain abnormalities (e.g., enlarged ventricles) and dopaminergic hypofunction leading to lesser antipsychotic responsiveness and to poor outcome. Type II reflected an underlying degenerative process or a developmental impairment. In

TABLE 11–4. ICD-10 diagnostic criteria for schizophrenia

I. Either at least one of the syndromes, symptoms, and signs listed under 1 below, or at least two of the symptoms and signs listed under 2 should be present for most of the time during an episode of psychotic illness lasting for at least 1 month (or at some time during most of the days):

1. At least one of the following must be present:

   A. Thought echo, thought insertion or withdrawal, or thought broadcasting.
   B. Delusions of control, influence, or passivity, clearly referred to body or limb movements or specific thoughts, actions, or sensations; delusional perception.
   C. Hallucinatory voices giving a running commentary on the patient's behavior, or discussing the patient among themselves, or other types of hallucinatory voices coming from some part of the body.
   D. Persistent delusions of other kinds that are culturally inappropriate and completely impossible.

2. Or at least two of the following:
   A. Persistent hallucinations in any modality, when occurring every day for at least 1 month, when accompanied by delusions without clear affective content, or by persistent overvalued ideas.
   B. Neologisms, breaks, or interpolations in the train of thought, resulting in incoherence or irrelevant speech.
   C. Catatonic behavior, such as excitement, posturing, or waxy flexibility, negativism, mutism, or stupor.
   D. "Negative" symptoms, such as marked apathy, paucity of speech, and blunting or incongruity of emotional responses.

II. Exclusion clauses:

If the patient also meets criteria for manic episode or depressive episode, the criteria listed under I(1) and I(2) above must have been met before the disturbance of mood developed.

The disorder is not attributable to organic brain disease, or to alcohol- or drug-related intoxication, dependence, or withdrawal.

Source. Reprinted from World Health Organization: *International Statistical Classification of Diseases and Related Health Problems*, 10th Revision. Geneva, World Health Organization, 1992. Used with permission.

contrast, patients with positive schizophrenia (type I schizophrenia) had normal brain structures, good response to treatment, and better outcomes. Andreasen and Olsen (1982) further elaborated the syndromal concept of schizophrenia by contributing definitive psychopathological descriptions of the two domains. They proposed that positive-symptom patients and negative-symptom patients can be classified into two distinct categories. However, this dichotomous typological approach was later found not to be valid because many patients could not be classified as belonging to either category and in fact showed features of both syndromes (Andreasen et al. 1990; Kay 1990).

A heuristically fruitful approach is to consider the positive and negative syndromes as representing different psychopathological dimensions rather than coexclusive subtypes of schizophrenia (Kay 1990). The two syndromes differ in their association with premorbid functioning, family history of illness, cognitive profile, and neurological signs. Longitudinal studies have generally shown that negative symptoms are more stable than positive symptoms and are less likely to improve over the course of the illness (Addington and Addington 1991; Kay et al. 1986; Lindenmayer et al. 1984, 1986; Pfohl and Winokur 1982).

Another important reason for the development and renewed research interest in the characteristics of positive and negative syndromes was the development of rating scales for the assessment of schizophrenia symptoms, which used the subdivision into positive and negative symptoms (see Andreasen 1982; Fenton and McGlashan 1992; Kay et al. 1987; Moller et al. 1994). These scales use highly operationalized and standardized items, with specifically defined levels of severity. They have to some degree supplanted the Brief Psychiatric Rating Scale (BPRS; Overall and Gorham 1962), an 18-item symptom scale that includes a more narrow set of schizophrenia symptoms. Andreasen (1982) and colleagues developed the Scale for the Assessment of Positive Symptoms (SAPS) and the Scale for the Assessment of Negative Symptoms (SANS), consisting of 35 and 29 items, respectively. The SAPS groups positive symptoms into five subscales of symptoms (hallucinations, delusions, bizarre behavior, positive formal thought disorder, and inappropriate affect) (Table 11–8), whereas the SANS includes five areas of negative symptoms (affective flattening or blunting, alogia, avolition-apathy, anhedonia-asociality, attention) (Table 11–9). Scoring of items is based on a 6-point scale from 0 (not present) to 5 (severe).

TABLE 11–5.   Subtypes of schizophrenia (DSM-IV-TR and ICD-10)

Paranoid schizophrenia	Primarily marked by delusions of persecution and/or grandeur and frequent auditory hallucinations. Generally does not include the degree of disorganization of speech/behavior seen in other subtypes. Individuals are tense, suspicious, and guarded. Associated features include anxiety, anger, aloofness, and argumentativeness. Onset often later compared with other schizophrenia subtypes; little or no impairment in neurocognitive functions (American Psychiatric Association 2000). DSM-IV-TR diagnostic criteria for paranoid schizophrenia include a preoccupation with one or more paranoid delusions, which may be systematized, or frequent auditory hallucinations along with no prominent symptoms of disorganized speech, disorganized behavior, or flat/inappropriate affect. ICD-10 diagnostic criteria are similar to those of the DSM-IV-TR but exclude paranoia and involutional paranoid state.
Disorganized or hebephrenic schizophrenia	Primarily marked by inappropriate affect, disorganized speech, and maladaptive behavior. Disorganized (hebephrenic) behavior can lead to significant interference with activities of daily living. DSM-IV-TR diagnostic criteria include disorganized speech, disorganized behavior, and flat/inappropriate affect and exclude catatonia and delusions and hallucinations that are systematized into a lucid theme. ICD-10 criteria are similar to DSM-IV-TR criteria but add that the disorganized/hebephrenic subtype should normally be diagnosed for the first time only in adolescents or young adults, with a period of 2–3 months of observation ensuring sustained characteristic features. ICD-10 also indicates that the premorbid personality of these individuals includes timid and solitary behavior.
Undifferentiated schizophrenia	Incorporates a combination of symptoms from other subtypes. Individuals should meet criterion A of DSM-IV-TR (American Psychiatric Association 2000, p. 312; see also Table 11–3 in this chapter) and should not have symptoms of catatonia or paranoid and disorganized schizophrenia. ICD-10, although following DSM-IV-TR criteria, includes the stipulation that undifferentiated schizophrenia should not satisfy the criteria for residual schizophrenia (described below) or postschizophrenia depression.
Residual schizophrenia	A state in which the individual is not currently suffering from severe delusions, hallucinations, or disorganized speech and behavior but lacks motivation and interest in day-to-day living. DSM-IV-TR diagnostic criteria include an absence of prominent delusions, hallucinations, disorganized speech, and grossly disorganized or catatonic behavior. It also specifies the existence of negative symptoms or two or more of the symptoms specified in criterion A (American Psychiatric Association 2000, p. 312; see also Table 11–3 in this chapter) present in an attenuated form (e.g., odd beliefs). ICD-10 adds as a requirement an absence of dementia or other organic brain disease or disorder and chronic depression or institutionalism that could explain the negative impairments.
Catatonic schizophrenia	Primarily marked by motor disturbances ranging from immobility to excessive meaningless activity. Dominated by psychomotor symptoms. DSM-IV-TR diagnosis includes two or more and ICD-10 specifies at least one of the following behaviors: stupor (marked reduction or suspended sensibility) or mutism, excitement not influenced by external stimuli, bizarre postures, meaningless resistance toward instructions or attempts to be moved, rigidity, waxy flexibility, and echolalia or echopraxia. Differential diagnosis includes brain disease, metabolic instability, substance abuse, or mood disorders such as bipolar disorder.

TABLE 11–6. Comparison of the DSM-IV-TR and ICD-10 diagnostic criteria for schizophrenia

	DSM-IV-TR	ICD-10
Duration of symptoms	≥1 month; prodromal or residual features for at least 6 months	≥1 month
Course	Deterioration should be present from a premorbid level of functioning	N/A
Characteristic symptoms: one present	Bizarre delusions (primary or secondary delusions) Voices commenting/conversing	Thought echo/insertion/withdrawal/broadcasting Delusions of control, delusional perception Voices commenting/conversing or coming from a part of the body Persistent impossible delusions
Other symptoms that are less specific: two present	Other delusions Other hallucinations Disorganized speech Grossly disorganized or catatonic behavior Negative symptoms	Other persistent hallucinations Thought-form disorder Catatonia Negative symptoms Significant personality change
Affective symptoms	Affective syndrome included if relatively brief	Affective symptoms, if present, must follow psychotic symptoms
Social/occupational dysfunction	One or more major areas of dysfunction (work, occupation, interpersonal)	N/A
Exclusion criteria	Schizoaffective or mood disorder Substance use or general medical condition Pervasive developmental disorder	Schizoaffective or mood disorder Drug intoxication or withdrawal Overt brain disease

TABLE 11–7. Research Diagnostic Criteria (RDC) for schizophrenia

A. During an active phase of the illness, at least two of the following are required for definite and one for probable diagnosis of schizophrenia:

   1. Thought broadcasting, insertion, or withdrawal
   2. Delusions of being controlled or influenced, other bizarre delusions, or multiple delusions
   3. Somatic, grandiose, religious, nihilistic, or other delusions without persecutory or jealous content lasting at least 1 week
   4. Delusions of any type if accompanied by hallucinations of any type for at least 1 week
   5. Auditory hallucinations in which either a voice keeps up a running commentary on the subject's behaviors or thoughts as they occur or two or more voices converse with each other.
   6. Nonaffective verbal hallucinations spoken to the subject
   7. Hallucinations of any type throughout the day for several days or intermittently for at least 1 month
   8. Definite instances of marked formal thought disorder (as defined in this manual) accompanied by either blunted or inappropriate affect, delusions or hallucinations of any type, or grossly disorganized behavior

B. Signs of the illness have lasted at least 2 weeks from the onset of a noticeable change in the subject's usual condition.

C. At no time during the active period of illness being considered has the subject met the full criteria for either probable or definite manic or depressive syndrome to such a degree that it was a prominent part of the illness.

Note. RDC included five subtypes of schizophrenia; prominent symptoms of each type were delusions and/or hallucinations in the paranoid type, marked formal thought disorder and inappropriate or blunted affect or not well-organized delusions or hallucinations in the disorganized type, and catatonic symptoms in the catatonic type.

Source. Reprinted from Spitzer RL, Endicott J, Robins E: "Research Diagnostic Criteria for a Selected Group of Functional Disorders." New York, New York State Psychiatric Institute, 1978.

TABLE 11–8. Scale for the Assessment of Positive Symptoms (SAPS) items

Hallucinations
1. Auditory hallucinations
2. Voices commenting
3. Voices conversing
4. Somatic and tactile hallucinations
5. Olfactory hallucinations
6. Visual hallucinations
7. Global rating of severity of hallucinations

Delusions
1. Persecutory delusions
2. Delusions of jealousy
3. Delusions of sin and guilt
4. Grandiose delusions
5. Religious delusions
6. Somatic delusions
7. Ideas and delusions of reference
8. Delusions of being controlled
9. Delusions of mind reading
10. Thought broadcasting
11. Thought insertion
12. Thought withdrawal
13. Global rating of the severity of the delusions

Bizarre behavior
1. Clothing and appearance
2. Social and sexual withdrawal
3. Aggressive and agitated behavior
4. Repetitive or stereotyped behavior
5. Global rating of the severity of bizarre behavior

Positive formal thought disorder
1. Derailment (loose associations)
2. Tangentiality
3. Incoherence (word salad)
4. Illogicality
5. Circumstantiality
6. Pressure of speech
7. Distractible speech
8. Clanging
9. Global rating of positive formal thought disorder

(Inappropriate affect: single item rating of degree of inappropriate affect)

Source. Reprinted from Andreasen NC: "Negative Symptoms in Schizophrenia: Definition and Reliability." *Archives of General Psychiatry* 39:784–788, 1982. Copyright 1982, American Medical Association. Used with permission.

Similarly, Kay and colleagues (1987) created the Positive and Negative Syndrome Scale (PANSS), consisting of three subscales measuring 7 positive, 7 negative, and 16 general psychopathology symptoms (Table 11–10). Items are scored from 1 to 7, with 1 being absent and 7 extreme. Both scales have developed precise operationalized item descriptions with defined levels of severity. They have shown excellent reliability and internal and external validity, resulting in their wide use in research and treatment studies.

More recently, it has become clear that the traditional positive-negative distinction of schizophrenic phenomenology is incomplete and must be enlarged to include other, in part nonoverlapping, syndromal domains, such as cognitive and affective symptoms. A number of studies have examined the symptom presentation of large samples of patients with schizophrenia using factor analysis of symptoms assessed with the newer symptom scales. These studies have resulted in a number of expanded syndromal models of schizophrenia. They range from the original two-dimensional model (positive-negative) to five-dimensional models and are associated with various levels of validity based on course, demographic, neurocognitive, and treatment response correlates (Table 11–11).

Most factor analyses based on the SAPS and the SANS have suggested a clustering of schizophrenia symptoms into three factors (Andreasen et al. 1995; Liddle 1987; Peralta et al. 1992): 1) positive or psychotic cluster (hallucinations, delusions, catatonic symptoms), 2) negative cluster (anhedonia, avolition, poverty of speech, blunted affect), and 3) disorganization cluster (disorganized speech, inappropriate affect, bizarre behavior). Using the PANSS, Lindenmayer and colleagues (1994) proposed a five-factor model of schizophrenia, consisting of a positive factor (delusions, hallucinatory behavior, grandiosity, unusual thought content, suspiciousness/persecution), a negative factor (blunted affect, emotional withdrawal, poor rapport, passive/apathetic social withdrawal, lack of spontaneity, active social avoidance), an excitement factor (excitement, hostility, uncooperativeness, poor impulse control), a cognitive factor (conceptual disorganization, difficulty with abstract thinking, disorientation, poor attention, preoccupation), and a depression/anxiety factor (anxiety, guilt feelings, tension, depression). This model has proved to be very robust across various phases of the illness, cross-culturally and longitudinally, as well as stable after antipsychotic treatments (Lindenmayer et al. 1995; Marder et al. 1997; Peralta et al. 1992; Toomey et al. 1997; White et al. 1997).

This dimensional approach has several important advantages over a categorical approach in the diagnosis, pathophysiology, and treatment of schizophrenia. It is highly unlikely that schizophrenic symptoms are caused by a single underlying single neurotransmitter or pathophysiological abnormality. It is heuristically more plausible that each psychopathological syndromal dimension relates to an underlying pathophysiological abnormality, which in turn may be associated to one or more liability genes. This approach also has the advantage of accommodating the apparent continuity of some clinical manifestations seen in disorders represented in the schizophrenia spectrum concept. For example, the diagnosis of schizotypal personality disorder is characterized by social and interpersonal deficits (negative symptoms) and cognitive distortions but does not rise to the full diagnosis of schizophrenia. The syndromal approach furthermore allows for the evaluation of treatment interventions on each one of the psychopathological domains separately and to define comorbidity phenomena more appropriately.

Refining the negative syndrome concept further, Carpenter and colleagues (1988, 1991) called attention to the differences between primary negative symptoms and secondary negative symptoms. Primary negative symptoms are thought to be expressions of the avolitional aspects of schizophrenia, to fluctuate less over the course of the illness, to be less responsive to situational changes, and to rarely remit (Carpenter and Kirkpatrick 1988). Secondary negative symptoms are reversible and often caused by drug effects (e.g., extrapyramidal symptoms), depression, or absence of stimulation. Carpenter and Kirkpatrick (1988) also proposed referring to primary negative symptoms as "deficit symptoms." They proposed that negative symptoms should be used as a descriptive term without implications concerning cause or duration. However, in clinical practice it may be difficult to reliably differentiate primary from secondary negative symptoms (Flaum and Andreasen 1995). It is likely that the underlying pathophysiological mechanisms are varied, although they may produce phenomenologically and clinically difficult to differentiate syndromes.

POSITIVE SYMPTOMS

CONCEPT OF POSITIVE SYMPTOMS

Positive symptoms of schizophrenia are symptoms that are in excess of or distortions of normal functions—specifically additions to normal thoughts, emotions, or behaviors (Weiden et al. 1999). Because of their relatively easier recognition and easier quantitative assessment, positive symptoms, more than negative symptoms, have been used in the past in diagnostic classificatory systems (e.g., as Schneiderian first-rank symptoms; Feighner criteria; Research Diagnostic Criteria for Schizophrenia). Positive symptoms can be present throughout the different phases of the disorder, from the prodromal phase to the acute psychotic phase and to a lesser degree in the more stable postpsychotic or residual phase. Positive symptoms are generally the targets of treatment with antipsychotic medications and are considered to be treatment responsive.

TABLE 11–9. Scale for the Assessment of Negative Symptoms (SANS) items

Affective flattening or blunting
1. Unchanging facial expression
2. Decreased spontaneous movements
3. Paucity of expressive gestures
4. Poor eye contact
5. Affective nonresponsivity
6. Lack of vocal inflections
7. Global rating of affective flattening

Alogia
1. Poverty of speech
2. Poverty of content of speech
3. Blocking
4. Increased latency response
5. Global rating of alogia

Avolition-apathy
1. Grooming and hygiene
2. Impersistence at work or school
3. Physical anergia
4. Global rating of avolition-apathy

Anhedonia-asociality
1. Recreational interests and activities
2. Sexual interest and activity
3. Ability to feel intimacy and closeness
4. Relationships with friends and peers
5. Global rating of anhedonia–asociality

Attention
1. Social attentiveness
2. Inattentiveness during mental status testing
3. Global rating of attention

Source. Reprinted from Andreasen NC: "Negative Symptoms in Schizophrenia: Definition and Reliability." *Archives of General Psychiatry* 39:784–788, 1982. Copyright 1982, American Medical Association. Used with permission.

Kurt Schneider (1959) sought to identify signs and symptoms that would be highly discriminating and pathognomonic for schizophrenia (Andreasen and Carpenter 1993; see Table 11–1 earlier in this chapter). Schneider's *first-rank symptoms* of schizophrenia are strongly suggestive of schizophrenia. Other symptoms, which occur frequently in schizophrenia and are important in the diagnosis of the illness but do not have the same close relationship to the illness as first-rank symptoms, were called *second-rank symptoms.*

DELUSIONS

Delusions are false beliefs about which a person is firmly convinced and is impervious to outside contradictory evidence. Delusions must be distinguished from a person's

TABLE 11–10.   Positive and Negative Syndrome Scale (PANSS) for Schizophrenia

Positive symptoms
1. Delusions
2. Conceptual disorganization
3. Hallucinatory behavior
4. Excitement
5. Grandiosity
6. Suspiciousness/persecution
7. Hostility

Negative symptoms
1. Blunted affect
2. Emotional withdrawal
3. Poor rapport
4. Passive/apathetic social withdrawal
5. Difficulty in abstract thinking
6. Lack of spontaneity and flow of conversation
7. Stereotyped thinking

General psychopathology symptoms
1. Somatic concern
2. Anxiety
3. Guilt feelings
4. Tension
5. Mannerism and posturing
6. Depression
7. Motor retardation
8. Uncooperativeness
9. Unusual thought content
10. Disorientation
11. Poor attention
12. Lack of judgment and insight
13. Disturbance and volition
14. Poor impulse control
15. Preoccupation
16. Active social avoidance

Source.   Reprinted from Kay SR, Fisz-Bein A, Opler LA: "The Positive and Negative Syndrome Scale (PANSS) for Schizophrenia." *Schizophrenia Bulletin* 13:261–274, 1987. Used with permission.

religious or cultural beliefs. Generally, the latter are also held by the group or community of people who form the individual's religious or cultural group and do not interfere with day-to-day functioning as delusions often do in patients with schizophrenia.

Fish (1984) proposed the concept of primary delusional experience as the underlying unifying construct, which forms the basis of paranoid delusions in schizophrenia. This is an abnormal consciousness of significance occurring in connection with a given experience. Examples of such phenomena are delusional mood, delusional states of consciousness, sudden delusional ideas, and delusional perceptions. In particular, delusional perception may be an important starting point for the development of a system of delusional ideas. An abnormal significance, usually in the sense of self-reference, despite the absence of any emotional or logical reason, is attributed to a normal perception (Fish 1984). For example, a patient observes that the traffic light is switching from green to red and immediately concludes that it means to him personally that an outside force is telling him to curb his homosexual interests. Such primary delusional experiences will then be expanded and elaborated into a group of secondary delusions. At times, these delusions will be highly systematized and complex, centering on one or two themes. Systematized delusions are usually seen in patients who are cognitively intact and who function quite well outside an acute episode. During those times these individuals tend to be able to hide their beliefs and show little interference in their daily functioning. On the other hand, during overtly psychotic phases, individuals holding false beliefs may act in unusual ways because of their beliefs or they may be fearful that they will be harmed.

Although delusions are often described as "fixed false beliefs," delusions in their mildest form may be questioned or doubted by the individual and persist for weeks to months (Andreasen 1984). The presence of bizarre delusions, which are entirely inconsistent with shared social realism and are illogical to most people, are recognized by DSM-IV-TR as being sufficient as a characteristic symptom (Cluster A) to qualify for schizophrenia, underlining the weight this symptom is attributed in the diagnosis of schizophrenia. Examples of bizarre delusions include a patient reporting his heart is missing or that aliens are seeking the patient to rule their planet.

Differential Diagnosis of Delusions

Paranoid disorders.   Delusions found in paranoid disorders are at times not easy to differentiate from those found in schizophrenia. These conditions include paranoia, shared paranoid disorder (folie à deux), and acute paranoid disorder. Paranoid delusions in these disorders are usually nonbizarre and center on one or two themes. These delusions may have been started by a small and/or real slight in the person's life and then become elaborated and embedded in a paranoid delusional system. These individuals often get involved in extensive letter writing campaigns, litigiousness, and legal actions to seek redress of perceived delusional wrongs.

These disorders are chronic except for the acute paranoid disorder, which has duration of less than 6 months. The person's functioning is usually not markedly impaired, but hostility and violence may at times be associated. There are no hallucinatory experiences or marked

TABLE 11–11. Syndromal models of schizophrenia

Model	Description	Reference(s)
Two-dimensional	Positive and negative dimensions, independent of each other	Crow et al. 1986
Three-dimensional	Positive and negative dimensions and symptoms of poor relating	Strauss et al. 1974
	Positive, negative, and disorganization dimensions, which include thought disorder, poor attention, and inappropriate affect	Arndt et al. 1991; Bilder et al. 1985; Liddle 1987
Four-dimensional	Positive, negative, excitement, and depression dimensions	Kay and Sevy 1990; Peralta et al. 1992
Five-dimensional	Positive, negative, excitement, depression/anxiety, and cognitive dimensions	Lindenmayer et al. 1994

thought disorders, and affect is usually well preserved. Delusions of jealousy may be included in which there are unconfirmed and unfounded thoughts that a person is being disloyal or treacherous within a relationship. The delusions are usually accompanied by attempts to find evidence to support the delusional belief. Individuals with delusions of jealousy are not satisfied until evidence is obtained, which can sometimes lead to violent episodes with a significant other (Soyka et al. 1991). Delusions of jealousy can also be seen in paranoid states caused by alcohol dependence.

Capgras syndrome. Capgras syndrome is named for its discoverer, the French psychiatrist Jean Marie Joseph Capgras (1873–1950). Individuals displaying this syndrome believe that people in their lives (e.g., family members, doctors, close friends) have been replaced by exact doubles. Those afflicted may even believe that they themselves are represented somewhere by a double they never see. The persons who are not replaced are always identified accurately. Capgras syndrome is also referred to as delusional misidentification, illusion of doubles, illusion of negative doubles, misidentification syndrome, nonrecognition syndrome, phantom double syndrome, and subjective doubles syndrome.

It has been reported that 35% of patients diagnosed with the Capgras syndrome or related substitution delusions have an organic etiology. Some of these etiologies involve failure of normal recognition processes following brain damage from a stroke, drug overdose, or some other central nervous system cause, although earlier reports hypothesized psychodynamic etiologies (Alexander et al. 1979; Ellis et al. 1997). Associated features of Capgras syndrome involve not only other functional psychoses such as schizophrenic conditions (e.g., paranoid schizophrenia) but also affective and organic-psychic disturbances.

Organic delusional syndrome. DSM-IV-TR places organic delusional syndrome (ICD-9-Clinical Modification [CM]; World Health Organization 1978) under psychotic disorder due to general medical condition with delusions. The psychotic disturbance is identifiable from history, physical examination, or laboratory results. The delusions are the unequivocal physiological corollary of a general medical condition. Whereas multiple delusions can be present in these syndromes, they are accompanied typically by significant cognitive symptoms, such as disorientation, confusion, and memory impairments, which will determine the correct diagnosis. In addition, hallucinatory experiences often complete the clinical picture. It is imperative to investigate the medical etiology of these disorders.

Affective disorder with psychotic features. Delusions in manic states or depressive states are usually mood-congruent—that is they are consistent with the underlying mood, both for the manic state (inflated worth, power, wealth) or the depressive state (guilt, death, deserving punishment).

Types of Delusions

Persecutory delusions. Individuals afflicted with persecutory delusions believe they are being conspired or discriminated against, threatened, or intentionally victimized. This can be by someone familiar to them (e.g., a family member, friend, doctor, or nurse), someone in the media (e.g., a television personality), a powerful external organization (e.g., the FBI, KGB, or CIA), religious figures such as the devil, or extraterrestrial forces such as aliens. Persecutory delusions are among the most common symptoms of schizophrenia, although they can also be seen in delusional disorder, psychotic depression, and organic delusional syndromes. Particularly, delusions with mood incongruent or idiosyncratic content are seen in patients with schizophrenia. Patients sometimes report opposite influences, resulting in a persecutory delusional conviction of being controlled by opposing outside forces, such as God and the devil, matter and antimatter, the sun and the moon, positive and negative electron charges. The persecutory content of delusions sometimes reflects the evolution of modern technology. Patients may be convinced that there are sophisticated electronic devices secretly hidden in all areas of their surroundings that spy on them and monitor their every movement.

Persecutory delusions can be vague, unstable, and few in number, or they can be numerous, systematized, and fully crystallized, demonstrating an internally coherent logic and dominating major aspects of the patient's life. These delusions can lead to inappropriate or irresponsible actions jeopardizing the safety of the patients or others.

EXAMPLE

A patient felt that he was under constant government surveillance through planted microphones and hidden cameras in the ceiling and was receiving through electronic devices irritating high-frequency tones affecting his ears and legs. These tones were interfering with his functioning and his relationships with other patients in the ward. In fact, he believed that all other patients were involved in this plot, which ultimately was designed to kill him because he was a spy.

Delusions of reference. Individuals with delusions of reference attach a personal meaning to the actions, remarks, and statements of other people and to objects or events when in fact there is none. A common example is an individual's belief that a television program is specifically directed at him or her. There is a conviction of certitude that the individual's observation is absolutely correct without the need of any corroboration by others or any other supporting evidence. In contrast, when a nondelusional individual is unsure that the remark, action, or statement is referring to him or her, the person will be suspicious and will be able to acknowledge that the idea is misguided. The content of a delusion of reference is often idiosyncratic and can be derogatory, persecutory, or enhancing of one's self-worth.

Delusions of being controlled. Individuals with delusions of control feel that an outside force or agency is controlling or manipulating their thoughts, feelings, or parts of their body. These delusions are also referred to as delusions of passivity and are often associated with somatic hallucinations. Patients may use them as delusional explanations of abnormal somatic sensations.

EXAMPLE

A patient responded to the question: Is somebody influencing your mind or your head? "Yes, they have a weapon that the CIA and the Defense Department use. They use microwaves. They send them inside your head. They are digital and they convert them from analog to digital. They pick up your thoughts and they change you to another person. That's what they work on, getting you lazy, taking away your stamina."

Thought insertion. Individuals with thought insertion believe that some of their thoughts are not their own but have been implanted by an outside agency. Often, there is a persecutory theme and a sense that their thoughts are controlled or manipulated by an outside agency. The condition differs from the symptoms of obsessive-compulsive patients, where patients may be distraught by recurrent intrusive thoughts but are certain that these thoughts originate from their own mind and not by an outside force. In schizophrenia, individuals misplace their own intentions and attribute them to an agency or to someone else (Frith 1992).

Thought withdrawal and thought broadcasting. The individual believes that thoughts have been taken out of his or her mind. Further, the individual can often trace the initial experience of a thought and then the incident of that thought being removed. In thought broadcasting, one's thoughts are passively transmitted to others, often through electronic or telepathic means.

Delusions of sin or guilt. Individuals with delusions of sin or guilt believe that they have committed a terrible crime. These delusions can manifest themselves as a minor error in the past that the individual believes may lead to a major disaster or divine retribution that can also affect his or her family. They may also be associated with grandiose ideas with the belief that the committed sin will destroy the whole world and also may be associated with delusions of nihilism. Hence, these individuals can also believe that they warrant punishment by society or by an outside delusional agency. The content of these delusions usually is bizarre and mostly mood incongruent. In contrast, delusions of sin and guilt that are seen in severe depressive episodes with psychotic symptoms are usually comprehensible and ego-syntonic (i.e., referring to a person's personality aspects, thoughts, or behaviors that are viewed by the person as acceptable). In persons with psychotic depression, these mood-congruent delusions are usually associated with vegetative symptoms of depression, ideas of hopelessness, worthlessness, and possibly suicidal ideation.

EXAMPLE

A patient believed that he had killed millions of Jews during World War II, although he was born after 1945. He stated that he felt he was worse than Hitler; in fact, he believed he was the greatest killer in the world and deserved punishment for his deeds.

Grandiose delusions. Individuals who experience delusions of grandiosity believe they have extraordinary powers, wealth, fame, or talents. They may think they are religious saviors, world leaders, or famous persons. Grandiose delusions in the extreme can affect behavior, be acted upon, and lead to irresponsible or dangerous and even deadly actions, such as believing that one has the ability to fly and stepping out of a window. Grandiose delusions are also seen in individuals with mania with psychosis. Other manic features, such as elated mood, hyperactivity and expansiveness, flight of ideas, and accelerated speech, will help in the differential diagnosis.

EXAMPLE

A patient answered to a question regarding whether he had any special talents: "I am very famous. I am known in London and Paris as an inventor; I have invented candy bars, elevator cleansers. They are writing a book about me."

Religious delusions. Religious delusions contain unusual preoccupations of a religious nature. Individuals are absorbed with religious subject matters that extend beyond the normal breadth of their cultural or religious background. These preoccupations are usually mood incongruous. Religious delusions can also be found in patients with depression with psychotic symptoms; however, delusions associated with psychotic depression must be manifested within an episode of major depression with the associated depressive symptoms and are mood congruous.

EXAMPLE

A female patient was intensely preoccupied with warding off imaginary sexual harassments to receive sanctification, which eventually would promote her to sainthood. She believed that Satan was sending her this task to challenge her mission to sanctification, which in turn would bring her closer to God.

Somatic delusions. Somatic delusions consist of preoccupations that a body part is diseased or malfunctions without objective medical evidence. The delusion can involve a false belief in a medical condition or physical deformity. These delusions are at times associated with kinesthetic hallucinations representing abnormal somatic perceptions supporting the delusional somatic belief. Somatic delusions must be differentiated from hypochondriacal preoccupations, which are exaggerated fears of somatic illness and tend not to be bizarre as in the case of schizophrenic somatic delusions. Further, hypochondriacal preoccupations are not attributed to external forces. In contrast to the hypochondriacal patient, the patient with schizophrenia reacts to rather significant but delusionally held medical morbidity remarkably calmly.

EXAMPLE

A patient answered to a question regarding his health: "Not good. I have my nostrils clogged, which is affecting my brain. A spear flew into my nose, made out of plastic, and went into my brain and has affected my mood; it made me down and depressed. They did it to torture me."

HALLUCINATORY EXPERIENCES

A hallucination is defined as a sensory perception in the absence of any externally generated stimulus or perception. Certain abnormal sensory perceptions are reported as distinct from actual hallucinations and could be called "prehallucinatory experiences." They include hypersensitivity to sound, light, smells, misperceptions of movements, and changes in the perception of people's faces or bodies. These abnormal perceptions are often seen during the prodromal phase of schizophrenia.

Auditory Hallucinations

Auditory hallucinations are the most common type of hallucinations observed in individuals with schizophrenia. Auditory hallucinations are usually voices that often comment on the person's everyday activities, that may be threatening, or, in rare cases, command the individual to execute an action (Andreasen et al. 1995; Mueser et al. 1990). Less frequently, the hallucinations are sounds other than voices. Voices may be heard from inside one's head or may appear to come from the outside. They may be perceived as being as clear as the voice of the interviewer, or less frequently, they are muffled and difficult to understand. Usually, their sentence structure is clear, although at times, when they consist of insults or accusations, they may be just short, monosyllabic words. Often voices are accusatory, hostile, or unfriendly. They consist of a string of sentences, may be continuous, and may occur every day. Occasionally, as with delusional beliefs of powerful opposite forces and at times associated with these beliefs, patients may report "good" and "bad" voices. The response to auditory hallucinations may vary. In acute stages of the illness, patients may be terrified. They may be seen to respond in an audible fashion to auditory hallucinations or, if in distress about them, to scream or yell at them. In more chronic stages of the illness patients will display little affect or emotional responses to what would appear to the interviewer to be rather terrifying voices. The execution of commands transmitted by auditory hallucinations is rare, although some patients will follow the instructions that can lead to suicidal or homicidal actions. Auditory hallucinations are reported by 50%–70% of patients with schizophrenia (Andreasen and Flaum 1991; Hoffman et al. 2003; Sartorius et al. 1974). Patients with schizophrenia rarely present auditory hallucinations in isolation. The hallucinations are usually associated with delusional interpretations, which may be attempts at explanation of abnormal perceptions or, conversely, be elaborations of a delusional paranoid system. In fact, single auditory hallucinations (elementary hallucination) should alert the clinician to look for another, nonschizophrenia diagnosis. Auditory hallucinations in patients with psychotic depression tend to consist of short sentences and are mood congruent.

Auditorization of thoughts refers to instances when individuals report that they hear their thoughts aloud in their head. They can clearly describe this phenomenon and at times are able to differentiate these loud thoughts from ordinary silent thoughts. It is possible that auditorization of thoughts is a precursor of auditory hallucinations.

An individual may experience auditory hallucinations that involve hearing voices of people commenting on his or her actions or conversing with each other. Typically, the comments are spoken in the third person; they may be simply commenting on the individual's moment-to-moment actions or, less frequently, arguing about the individual.

Visual Hallucinations

Individuals with visual hallucinations observe people, shapes, colors, and objects that are not actually present. Visual hallucinations are less frequent in individuals with schizophrenia compared with those with delirium. These hallucinations tend to be associated with delusional interpretation of threatening or persecutory themes, or, in the context of religious delusions, they are seen as visions of religiously meaningful figures. The major differential diagnosis is with visual hallucinations encountered in organic and delirious states. The latter hallucinations are more elementary in nature, often represent animals, and may be accompanied by tactile hallucinations. The presence of significant cognitive impairment (e.g., disorientation) will help to rule in an organic etiology.

Another type of abnormal visual perception that occurs rarely in schizophrenia patients is flashbacks, which are spontaneous visual hallucinations. Flashbacks may take the form of pictures, sounds, smells, body sensations, or the presence of unusual sensations. Studies have shown that flashbacks occur in some schizophrenic patients with a history of drug abuse (Degenhardt and Hall 2002; Lerner et al. 2002; Linszen et al. 1994).

Lilliputian hallucinations are visual hallucinations whereby the patient experiences seeing people who appear reduced in size or dwarfed. Lilliputian hallucinations are rare and seen in about 5% of patients with schizophrenia (Goodwin et al. 1971). They are mostly seen in patients with alcoholic, organic (Cohen et al. 1994), or toxic psychosis (Lewis 1961), particularly psychosis caused by anticholinergic drug toxicity (Asaad 1990).

Somatic and Tactile Hallucinations

Somatic and tactile hallucinations involve physical sensations, for example, of being touched by another person, object, or animal, or a perception that one's body has been altered in some way. These hallucinations are also known as *haptic* or *kinesthetic hallucinations* and consist of the perception of heat, cold, or electricity shocks. The individual can experience somatic passivity, in which the patient believes that an outside agent has caused him or her to be a passive receiver of unwanted bodily sensations, for example a burning sensation in the brain or a sensation of being raped.

Olfactory Hallucinations

Olfactory hallucinations are sensations, such as unusual smells, that no one else experiences. Often, olfactory hallucinations are related to gustatory hallucinations, in which the individual may describe unusual tastes like sweet, salty, bitter, or odd flavors (Carter 1992). These hallucinations are often associated with a persecutory theme, in which unpleasant or poisonous smells are sent to the individual in a malevolent or persecutory fashion. Olfactory hallucinations can also be seen in temporal lobe epilepsy ("uncinate fits"), in which they are usually accompanied by an altered state of consciousness with altered perception and occurring in a paroxysmal context.

BIZARRE BEHAVIOR

Some individuals with schizophrenia behave in unusual and eccentric ways or transgress social mores. For example, they may talk to themselves, walk backward, laugh suddenly without explanation, make unnatural faces, mimic behaviors, masturbate in public, engage in repetitive behaviors, or express manneristic speech patterns. Occasionally, bizarre behavior may also be shown by individuals who maintain a rigid posture for an extensive period of time. Bizarre behavior is generally found in individuals with disorganized or catatonic schizophrenia.

Clothing and Appearance

Patients may dress in an uncommon manner or modify their appearance in an eccentric fashion. More often, they neglect their appearance, which results in disheveled clothing, an unkempt look, and lack of personal hygiene. Patients often may not be able to gauge the outside temperature accurately and therefore overdress during warm temperatures.

Social and Sexual Behavior

Individuals' social and sexual behavior may at times represent a deviation from the norm. For example, urinating or masturbating in public, mimicking the behaviors of others, and spontaneous laughter or sudden outbursts may occur.

Motor Behavior

Bizarre motor behavior can involve unusual mannerisms, grimacing, or rocking movements. Stereotyped and ritualistic movements can be observed. Catatonic motor behavior is an extreme form of bizarre behavior that can include maintaining a rigid or unnatural posture with an awkward, stilted, disorganized appearance, and resisting efforts to be moved or engaging in purposeless and unstimulated motor activity. Waxy flexibility, a rare form of catatonic motor behavior, consists of maintenance of bizarre postures that the examiner has induced in the patient. An important differential diagnostic issue in assessing stereotyped movements is the recognition of involuntary movements caused by tardive dyskinesia. These neurological involuntary movements may look purposeless, repetitive, and stereotypical, but they have characteristic features and are usually located in the extremities or lingual and perioral areas.

Inappropriate Affect

This affective dysfunction is at times incorrectly subsumed under flat affect; however, it reflects not an absence of affect, but rather a discoordination or incongruity of affect. Affect expression is misplaced and does not correspond to the ideational content the person is expressing at the time. Sudden and unexpected discharges of affect may occur. The patient may smile while talking about a sad topic or may unexpectedly burst out in anger when discussing a minor psychological insult.

NEGATIVE SYMPTOMS

CONCEPT OF NEGATIVE SYMPTOMS

Bleuler (1950) and Kraepelin (1919) considered emotional blunting and lack of outward emotional display fundamental features of schizophrenia. Both of these features are considered to be examples of negative symptoms. Kraepelin postulated that the distinct and varied symptomatology of schizophrenia may be divided into "two principal groups of disorders which characterize the malady"—one marked by a "loss of inner unity of the activities of intellect, emotion and volition in themselves and among one another," and the other marked by "a weakening of those emotional activities which permanently form the mainsprings of volition"—pointing in an anticipatory fashion to a disorganization dimension and a negative symptom dimension seen in schizophrenia. Following the Jacksonian model, negative symptoms can be seen as a decrease or loss of normal functions, such as a loss of energy and motivation, and a loss of emotional display of affect.

Negative symptoms are a frequent and persistent characteristic of schizophrenia. They can emerge as early as during the prodromal stage of the disorder, long before the presentation of the first psychotic episode (Hafner et al. 1995). It is now generally accepted that there are primary and secondary negative symptoms (Carpenter and Kirkpatrick 1988; Tandon and Greden 1989). *Primary negative symptoms* are deficit symptoms, which may precede psychosis onset and usually persist between the episodes. These symptoms include primary anhedonia, flattening and narrowing of affect, poverty of speech, avolition, and reduced social activity (Carpenter and Kirkpatrick 1988). From a longitudinal standpoint, the following components of primary negative symptoms have been conceptualized (Miller and Tandon 2001):

- **Premorbid negative symptoms:** these symptoms exist before psychosis onset and are related to poor premorbid functioning.
- **Psychotic phase:** during this phase the individual exhibits unstable negative symptoms that coexist with positive symptoms during periods of psychotic exacerbation.
- **Postpsychotic deterioration component:** persistent negative symptoms after a psychotic episode and represent a degeneration from premorbid levels of functioning.

Secondary negative symptoms are "nondeficit" symptoms and are assumed to correlate with psychotic episodes, depression or demoralization, and medication side effects (Carpenter et al. 1991). Secondary negative symptoms usually respond to treatment of the underlying cause.

COURSE OF NEGATIVE SYMPTOMS

Crow (1981) predicted that negative symptoms would be stable because he theorized that they are associated with structural brain changes. Indeed, studies generally show that negative symptoms are more stable than positive symptoms over time and are less likely to improve over the course of illness (Addington and Addington 1991; Hull et al. 1997; Pfohl and Winokur 1982). In a longitudinal study of symptoms, Arndt and colleagues (1995) found that negative symptoms were already prominent at the time of patients' first episode and remained relatively stable for approximately 2 years in which the patients were followed. Hafner et al. (1999), exploring five SANS measures of negative symptoms, found that in a sample of 115 first episodes of schizophrenia, alogia, attention, affect, abulia, and anhedonia persisted over a 5-year period. Similarly, Amador and colleagues (1999) presented evidence for a high degree of stability of primary negative symptoms over an approximate 4-year follow-up period.

NEUROCOGNITIVE CORRELATES

Many studies have examined the correlation between performance on certain neuropsychological tests and positive or negative symptoms. It appears that cognitive impairment is largely independent of positive symptoms, particularly delusions and hallucinations. In contrast, negative symptoms are associated with impairment of general intellectual ability and executive function, including verbal fluency and performance in working memory tasks such as the Wisconsin Card Sorting Test. Patients with prominent negative symptoms have been shown to perform poorly on backward masking tests (Braff et al. 1991; Green et al. 1994) and on other measures from standard neuropsychological batteries (Addington et al. 1991a; Lindenmayer et al. 1997; Perry and Braff 1998). The pathophysiology of primary negative symptoms is further described in Chapter 6, "Neurochemical Theories," of this book.

SPECIFIC NEGATIVE SYMPTOMS

Blunted or Flat Affect

Blunted or flat affect is characterized by an absence and diminution of emotional reaction to stimuli. Some affected individuals show fewer emotions (e.g., anger, plea-sure, sadness), whereas others exhibit a total lack of facial expression (Salem and Kring 1999). However, despite this lack of affect these individuals report sensations of positive and negative emotions (Kring and Neale 1996). An important differential diagnosis is pseudoparkinsonism (masked facies) induced by antipsychotic medication. Other aspects of pseudoparkinsonism may be helpful in differentiating it from blunted affect, such as a resting tremor (4–5 cycles per second), bradykinesia, absence of blinking, and at times drooling.

Decreased spontaneous movements.   The individual shows decreased spontaneous movements and may maintain the same posture, with fewer shifts in body position for some time when sitting. Movements of limbs when walking are reduced.

Paucity of expressive gestures.   The individual is unable to show emotion by the use of gestures when responding to stimuli. For example, there is paucity in the use of hand gestures in conjunction with speech to emphasize or enhance the meaning of accompanying speech.

Poor eye contact.   The individual avoids direct eye contact or may appear to be staring when responding verbally.

Lack of vocal inflections.   The individual lacks vocal inflections and is unable to show emotions by varying the tone of voice. Speech is characterized by a monotonic quality, and words are not emphasized (Andreasen 1983).

Poor Rapport

Signs of poor rapport include avoidance of eye contact, lack of responsiveness to questions, and reduced verbal and nonverbal communication of personal information with others. Individuals with poor rapport show a lack of interpersonal empathy, a reduced interaction in conversation, and a lack or total avoidance of interactions with others.

Passive/Apathetic Social Withdrawal

Individuals with passive or apathetic social withdrawal have fewer social interactions with others, which can eventually result in a lack of speech (alogia).

Reduced sexual interests and activities.   There is a lack of or impairment of sexual interests and activities. Individuals may report minimal sexual drive or express a lack of enjoyment from sexual activities (Andreasen 1983).

Inability to feel intimacy and closeness.   The individual is unable to form a close relationship with others, and there is an inability to recognize others' emotional needs (Mueser et al. 1996). This results in a lack of mutuality in relationships.

Reduced relationship with friends and peers. The individual's interaction with others may be brief and superficial. There may be few or no friends, and most of the time is spent isolated from others.

Stereotyped Thinking

Individuals with stereotyped thinking show repetitive or barren thoughts that may infringe and interfere with their thinking. They maintain rigid beliefs that may appear unreasonable or excessive. Conversations revolve around a recurrent theme, and the individual is unable to shift to a new topic. There is an impoverishment in the amount of nuances and intermediate positions between extreme statements. At the extreme, the individual's conversation is limited to only a few topics or to repetitive and rigid demands or statements that severely impair the amount and content of conversation.

Alogia

Alogia refers to deficient fluency or productivity of thought and speech associated with avolition or apathy.

Poverty of speech. Poverty of speech is a type of alogia, in which the individual demonstrates a restriction in the amount of spontaneous speech. The individual responds to questions with brief, concrete and unembellished answers. In some instances, the individual does not respond to questions or responses are monosyllabic. Leading questions are constantly needed by the interviewer to proceed with the conversation. Harvey and colleagues (1997) suggest that poverty of speech is more common and more severe in geriatric patients with schizophrenia, perhaps as a result of cognitive and biological factors.

Poverty of content of speech. The individual's speech is adequate in amount but expresses little information because it is vague, excessively abstract or concrete, repetitive, or stereotyped.

Increased latency of response. Individuals take a longer time to respond to questions than normal and may appear distant or preoccupied when asked a question.

Avolition and Apathy

Avolition and apathy appear as a distinctive lack of energy, drive, or interest. Individuals show a lack of motivation in

completing tasks and a lack of initiative or goals. Individuals have few interests and reduced investment in personal activities. When asked about current world events, such individuals may only be partially aware of events and know only limited details about them. These individuals participate in few or no activities or only engage in passive activities such as watching television.

EXAMPLE

Patients with chronic schizophrenia on an inpatient ward in New York City were exposed to both ample television and newspaper coverage of the World Trade Center attack in New York on September 11, 2001. During ward discussions in the aftermath of the tragedy it became clear that patients took relatively little notice of the event, that their emotional response was limited, and that there were few spontaneous verbal expressions about this event.

An important differential diagnostic concern is anhedonia found in states of depression. Anhedonia associated with depression is accompanied by the usual symptoms of depression, such as ideas of hopelessness, worthlessness, and helplessness, together with the vegetative signs of depression.

Grooming and hygiene. The individual displays a lack of interest in grooming and hygiene. This trait is characterized by sloppy, obsolete, blemished attire, infrequent daily hygienic activities such as washing hands, combing hair, and brushing teeth.

Impersistence at work or school. The individual has difficulty seeking or maintaining employment or does not complete tasks in school or work.

Physical anergia. The individual has a tendency to be physically inert. Upon encouragement, the individual participates briefly and then reverts to immobility. The individual shows a lack of drive or spontaneous activity.

DEFICIT STATES OF SCHIZOPHRENIA: CLINICAL CORRELATES

Deficit schizophrenia was introduced to distinguish a relatively homogeneous subgroup of patients within schizophrenia. Deficit schizophrenia is characterized by persistent primary negative symptoms such as restricted affect, diminished emotional range, poverty of speech, curbing of interests, and reduced sense of purpose and social drive. Kirkpatrick and colleagues (2001) found that deficit schizophrenia exists among 15% of first-episode individ-

TABLE 11–12. Schedule for Deficit Syndromes

Criterion 1

At least two of the following six negative symptoms must be present:

A. Restricted affect
  1. Relatively expressionless face or an unchanging facial expression.
  2. Reduced expressive gestures
  3. Diminished modulation of the voice, which supplements the spoken content (for example, changes in speed, volume, and inflection of speech).

B. Diminished emotional range and inability to experience pleasure (a patient who fails to exhibit pleasure because of feeling tortured by auditory hallucinations would not be considered to have diminished emotional range).

C. Poverty of speech
  The deliberate withholding of speech, for instance, on the basis of persecutory beliefs or a relatively normal reticence with strangers, would not be considered primary poverty of speech.

D. Curbing of interests
  The patient may display a diminished range of interests or a diminished depth of interests; either impairment may be considered pathological. However, a great depth of interest in a narrow range of topics will usually not be considered a curbing of interests.

E. Diminished sense of purpose
  1. The degree to which the patient posits goals for his or her life
  2. The extent to which the patient fails to initiate or sustain goal-directed activity due to inadequate drive.
  3. The amount of time passed in aimless activity regardless of the relevancy of the goal.

F. Diminished social drive
  The degree to which the person seeks or wishes for social interaction. The avoidant patient, who longs for social contact and fitfully seeks it but is made uncomfortable by it, is not considered to have diminished social drive.

Criterion 2

Some combination of two or more of the negative symptoms listed above have been present for the preceding 12 months and were always present during periods of clinical stability (including chronic psychotic states). These symptoms may or may not be detectable during transient episodes of acute psychotic disorganization or decompensation.

Criterion 3

The negative symptoms above are primary or idiopathic, i.e., not secondary to factors other than the disease process. Such factors include

A. Anxiety
B. Drug effect
C. Suspiciousness (and other psychotic symptoms)
D. Mental retardation
E. Depression

Criterion 4

The patient meets DSM criteria for schizophrenia.

Source. Reprinted from Kirkpatrick B, Buchanan RW, McKenney PD, et al.: "The Schedule for the Deficit Syndrome: An Instrument for Research in Schizophrenia." *Psychiatry Research* 30:119–123, 1989. Used with permission.

uals and among 25%–30% of those with chronic schizophrenia. The clinical features of schizophrenic deficit states refer to the cohesive and idiopathic set of signs and symptoms as presented in the Schedule for Deficit Syndromes (Table 11–12) (Kirkpatrick et al. 1989). For a description of the neurological, neuropsychological, and morphological correlates of deficit syndrome in schizophrenia, please refer to Chapter 5, "Neurodevelopmental Theories," of this volume.

COGNITIVE SYMPTOMS: CONCEPTUAL DISORGANIZATION/ FORMAL THOUGHT DISORDER

Schizophrenic thought disorder is often included under the rubric of positive symptoms, although recent research suggests that it represents an independent dimension of symptomatology in schizophrenia (Andreasen and Olsen 1982;

Kay 1990; Liddle 1987; Lindenmayer et al. 1994; Peralta et al. 1992; Thompson and Meltzer 1993). This discrete dimension has been variably called "disorganization factor," "cognitive factor," or "thought disorder factor."

Symptoms that contribute to the SAPS disorganization factor are disorganized speech, inappropriate affect, and bizarre behavior. Symptoms contributing to the PANSS cognitive factor are conceptual disorganization, difficulty in abstract thinking, disorientation, poor attention, and preoccupation.

DEFINITIONS AND CLASSIFICATION

Disturbance of thinking is a cardinal and almost constant symptom of schizophrenia. It describes a persistent underlying disturbance of conscious thought and is recognized largely by its effects on speech and writing. Bleuler (1911/1950) believed that "peculiar association disturbances" were fundamental features of schizophrenia.

There is an abundant literature on the formal thought and language pathology in schizophrenia. It can be grouped into pathology of word use and pathology of sentence use. According to Oppenheimer (1971), "A word evolves from the lowest level of its meaningless sound quality to the highest level of its metaphorical meaning. Between these levels are, in descending order, connotation, denotation, and verbalization" (p. 228). In schizophrenia there can be deficits in any one of these levels of word formation, such as desymbolization of words, expansions of the meaning of a word, conceptual contaminations, and neologisms. In pathological use of sentences, patients may not be able to exclude words or ideas that belong to different semantic categories, resulting in a disorganized structure of the sentence appearing as loosening of associations. Adherence to the appropriate mental set or context of a sentence may be incomplete and results in tangentiality.

Thought disorders have been grouped into two categories by Andreasen (1982) and Cutting and Murphy (1988): 1) intrinsic disturbance of thinking (e.g., concreteness) and 2) disordered language and speech (e.g., derailment or tangentiality).

MECHANISMS OF THOUGHT DISORDER

Thought disorder is not a unitary concept; it can be better conceptualized in terms of its multidimensional makeup (Cuesta and Peralta 1999). Recent attempts to understand the cognitive underpinnings of thought disorder in schizophrenia have focused on abnormalities in attention, on problems in the use of contextual cues, and on impairments of executive functions.

Attention Impairment

Thought disorder has been shown to involve attention deficits, which may include distractibility, disorganization, and cognitive disinhibition. It has also been reported that individuals with schizophrenia are unable to maintain attention during language production (Liddle 1987). Nuechterlein and colleagues (1986) found that impairments on a difficult version of the Continuous Performance Test (CPT) were associated with measures of thought disorder in the posthospitalization period of schizophrenic patients. They also reported that signal discrimination deficits in situations demanding high levels of processing were stable susceptibility factors for negative symptoms and certain forms of thought disorder. However, some accepted tests of attention may actually measure response preparation or working memory rather than distractibility (Servan-Schreiber 1996), rendering the relationship of thought disorder and attention impairments a complex one. In addition, patients with attention-deficit/hyperactivity disorder, who usually exhibit impulsivity and distractibility, do not exhibit thought disorder (Servan-Schreiber et al. 1996).

There has been considerable work on latent inhibition and schizophrenia, which is the repeated pre-exposure to a stimulus without reinforcement consequences in which the learning of subsequent associations of the stimulus is retarded (Escobar et al. 2002). Following preliminary research in animals and children, reduced latent inhibition was proposed as a model of the attentional deficit in schizophrenia (Lubow et al. 1982). Schizophrenia patients who express abnormal attentional processes do not develop latent inhibition because they do not stop attending to the conditioned stimulus (repeated pre-exposed stimulus) (Mackintosh 1975) or they do not become inattentive to it (Lubow 1989). Cognitive tests such as the lexical decision task (LDT [visual]) have been used to test the latent inhibition and semantic activation in schizophrenic patients who were assessed for thought disorder. Manschreck and colleagues (1988) used an LDT to test the theory of augmented semantic activation and found that schizophrenic patients with thought disorder had quicker response times than non-thought-disordered schizophrenic patients.

Contextual Difficulties

It has been suggested that reduced sensitivity to linguistic context (both in semantic and syntactic aspects) may lead to thought disorder. For example, although schizophrenic patients without thought disorder were able to recall sentence-like passages better than random strings of words, schizophrenic patients with thought disorder benefited less from the added phrase structure (Maher et al. 1980; Speed et al. 1991). Still more evidence has come from a recent report that facilitation in recognition of words that are preceded by a consistent compared with an inconsistent sentence context was more impaired in individuals with thought disorder than in those without (Kuperberg et al. 1998), pointing to the difficulty in recognizing contextual cues by thought-disordered individuals.

Additional evidence for defects in the contextual processing comes from studies using list-learning tasks. For example, when learning a list of words, healthy subjects achieve a better recall rate if the list can be organized into semantic categories (context) than if it consists of a sequence of unrelated words. Words are recalled within category groups, thus reflecting the organization of memory storage. Patients with schizophrenia produce largely unorganized verbal material during list learning tasks (Koh et al. 1973). When asked to classify the words to be learned before performing the learning task, however, patients and normal subjects apparently use similar semantic categories. It has also been observed that patients with schizophrenia and control subjects produce similar recall performance (Koh et al. 1974; Russel and Beekhius 1976). Therefore, it can be hypothesized that the impairment is not caused by structural damage to the lexical memory system but to a failure to use encoding strategies spontaneously. It is likely that these strategies also intervene during recall because schizophrenic patients' performances only match those of control subjects when categorical clues are provided during both encoding and recall (Larsen and Fromholt 1976; Mac-Clain 1983).

More recent research by Goldberg and Weinberger (2000) involving the degree of priming and medication status found that thought disorder may be related to a specific abnormality in the semantic system, involving not the integrity of representations but access to connectivity among representations. The studies based on the behavioral measures provided rather conclusive evidence that schizophrenia patients with thought disorder are impaired in sentence-level context processing.

Finally, the role of impairments in executive functions underlying thought disorder is illustrated in detail in Chapter 13, "Neurocognitive Impairments," of this book.

MEASUREMENT OF THOUGHT DISORDER

Careful listening to patients' word productions and sentence construction allows for assessing thought disorder. Difficulty in abstract thinking and concrete thinking can

be measured with proverb interpretations and similarities. Proverb interpretation challenges the individual's ability in abstract-symbolic thinking, in shifting of sets, and in the ability to generalize. The task of establishing similarities reveals difficulties in classification and categorization. Object-sorting tasks can be used to assess overinclusion; an overinclusive reply would include too many or unsuitable items within a group of items. The thought disorder index evaluates the verbal productions of schizophrenic patients in an unstructured interaction (Hurt et al. 1983).

The assessment of thought, language, and communication (Andreasen 1979a, 1979b) offers a clinical rating for a series of different types of thought disorders. In addition, the SAPS (Andreasen 1982), the SANS (Andreasen 1982), and the PANSS (Kay et al. 1987), frequently used to assess symptoms in schizophrenia research, provide for some measures of thought disorder.

TYPES OF THOUGHT DISORDERS

Derailment (Loosening of Associations)

Derailment occurs when an individual's speech shows loss of logical or meaningful connections between words or sentences. The relationship between sentences may be indirect or may not be present at all. The individual is also unaware of the lack of association between sentences.

EXAMPLE

A patient responded to the request to interpret the proverb "Don't cry over spilt milk": "I believe you should release the tension now of all milk on the ground. I think you should cry over spilt milk. I think you should release yourself after all that milk is on the ground. You should let it out in tears. You know you hold it inside and you could explode a lot, all of these little things kept inside."

Tangentiality

Tangentiality is a disruption in the associative thought process in which one tends to deviate readily and gradually from the topic under discussion to other topics, which arise in the course of associations, but connections are still recognizable by the listener.

EXAMPLE

A patient complained about a supervisor who she felt made homosexual advances to her: "She was a pervert homosexual, and she said I was her red painted lady in the closet, and that I knew nothing about this world. But I went to the library and found the red Bible and read up on it, in a hurry. And it was a lie."

Incoherence

Incoherence refers to sentence patterns that are unintelligible and incomprehensible because of total loss of logical connections. At times there are periods of coherent parts that are incorporated in an incoherent sentence. Incoherence can also occur at a semantic level, in which words are substituted in a phrase or sentence and the meaning is distorted. Conjunctions and adjectives can also be deleted (Andreasen 1984). In extreme situations, incoherence can also be referred to as *word salad*.

EXAMPLE

A patient is asked, "How do you feel today?" The patient responds, "I'm feeling that people say doctors are wrong. In Europe, there was a meeting. The president of the United States, it was AIDS. But in Iraq the man pulled it out with the money under the train tracks. Save yourself, help yourself." The patient is unable to join the associated concepts of each sentence into one coherent response that would convey a comprehensible meaning to the listener. The patient shifts sets inappropriately, and there is no relationship among sentences. The patient is unable to include any logical causality.

Illogicality

Individuals who show illogicality respond to questions without a logical rationalization. Examples are non sequiturs, in which the individual formulates an illogical response to a logical question, and faulty inductive inferences, in which the patient makes conclusions based on incoherent assertions (Andreasen 1984).

Circumstantiality

Circumstantiality refers to a disturbance in the thought process, in which one gives an unwarranted amount of details, which are frequently tangential, elaborate, and irrelevant, and in which the patient finds it difficult to make a direct statement or give a direct answer to a question. Circumstantial speech eventually returns to the original topic.

EXAMPLE

In the following example the patient uses circumstantiality and tangentiality in response a question on his overall life philosophy. "You have to be modern and you have to be sophisticated, you have to have a girlfriend, you have to go to church. You have to have your name in the Bible. You go out with your wife or fiancée. And you have to learn, should be married, and be a good neighbor."

Clanging

Clanging consists of usage of the sound of a word or its phonetic resemblance (clang equivalence) rather than its meaning, which is substituted for the correct word. Some individuals speak only in rhymes, and others will engage in repetitive speech (Capleton 1996) as a substitute for logical associations.

EXAMPLE

A patient explained: "We function as liberal Jews, however, we speak British, not Yiddish."

Neologism

Neologism is another well-recognized pathology of word use, in which a new nonsensical word is created that often is a condensation or combination of two different words. This is in contrast to the creative use of neologisms in everyday language, which elicits in the listener amusement or understanding.

EXAMPLE

A patient who considered himself to be overweight, reported to have an "altership." Asked about its meaning, he explained: "It is me at 177 pounds; then I will be Sonny Boy, a rock star."

Difficulty in Abstract Thinking

Difficulty in abstract thinking is reflected in impairment of symbolic ability to think beyond concrete and egocentric thinking, which leads to difficulties in proverb interpretation and in generalizations. There may be the inverse tendency to be overly abstract and to use stilted or manneristic language. In mental status exams, proverb interpretations are commonly used to evaluate an individual's ability to think abstractly.

EXAMPLE

In interpreting the proverb "Don't cry over spilt milk," a patient stated: "Don't cry over spilt milk are the decisions we make about the decision-making process. The essence of men making decisions." In another example of overly abstract, stilted speech, a patient stated that "The barrister comported himself utterly brusque when I previously inspected his interface with his patron."

Echolalia

Some schizophrenia patients exhibit echolalia by repeating words, phrase, fragments or sounds that were presented to them. Related to this is echopraxia, in which the individual repeats or imitates observed gestures or physical expressions.

Thought Blocking

Thought blocking refers to cessation or complete interruption in the flow of the stream of thought. It can be interrupted suddenly, and there is a disruption in the flow of conversation. Thought blocking can be recognized when disruptions in speech are abrupt, prominent, and continual. The patient may describe it as a sudden and inclusive "draining of the brain."

POOR ATTENTION

Patients with schizophrenia often present poor concentration, distractibility from internal or external stimuli, and difficulties in shifting focus to new stimuli. Patients will exhibit impaired attention, particularly in the acute psychotic phase. Scanning the environment during a clinical interview rather than focusing on the interviewer's questions may be seen during the interview. It may be difficult for the individual to follow a more complex set of questions, and he or she may lose track of the interviewer's question. In another situation, the individual may not be able to respond to a new topic being introduced in the interview and will continue to talk about the previous topic, totally oblivious to the new inquiry.

EXCITEMENT SYMPTOMS

Symptoms contributing to this domain of psychopathology of schizophrenia are hostility, excitement, uncooperativeness, and poor impulse control. We address in this section predominantly the symptoms of hostility and aggression.

HOSTILITY AND AGGRESSION

Hostility and aggression in schizophrenia involve verbal and nonverbal expressions of anger and resentment, including sarcasm, passive-aggressive behavior, verbal abuse and assaultiveness, irritability, suspicion, and uncooperativeness (Volavka 2002). Hostility/aggression in schizophrenia is difficult to predict (Monahan et al. 2000; Steadman et al. 1998; Wallace et al. 1998) and can be both a trait and state phenomenon.

Epidemiology

The probability of violent behavior among patients with mental disorders is greater than that of the general population. There is an increased risk of violence among schizophrenia patients based on examination of criminal records (Hodgins 1992; Wessely et al. 1994), results of a twin study (Coid et al. 1993), and data from persons who committed homicide (Eronen et al. 1996). Although patients with mental disorders certainly do not carry out most violent crimes, they are at increased jeopardy for committing them (Citrome and Volavka 1999). Evidence exists for an increased incidence of hostile and aggressive behavior in schizophrenia, estimated at two to 10 times that of the general population (Hafner and Boker 1982; Wessely 1997). Results of the Epidemiologic Catchment Area project reported that the probabilities of violent behavior in patients with schizophrenia were 5.3 times greater for males and 5.9 times greater for females than in individuals with no diagnosed mental disorder (Regier et al. 1990).

Hostility and aggressive behaviors in patients with schizophrenia have also been studied across different cultures. The World Health Organization conducted a study across several different countries and found that the incidence rate of aggression among 1,017 patients with schizophrenia was 20.6%, with the rate three times higher in developing countries such as Colombia, India, and Nigeria (31.5%) compared with developed countries, such as Denmark, Ireland, Japan, the United States, the United Kingdom, and the former countries of the U.S.S.R. (10.5%) (Volavka et al. 1997).

Causes of Aggressive Behavior in Schizophrenia

Causes of aggressive behavior are complex and multifactorial. Some important underlying causes are the presence of comorbid substance abuse, substance dependence, and intoxication (Citrome and Volavka 2001; Steadman et al. 1998). In addition, the disease process itself produces hallucinations and delusions, which may provoke violence (Citrome and Volavka 1999). Krakowski and Czobor (1997), in a study examining psychosis and ward turmoil in schizophrenic inpatients, reported that persistent violence, in contrast to episodic violence, was associated with frontal lobe neurocognitive deficits. Episodic violence was associated with significant florid positive symptoms and tended to abate as positive symptoms improved. Such episodic violence can be related to delusional perceptions that other people are persecuting the individual, against which the individual has to defend him- or herself with a preemptive aggressive act. Environmental factors that are associated with aggressive behavior include a chaotic or unstable home or hospital situation, which may encourage maladaptive aggressive behaviors (Owen et al. 1998). Researchers have also examined biological determinants of aggressive behavior, which are further presented in Chapter 12, "Co-occurring Substance Use and Other Psychiatric Conditions," of this book.

Assessment

Aggression can be clinically assessed by means of the Overt Aggression Scale (Yudofsky et al. 1986) or the excitement factor of the PANSS, whose other symptoms are hostility, uncooperativeness, and poor impulse control. In most studies aggression is measured by using data from different sources (Swanson et al. 2000). Steadman and colleagues (2000) have proposed an actuarial tool for assessing the risk of violence, which has been evaluated in civil psychiatric patients (Monahan et al. 2000). Besides the clinical interview and specific psychopathological scales, a number of other diagnostic instruments can be used to assess aggression and the risk for violence in psychiatric patients. Examples are the Buss-Durkee Hostility Inventory (Buss and Durkee 1957), with its subscales (including physical aggression), and the Brown-Goodwin assessment for lifetime history of aggression (Brown et al. 1979).

Differential Diagnosis

One of the most important differential diagnoses of violent behaviors in patients with schizophrenia is substance abuse and withdrawal. Substance abuse enhances the probability of aggressive behavior substantially more than schizophrenia alone (Swanson 1994). Aggressive and violent behavior in patients can be triggered by alcohol, cocaine, phencyclidine (PCP), or amphetamine intoxication (Smith and Hucker 1994; Swanson 1994). Additionally, withdrawal from abused substances can lead to hostility and aggressive behavior (Citrome and Volavka 1999; Verhayden et al. 2003). Other less frequent differential diagnostic considerations are medical conditions. Brain injuries, brain tumors, and rarely temporal lobe epilepsies or metabolic disturbances may lead to aggressive behavior in a patient who does not have a prior history of continuous aggressive tendencies.

DEPRESSION AND ANXIETY

DEPRESSION

Symptoms that contribute to this domain of psychopathology in schizophrenia are anxiety, depression, guilt feelings, and tension. Although not uncommon, these symptoms tend to be associated with specific phases of the illness.

In addition, they may be at times secondary to the primary symptoms of the disorder and can be conceptualized as emotional responses to very unusual experiences such as hallucinations or delusions.

Depressive Symptoms in the Course of Schizophrenia

Mood disorders are nosologically discrete from schizophrenia; however, depressive symptoms can be seen throughout the course of schizophrenia (Bleuler 1911/1950). Bottlender and colleagues (2000) found depressive symptoms to be frequent among first-episode patients. The ability to distinguish schizophrenia from depression is most difficult early in the course of schizophrenic illness. The prodrome of schizophrenia can resemble depression, and some of the symptoms required in DSM-IV-TR for a major depressive episode (e.g., anhedonia, attention difficulties, psychomotor abnormalities) are common in schizophrenia as well (Andreasen and Flaum 1991). Other differential diagnostic issues to consider include schizoaffective disorder, negative symptoms of schizophrenia, and symptoms of pseudoparkinsonism due to antipsychotic medication effects. Siris (1995) reviewed 30 studies of depression in schizophrenia and found incidence rates ranging from 7% to 65%, with a modal rate of 25% (Hirsch and Jolley 1989; Johnson 1988).

Depressive symptoms do not appear to be entirely a response to the course of chronic schizophrenia, because these symptoms can be present in all phases of schizophrenia: during first episodes (Koreen et al. 1993), chronic illness (Leff 1990), relapse, and remission in individuals receiving maintenance neuroleptics (Van Putten 1975). Depression can precede psychosis as prepsychotic depression (Green et al. 1990; McGlashan and Carpenter 1976; Roth 1970) or depression in the course of schizophrenia can be assessed as a result of recovery from an acute psychotic episode (postpsychotic depression). Traditional research has regarded the presence of affective symptoms during the course of schizophrenia to be a positive predictive factor (Roth 1970; Valliant 1964). Recent research, however, has reported that depression in the course of chronic schizophrenia may also display a distinct morbidity and mortality profile that includes poor outcome, reduced social adjustment (Carpenter et al. 1988), increased rates of relapse (Birchwood et al. 1993), treatment noncompliance (Hogarty et al. 1995; Van Putten 1974) and increased risk of suicide (Drake et al. 1986; Miles 1977; Roy et al. 1983; Westermeyer et al. 1991).

The development of depressive symptoms with chronic schizophrenia has been linked to a higher likelihood for potential relapse (Hertz and Melville 1980; Johnson 1988;

Mandel et al. 1982). Depression occurring more than 1 year following recovery from an acute psychotic relapse is related to an increased risk of relapse, while depression that appears in the first year following an acute psychotic episode is not associated with relapse (Koreen et al. 1993).

Postpsychotic Depressive Disorder

Postpsychotic depression represents both a reaction to the realization of the damage the illness has caused and a reaction of distress to the symptoms of the illness. It occurs in approximately 25% of psychotic patients (Jeczmein et al. 2001) and is characterized by significant anhedonia. McGlashan and Carpenter (1976) were the first to present postpsychotic depressive disorder as a syndrome in itself, which was subsequently defined in DSM-IV as a separate diagnostic entity.

Siris (1990) has argued that postpsychotic depression has been used to describe clinically diverse types of patients. In one group of individuals, depressive symptoms are clearly present during an acute psychotic episode and resolve as the positive symptoms resolve, although sometimes more slowly (also referred to as "revealed depression"). In other individuals, significant depressive symptoms appear after the acute episode has resolved. The main clinical symptoms are depressed affect and generalized motor slowness (Jeczmien et al. 2001). Also, Cutler and Siris (1991) reported that approximately one-quarter of patients with schizophrenic and postpsychotic depression experience panic attacks, indicating that symptoms of anxiety may be part of the clinical profile of postpsychotic depressive disorder. Further studies (Shuwall and Siris 1994) indicated that in postpsychotic depression, the presence of psychosis and anxiety is linked with a higher level of suicidal ideation regardless of the level of depression. Patients with postpsychotic depressive disorder can also suffer from negative symptoms, and this makes the distinction between the two phenomena sometimes difficult.

Differentiating Depressive Symptoms From Negative Symptoms

Several studies have suggested that depression may be associated with negative symptoms (Fitzgerald et al. 2002; Kulhara et al. 1989; Norman et al. 1998; Sax et al. 1996). Overlapping features of depressive symptoms and negative symptoms include reduced social and personal interests, reduced pleasure, diminished energy, and loss of motivation, together with psychomotor retardation (Andreasen and Olsen 1982; Bermanzohn and Siris 1992; Carpenter et al. 1985; Crow 1980; Hausmann and Fleischhacker 2002; Lindenmayer and Kay 1989; Romney and Candido

2001; Siris 2000). Distinguishing features of depressive symptoms and negative symptoms can be identified: distinct sad mood, disturbance in sleep and appetite, guilt, hopelessness, or suicidal thoughts suggest depression, while blunted affect suggests negative symptoms (Barnes et al. 1989; Kibel et al. 1993; Kuck et al. 1992; Lindenmayer et al. 1991; Müller et al. 2001; Norman and Malla 1991). It is important to identify the entire syndrome rather than to measure discrete symptoms that can occur in both negative symptoms and depression.

Differentiating Depressive Symptoms in Schizophrenia From Schizoaffective Disorder

Differentiating schizoaffective disorder from depression in schizophrenia entails longitudinal assessment of symptoms and symptom development. The term *schizoaffective disorder* was used to describe individuals showing an overlap of features of schizophrenia and affective disorder (Norman and Malla 1991). More recently, schizoaffective disorder has been classified distinctively according to different diagnostic systems (Barnes et al. 1989; Kibel et al. 1993; Kuck et al. 1992), which has affected disparities between schizoaffective disorder and depression in schizophrenia. Operationalized criteria such as those in ICD-10 (World Health Organization 1992) specify schizophrenic depressive symptoms (called *postschizophrenic depression*), whereby the individual has some schizophrenic symptoms with prominent depressive symptoms that are distressing and fulfill at least one criterion of a depressive episode. ICD-10 diagnostic criteria for schizoaffective disorder specify that individuals have both definite prominent schizophrenic and simultaneously definite affective symptoms. In DSM-IV-TR, schizoaffective disorder refers to individuals in whom a full affective syndrome corresponds with the complete psychotic syndrome but who also have considerable episodes of psychosis in the absence of an affective syndrome.

In spite of these specific definitions, discussion persists as to whether schizoaffective disorder should be considered a subtype of schizophrenia, a subtype of affective disorder, a distinct entity with dimensions between schizophrenia and affective disorder, a co-occurrence of two distinct diatheses, or an erroneous concept altogether (Siris 2000).

Measurement of Depression in Schizophrenia

Assessment of depression in schizophrenia can be performed using the Calgary Depression Rating Scale for Schizophrenia (CDSS), which, because of its proven reliability and validity, is the standard assessment instrument to measure depression in schizophrenia (Addington et al. 1990, 1991b; Müller et al. 2005).

SUICIDE AND SELF-INJURY

Suicide

The occurrence of suicide attempts during the course of schizophrenia is a serious complication of the illness. Studies estimate that 9%–24% of individuals with schizophrenia will die by suicide (Caldwell and Gottesman 1992; Siris et al. 1993). Bleuler (1911/1950) suggested that the suicidal drive is "the most serious of schizophrenic symptoms" (as cited in Meltzer 1999). Further, an estimated 3,600 patients with schizophrenia commit suicide each year in the United States alone (Meltzer 1999), a rate more than 20 times higher than the general population (Allebeck 1989; Black 1988; Meltzer et al. 2000). It has been reported that up to 40% of patients diagnosed with schizophrenia will have at least one suicide attempt in the course of their illness (Meltzer et al. 2000; Planansky and Johnston 1971).

Given the clinical relevance of suicide attempts in the course of schizophrenia, several studies have investigated the clinical variables associated with suicidal behavior. Male gender, younger age, unemployment, presence of depressive symptoms (particularly hopelessness), a positive family history for suicide attempts, comorbid substance abuse, lack of a supportive environment, and a longer duration of untreated psychosis have been associated with increased suicide risk in patients with schizophrenia (Black et al. 1988; Breier and Astrachan 1984; Caldwell and Gottesman 1990; Heila et al. 1997; Siris 2001). Substance and drug use is another important risk factor for suicidal behavior. Heila and colleagues (1997) reported that substance use, particularly alcohol, is a specific risk factor in older males with schizophrenia. Social dysfunction is an additional risk factor. Socially isolated and unemployed males have been found to be more at risk of suicide (Drake et al. 1984), although the existence of social factors may also suggest disease progression as a risk factor. Other studies (Adam et al. 1982; Peuskens et al. 1997) have examined the relationship of loss and suicide attempts and completion in patients with schizophrenia. They yielded varying results with no clear-cut validation of loss leading to suicidal tendencies. Continually depressed mood—specifically hopelessness and psychomotor instability—was significantly associated with suicide in a prospective study examining 104 schizophrenic patients, 15 of whom committed suicide (Drake et al. 1986). Also, Gupta and colleagues (1998), in a study investigating 336 schizophrenia patients and patients with schizoaffective disorder, found that 98 patients with a history of attempted suicide had exhibited a significantly higher mean number of lifetime depressive episodes compared with 238 patients with no prior suicidal history. Kaplan and Harrow (1996) have provided prospective evidence that the construct of poor overall function, poor social and work function, and poor quality of life are predictive risk factors for later suicide.

Self-Injury

The National Mental Health Association (Contero and Lader 1998) describes self-injury as self-mutilation, self-harm, or self-abuse. This behavior is defined as the deliberate, repetitive, impulsive, nonlethal harming of oneself. Self-injury includes 1) cutting, 2) scratching, 3) picking at scabs or interfering with wound healing, 4) burning, 5) punching self or objects, 6) infecting oneself, 7) inserting objects in body openings, 8) bruising or breaking bones, 9) some forms of hair-pulling, as well as other various forms of bodily harm. These behaviors are relatively uncommon in patients with schizophrenia but can lead to significant dangers in patients' health when they do occur. Examples include burning the skin with an iron or cigarette, cutting off a finger, enucleating an eye, or cutting the skin with a knife or razor in a ritualistic manner. Genital self-mutilation is a rare, severe form of self-injurious behavior. It is usually seen in schizophrenia as being the result of delusions and hallucinations (Becker and Hartmann 1997; Martin and Gattaz 1991; Mishra and Kar 2001). Specific risk factors of genital self-mutilation include command hallucinations, religious delusions (Bhargava et al. 2001), substance abuse, and social isolation (Tobias et al. 1988).

ANXIETY

Although anxiety is common during the prodromal and the acute psychotic phase, it is less prominent during the chronic stages of the illness. During the prodromal phase, even before the presentation of delusional or hallucinatory manifestations, anxiety can be a very common feature. *Anxiety* is defined as a feeling of apprehension caused by the anticipation of danger, which may be internal and external, or it can be a response to a threat that is vague or unknown. Anxiety can arise as a component of psychosis. For example, a patient with schizophrenia may become hypervigilant as a reaction to delusional perception and hallucinations. Fish (1984) indicated that anxiety is usually associated with persecutory delusions and hallucinations during the acute onset of psychosis. Thus, the sudden onset of hallucinations can generate marked depression and anxiety. An important differential diagnosis is the iatrogenic anxiety of akathisia induced by antipsychotic treatment. The timing of onset of the predominant motor restlessness in the legs associated with the antipsychotic treatment may help clarify the diagnosis.

It has been reported that approximately 45% of patients with schizophrenia may also have an anxiety disorder (Pallanti et al. 2003). Studies have shown that alcohol abuse in patients with schizophrenia can produce anxiety symptoms (Drake and Wallach 1989; Strakowski et al. 1994). Similarly, marijuana use in schizophrenia patients is associated with increased symptoms of anxiety (Ziedonis and Nickou 2001, p. 198).

As with depression, anxiety is occasionally an early precursor of a psychotic relapse (Docherty et al. 1978). Jorgensen (1998) examined anxiety as one of several warning signs of recurrence of psychotic symptoms in 131 patients with schizophrenia. Results showed that delusional formation correlated with anxiety and early signs of psychosis measures.

The impact of anxiety and depression on the quality of life in schizophrenic patients has been studied more recently, showing that patients exhibiting anxiety symptoms show impairment in their quality of life that is independent of depressive symptoms (Goodwin et al. 2001; Huppert et al. 2001; Wetherell et al. 2003).

Comorbid Anxiety Disorders and Schizophrenia

Patients with schizophrenia may have significant difficulty in social interactions associated with social anxiety. *Social anxiety disorder*, or social phobia, is a state characterized by an acute and continual fear of social situations in which the person fears degradation or embarrassment in the presence of others. Penn and colleagues (1994) conducted one of the first major studies on social anxiety in a population of patients with schizophrenia. They found that positive symptoms correlated with increased self-reports of social anxiety, whereas negative symptoms correlated with specific behavioral indicators of social anxiety, such as speech rate and fluency. Cosoff and Hafner (1998), using a structured diagnostic interview to assess anxiety in 100 successively admitted patients with a psychotic disorder (60 of whom were diagnosed with schizophrenia), found that 17% of patients with schizophrenia had social anxiety disorder, 13% had obsessive-compulsive disorder (OCD), and 12% had generalized anxiety disorder. For the schizophrenic subjects who displayed comorbid anxiety, approximately 50% reported that the anxiety disorder occurred before the onset of psychosis by several years. More recently, elevated rates of social anxiety disorder in clinical samples of patients with schizophrenia ranging from 6.0% to 42.8% have been reported (Pini et al. 2003).

DIFFERENTIAL DIAGNOSIS OF SCHIZOPHRENIA

Aspects of the positive, negative, and cognitive symptom dimensions are not unique to schizophrenia; they can be found in other psychotic, neurological, and medical disorders as well (Maziade et al. 1995; Rotakonda et al. 1998; Serretti et al. 1996). The diagnosis of schizophrenia is not easy to establish, particularly when patients present with a first psychotic episode. It should be emphasized that no single feature (e.g., family history, cross-sectional symptomatology) can determine a diagnosis of schizophrenia. A comprehensive history of symptom development, family history, careful clinical interview exploring all symptom dimensions, and review of any physical signs, together with laboratory assessments, will be necessary to arrive at an accurate diagnosis. In terms of symptom presentation, formal thought disorders and affect disorders are characteristic features of schizophrenia. At times, the diagnosis may not be clear in the beginning of the disorder, and there may be need for an extended observation period to examine the stability and course of symptoms. In general, the reliability of differentiating schizophrenia from other psychotic disorders is strengthened by the guidelines presented in DSM-IV-TR or ICD-10 (see Tables 11–3 and 11–4).

The clinical presentation, course, and outcome of psychotic and other symptoms are the major factors that differentiate schizophrenia from other psychotic disorders. The following psychiatric illnesses must be excluded before diagnosing schizophrenia:

SCHIZOPHRENIFORM DISORDER

DSM-IV-TR requires the duration for schizophreniform disorder to be at least 1 month but less than 6 months (American Psychiatric Association 2000, p. 317). Hence, schizophreniform disorder is likely to be diagnosed in patients who have an abrupt rather than insidious onset and who have good premorbid adjustment. The most important distinctions between the two disorders are mode of onset and duration of symptoms.

SCHIZOAFFECTIVE DISORDER

Schizoaffective disorder is characterized by an uninterrupted period of illness during which there is at some time either a major depressive episode, a manic episode, or a mixed episode that meets the respective full criteria together with symptoms that meet criterion A for schizophrenia for at least 1 month (see Table 11–4). Schizoaffective disorder differs from schizophrenia in that both the required affective symptoms and the features of schizophrenia are prominent and co-occur (Tsuang et al. 1985). Patients with schizoaffective disorder may also have a relatively abrupt onset of illness and do not meet the social/occupational dysfunction criteria required for a diagnosis of schizophrenia as specified in DSM-IV-TR. Patients should show at least two of the following: delusions, hallucinations, disorganized speech, grossly disorganized or catatonic behavior, and negative symptoms (such as alogia, blunted affect, avolition) during the period of illness. DSM-IV-TR specifies that during the episode of illness there have to be delusions and hallucinations for at least 2 weeks that occur in the absence of prominent mood symptoms (p. 322). Both bipolar and depressive schizoaffective subtypes have been defined.

AFFECTIVE DISORDERS

Mood disorders such as bipolar affective disorder and depressive disorder with psychotic features are diagnosed when there are psychotic symptoms that occur only during periods of diagnosable mood disturbance. For example, bipolar patients with mania may display a wide variety of psychotic symptoms such as hallucinations, paranoid delusions, and formal thought disorder (Csernansky 2002). Inflated self-esteem and grandiose ideas may expand into delusions of grandiosity, and irritability and suspiciousness into delusions of persecution. Patients with schizophrenia will usually have delusions with mood-incongruent and bizarre content, whereas patients with major depressive episodes or bipolar manic episodes may experience hallucinations, and/or delusions, which are usually mood congruent. Also, the presence or absence of Schneiderian first-rank symptoms may provide some diagnostic guidance.

DELUSIONAL DISORDER

Delusional or paranoid disorder can be frequently confused with schizophrenia. The age at onset of delusional disorder is later than that for schizophrenia, and there is typically less deterioration in occupational and social functioning. Another distinction between delusional disorder and schizophrenia is that in the former there is a well-articulated, nonbizarre delusional system with only one or two themes. Thus, the diagnosis of delusional disorder does not include hallucinations, disorganized behavior, or negative symptoms (Csernansky 2002).

BRIEF PSYCHOTIC DISORDER

Brief psychotic disorder has a rapid onset, generally following a major stressor. Individuals with brief psychotic disorder are characterized by one (or more) positive symptoms such as delusions, hallucinations, disorganized speech, or grossly disorganized or catatonic behavior. Symptoms of brief psychotic disorder occur shortly after or in response to a psychotic stressor such as trauma. A distinctive feature of brief psychotic disorder from schizophrenia is that symptoms can only last from 1 day to 1 month and that the individual shows a full return to premorbid level of functioning.

SHARED PSYCHOTIC DISORDER

Shared psychotic disorder (folie à deux) is a delusional disorder in which an individual develops delusions as a result of a relationship with another individual who has been diagnosed with a psychotic disorder, usually schizophrenia, with prominent delusions. This occurs generally in a long-standing, close relationship that has been fairly socially isolated, with the initially healthy person being the more passive partner. The content and nature of the delusions are very similar between the two individuals and can be very bizarre. The close relationship and the similarity of the delusional material of the two individuals are the differentiating features from schizophrenia.

OBSESSIVE-COMPULSIVE PERSONALITY DISORDER

The essential feature of obsessive-compulsive personality disorder (OCPD) is a "preoccupation with order, perfectionism, and mental and interpersonal control, at the expense of flexibility, openness, and efficiency" (American Psychiatric Association 2000, p. 725). Patients recognize that their preoccupation with orderliness is internally motivated, and there are no well-formed delusions or hallucinations or a thought disorder. OCPD should not be confused with OCD. The American Psychiatric Association (2000, pp. 725; see also pp. 457–458) defines OCPD as a personality disorder, whereas OCD is an anxiety disorder. The main difference between OCD and OCPD lies in the degree of life-impairment. Although some schizophrenic delusions may resemble obsessions seen in OCD, people experiencing delusions do not have insight into their content (O'Dwyer and Marks 2000). DSM-IV-TR suggests that when the obsession in OCD reaches "delusional proportions," delusional disorder or psychotic disorder not otherwise specified should be diagnosed in addition to OCD (p. 461). On the other hand, ICD-10 states that obsessive symptoms in the presence of schizophrenia should be regarded as part of the disorder.

SCHIZOTYPAL PERSONALITY DISORDER

Schizotypal personality disorder is characterized by social and interpersonal deficits evidenced by reduced competence for relationships, cognitive distortions, and unconventional behavior. Individuals with this disorder may have bizarre forms of thinking and perceiving and often seek isolation from others. Schizotypal personality disorder generally begins in early adulthood and presents in a variety of contexts, as indicated by five (or more) of the following symptoms (American Psychiatric Association 2000, p. 701):

1. Ideas of reference (excluding delusions of reference)
2. Odd beliefs or magical thinking that influences behavior and is inconsistent with subcultural norms
3. Unusual perceptual experiences, including bodily illusions
4. Odd thinking and speech
5. Suspiciousness or paranoid ideation
6. Inappropriate or constricted affect
7. Behavior or appearance that is odd, eccentric, or peculiar
8. Lack of close friends or confidants other than first-degree relatives
9. Excessive social anxiety that does not diminish with familiarity and tends to be associated with paranoid fears rather than negative judgments about self

In contrast to schizophrenia, schizotypal personality disorder does not involve delusions or hallucinations, and there is no deterioration in social and occupational functioning.

BODY DYSMORPHIC DISORDER

The main characteristic feature of body dysmorphic disorder (BDD) is a preoccupation with an alleged deficiency in one's physical body shape. Patients with BDD may display disproportionate distress about an insignificant imperfection or have persistent, anxiety-provoking feelings concerning a minor flaw. Underlying this distress is a persistent distortion of one's body scheme, which may take on delusional proportions. Patients with BDD are most regularly focused on head and face but may also involve any other body part. At times, an individual with BDD may avoid contact with others to prevent his or her defect from being observed by other people (Veale et al. 1996). Although rare childhood cases have been reported, most people develop BDD in their early or middle teens (Phillips 1996). Individuals with BDD do not experience hallucinations and disorganized thinking. They do not assign the cause of their distorted body image to outside malevolent forces as patients with schizophrenia often do.

PSYCHOTIC DISORDERS DUE TO MEDICAL CONDITIONS

It is important to differentiate psychosis caused by head trauma, brain tumors, multiple sclerosis, Huntington's disease, or Wilson's disease from schizophrenia. In these disorders, cognitive symptoms such as disorientation, short-term memory loss, and confusion will predominate the clinical picture. A full neurological and medical examination will assist with the diagnosis. Also, adverse effects to medications can manifest as psychotic symptoms. For example, symptoms of psychosis can occur during treatment with L-dopa, anticholinergics, and corticosteroids (Guggenheim and Babigian 1974; Rudick et al. 1997).

SUBSTANCE-INDUCED PSYCHOTIC DISORDERS

The main characteristics of substance-induced psychotic disorders are the presence of prominent hallucinations and delusions, which are thought to be directly related to the physiological effects of a substance. There has to be evidence, based on history, physical examination, and laboratory findings, that the disorder arises in the context of substance withdrawal or intoxication. Usually, the disorder lasts as long as there is use of the substance (onset during intoxication) or can begin after the individual has stopped using substances (onset during withdrawal). Hallucinogens such as lysergic acid diethylamide (LSD) and stimulants such as methamphetamine, amphetamine, cocaine, and PCP can generate visual and auditory hallucinations. Alcohol hallucinations, which tend to be visual and kinesthetic, differ from those seen in schizophrenia in that they occur only after extended use of alcohol and usually last for a short period of time (Csernansky 2002). Moreover, alcohol-related hallucinations are not associated with a family history of schizophrenia, and generally individuals are aware that their hallucinations are not real, which is characteristically not the case with individuals with schizophrenia (Csernansky 2002).

SUBTYPES OF SCHIZOPHRENIA

The subtypes of schizophrenia are distinguished by the prevalent symptomatology. Initially, Kraepelin (1919) divided "dementia praecox" into three clinical subtypes: hebephrenic, catatonic, and paranoid. He later expanded on these three subtypes to include several other categories, yet emphasized that the subgrouping of different clinical descriptions was of restricted clinical value (pp. 89–180). Currently, there are various subtypes of schizophrenia as specified by the particular diagnostic system. Table 11–5 presents the most dominant subtypes occurring in schizophrenia patients, which include paranoid, disorganized (hebephrenic), catatonic, undifferentiated, and residual schizophrenia.

CONCLUSION

Schizophrenia is a disorder with a significant heterogeneous presentation of a variety of symptoms that can affect virtually all areas of psychological functioning and which are best understood to represent separate psychopathological syndromal domains. These major symptom domains include positive, negative, cognitive, excitement, and depression/anxiety symptoms and are found in each patient with schizophrenia to a variable extent. Each of these domains will affect patients' instrumental, social, and occupational functioning to various degrees and can lead to significant overall functional impairment. Recognizing and identifying the specific pathophysiological processes underlying each of these domains, together with their distinct dysregulated neuronal circuitry and susceptibility genes, will help identify underlying endophenotypes. This process will in turn lead to a better understanding of underlying illness mechanisms and in the development of better approaches in the treatment of this complex disorder.

REFERENCES

Adam K, Bouckoms A, Steiner D: Parental loss and family stability in attempted suicide. Arch Gen Psychiatry 39:1081–1085, 1982

Addington J, Addington D: Positive and negative symptoms of schizophrenia: their course and relationship over time. Schizophr Res 5:51–59, 1991

Addington D, Addington J, Schissel B: A depression rating scale for schizophrenics. Schizophr Res 3:247–251, 1990

Addington J, Addington D, Maticka-Tyndale E: Cognitive functioning and positive and negative symptoms in schizophrenia. Schizophr Res 5:123–134, 1991a

Addington A, Addington J, Maticka-Tyndale E, et al: Reliability and validity of a depression rating scale for schizophrenics. Schizophr Res 6:201–208, 1991b

Alexander MP, Stuss DT, Benson DF: Capgras syndrome: a reduplicative phenomenon. Neurology 29:334–339, 1979

Allebeck P: Schizophrenia: a life-shortening disease. Schizophr Bull 15:81–89, 1989

Amador XF, Kirkpatrick B, Buchanan RW, et al: Stability of the diagnosis of deficit syndrome in schizophrenia. Am J Psychiatry 156:637–639, 1999

American Psychiatric Association: Diagnostic and Statistical Manual of Mental Disorders, 2nd Edition. Washington, DC, American Psychiatric Association, 1968

American Psychiatric Association: Diagnostic and Statistical Manual of Mental Disorders, 3rd Edition. Washington, DC, American Psychiatric Association, 1980

American Psychiatric Association: Diagnostic and Statistical Manual of Mental Disorders, 3rd Edition, Revised. Washington, DC, American Psychiatric Association, 1987

American Psychiatric Association: Diagnostic and Statistical Manual of Mental Disorders, 4th Edition. Washington, DC, American Psychiatric Association, 1994

American Psychiatric Association: Diagnostic and Statistical Manual of Mental Disorders, 4th Edition, Text Revision. Washington, DC, American Psychiatric Association, 2000

Andreasen N: Thought, language, and communication disorders, I: clinical assessment, definition of terms, and evaluation of their reliability. Arch Gen Psychiatry 36:1315–1321, 1979a

Andreasen N: Thought, language, and communication disorders, II: diagnostic significance. Arch Gen Psychiatry 36:1325–1330, 1979b

Andreasen NC: Negative symptoms in schizophrenia: definition and reliability. Arch Gen Psychiatry 39:784–788, 1982

Andreasen NC: Scale for the Assessment of Negative Symptoms (SANS). Iowa City, University of Iowa, 1983

Andreasen NC: Scale for the Assessment of Positive Symptoms (SAPS). Iowa City, University of Iowa, 1984

Andreasen NC: The Comprehensive Assessment of Symptoms and History (CASH). Iowa City, University of Iowa, 1985

Andreasen NC, Carpenter WT Jr: Diagnosis and classification of schizophrenia. Schizophr Bull 19:199–214, 1993

Andreasen NC, Flaum M: Schizophrenia: the characteristic symptoms. Schizophr Bull 17:27–49, 1991

Andreasen NC, Olsen S: Negative v positive schizophrenia: definition and validation. Arch Gen Psychiatry 39:789–794, 1982

Andreasen NC, Swayze VW, Flaum M, et al: Ventricular enlargement in schizophrenia evaluated with computed tomographic scanning: effects of gender, age, and stage of illness. Arch Gen Psychiatry 47:1008–1015, 1990

Andreasen NC, Arndt S, Alliger R, et al: Symptoms of schizophrenia: methods, meanings, and mechanisms. Arch Gen Psychiatry 52:341–351, 1995

Arndt S, Alliger R, Andreasen NC: The distinction of positive and negative symptoms: the failure of a two-dimensional model. Br J Psychiatry 158:317–322, 1991

Arndt S, Andreasen NC, Flaum M, et al: A longitudinal study of symptom dimensions in schizophrenia: prediction and patterns of change. Arch Gen Psychiatry 52:352–360, 1995

Asaad G: Hallucinations in Clinical Psychiatry: A Guide for Mental Health Professionals. New York, Brunner/Mazel, 1990

Barnes TR, Curson DA, Liddle PF, et al: The nature and prevalence of depression in chronic schizophrenic inpatients. Br J Psychiatry 154:486–491, 1989

Beck AT, Ward CH, Mendelson M: A study of consistency of clinical judgments and ratings. Am J Psychiatry 119:351–357, 1962

Becker H, Hartmann U: [Genital self-injury behavior: phenomenologic and differential diagnosis considerations from the psychiatric viewpoint]. Fortschr Neurol Psychiatr 65:71–78, 1997

Bermanzohn PC, Siris SG: Akinesia: a syndrome common to parkinsonism, retarded depression, and negative symptoms of schizophrenia. Compr Psychiatry 33:221–232, 1992

Bhargava CS, Sethi S, Vohra AK: Klingsor syndrome: a case report. Indian J Psychiatry 43:349–350, 2001

Bilder RM, Mukherjee S, Rieder RO, et al: Symptomatic and neuropsychological components of defect states. Schizophr Bull 11:409–419, 1985

Birchwood M, Mason R, Macmillan F, et al: Depression, demoralization and control over psychotic illness: a comparison of depressed and non-depressed patients with a chronic psychosis. Psychol Med 23:387–395, 1993

Black DW: Mortality in schizophrenia: the Iowa record-linkage study: a comparison with general population mortality. Psychosomatics 29:55–60, 1988

Black DW, Winokur G, Nasrallah A: Effect of psychosis on suicide risk in 1,593 patients with unipolar and bipolar affective disorders. Am J Psychiatry 145:849–852, 1988

Bleuler E: Dementia Praecox or the Group of Schizophrenias (1911). Translated by Zitkin J. New York, International Universities Press, 1950

Bottlender R, Strauss A, Moller HJ: Prevalence and background factors of depression in first admitted schizophrenic patients. Acta Psychiatr Scand 101:153–160, 2000

Braff DL, Heaton RK, Kuck J, et al: The generalized pattern of neuropsychological deficits in outpatients with chronic schizophrenia with heterogeneous Wisconsin Card Sorting Test results. Arch Gen Psychiatry 48:891–898, 1991

Breier A, Astrachan BM: Characterization of schizophrenic patients who commit suicide. Am J Psychiatry 141:206–209, 1984

Brown GL, Goodwin FK, Ballenger JC, et al: Aggression in humans: correlates with cerebrospinal fluid amine metabolites. Psychiatry Res 1:131–139, 1979

Buss AH, Durkee A: An inventory for assessing different kinds of hostility. J Consult Psychol 21:343–349, 1957

Caldwell CB, Gottesman II: Schizophrenics kill themselves too: a review of risk factors for suicide. Schizophr Bull 16:571–589, 1990

Caldwell CB, Gottesman II: Schizophrenia: a high-risk factor for suicides: clues to risk reduction. Suicide Life Threat Behav 22:479–493, 1992

Capleton RA: Cognitive function in schizophrenia: association with negative and positive symptoms. Psychol Rep 78:123–128, 1996

Carpenter WT Jr, Kirkpatrick B: The heterogeneity of the long-term course of schizophrenia. Schizophr Bull 14:645–652, 1988

Carpenter WT Jr, Strauss JS, Bartko JJ: Flexible system for the diagnosis of schizophrenia: report from WHO International Pilot Study of Schizophrenia. Science 182:1275–1278, 1973

Carpenter WT, Heinrichs DW, Alphs LD: Treatment of negative symptoms, Schizophr Bull 11:440–452, 1985

Carpenter WT Jr, Buchanan RW, Brier A, et al: Psychopathology and the question of neurodevelopmental or neurodegenerative disorder. Schizophr Res 5:192–194, 1991

Carter JL: Visual, somatosensory, olfactory and gustatory hallucinations: the interface of psychiatry and neurology. Psychiatr Clin North Am 15:347–358, 1992

Citrome L, Volavka J: Schizophrenia: violence and comorbidity. Curr Opin Psychiatry 12:47–51, 1999

Citrome L, Volavka J: Aggression and violence in patients with schizophrenia, in Schizophrenia and Comorbid Conditions: Diagnosis and Treatment. Edited by Hwang MY, Bermanzohn PC. Washington, DC, American Psychiatric Press, 2001, pp 149–185

Cohen MA, Alfonso CA, Haque MM: Lilliputian hallucinations and medical illness. Gen Hosp Psychiatry 16:141–143, 1994

Coid B, Lewis SW, Revely AM: A twin study of psychosis and criminality. Br J Psychiatry 162:87–92, 1993

Contero K, Lader W: Self-injury. November 1998. Available at: http://www.nmha.org/infoctr/factsheets/selfinjury.cfm. Accessed May 23, 2005.

Cosoff SJ, Hafner RJ: The prevalence of comorbid anxiety in schizophrenia, schizoaffective disorder and bipolar disorder. Aust N Z J Psychiatry 32:67–72, 1998

Crow TJ: Molecular pathology of schizophrenia: more than one disease process? Br Med J 280:66–68, 1980

Crow TJ: Positive and negative symptoms and the role of dopamine. Br J Psychiatry 139:251–254, 1981

Crow TJ: The two-syndrome concept: origins and current status. Schizophr Bull 11:471–486, 1985

Crow TJ. MacMillan JF, Johnson AL, et al: The Northwick Park study of first episodes of schizophrenia, II: a randomized controlled trial of prophylactic neuroleptic treatment. Br J Psychiatry 148:120–127, 1986

Csernansky JG: Schizophrenia: A New Guide for Clinicians. New York, Marcel Dekker, 2002

Cuesta MJ, Peralta V: Thought disorder in schizophrenia: testing models through confirmatory factor analysis. Eur Arch Psychiatry Clin Neurosci 249:55–61, 1999

Cutler JL, Siris SG: "Panic-like" symptomatology in schizoaffective patients with postpsychoatic depression: observations and implications. Compr Psychiatry 32:465–473, 1991

Cutting J, Murphy D: Schizophrenic thought disorder: a psychological organic interpretation. Br J Psychiatry 152:310–319, 1988

Degenhardt L, Hall W: Cannabis and psychosis. Current Psychiatry Reports 4:191–196, 2002

Docherty JP, Van Kammen DP, Siris SG, et al: Stages of onset of schizophrenic psychosis. Am J Psychiatry 135:420–426, 1978

Drake RE, Gates C, Cotton PG, et al: Suicide among schizophrenics: who is at risk? J Nerv Ment Dis 172:613–617, 1984

Drake RE, Gates C, Cotton PG: Suicide among schizophrenics: a comparison of attempters and completed suicides. Br J Psychiatry 149:784–787, 1986

Drake RE, Wallach MA: Substance abuse among the chronic mentally ill. Hosp Community Psychiatry 40:1041–1046, 1989

Ellis HD, Young AW, Quayle AH, et al: Reduced autonomic responses to faces in Capgras delusion. Proc Biol Sci 264:1085–1092, 1997

Endicott J, Spitzer RL: A diagnostic interview: the Schedule for Affective Disorders and Schizophrenia. Arch Gen Psychiatry 35:837–844, 1978

Eronen M, Hakola P, Tiihonen J: Mental disorders and homicidal behavior in Finland. Arch Gen Psychiatry 53:497–501, 1996

Escobar M, Oberling P, Miller RR: Associative deficit accounts of disrupted latent inhibition and blocking in schizophrenia. Neurosci Biobehav Rev 26:203–216, 2002

Feighner JP, Robbins E, Guze SB, et al: Diagnostic criteria for psychiatric research. Arch Gen Psychiatry 26:57–63, 1972

Fenton WS, McGlashan TH: Testing systems for assessment of negative symptoms in schizophrenia. Arch Gen Psychiatry 49:179–184, 1992

First MB, Spitzer RL, Gibbon M, et al: Structured Clinical Interview for DSM-IV Axis I Disorders (SCID-1). Washington, DC, American Psychiatric Association, 1997

Fish F: Schizophrenia, 3rd Edition. Edited by Hamilton M. Baltimore, MD, Williams & Wilkins, 1984

Fitzgerald PB, Rolfe TJ, Berwer K, et al: Depressive, positive, negative and parkinsonian symptoms in schizophrenia. Aust N Z J Psychiatry 36:340–346, 2002

Flaum M, Andreasen N: The reliability of distinguishing primary versus secondary negative symptoms. Compr Psychiatry 36:421–427, 1995

Frith CD, Friston KJ, Liddle PF, et al: PET imaging and cognition in schizophrenia. J R Soc Med 85:222–224, 1992

Goldberg TE, Weinberger DR: Thought disorder in schizophrenia: a reappraisal of older formulations and an overview of some recent studies. Cognitive Neuropsychiatry 5:1–19, 2000

Goodwin DW, Alderson P, Rosenthal R: Clinical significance of hallucinations in psychiatric disorders: a study of 116 hallucinatory patients. Arch Gen Psychiatry 24:76–80, 1971

Goodwin R, Stayner DA, Chinman MJ, et al: Impact of panic attacks rehabilitation and quality of life among persons with severe psychotic disorders. Psychiatr Serv 52:920–924, 2001

Green MF, Nuechterlein KH, Ventura J, et al: The temporal relationship between depressive and psychotic symptoms in recent onset schizophrenia. Am J Psychiatry 147:179–182, 1990

Green MF, Nuechterlein KH, Mintz J: Backward masking in schizophrenia and mania: specifying the visual channels. Arch Gen Psychiatry 51:945–951, 1994

Guggenheim FG, Babigian HM: Catatonic schizophrenia: epidemiology and clinical course: a 7-year register study of 798 cases. J Nerv Ment Dis 158:291–305, 1974

Gupta S, Black DW, Arndt S, et al: Factors associated with suicide attempts among patients with schizophrenia. Psychiatr Serv 49:1353–1355, 1998

Hafner H, Boker W: Crimes of Violence by Mentally Abnormal Offenders. Cambridge, UK, Cambridge University Press, 1982

Hafner H, Nowotny B, Loftler W, et al: When and how does schizophrenia produce social deficits? Eur Arch Psychiatry Clin Neurosci 246:17–28, 1995

Hafner H, Loffler W, Maurer K, et al: Depression, negative symptoms, social stagnation, and social decline in the early course of schizophrenia. Acta Psychiatr Scand 100(2):105–118, 1999

Harvey PD, Lombardi J, Leibman M, et al: Age related differences in formal thought disorder in chronically hospitalized schizophrenic patients: a cross sectional study across nine decades. Am J Psychiatry 154:205–210, 1997

Hausmann A, Fleischhacker WW: Differential diagnosis of depressed mood in patients with schizophrenia: a diagnostic algorithm based on a review, Acta Psychiatr Scand 106:83–96, 2002

Heila H, Isometsa ET, Henriksson KV, et al: Suicide and schizophrenia: a nationwide psychological autopsy study on age and sex specific clinical characteristics of 92 suicide victims with schizophrenia. Am J Psychiatry 154:1235–1242, 1997

Hertz MI, Melville C: Relapse in schizophrenia. Am J Psychiatry 137:801–805, 1980

Hirsch SR, Jolley AG: The dysphoric syndrome in schizophrenia and its implications for relapse. Br J Psychiatry Suppl 5:46–50, 1989

Hoch P, Polantin P: Pseudoneurotic forms of schizophrenia. Psychiatr Q 23:248–276, 1949

Hodgins S: Mental disorder, intellectual deficiency, and crime: evidence from a birth cohort. Arch Gen Psychiatry 49:476–483, 1992

Hoffman RE, Hawkins KA, Gueorguieva R, et al: Transcranial magnetic stimulation of left temporoparietal cortex and medication-resistant auditory hallucinations. Arch Gen Psychiatry 60:49–56, 2003

Hogarty GE, McEvoy JP, Ulrich RF, et al: Pharmacotherapy of impaired affect in recovering schizophrenic patients. Arch Gen Psychiatry 52:29–41, 1995

Hull JW, Smith TE, Anthony DT, et al: Patterns of symptom change: a longitudinal analysis. Schizophr Res 24:17–18, 1997

Huppert JD, Weiss KA, Lim R, et al: Quality of life in schizophrenia: contributions of anxiety and depression. Schizophr Res 51:171–180, 2001

Hurt SW, Holzman PS, Davis JM: Thought disorders: the measurement of its changes. Arch Gen Psychiatry 40:1281–1285, 1983

Jackson JH: Remarks on evolution and dissolution of the nervous system. J Med Sci 33:25–48, 1887–1888

Jeczmien P, Levkovitz Y, Weizman A, et al: Postpsychotic depression in schizophrenia. Isr Med Assoc J 3:589–592, 2001

Johnson DAW: The significance of depression in the prediction of relapse in chronic schizophrenia. Br J Psychiatry 152:320–323, 1988

Jorgensen P: Schizophrenic delusions: detection of warning signals. Schizophr Res 32:17–22, 1998

Kaplan KJ, Harrow M: Positive and negative symptoms as risk factors for later suicidal activity in schizophrenics vs depressives. Suicide Life Threat Behav 26:105–121, 1996

Kasanin J: The acute schizoaffective psychoses. Am J Psychiatry 113:97–126, 1933

Kay SR: Positive-negative assessment in schizophrenia: psychometric issues and scale comparison. Psychiatr Q 61:163–168, 1990

Kay SR, Sevy S: Pyramidical model of schizophrenia. Schizophr Bull 16:537–545, 1990

Kay SR, Opler LA, Fiszbein A: Significance of positive and negative syndromes in chronic schizophrenia. Br J Psychiatry 149:439–448, 1986

Kay SR, Fisz-Bein A, Opler LA: The positive and negative syndrome scale (PANSS) for schizophrenia. Schizophr Bull 13:261–274, 1987

Kibel DA, Laffont I, Liddle PF: The composition of the negative syndrome of chronic schizophrenia, Br J Psychiatry 62:744–750, 1993

Kirkpatrick B, Buchanan RW, McKenney PD, et al: The Schedule for the Deficit Syndrome: an instrument for research in schizophrenia. Psychiatry Res 30:119–123, 1989

Kirkpatrick B, Buchanan RW, Ross DE, et al: A separate disease within the syndrome of schizophrenia. Arch Gen Psychiatry 58:165–171, 2001

Koh S, Kayton L, Berry R: Mnemonic organization in young nonpsychotic schizophrenics. J Abnorm Psychol 81:299–310, 1973

Koh S, Kayton L, Schwartz C: The structure of word-storage in the permanent memory of nonpsychotic schizophrenics. J Consult Clin Psychol 42:879–887, 1974

Koreen AR, Siris SG, Chakos M, et al: Depression in first-episode schizophrenia. Am J Psychiatry 150:1643–1648, 1993

Kraepelin E: Dementia Praecox and Paraphrenia. Translated by Barclay RM. New York, Robert E Krieger Publishing Company, 1919

Krakowski M, Czobor P: Violence in psychiatric patients: the role of psychosis, frontal lobe impairment, and ward turmoil. Compr Psychiatry 38:230–236, 1997

Kring AM, Neale JM: Do schizophrenic patients show a disjunctive relationship among expressive, experiential, and psychophysiological components of emotion? J Abnorm Psychol 105:249–257, 1996

Kuck J, Zisook S, Moranville JT, et al: Negative symptomatology in schizophrenic outpatients. J Nerv Ment Dis 180:510–515, 1992

Kulhara P, Avasthi A, Chadda R, et al: Negative and depressive symptoms in schizophrenia. Br J Psychiatry 154:207–211, 1989

Kuperberg GR, McGuire PK, David AS: Reduced sensitivity to linguistic context in schizophrenic thought disorder: evidence from on-line monitoring for words in linguistically anomalous sentences. J Abnorm Psychol 107:423–434, 1998

Larsen S, Fromholt P: Mnemonic organization and free recall in schizophrenia. J Abnorm Psychol 85:61–65, 1976

Leff J: Depressive symptoms in the course of schizophrenia, in Depression in Schizophrenia. Edited by DeLisi LE. Washington, DC, American Psychiatric Press, 1990, pp 1–23

Lerner AG, Shufman E, Kodesh A, et al: Risperidone-associated, benign transient visual disturbances in schizophrenic patients with a past history of LSD abuse. Isr J Psychiatry Relat Sci 39:57–60, 2002

Lewis DJ: Lilliputian hallucinations in the functional psychoses. Can Psychiatr Assoc J 6:177–201, 1961

Liddle PF: The symptoms of chronic schizophrenia: a re-examination of the positive-negative dichotomy. Br J Psychiatry 151:145–151, 1987

Lindenmayer JP, Kay SR: Depression, affect, and negative symptoms in schizophrenia, Br J Psychiatry 5 (suppl 7):108–114, 1989

Lindenmayer JP, Kay SR, Opler L: Positive and negative subtypes in acute schizophrenia. Compr Psychiatry 2594:445–464, 1984

Lindenmayer JP, Kay SR, Freidman C: Negative and positive syndromes after the acute phase: a prospective follow-up. Compr Psychiatry 27:276–286, 1986

Lindenmayer JP, Grochowski S, Kay SR: Schizophrenic patients with depression: psychopathological profiles and the relationship with negative symptoms. Compr Psychiatry 32:528–533, 1991

Lindenmayer JP, Bernstein-Hyman R, Grochowski S: Five-factor model of schizophrenia: initial validation. J Nerv Ment Dis 182:631–638, 1994

Lindenmayer JP, Bernstein-Hyman R, Grochowski S, et al: Psychopathology of schizophrenia: initial validation of a 5-factor model. Psychopathology 28:22–31, 1995

Lindenmayer JP, Negron AE, Shah S, et al: Cognitive deficits and psychopathology in elderly schizophrenic patients. Am J Geriatr Psychiatry 5:31–42, 1997

Linszen DH, Dingemans PM, Lenior ME: Cannabis abuse and the course of recent onset schizophrenic disorders. Arch Gen Psychiatry 51:273–279, 1994

Lubow RE: Latent Inhibition and Conditioned Attention Theory. Cambridge, UK, Cambridge University Press, 1989

Lubow RE, Weiner I, Feldon J: An animal model of attention, in Behavioral Models and the Analysis of Dry Action. Edited by Speigelstein MY, Levy A. New York, Elsevier, 1982, pp 89–107

MacClain L: Encoding and retrieval in schizophrenics' free recall. J Nerv Ment Dis 171:471–479, 1983

Mackintosh NJ: A theory of attention: variations in the associability of stimuli with reinforcement. Psychol Rev 82: 276–98, 1975

Maher BA, Manschreck TC, Rucklos ME: Contextual constraint and the recall of verbal material in schizophrenia: the effect of thought disorder. Br J Psychiatry 137:69–73, 1980

Mandel MR, Severe JB, Schooler NR, et al: Development and prediction of postpsychotic depression in neuroleptic-treated schizophrenics. Arch Gen Psychiatry 39(2):197–203, 1982

Manschreck T, Maher BA, Milavetz JJ, et al: Semantic priming in thought disordered schizophrenic patients. Schizophr Res 1:61–66, 1988

Marder SR, Davis JM, Chouinard G: The effects of risperidone on the five dimensions of schizophrenia derived by factor analysis: combined results of the North American trials. J Clin Psychiatry 58:538–546, 1997

Martin T, Gattaz WF: Psychiatric aspects of male genital self-mutilation. Psychopathology 24:170–178, 1991

Maziade M, Roy MA, Martinez M, et al: Negative, psychotism, and disorganized dimensions in patients with familial schizophrenia or bipolar disorder: continuity and discontinuity between the major psychosis. Am J Psychiatry 152:1458–1463, 1995

McGlashan TH, Carpenter WT: Postpsychotic depression in schizophrenia. Arch Gen Psychiatry 33:231–239, 1976

McGorry PD, Edwards J, Mihalopoulos C, et al: EPPIC: an evolving system of early detection and optimal management. Schizophr Bull 22:305–326, 1996

Meltzer HY: Suicide and schizophrenia: clozapine and the InterSePT study. J Clin Psychiatry 60 (suppl 12):47–50, 1999

Meltzer HY, Anand R, Alphs L: Reducing suicide risk in schizophrenia: focus on the role of clozapine. CNS Drugs 14: 355–365, 2000

Miles CP: Conditions predisposing to suicide. J Ment Dis 164: 231–246, 1977

Miller DD, Tandon R: The biology and pathophysiology of negative symptoms, in Negative Symptom and Cognitive Deficit Treatment Response in Schizophrenia. Edited by Keefe RSE, McEvoy JP. Washington, DC, American Psychiatric Press, 2001, pp 163–186

Mishra B, Kar N: Genital self amputation for urinary symptoms relief or suicide? Indian J Psychiatry 43:342–344, 2001

Moller HJ, Van Praag HM, Aufdembrinke B, et al: Negative Symptoms in schizophrenia: considerations for clinical trials: working group on negative symptoms in schizophrenia. Psychopharmacology (Berl) 115:221–228, 1994

Monahan J, Steadman HJ, Appelbaum PS, et al: Developing a clinically useful actuarial tool for assessing violence risk. Br J Psychiatry 176:312–319, 2000

Mueser KT, Yarnold PR, Levinson DF, et al: Prevalence of substance abuse in schizophrenia: demographic and clinical correlates. Schizophr Bull 16:31–56, 1990

Mueser KT, Doonan R, Penn DL, et al: Emotion recognition and social competence in chronic schizophrenia. J Abnorm Psychol 105:271–275, 1996

Müller MJ, Szegedi A, Wetzel H, et al: Depressive factors and their relationships with other symptom domains in schizophrenia, schizoaffective disorder and psychotic depression, Schizophr Bull 27:9–28, 2001

Müller MJ, Brening H, Gensch C, et al: The Calgary Depression Rating Scale for schizophrenia in a healthy control group: psychometric properties and reference values. J Affect Disord 88(1):69–74, 2005

Norman RMG, Malla AK: Dysphoric mood and symptomatology in schizophrenia. Psychol Med 21:897–903, 1991

Norman RMG, Malla AK, Cortese L, et al: Aspects of dysphoria and symptoms of schizophrenia, Psychol Med 28:1433–1441, 1998

Nuechterlein KH, Edell WS, Norris M: Attentional vulnerability indicators, thought disorder, and negative symptoms. Schizophr Bull 12:408–426, 1986

O'Dwyer AM, Marks I: Obsessive-compulsive disorder and delusions revisited. Br J Psychiatry 176:281–284, 2000

Oppenheimer H: Clinical Psychiatry: Issues and Challenges. New York, Harper & Row, 1971

Overall JE, Gorham DR: The brief psychiatric rating scale. Psychol Rep 10:799–812, 1962

Owen C, Tarantello C, Jones M, et al: Violence and aggression in psychiatric units. Psychiatr Serv 49:1452–1457, 1998

Pallanti S, Quercioli L, Hollander E: Assessment and characterization of social anxiety in schizophrenia (S53C), in 2003 New Research Program and Abstracts, American Psychiatric Association 156th Annual Meeting, San Francisco, CA, May 17–22, 2003

Penn DL, Hope DA, Spaulding W, et al: Social anxiety in schizophrenia. Schizophr Res 1:277–284, 1994

Peralta V, De Leon J, Cuesta MJ: Are there more than two syndromes in schizophrenia? A critique of the positive-negative dichotomy. Br J Psychiatry 161:335–343, 1992

Perry W, Braff DL: A multimethod approach to assessing perseverations in schizophrenic patients. Schizophr Res 33:69–77, 1998

Peuskens J, Dehert M, Cosyns P, et al: Suicide in young schizophrenic patients during and after inpatient treatment. Int J Ment Health 25:39–44, 1997

Pfohl B, Winokur G: The evolution of symptoms in institutionalized hebephrenic/catatonic schizophrenics. Br J Psychiatry 141:567–572, 1982

Phillips KA: Body dysmorphic disorder: diagnosis and treatment of imagined ugliness. J Clin Psychiatry 57:61–65, 1996

Pini S, Dell'osso L, Saettoni M, et al: Interpersonal sensitivity, social anxiety disorder, and insight into illness in psychotic patients (S93E), in 2003 New Research Program and Abstracts, American Psychiatric Association 156th Annual Meeting, San Francisco, CA, May 17–22, 2003

Planansky K, Johnston R: The occurrence and characteristics of suicidal preoccupation and acts in schizophrenia. Acta Psychiatr Scand 47:473–483, 1971

Regier DA, Farmer ME, Rae DS: Comorbidity of mental disorders with alcohol and other drug abuse: results from the Epidemiologic Catchment Area (ECA) Study. JAMA 264:2511–2518, 1990

Robbins LN, Helzer JE, Croughan J, et al: National Institute of Mental Health Diagnostic Interview Schedule: its history, characteristics, and validity. Arch Gen Psychiatry 38:381–389, 1981

Romney DM, Candido CL: Anhedonia in depression and schizophrenia: a reexamination. J Nerv Ment Dis 189:735–740, 2001

Rotakonda S, Gorman JM, Yale SA, et al: Characterization of psychotic conditions: use of the domains of psychopathology model. Arch Gen Psychiatry 55:75–81, 1998

Roth S: The seemingly ubiquitous depression following acute schizophrenic episodes: a neglected area of clinical discussion. Am J Psychiatry 127:91–98, 1970

Roy A, Thompson R, Kennedy S: Depression in chronic schizophrenia. Br J Psychiatry 142:465–470, 1983

Rudick RA, Cohen JA, Weinstock-Guttman B, et al: Management of multiple sclerosis. N Engl J Med 337:1604–1611, 1997

Russel P, Beekhuis M: Organization in memory: a comparison of psychotics and normals. J Abnorm Psychol 85:527–534, 1976

Salem JE, Kring AM: Flat affect and social skills in schizophrenia: evidence for their independence. Psychiatry Res 87:159–167, 1999

Sartorius N, Shapiro R, Jablensky A: The international pilot study of schizophrenia. Schizophr Bull 1:21–35, 1974

Sax KW, Strakowski SM, Keck PEJ, et al: Relationship among negative, positive, and depressive symptoms in schizophrenia and psychotic depression. Br J Psychiatry 168:68–71, 1996

Schneider K: Clinical Psychopathology. Translated by Hamilton MW. New York, Grune & Stratton, 1959

Schneider K: Primary and secondary symptoms in schizophrenia, in Themes and Variations in European Psychiatry. Edited by Hirsch SR, Shepard M. Bristol, UK, John Wright, 1974, pp 40–46

Serretti A, Macciardi F, Smeraldi E: Identification of symptomologic patterns common to major psychoses: proposal for a phenotype definition. Am J Med Genet Neuropsychiatr Genet 67:393–400, 1996

Servan-Schreiber D, Cohen JD, Steingard S: Schizophrenia deficits in processing of context: a test of a theoretical model. Arch Gen Psychiatry 53:1105–1112, 1996

Shuwall M, Siris SG: Suicidal ideation in postpsychotic depression. Compr Psychiatry 35:132–134, 1994

Siris SG: Depressive symptoms in the course of schizophrenia, in Depression in Schizophrenia. Edited by DeLisi LE. Washington, DC, American Psychiatric Press, 1990, pp 3–23

Siris SG: Depression and schizophrenia, in Schizophrenia. Edited by Hirsch SR, Weinberger DR. Oxford, England, Blackwell Science, 1995, pp 128–145

Siris SG: Depression in schizophrenia: perspective in the era of "atypical" antipsychotic agents. Am J Psychiatry 157:1379–1389, 2000

Siris SG: Suicide and schizophrenia. J Psychopharmacol 15:127–135, 2001

Siris SG, Adan F, Cohen M, et al: Postpsychotic depression and negative symptoms: an investigation of syndromal overlap. Am J Psychiatry 145:1532–1537, 1988

Siris SG, Mason SE, Shuwall MA: Histories of substance abuse, panic and suicidal ideation in schizophrenic patients with histories of post-psychotic depressions. Prog Neuropsychopharmacol Biol Psychiatry 17:609–617, 1993

Smith J, Hucker S: Schizophrenia and substance abuse. Br J Psychiatry 165:13–21, 1994

Soyka M, Naber G, Volcker A: Prevalence of delusional jealousy in different psychiatric disorders: an analysis of 93 cases. Br J Psychiatry 158:549–553, 1991

Speed M, Toner B, Shugar G, et al: Thought disorder and verbal recall in acutely psychotic patients. J Clin Psychol 47:735–744, 1991

Spitzer RL, Fleiss JL: A re-analysis of the reliability of psychiatric diagnosis. Br J Psychiatry 125:341–347, 1974

Spitzer RL, Williams JBW: Structured Clinical Interview for DSM-II (SCID). New York, Biometrics Research Division, New York State Psychiatric Institute, 1984

Spitzer RL, Endicott J, Robins E: Research Diagnostic Criteria for a Selected Group of Functional Disorders. New York, New York State Psychiatric Institute, 1978

Steadman HJ, Mulvey EP, Monahan J, et al: Violence by people discharged from acute psychiatric inpatient facilities and by others in the same neighborhoods. Arch Gen Psychiatry 55:1–9, 1998

Steadman HJ, Silver E, Monahan J, et al: A classification tree approach to the development of actuarial violent risk assessment tools. Law Hum Behavior 24:83–100, 2000

Strakowski SM, Tohen M, Flaum M, et al: Substance abuse in psychotic disorders: associations with affective syndromes: DSM-IV Field Trial Work Group. Schizophr Res 14:73–81, 1994

Strauss JS, Carpenter WT Jr, Bartko JJ: The diagnosis and understanding of schizophrenia, Part III: speculations on the processes that underlie schizophrenic symptoms and signs. Schizophr Bull 11:61–69, 1974

Swanson J: Mental disorder, substance abuse and community violence: an epidemiological approach, in Violence and Mental Disorder: Developments in Risk Assessment. Edited by Monahan J, Steadman H. Chicago, IL, University of Chicago Press, 1994, pp 101–136

Swanson JW, Swartz MS, Borum R, et al: Involuntary outpatient commitment and reduction of violent behaviour in persons with severe mental illness. Br J Psychiatry 176:324–331, 2000

Tandon R, Greden J: Cholinergic hyperactivity and negative schizophrenic symptoms. Arch Gen Psychiatry 46:745–753, 1989

Thompson PA, Meltzer HY: Positive, negative, and disorganization factors from the Schedule for Affective Disorders and Schizophrenia and the Present State Examination: a three-factor solution. Br J Psychiatry 163:344–351, 1993

Tobias CR, Turns DM, Lippmann S, et al: Evaluation and management of self-mutilation. South Med J 81:1261–1263, 1998

Toomey R, Kremen WS, Simpson JC, et al: Revisiting the factor structure for positive and negative symptoms: evidence from a large heterogeneous group of psychiatric patients. Am J Psychiatry 154:371–377, 1997

Tsuang MT, Kendler KK, Gruenberg AM: A DSM-III schizophrenia: is there evidence for familial transmission? Acta Psychiatr Scand 71:77–83, 1985

Valliant GE: Prospective prediction of schizophrenic remission. Arch Gen Psychiatry 11:509–518, 1964

Van Putten T: Why do schizophrenic patients refuse to take their drugs? Arch Gen Psychiatry 31:67–72, 1974

Van Putten T: Why do patients with manic-depressive illness stop their lithium?
Compr Psychiatry 16(2):179–183, 1975

Veale D, Boocock A, Gournay K, et al: Body dysmorphic disorder: a survey of fifty cases. Br J Psychiatry 169:196–201, 1996

Verheyden SL, Maidment R, Curran HV: Quitting ecstasy: an investigation of why people stop taking the drug and their subsequent mental health. J Psychopharmacol 17:371–378, 2003

Volavka J: Neurobiology of Violence, 2nd Edition. Washington, DC, American Psychiatric Publishing, 2002

Volavka J, Laska E, Baker S, et al: History of violent behaviour and schizophrenia in different cultures: analyses based on the WHO study on Determinants of Outcome of Severe Mental Disorders. Br J Psychiatry 171:9–14, 1997

Wallace C, Mullen P, Burgess P, et al: Serious criminal offending and mental disorder: case linkage study. Br J Psychiatry 172: 477–484, 1998

Weiden P, Scheifler P, Diamond R, et al: Breakthroughs in Antipsychotic Medications. New York, WW Norton, 1999

Wessely S: The epidemiology of crime, violence and schizophrenia. Br J Psychiatry 170 (suppl 32):8–11, 1997

Wessely S, Castle D, Douglas AJ, et al: The criminal careers of incident cases of schizophrenia. Psychol Med 24:483–502, 1994

Westermeyer JF, Harrow M, Marengo JT: Risk for suicide in schizophrenia and other psychotic and nonpsychotic disorders. J Nerv Ment Dis 179:259–266, 1991

Wetherell JL, Barton BW, Thorp SR, et al: Anxiety symptoms and quality of life in middle-aged and older outpatients with schizophrenia and schizoaffective disorder. J Clin Psychiatry 63:1476–1482, 2003

White L, Harvey PD, Opler L, et al: Empirical assessment of the factorial structure of clinical symptoms in schizophrenia: a multisite, multimodel evaluation of the factorial structure of the Positive and Negative Syndrome Scale. The PANSS Study Group. Psychopathology 30:263–274, 1997

Wing J: A standard form of psychiatric Present-State Examination and a method for standardizing the classification of symptoms, in Psychiatric Epidemiology: An International Symposium. Editing by Hare EH, Wing JK. London, Oxford University Press, 1970, pp 93–108

Wing J, Nixon J: Discriminating symptoms in schizophrenia: a report from the international pilot study of schizophrenia. Arch Gen Psychiatry 32:853–859, 1975

World Health Organization: International Classification of Diseases, 9th Revision, Clinical Modification. Ann Arbor, MI, Commission on Professional and Hospital Activities, 1978

World Health Organization: International Statistical Classification of Diseases and Related Health Problems, 10th Revision. Geneva, World Health Organization, 1992

Yudofsky SC, Silver JM, Jackson W, et al: The Overt Aggression Scale for the objective rating of verbal and physical aggression. Am J Psychiatry 143:35–39, 1986

Ziedonis D, Nickou C: Substance abuse in patients with schizophrenia, in Schizophrenia and Comorbid Conditions: Diagnosis and Treatment. Edited by Hwang MY, Bermanzohn PC. Washington, DC, American Psychiatric Press, 2001, pp 187–221

CO-OCCURRING SUBSTANCE USE AND OTHER PSYCHIATRIC DISORDERS

MARY F. BRUNETTE, M.D.

DOUGLAS L. NOORDSY, M.D.

ALAN I. GREEN, M.D.

More than half of all patients with schizophrenia experience at least one co-occurring (i.e., comorbid) psychiatric disorder (Bermanzohn et al. 2000; Bland et al. 1987; Cassano et al. 1998); moreover, such co-occurring disorders often have a deleterious effect on the course of schizophrenia (Bermanzohn et al. 2000; Bland et al. 1987; Cassano et al. 1998). Detection and optimal treatment of such co-occurring disorders in this patient population are essential if patient outcomes are to be optimized.

Some co-occurring conditions may have a genetic link to schizophrenia, and research aimed at establishing whether patients with schizophrenia are at increased risk for certain disorders may expand our understanding of the causes of schizophrenia (see Chapter 3, "Genetics"). Thus far, the best example of this notion involves adults who have the velocardiofacial syndrome. People with this condition, which is associated with small deletions of chromosome region 22q11, are more likely to receive diagnoses of schizophrenia and bipolar disorders than are those without the syndrome (Murphy et al. 1999). Moreover, 22q11 contains the gene for catechol-O-methyltransferase, an enzyme involved in the degradation of dopamine (Grossman et al. 1992), a neurotransmitter thought to play an important role in the expression of psychotic symptoms (Carlsson 1988). Interestingly, more recent studies have suggested that polymorphisms of the catechol-O-methyltransferase gene may impair prefrontal cognitive function and increase the risk for psychotic symptoms (Egan et al. 2001).

Co-occurring disorders also may provide clues about the neurobiology of schizophrenia itself. For example, Green and colleagues (1999) proposed a neurobiological hypothesis to explain the high rates of substance use disorders observed in patients with schizophrenia. This hypothesis suggests that dysfunctional dopamine-mediated mesocorticolimbic brain reward pathways may underlie the symptoms of schizophrenia and the high vulnerability to substance abuse in these individuals.

Although medications and psychosocial interventions are effective for the treatment of symptoms of schizophrenia and its associated cognitive deficits, identifying and treating co-occurring conditions in patients with schizophrenia remain major clinical challenges. In this chapter, we address many important co-occurring symptoms and disorders: substance use, depressive disorder, suicide, panic, social phobia, trauma and posttraumatic stress disorder (PTSD), and obsessive-compulsive disorder (OCD).

SUBSTANCE USE DISORDERS

Prevalence and Etiology

The lifetime prevalence of alcohol or drug use disorders (referred to in this chapter by the generic term *substance use disorders*) in patients with schizophrenia is surprisingly high. The Epidemiologic Catchment Area study reported a lifetime prevalence of 47% for substance use disorders in people with schizophrenia as compared with 16% of the general population (Regier et al. 1990). The National Comorbidity Study reported a lifetime substance use disorder comorbidity of 59% in the population with schizophrenia (Kendler et al. 1996a). Alcohol is the most commonly abused substance in patients with schizophrenia, followed by cannabis (Drake and Mueser 1996; Mueser et al. 1990; Selzer and Lieberman 1993), which was reported to occur in more than 50% of first-episode patients in one sample (Rolfe et al. 1999). In addition, most people with schizophrenia are dependent on nicotine (58%–90%) (Dalack et al. 1998; Hughes et al. 1986), a rate approximately three times that in the general U.S. population (Centers for Disease Control 2004).

Substance use disorders complicate the course of illness and treatment of patients with schizophrenia, even when the substance use pattern is rather modest. For these individuals, regular use of even small amounts of alcohol can have negative effects (Drake and Wallach 1993). Substance use is associated with treatment nonadherence; suicidality; hospitalization; homelessness; victimization; violence; increased risk for HIV, hepatitis B, and hepatitis C infection; and lower functioning in general (Brady et al. 1990; Drake and Mueser 1996; Drake et al. 1989; Hurlburt et al. 1996; Lysaker et al. 1994; Neria et al. 2002; Owen et al. 1996; Rosenberg et al. 2001a). Moreover, substance use disorders in first-episode patients may complicate assessment of the psychosis and delay treatment (J. Addington and Addington 2001; Green et al. 2004).

Many theories have been developed to explain the increased prevalence of substance use disorders in people with schizophrenia. The stress-vulnerability model proposes that a genetic vulnerability, modified by early environmental events, interacts with later environmental stressors to precipitate either the onset or the relapse of a psychiatric or substance use disorder. Vulnerability to

schizophrenia and substance use disorders may be related to each other in this model, and substance use may serve as the environmental stressor that precipitates onset of psychosis in vulnerable individuals (Deganhardt et al. 2003). The stress-vulnerability model is supported by data indicating that use of cannabis is associated with an earlier onset of schizophrenia (Green et al. 2004); that patients with schizophrenia are highly sensitive to the detrimental effects of low doses of substances, such as amphetamine (Lieberman et al. 1987) and alcohol (Drake and Wallach 1993); and that these patients experience negative clinical effects, such as relapse, following use of small quantities of substances (Drake et al. 1989; Treffert 1978).

Several authors have proposed a "self-medication" hypothesis, suggesting that substances are used to lessen symptoms of the psychotic disorder or to reduce side effects of antipsychotic medications (Khantzian 1997; Siris 1990). Although some research indicates that substance use may decrease negative symptoms and medication-induced extrapyramidal side effects (J. Addington and Addington 1998; Buckley et al. 1994; Glynn and Sussman 1990; Kavanagh et al. 2004; Lysaker et al. 1994; Yang et al. 2002), the bulk of the research in this area does not support a causal relation between substance use and level of psychiatric symptoms (J. Addington and Addington 1998; Brunette et al. 1997; Buchanan et al. 1997; Hamera et al. 1995; Mueser et al. 1990; Soni and Brownlee 1991). Moreover, first-episode patients have high rates of substance use disorders prior to exposure to antipsychotic medications and their side effects (J. Addington and Addington 2001; Green et al. 2002, 2004; McEvoy and Brown 1999; Veen et al. 2004), and first-episode patients with a history of substance abuse report fewer negative symptoms than do those without such a history (Green et al. 2004).

A family history of substance use disorder may increase the risk for substance use disorders in patients with schizophrenia (Noordsy et al. 1994), but family history alone does not explain the overall increased prevalence. Family, twin, and genetic studies thus far indicate that the biological (presumed genetic) vulnerability for one disorder is different from the vulnerability for the other. Thus, the presence of schizophrenia in a family member does not appear to increase the risk for substance use disorder in other family members without schizophrenia, and the presence of a substance use disorder in a family member does not increase the rest of the family's risk for schizophrenia (Bidaut-Russell et al. 1994; Jones and Cannon 1998; Kendler 1985; Kendler et al. 1985, 1996b, 1996c).

Nevertheless, the biological vulnerability to substance abuse in schizophrenia may be an inherent part of the neurobiology of schizophrenia (Green et al. 1999; Stone et al. 2001). Green and colleagues (1999) proposed a neu-

TABLE 12–1. Principles of integrated dual-disorder treatment for patients with schizophrenia

Integration of mental health and substance use disorder treatments

Stagewise treatment that is tailored to the patient's motivation for change

Comprehensive services that include medication management, psychosocial rehabilitation, skills training, and residential and vocational services

Long-term perspective

robiological formulation suggesting that the high rates of comorbid substance use disorders in patients with schizophrenia may relate to a deficiency in the dopamine-mediated mesocorticolimbic brain reward circuits and to the ability of substances of abuse to ameliorate this deficiency. Chambers and colleagues (Chambers and Self 2002; Chambers et al. 2001) subsequently described a similar theory, proposing that dysfunctions of the hippocampal and prefrontal areas, as well as other components of the brain reward circuit, form the neurobiological basis for high rates of co-occurring substance use disorders in schizophrenia. Although the heightened vulnerability to substance use disorders in people with schizophrenia is likely multidetermined, the confluence of findings from neuroanatomical, neuropsychological, and neuropharmacological studies is consistent with the reward system dysfunction model (Chambers et al. 2001; Dervaux et al. 2001; Green et al. 1999). In patients with schizophrenia, this model suggests that alcohol and drug use may enhance the functioning of the brain reward circuit by acting to improve the "signal detection" capability of dopamine-rich pathways (Fadda et al. 1989; Goeders and Smith 1986; Green et al. 1999), resulting in a subjective improvement in how patients feel despite having a negative effect on the illness course.

DETECTION AND MANAGEMENT

Co-occurring substance use disorders usually are underdetected and undertreated in mental health settings (Ananth et al. 1989), where the traditional separation between mental health and substance abuse training programs and service-delivery systems leads to a lack of knowledge about co-occurring disorders and inconsistent commitment to the treatment of the substance abuse component (Ridgely et al. 1990). Given the substantial lifetime vulnerability of patients with schizophrenia for substance use disorders, clinicians should discuss substance use with all patients at regular intervals over time. Screening and assessment can

be assisted through the use of standardized measures, especially instruments specifically developed for patients with mental illness (e.g., Dartmouth Assessment of Lifestyle Instrument [Rosenberg et al. 1998], Alcohol Use Scale [Mueser et al. 1995], and Drug Use Scale [Mueser et al. 1995]). Clinicians should supplement their observation of behaviors consistent with substance use (e.g., frequent missed appointments and financial or legal problems) with collateral information from family members, case managers, and significant others. A functional analysis of substance use incorporates the patient's view of both the positive and the negative aspects of substance use and actively involves the patient in the assessment process while simultaneously providing the foundation for cognitive-behavioral substance abuse counseling. A nonjudgmental attitude reinforces honest communication about substance use and improves detection and treatment (Miller and Rollnick 2002).

In a review of 26 controlled studies of outpatient and residential programs, Drake and colleagues (2004) emphasized that integrating the treatment of the psychotic and the substance use disorders, thereby allowing for the coordination of pharmacotherapy, psychosocial treatments, and substance abuse counseling into one comprehensible package, results in improved patient outcomes (Barrowclough et al. 2001; Blankertz and Cnaan 1994; Drake et al. 1998). Important components of the effective integrated treatment of dual disorders include 1) staged interventions that are tailored to the patient's motivation for change (e.g., assertive outreach and motivational interviewing); 2) comprehensive services (e.g., medication management, rehabilitation, and social support interventions); and 3) a long-term perspective (Drake et al. 2004) (Table 12–1). One such treatment program, Integrated Dual Disorder Treatment (Brunette et al. 2002; Mueser et al. 2003a), recommends that multidisciplinary teams provide the components of integrated care by using case management, individual counseling, treatment groups, and family interventions. It is also important to ensure that these patients have access to residential services and vocational supports.

Research on the optimal pharmacotherapy for dual-diagnosis patients has not yet established a standardized treatment approach that can meet the needs of all or even most patients (Krystal et al. 1999; Noordsy and Green 2003; Wilkins 1997). However, it is clear that antipsychotic agents decrease symptoms of schizophrenia and improve overall functioning in these patients; moreover, some agents may even reduce substance use. Optimally, medications serve to enhance a patient's ability to participate in psychosocial treatments and thus facilitate recovery from both disorders (Noordsy et al. 2002).

Although first-generation antipsychotic medications are effective for psychosis, patients with co-occurring substance abuse tend to continue to use substances and experience poor outcomes while taking them (Drake et al. 1989; Salyers and Mueser 2001). Research on the effect of second-generation antipsychotics is in its infancy but appears to suggest that some of these medications may be particularly helpful for these patients. Five preliminary studies suggested that the second-generation antipsychotic clozapine may be helpful in treating substance use disorders (Buckley et al. 1999; Drake et al. 2000; Green et al. 2003; Lee 1998; Zimmet et al. 2000). Two of three recent studies showed striking reductions (approximately 80% reduction) in the use of substances in dual-disorder patients who took clozapine (Drake et al. 2000; Zimmet et al. 2000). The most recent study reported abstinence from alcohol and cannabis (a more rigorous outcome) in 54% of the clozapine users compared with 13% of the risperidone users with dual disorders (Green et al. 2003). Additionally, three studies suggested that clozapine helps patients with schizophrenia reduce cigarette smoking (George et al. 1996; McEvoy et al. 1995, 1999).

Research on the effect of risperidone is even more preliminary and has produced mixed results, but it appears that risperidone may be less effective than clozapine in reducing substance use in patients with schizophrenia (Albanese 2001; Green et al. 2003; Smelson et al. 2002). The research on olanzapine is also mixed. Two case reports (Longo et al. 2002; Tsuang et al. 2002) and a small study (Littrell et al. 2001) suggested that it may help patients with schizophrenia reduce cocaine use, but another naturalistic prospective study reported that it was not more effective than first-generation agents (Noordsy et al. 2001). One report of the use of quetiapine in psychiatric patients with comorbid stimulant abuse showed decreased stimulant craving but not drug use (Brown et al. 2002). Two studies suggested that second-generation antipsychotics are more effective than first-generation antipsychotics for smoking cessation when used in combination with a nicotine patch and psychosocial treatments (George et al. 2000) or when used with bupropion and psychosocial treatments (George et al. 2002) in this population. To our knowledge, no reports have been published on the effect of ziprasidone or aripiprazole on substance abuse in patients with schizophrenia.

Green and colleagues (1999) suggested that clozapine may be uniquely effective for patients with schizophrenia and substance use disorders because of its unusual pharmacological profile. Clozapine potently blocks α_2-noradrenergic receptors, increases norepinephrine levels, and weakly blocks dopamine$_2$ receptors, which may allow it to normalize the signal detection capability of dysfunctional mesocorticolimbic brain reward circuits (Green et

al. 1999). Clearly, more studies are required to assess the effects of novel antipsychotics in this population.

Other medications demonstrated to be effective for the treatment of substance abuse in the general population show some promise for patients with schizophrenia. For example, bupropion, an antidepressant approved by the U.S. Food and Drug Administration (FDA) for smoking cessation, was shown to be helpful for smoking cessation in three small groups of patients with schizophrenia (Evins et al. 2001; George et al. 2002; Weiner et al. 2001). The tricyclic antidepressants desipramine and imipramine have been shown in small, preliminary studies to have a potential role in treating patients with comorbid substance abuse, especially those with a cocaine use disorder (Siris et al. 1993; Ziedonis et al. 1992), but further research is needed. Disulfiram has been used with safety and some success to decrease alcohol use in this patient population (Kofoed et al. 1986), although it must be used with caution because of its potential ability to increase psychosis (Kingsbury and Salzman 1990). A retrospective, uncontrolled study of disulfiram in 33 patients with alcoholism and severe mental illness showed a 64% rate of sustained remission from alcoholism (Mueser et al. 2003b). Four preliminary studies (Dougherty 1997; Maxwell and Shinderman 1997, 2000; Petrakis et al. 2004) reported that naltrexone, an agent that has been shown to reduce drinking in people with alcohol use disorders in the general population (O'Malley et al. 1992; Volpicelli et al. 1992), may have some value in decreasing alcohol use in patients with comorbid schizophrenia as well.

Pharmacotherapy for patients with co-occurring schizophrenia and substance use disorders should include medications to treat both the mental illness and the substance use disorder, taking care to prescribe medications that are safe in the context of substance use. Although dangerous interactions between psychotropic medication and substances of abuse are of real concern, they seem to be rare (for a review of potential interactions, see Mueser et al. 2003a). The second-generation antipsychotic agents are generally safer and have fewer side effects than older medications and may be more useful than first-generation agents in this population. Clozapine, despite its potential side effects, shows the most promise. Prescription benzodiazepine use is controversial in persons with primary substance use disorders, but the practice appears to be common for people with dual disorders (Clark et al. 2004). Because these medications do not appear to improve outcomes and are associated with the development of benzodiazepine use disorders (Brunette et al. 2003), they probably should be avoided in these patients.

A shared decision-making approach to prescribing medications that may be likely to support the patient's progress

TABLE 12–2.   Co-occurring substance use and other psychiatric disorders in schizophrenia

Co-occurring disorder	Estimated lifetime prevalence (%)	Recommended treatments
Substance use disorders	47–59	Second-generation antipsychotics, with more evidence for clozapine; medications for substance use disorders; integrated treatments for mental illness and substance use disorders
Depressive disorders	Up to 81	Second-generation antipsychotics; addition of antidepressant medication; psychosocial treatments for depression
Panic disorder	6–30	Case reports suggest addition of antipanic medications and cognitive-behavioral therapy
Social phobia	15–40	Case reports suggest addition of antidepressants and cognitive-behavioral therapy
Posttraumatic stress disorder	14–43	Consider treatments effective in general population: antidepressant medications and cognitive-behavioral therapy
Obsessive-compulsive disorder	4–24	Case reports suggest addition of serotonin reuptake inhibitors and cognitive-behavioral therapy

toward recovery from both disorders is useful (Noordsy et al. 2000). Importantly, clinicians should encourage patients to take antipsychotics and other appropriate psychotropic medication, despite ongoing substance use, in order to stabilize the mental illness and to facilitate participation in substance abuse counseling. Comprehensive, integrated psychosocial and psychopharmacological treatments of both the psychotic and the substance use disorders delivered by multidisciplinary teams are recommended (Drake et al. 2001; Mueser et al. 2003a) (Table 12–2), but further research is needed to clarify effective psychopharmacology for this group of patients.

DEPRESSIVE DISORDERS

PREVALENCE AND OUTCOME

Although schizophrenia is viewed primarily as a psychotic disorder, patients with schizophrenia experience a variety of depressive states, ranging from dysphoria to major depression. The National Comorbidity Study (Kendler et al. 1996a), as well as other studies (Bland et al. 1987; Hafner et al. 1999; Koreen et al. 1993; Martin et al. 1985), reported a lifetime risk of depression in patients with schizophrenia of up to 81%, with the point prevalence of major depression ranging from 10% to 30% (Baynes et al. 2000; Delahanty et al. 2001; Hafner et al. 1999; Herbener and Harrow 2002; Jin et al. 2001; Messias et al. 2001). Depression can be a symptom of the prodromal period prior to onset of psychotic symptoms (Hafner et al. 1999), and it can be an integral component of an acute episode of schizophrenia (McGlashan and Carpenter 1976; Sax et al. 1996). For example, although 50%–80% of patients with first-episode schizophrenia have depressive symptoms prior to or during their first psychotic episode, nearly all of the depressive symptoms resolve as the psychosis remits (J. Addington et al. 2003; Hafner et al. 1999; Koreen et al. 1993; Oosthuizen et al. 2002; Tollefson et al. 1999). Others have observed that depression can occur as a postpsychotic syndrome after the resolution of psychosis (Birchwood et al. 2000) and can be seen as a response to psychosis (Sax et al. 1996). Furthermore, depression commonly occurs during the process of decompensation into a new psychotic episode (Malla and Norman 1994; Subotnik and Nuechterlein 1988; Tollefson et al. 1999). Although women in the general population are more likely to experience depressive symptoms and syndromes than are men, the evidence is mixed as to whether women with schizophrenia are at higher risk for depression than are men with schizophrenia (D. Addington et al. 1996; Brunette et al. 1997; Hafner et al. 1999; Jin et al. 2001; McGlashan and Bardenstein 1990; Messias et al. 2001; Oosthuizen et al. 2002).

The prognostic significance of depressive symptoms in patients with schizophrenia depends in part on the timing of the symptoms (Siris 1991). Some (Hafner et al. 1999; Oosthuizen et al. 2002) but not all (Baynes et al. 2000) investigators have found that depressive symptoms in the early phase of the disorder predict lower levels of negative symptoms later. Moreover, depression during psychosis predicts good outcome (Emsley et al. 1999; McGlashan and Carpenter 1976; Oosthuizen et al. 2002), whereas depression during remission of psychosis predicts poor outcome (Bartels and Drake 1988; Mandel et al. 1982; Siris 1991). Depression over the course of chronic schizophrenia is associated with a risk of relapse of psychosis (Mandel et al. 1982), readmission (Shepherd et al. 1989), worse functioning (Jin et al. 2001), lower quality of life (Delahanty et al. 2001), and suicide (Drake et al. 1986), and relatives report more distress over this symptom cluster than over others (Boye et al. 2001).

DETECTION AND MANAGEMENT

Patients with schizophrenia may experience a variety of depressive states, ranging from symptoms to syndromes that must be distinguished from the negative symptoms of schizophrenia and from medication-induced side effects. Determining the temporal appearance, duration, quality, and severity of depressive symptoms is necessary for diagnosis and formulation of an appropriate treatment plan. Assessment of co-occurring substance use disorder (Scheller-Gilkey et al. 2002) and family history of depressive disorders (Subotnik et al. 1997), which are more common in patients with co-occurring depressive syndromes, also may be helpful in this process. Depressive syndromes tend to be underidentified in patients with schizophrenia, especially in African American patients (Delahanty et al. 2001; Elk et al. 1986).

Symptoms of depression are common during exacerbations of psychosis (Baynes et al. 2000; Hafner et al. 1999; Jin et al. 2001; Oosthuizen et al. 2002) and usually improve as the psychosis remits (Birchwood et al. 2000; Hafner et al. 1999; Koreen et al. 1993; Tollefson et al. 1999). Postpsychotic depression classically emerges after the resolution of psychotic symptoms and is most common after the first episode of schizophrenia (Birchwood et al. 2000; Koreen et al. 1993). In patients with schizoaffective disorder, depressed type, symptoms of depression are present concurrently with psychosis for a substantial proportion of the total duration of the psychotic illness.

Other clinically significant depressive phenomena, such as dysphoria and demoralization, occur frequently in patients with schizophrenia (Iqbal et al. 2000; Siris 2000a). Dysphoria, which includes symptoms of depression and anxiety, may occur at any point in the illness and seems to be associated with psychosocial stress (C.C. Schwartz and Myers 1977) and positive symptoms (Lysaker et al. 1995). Demoralization, which occurs as patients struggle with their illness and its effect on their functioning (Siris 2000a), seems to be associated with high performance expectations and better insight into the illness, as well as with hopelessness, low self-esteem, and suicidal thoughts (Bartels and Drake 1988). Classic vegetative symptoms of depression may not be present in pa-

tients with demoralization and dysphoria (Bartels and Drake 1988). Some patients develop a sense of hopelessness, helplessness, and external locus of control, phenomena that Hoffman and colleagues (2000) found to be more powerful predictors of poor outcome in rehabilitation than depressive symptoms per se.

Symptoms of depression in patients with schizophrenia can be mistaken for negative symptoms, including affective flattening, alogia, avolition, apathy, anhedonia, and asociality (Birchwood et al. 2000; Sax et al. 1996; Siris 2000a), or for medication side effects, such as sedation, akinesia, and other extrapyramidal symptoms, particularly parkinsonism (Norman et al. 1998; Siris 1987). Although some authors suggest that depression may overlap with or worsen negative symptoms (Brebion et al. 2000; Siris et al. 1988), others suggest that no relation exists (Barnes et al. 1989; Baynes et al. 2000; Bottlender et al. 2000; Zisook et al. 1999) or that depressive symptoms early in the course of illness predict lower levels of negative symptoms later (Hafner et al. 1999; Oosthuizen et al. 2002). Key features of depression that distinguish it from negative symptoms include the presence of depressed mood, nondelusional guilt, and neurovegetative symptoms. By contrast, flat affect and anhedonic indifference without mood changes are more characteristic of negative symptoms than depression (Herbener and Harrow 2002; McGlashan and Carpenter 1976). Cognitive impairment, another relatively independent aspect of schizophrenia (Tamminga et al. 1998), has been shown to correlate with depressive symptoms and syndromes (Brebion et al. 1997, 2000; Holthausen et al. 1999).

Second-generation antipsychotic medications, now often considered the first line of treatment for schizophrenia psychosis, may improve depressive symptoms related to acute psychosis (Siris 2000a). Although published clinical trials of second-generation antipsychotics were not designed to assess the effect of antipsychotics on major depression in patients with schizophrenia, they have reported reductions in affective subscores derived from broad symptom measures, such as the Brief Psychiatric Rating Scale (BPRS). Five of these studies suggested that second-generation antipsychotics may be more effective than first-generation agents in treating acutely psychotic patients with schizophrenia and depression symptoms (Azorin 1995; Banov et al. 1994; Emsley et al. 2003; Marder et al. 1997; Tollefson et al. 1998). Additionally, Tollefson and colleagues (1997) reported that people taking olanzapine experienced greater reductions in a depression measure than did people taking haloperidol. By contrast, several studies reported that risperidone treatment does not improve symptoms of depression more than haloperidol (Moller et al. 1995; Peuskens 1995), and one study reported that haloperidol treatment results in more improvement than risperidone (Ceskova and Cvesta 1993).

The results of controlled studies of the adjunctive use of antidepressant medications with antipsychotics have been mixed: 9 of 17 studies reported improvement compared with placebo or a comparison medication, and 8 showed no advantage of adding an antidepressant to the medication treatment (D. Addington et al. 2002; Becker 1983; Dufresne et al. 1988; Hogarty et al. 1995; Johnson 1981; Kirli and Caliskan 1998; Kramer et al. 1989; Kurland and Nagaraju 1981; Mulholland et al. 2000; Muller-Siecheneder et al. 1998; Prusoff et al. 1979; Singh et al. 1978; Siris et al. 1987, 1989a, 1992; Vlokh et al. 2000; Waehrens and Gerlach 1980). Unfortunately, many of the studies of the addition of an antidepressant (e.g., tricyclic antidepressants, serotonin reuptake inhibitors, or bupropion) to the antipsychotic treatment regimen to treat depression in schizophrenia were limited by small sample size and consequently had low power.

Psychosocial interventions are effective for the treatment of depression in the general population but have not been carefully studied in patients with schizophrenia. Interventions that may be helpful include problem-solving training, coping skills training, cognitive therapy, exercise, family therapy, and support (Siris 1990, 2000b). For people who are demoralized and hopeless, interventions geared toward developing meaningful daytime activities can be helpful (Provencher et al. 2002).

The management of depressive symptoms in patients with schizophrenia depends on when such symptoms appear during the disorder as well as on their severity and their persistence. Treatment may include pharmacological and psychosocial interventions (Siris 2000b). For brief depressive reactions to stressful life events, supportive counseling and monitoring may be effective. If symptoms persist or are severe, further interventions should be considered. If patients are taking first-generation antipsychotic medications, symptoms should be carefully differentiated from neurological side effects, and a trial of dose reduction or a switch to a second-generation agent should be considered to reduce the side effects that can mimic depression (Hogarty et al. 1995). Because depressive symptoms may herald psychotic relapse, the patient should be monitored carefully for the emergence or exacerbation of psychosis. If the depression is part of a psychotic exacerbation, the antipsychotic medication should be increased or replaced with another agent in the hope that it will be more efficacious. If depressive symptoms persist or worsen in the absence of a psychotic exacerbation, use of an antidepressant medication or a switch to a second-generation antipsychotic medication can be considered. Clearly, further research is needed to establish effective interventions for depressive disorders in schizophrenia.

SUICIDE

PREVALENCE AND RISK FACTORS

Suicide is the leading cause of premature death in people with schizophrenia (Black et al. 1985; Osby et al. 2000). Nearly 50% of patients with schizophrenia attempt suicide, and their lifetime risk of death by suicide is close to 10% (Inskip et al. 1998; Tsuang et al. 1999), a rate 10-fold higher than in the general population (Baxter and Appleby 1999). Suicide in patients with schizophrenia has been associated with depression, anxiety, hopelessness, and a sense of failure (Bartels et al. 1992; Drake and Cotton 1986; Drake et al. 1985; Funahashi et al. 2000; Heila et al. 1997; Saarinen et al. 1999; Westermeyer et al. 1991). Drake and Cotton (1986) found that patients with schizophrenia who succeeded in a suicide attempt were more depressed and isolated than were those who did not succeed. Moreover, suicide can be a "nonpsychotic reaction to a severe illness" (Drake et al. 1985), a notion that is supported by data showing a relation between higher levels of awareness and increased suicide risk in these patients (Amador et al. 1996).

One of the strongest predictors of suicide in people with schizophrenia is a history of previous suicide attempts (Alleback et al. 1987; Burgess et al. 2000; Nordentoft et al. 2002; Rossau and Mortensen 1997; Roy 1982). As in the general population, men are at higher risk than women (Rossau and Mortensen 1997), and patients who attempt or commit suicide score higher on impulsivity scales (Dervaux et al. 2001). The risk of suicide is elevated for 3 months after discharge from a psychiatric hospitalization (Heila et al. 1999; Rossau and Mortensen 1997; Roy 1982), even in patients who were rated as "improved" during the hospitalization (Drake et al. 1986).

An earlier age at onset (Gupta et al. 1998) and poor overall functioning (Kaplan and Harrow 1996) are risk factors for suicide in patients with schizophrenia. The early phase and active phases of the illness (Baxter and Appleby 1999; Heila et al. 1997; Osby et al. 2000; Westermeyer et al. 1991) are times of increased risk, although suicide can occur throughout the course of the illness (Heila et al. 1997). Patients with prominent negative symptoms may have a somewhat reduced risk for suicide as compared with patients with mostly positive symptoms (Fenton et al. 1997). Recent stressful life events or losses are present in most cases of suicide (Funahashi et al. 2000; Heila et al. 1999; Saarinen et al. 1999). Although substance abuse is an established risk factor for suicide in the general population (Weiss and Hufford 1999), the evidence is mixed as to whether it is a risk factor among patients with schizophrenia (Alleback et al. 1987; Drake and

Cotton 1986; Gupta et al. 1998; Meltzer 2002). Impulsivity is higher in persons with schizophrenia and substance use disorder (Dervaux et al. 2001), which may account for some reports of increased risk for suicide in persons with comorbid schizophrenia and substance abuse (Funahashi et al. 2000; Gut-Fayand et al. 2001).

DETECTION AND MANAGEMENT

The detection of suicidal ideation and prevention of suicide in patients with schizophrenia can be difficult, in part because many suicide attempts are impulsive (Alleback et al. 1987; Gut-Fayand et al. 2001), but also because patients may use highly lethal methods (Breier and Astrachan 1984; Heila et al. 1997) and give no advance disclosure (Earle et al. 1994). Opportunities to intervene do exist, however. Most patients with schizophrenia who commit suicide have been seen by a health care professional within 3 months prior to committing suicide (Heila et al. 1997). Roy (1982) and colleagues reported that more than half of the psychiatric patients who had completed suicide had been seen the week before their suicide.

Harkavy-Friedman and Nelson (1997) suggested that both psychosocial and biological issues should be addressed carefully when working with schizophrenic patients presenting with suicidal thoughts or behavior. Listening and responding to the patient's reports of distress is crucial (Cohen et al. 1990). Burgess and colleagues (2000) pointed out that increasing the level of supervision and support, as well as ensuring continuity of care across systems, is essential for suicide prevention. Hospitalization can maintain safety with monitoring, structure, and support as well as provide an opportunity for intensive review and adjustment of psychopharmacological treatments to address symptoms of psychosis and depression. However, because discharge from the hospital can lead to social isolation, increased stress, and higher suicide risk (Drake et al. 1986), follow-up treatment and supports should be in place prior to discharge. When the patient is discharged, engagement into treatment should be assured; intensive outreach, such as with assertive community treatment, may be required to engage patients with schizophrenia (Burgess et al. 2000).

Adequate psychopharmacological treatment of psychosis is essential. In a study of 88 patients with schizophrenia who died by suicide, Heila et al. (1999) found that more than half either had been prescribed inadequate doses of antipsychotic medication or had not been compliant with treatment; and an additional 23% had been judged nonresponsive to medication treatment. Psychoeducation and close monitoring may increase compliance with pharmacological treatment. Studies suggest that clozapine may decrease suicidal ideation, suicide attempts, and suicide completion in persons with schizophrenia more effectively than first-generation antipsychotic medications (Meltzer and Okayli 1995; Reid et al. 1998; Walker et al. 1997). Moreover, Meltzer and colleagues (2003) found that clozapine was more effective in decreasing suicidality than olanzapine in a large international trial of high-risk patients.

Optimal treatment for patients with schizophrenia who are at risk for suicide includes careful assessment of risk factors for suicide, the use of active outreach to engage patients in treatment and reduce isolation, psychosocial rehabilitation and skills training to improve coping skills, and effective pharmacotherapy.

ANXIETY SYMPTOMS AND DISORDERS

Anxiety symptoms and disorders are common in patients with schizophrenia. For example, in a study of 80 consecutive inpatients with schizophrenia and schizoaffective disorder, 44% had a diagnosis of a co-occurring anxiety disorder (Cosoff and Hafner 1998), and in the National Comorbidity Study, 71% of the people in the community with schizophrenia had a co-occurring anxiety disorder (Kendler et al. 1996a). In diagnosing a co-occurring anxiety disorder, anxiety symptoms occurring during psychotic episodes must be differentiated from paranoia, reactions to delusions, and agitation related to psychosis. For example, Bayle and colleagues (2001) noted that panic attacks were related to paranoid ideas in patients with the paranoid subtype of schizophrenia. Additionally, anxiety must be differentiated from antipsychotic medication–induced side effects, such as akathisia, as well as other comorbid syndromes, such as substance-induced symptoms (e.g., cocaine intoxication or alcohol withdrawal) and depressive disorders (Zisook et al. 1999). Comorbid anxiety disorders in patients with schizophrenia tend to be underdiagnosed, and therefore undertreated, especially in ethnic or racial minorities (Dixon et al. 2001). Female gender, higher level of education, and marriage have been associated with diagnosis and treatment of anxiety and depressive disorders in patients with schizophrenia (Dixon et al. 2001).

In this section, we review the literature on panic, social phobia, trauma and PTSD, and obsessive-compulsive symptoms in patients with schizophrenia. Although three studies have noted that generalized anxiety disorder occurs in up to 31% of patients with schizophrenia (Cosoff and Hafner 1998; Kendler et al. 1996a; Tibbo et al. 2003), very little is known about this disorder in these patients, and it is not discussed further here.

PANIC ATTACKS AND PANIC DISORDER

Prevalence and Outcome

Up to 45% of patients with schizophrenia experience panic attacks (Argyle 1990; Bayle et al. 2001; Bermanzohn et al. 2000; Bland et al. 1987; Craig et al. 2002; Goodwin et al. 2002; Labbate et al. 1999; Moorey and Soni 1994; Tibbo et al. 2003). Full panic disorder, with recurring spontaneous panic attacks and associated disability, occurs in 6%–33% of schizophrenia patients (Argyle 1990; Bermanzohn et al. 2000; Cosoff and Hafner 1998; Kendler et al. 1996a; Labbate et al. 1999; Pallanti et al. 2004; Stratkowsky et al. 1993; Tibbo et al. 2003). The large National Comorbidity Study found that 26% of patients with schizophrenia had panic disorder (Kendler et al. 1996a). Panic symptoms and panic disorder can develop before, during, or after the onset of the psychotic disorder (Bayle et al. 2001; Craig et al. 2002).

A recent report showed a relation between psychoticism and panic in adolescents, suggesting that panic could be a part of the prodrome of schizophrenia (Goodwin et al. 2004). Patients with schizophrenia and co-occurring social phobia or depression also have been noted to have panic symptoms (Bermanzohn et al. 1997; Cutler and Siris 1991). Patients with schizophrenia and panic attacks are more likely to be female, Caucasian, and married as well as to have less education (Goodwin et al. 2002) compared with patients with schizophrenia who do not experience panic.

The effect of panic on the course of schizophrenia and its relation to positive symptoms of psychosis remain poorly understood. Panic has been associated with comorbid depression and suicidal ideation in patients with schizophrenia (Bermanzohn et al. 2000; Cutler and Siris 1991; Goodwin et al. 2002), as in patients with primary panic disorder in the general population (Ballenger 1998). Anxiety and panic can be seen as a reaction to psychotic symptoms, such as delusional fears (Bayle et al. 2001), but research reports conflict as to whether panic is associated with positive symptoms of psychosis (Craig et al. 2002; Cutler and Siris 1991).

Detection and Management

Patients with schizophrenia and panic experience the full spectrum of classic panic symptoms (Goodwin et al. 2002). Goodwin and colleagues (2002) reported that trembling, feelings of unreality, and fear of dying are particularly prominent symptoms. Although patients with schizophrenia and panic are more likely to seek mental health and medical treatment than are patients with schizophrenia who do not have panic symptoms (Goodwin et al.

2002), panic is dramatically underrecognized in these patients (Craig et al. 2002).

Cognitive-behavioral therapy (CBT) is effective for the treatment of panic disorder in the general population (Barlow et al. 2000) and has been modified for use in treating schizophrenia (Hofmann et al. 2000). In a small, uncontrolled pilot study of CBT for panic in patients with schizophrenia, Arlow and colleagues (1997) attempted a 16-week CBT program, including psychoeducation, cognitive restructuring, and in vivo exposure. They found that 73% of the patients were able to complete treatment; of those who completed the treatment, 75% experienced symptom improvement.

Although antipsychotic medications generally reduce anxiety (as measured by subscales of symptom rating measures, such as the Positive and Negative Syndrome Scale for Schizophrenia) (Marder et al. 1997), no studies have assessed the effect of antipsychotic medications on panic per se. Moreover, although antidepressants and benzodiazepines are effective medications for patients with primary panic disorder in the general population, no controlled studies have assessed their effectiveness for panic disorder in patients with schizophrenia. A report of two patients showed that panic symptoms that had not responded to antipsychotic medication did respond to imipramine augmentation of fluphenazine (Siris et al. 1989b). In one of these patients, the symptoms recurred after withdrawal of imipramine and then remitted once again with reinstitution of imipramine. In addition, two small studies showed that benzodiazepines reduced panic attacks in 10 patients with schizophrenia (Argyle 1990; Kahn et al. 1988), and psychotic symptoms improved as the panic improved. In 7 of the patients, the panic attacks recurred when the benzodiazepine was withdrawn (Kahn et al. 1988). Further research is needed to assess the effect of panic disorder on patients with schizophrenia and the effectiveness of treatments.

SOCIAL PHOBIA

Prevalence and Outcome

Many patients with schizophrenia have social anxiety and resulting social dysfunction (R.L. Morrison and Bellack 1987). A full social phobia syndrome was found in 15%–36% of small groups of patients with schizophrenia and schizoaffective disorders (Argyle 1990; Cosoff and Hafner 1998; Pallanti et al. 2004; Tibbo et al. 2003) and in 40% of the patients with schizophrenia in the National Comorbidity Study (Kendler et al. 1996a).

One study suggested that social phobia in patients with schizophrenia is associated with poor outcomes: Pallanti and colleagues (2004) found that patients with co-morbid social phobia had lower scores on social adjustment and quality of life, as well as more suicide attempts, although symptoms of psychosis were not different between schizophrenia patients with and without social phobia. Theoretically, social anxiety and avoidance could impede participation in individual or group-based rehabilitation, but no studies have prospectively assessed the effect of such symptoms on the course and outcome in schizophrenia. Additionally, although impairment in social function, one of the hallmarks of schizophrenia, is generally thought to be caused by deficits in cognitive processes and social perception (Penn et al. 1997), research has yet to assess the relation between social anxiety, cognition, and social perception in schizophrenia.

Detection and Management

Patients with schizophrenia and social anxiety show levels of social fear (Penn et al. 1994) and social phobia (Pallanti et al. 2004) similar to those in persons with primary social phobia. However, social anxiety and fear of social situations may be confused with the avoidance and withdrawal associated with psychotic symptoms (Pallanti et al. 2004; Penn et al. 1994) and must be carefully delineated from paranoia, withdrawal, and apathy. The key identifying features of social phobia are *fear of social situations* in which the individual might be scrutinized by others and *avoidance* of those situations or *endurance* of them only with intense anxiety. Evidence of embarrassment regarding scrutiny, rather than fear of persecution, will help identify patients with schizophrenia and social fear.

CBT, which usually includes education, cognitive restructuring, social skills training, and gradual exposure to feared social situations, is effective for patients with primary social phobia in the general population (Taylor 1996), but only one study thus far has tested a cognitive-behavioral group treatment program for schizophrenia patients with social phobia (Halperin et al. 2000). The authors reported that mean scores of social anxiety and depression improved in the treatment group as compared with the control group, suggesting that this intervention may be promising for patients with schizophrenia. Social skills training and other rehabilitation efforts for patients with schizophrenia and social anxiety should incorporate education and gradual exposure to feared social situations (Heinssen and Glass 1990; Penn et al. 1994).

Regarding pharmacological interventions, antipsychotics alone may not always be helpful. Pallanti and colleagues (1999) described 12 patients taking clozapine whose social phobia symptoms became clinically detectable when their psychosis remitted during clozapine treat-ment. The same group suggested that serotonin reuptake inhibitors, which are effective for the treatment of social phobia in the general population (Blanco et al. 2003), may be helpful for patients with schizophrenia and social phobia (Pallanti et al. 1999), but no controlled trials have been completed. Further studies are needed to assess the effect and interactions of social phobia on patients with schizophrenia, as well as to systematically test behavioral and pharmacological treatments.

TRAUMA AND POSTTRAUMATIC STRESS DISORDER

Prevalence and Outcome

Patients with schizophrenia experience high rates of childhood and adult trauma (e.g., physical or sexual assault). Lifetime trauma (during childhood or adulthood) is very common, reported by 85%–98% of the patients with schizophrenia (Gearon et al. 2003; Goodman et al. 1995, 2001; Hutchings and Dutton 1993; Jacobson and Richardson 1987; Mueser et al. 1998); approximately half (34%–65%) of the patients with schizophrenia report childhood physical or sexual abuse (Darves-Bornoz et al. 1995; Goodman et al. 2001; Greenfield et al. 1994; Ross et al. 1994). Sexual assault in both childhood and adulthood in patients with schizophrenia is reported more frequently by women than by men, but total lifetime rates of any assault do not differ between women and men (Goodman et al. 2001).

PTSD is classified in DSM-IV-TR (American Psychiatric Association 2000) as an anxiety disorder that includes three symptom clusters: reexperiencing of the trauma, avoidance of stimuli associated with the trauma, and persistent symptoms of hyperarousal. PTSD has been reported in 9% of the general population overall and in 20% of women and 8% of men who have experienced trauma (Kessler et al. 1995). Studies of patients with schizophrenia report higher rates of PTSD, ranging between 14% and 43% (Craine et al. 1988; Fenton 2001; Frame and Morrison 2001; Kendler et al. 1996a; Mueser et al. 1998, 2004; Neria et al. 2002), with most studies reporting a rate between 30% and 40%. Among patients with schizophrenia who have reported a history of trauma, 27%–66% develop PTSD (Craine et al. 1988; Gearon et al. 2003; Mueser et al. 1998; Neria et al. 2002). More trauma experiences and childhood sexual abuse are significant predictors of the development of PTSD in this group (Gearon et al. 2003; Mueser et al. 1998; Neria et al. 2002).

Like people in the general population, patients with schizophrenia who have experienced trauma report more symptoms of anxiety, depression, suicidality, and dissociation than do those who have not experienced trauma

(Goodman and Dutton 1996; Goodman et al. 1997; Priebe et al. 1998; Read and Argyle 1999; R.C. Schwartz and Cohen 2001). The evidence is mixed as to whether the presence or severity of PTSD symptoms worsens psychosis (Lysaker et al. 2001a; Priebe et al. 1998; Resnick et al. 2003). However, a history of trauma and PTSD is associated with worse role function (Lysaker et al. 2001b), substance abuse (Goodman et al. 2001; Neria et al. 2002), homelessness (Goodman et al. 2001), lower quality of life, and less employment (Priebe et al. 1998).

Most patients with schizophrenia who have experienced one trauma report experiencing multiple traumas (Gearon et al. 2003; Goodman et al. 1995, 2001). The effect of trauma seems to be additive in that a history of more trauma experiences and reports of recent trauma are associated with increased mood, anxiety, and psychotic symptoms (Goodman et al. 1997) and an increased likelihood of PTSD (Gearon et al. 2003; Mueser et al. 1998; Neria et al. 2002). Additionally, Swanson and colleagues (2002) found that when they controlled for other factors, the experience of recurrent violent victimization in combination with substance abuse and a currently violent environment accounted for 30% of the likelihood that a person with severe mental illness was recently violent.

Detection and Management

Because trauma and PTSD are so common in patients with schizophrenia and are associated with a variety of negative outcomes, clinicians should ask about trauma, assess the patient for the presence of PTSD symptoms, and address the symptoms and functional correlates of trauma and PTSD. Despite concerns to the contrary, people with severe mental illness appear able to report trauma and PTSD symptoms reliably (Goodman et al. 1999). As reviewed earlier, many patients with schizophrenia and a trauma history also experience symptoms of anxiety, depression, suicidality, dissociation, hostility, and somatization, as well as substance abuse and violent behavior (Goff et al. 1991; Goodman et al. 1997; Holowka et al. 2003; Read and Argyle 1999; R.C. Schwartz and Cohen 2001; Swanson et al. 2002).

People who have been traumatized benefit from additional services, including education about trauma and its sequelae, training and support to enhance their current safety, and assistance to secure safe housing (Harris 2003). Developing a therapeutic alliance with traumatized patients can be difficult because of the patient's severity of symptoms (including avoidance), lower self-esteem, and overall lower ability to trust (Goodman and Dutton 1996) and because patients may have already experienced negative responses when they previously reported their victimization experience (Marley and Buila 1999). Clinicians therefore should take care to be respectful and to assume a supportive stance when discussing trauma with patients. CBT is helpful for people with primary PTSD in the general population (Harvey et al. 2003) and is being adapted for patients with schizophrenia (Rosenberg et al. 2001b) but has not yet been studied. Although antidepressants reduce PTSD symptoms (Albucher and Liberzon 2002), these drugs have not been studied in patients with schizophrenia and co-occurring PTSD. Further research is necessary to clarify how trauma and PTSD affect the course and treatment of schizophrenia and to assess interventions to reduce PTSD symptoms and prevent or reduce the negative sequelae of trauma in patients with schizophrenia.

OBSESSIVE-COMPULSIVE DISORDER AND SYMPTOMS

Prevalence and Outcome

Symptoms of OCD are common in patients with schizophrenia. Obsessive-compulsive symptoms have been documented in up to 59% of schizophrenia patients (Bland et al. 1987; Cassano et al. 1998; Cosoff and Hafner 1998; Craig et al. 2002; Eisen et al. 1997; Fenton and McGlashan 1986; Tibbo et al. 2000), although most contemporary studies report obsessive-compulsive symptoms in 10%–26% of adolescent (Fabisch et al. 2001; Nechmad et al. 2003) and adult patients with schizophrenia (Berman et al. 1995a; Cassano et al. 1998; Craig et al. 2002). Full OCD with obsessions and compulsions not related to delusions has been documented in 4%–24% of inpatients and outpatients with schizophrenia (Cosoff and Hafner 1998; Craig et al. 2002; Eisen et al. 1997; Ohta et al. 2003; Pallanti et al. 2004; Poyurovsky et al. 2001), a rate clearly higher than the general population rate of approximately 1% (Horwath and Weissman 2000). Obsessive-compulsive symptoms may precede the onset of psychosis, begin at or after the onset of schizophrenia, or occur transiently over time (Craig et al. 2002; Hwang and Opler 2000). Obsessive-compulsive symptoms are important to identify because they may have prognostic significance and may respond to specialized treatments as discussed in the following subsection.

Although obsessions and compulsions in patients with schizophrenia are similar to those in patients without psychosis (e.g., contamination/washing, harm/checking) (Eisen et al. 1997; Fenton and McGlashan 1986; Ohta et al. 2003; Poyurovsky et al. 2001), distinguishing between delusions, preoccupations, and obsessions can be difficult in patients with thought disorders (Eisen et al. 1997).

Classically, *delusions* are described as fixed, false beliefs that are ego-syntonic and actively embraced by the patient, whereas *obsessions* are ego-dystonic and recognized as pathological intrusions (Hwang and Opler 2000). However, this distinction does not always hold true in clinical interviews of patients with primary OCD or in patients with psychosis. About 15% of the patients with primary OCD have poor insight (Attiullah et al. 2000; Marazziti et al. 2002); moreover, there appears to be a continuum of insight in patients with schizophrenia, and for some patients, obsessions and delusions may be overlapping (Bermanzohn et al. 1997).

Several studies suggested that obsessive-compulsive symptoms in patients with schizophrenia may be associated with poor outcomes. Patients with obsessive-compulsive symptoms tend to be more socially isolated, to be less treatment responsive, and to have longer hospitalizations than do patients without this symptom complex (Berman et al. 1995a; Fenton and McGlashan 1986; Hwang et al. 2000). Moreover, research suggests an association between obsessive-compulsive symptoms and poorer neurocognitive dysfunction in schizophrenia (Berman et al. 1998; Hwang and Opler 2000; Lysaker et al. 2000; Schmidtke et al. 1998), but research regarding psychotic symptoms is mixed. Three studies found that patients with schizophrenia and obsessive-compulsive symptoms have higher levels of psychotic symptoms (Hwang et al. 2000; Lysaker et al. 2000; Nechmad et al. 2003), whereas five studies found that patients with schizophrenia and obsessive-compulsive symptoms have levels of positive and negative symptoms similar to those in patients without obsessive-compulsive symptoms (Berman et al. 1998; Craig et al. 2002; Ohta et al. 2003; Poyurovsky et al. 1999a, 2001).

Because most studies of people with schizophrenia and co-occurring obsessive-compulsive symptoms do not indicate whether the obsessive-compulsive symptoms were adequately treated, it is unclear whether the poor prognosis, more severe symptoms, and cognitive dysfunction would persist if these patients received adequate psychopharmacological or behavioral treatments for their obsessive-compulsive symptoms. In addition, it is unclear whether the obsessive-compulsive symptoms are related causally to OCD or whether they represent characteristics of a distinct subtype of schizophrenia (Berman et al. 1999). Craig and colleagues (2002) noted that obsessive-compulsive comorbidity is as common among patients with schizophrenia as among patients with bipolar or depressive disorders, suggesting that OCD could be a separate comorbid condition unrelated to schizophrenia per se.

Obsessive-compulsive symptoms in persons with schizophrenia may have heterogeneous causes. Some authors have suggested that a supersensitivity of serotonin receptors may occur during antipsychotic treatment, causing transient obsessive-compulsive symptoms (Baker et al. 1992; Kopala and Honer 1994; D. Morrison et al. 1998; Poyurovsky et al. 1996, 1998), although this phenomenon has not been shown in a controlled trial (Baker et al. 1996), and other case reports show the development of obsessive-compulsive symptoms after abrupt clozapine withdrawal and resolution of obsessive-compulsive symptoms with reinitiation of clozapine (Poyurovsky et al. 1998). Furthermore, several studies found that obsessive-compulsive symptoms predated psychotic symptoms in more than half of the patients with co-occurring obsessive-compulsive symptoms and schizophrenia (Craig et al. 2002; Hwang and Opler 2000; Ohta et al. 2003). Further research is needed to understand the cause and effect of OCD on patients with schizophrenia.

Detection and Management

Although the types of obsessions and compulsions experienced by patients with schizophrenia are similar to those found in classic OCD—contamination obsessions, handwashing rituals, and counting and checking compulsions (Tibbo et al. 2000)—obsessive-compulsive symptoms are typically underdiagnosed and undertreated (Craig et al. 2002). Most contemporary studies have reliably used the Yale-Brown Obsessive Compulsive Scale (Goodman et al. 1989) to detect the obsessive-compulsive symptoms in these patients.

First-generation antipsychotic medications used alone appear to be ineffective in the treatment of obsessive-compulsive symptoms in patients with schizophrenia (Poyurovsky et al. 2000), although serotonin reuptake inhibitors added adjunctively to first-generation antipsychotics may be effective (Berman et al. 1995b). A review (Chang and Berman 1999) of several small (and mostly open-label) trials that used adjunctive clomipramine, imipramine, or fluoxetine reported that 67% of the patients showed improvement in obsessive-compulsive symptoms with no worsening of psychosis, whereas 19% showed worsening of psychosis. Similar results were found in a 12-week case series of 10 patients who received fluvoxamine augmentation (Poyurovsky et al. 1999b). In a small double-blind, crossover study comparing adjunctive clomipramine with placebo, Berman and colleagues (1995b) showed that clomipramine augmentation of first-generation antipsychotics was superior to placebo augmentation for reducing obsessions and compulsions, and overall symptoms of psychosis improved as well.

Although second-generation antipsychotic medications are used to augment serotonin reuptake inhibitors for treatment-refractory primary OCD in the general population (Mohr et al. 2002; Pfanner et al. 2000), research regarding the use of second-generation antipsychotic medications alone in patients with schizophrenia and obsessive-compulsive symptoms is limited (Fenton 2001). Although one report suggested that the second-generation antipsychotic risperidone may enhance treatment response (McDougle et al. 2000), other reports suggested that second-generation antipsychotic medications occasionally increase obsessive-compulsive symptoms (Patel et al. 1997; Strous et al. 1999a). Serotonin reuptake inhibitors used in combination with second-generation antipsychotics have been reported to reduce obsessive-compulsive symptoms in case reports of patients with schizophrenia (Patel et al. 1997; Poyurovsky et al. 2003; Strous et al. 1999b). If the addition of one serotonin reuptake inhibitor is not effective, another may be tried (Poyurovsky et al. 2003). Because some serotonin reuptake inhibitors can increase levels of some antipsychotics in the blood as a result of a decreased rate of antipsychotic metabolism, this combination should be used carefully. Controlled trials are needed to assess the effect of both second-generation antipsychotic medications and adjunctive serotonin reuptake inhibitors for obsessive-compulsive symptoms in schizophrenia.

CBT, composed of systematic exposure to obsessions and response (compulsion) prevention, is effective for the treatment of primary OCD in the general population (van Balkom et al. 1998) but has not been systematically studied in patients with schizophrenia and co-occurring obsessive-compulsive symptoms. The potential value of CBT in patients with schizophrenia may be influenced by each individual's level of cognitive function and insight (Goff 1999). More research is necessary to clarify the clinical correlates, prognostic significance, and optimal treatment strategies for obsessive-compulsive symptoms and OCD in patients with schizophrenia.

CONCLUSION

Co-occurring disorders, such as substance abuse, major depression, and anxiety disorders, are common in patients with schizophrenia and are associated with a more difficult course of illness. These co-occurring disorders can be reliably identified, if clinicians look for them. Treatment protocols for some co-occurring disorders have been established, while for others further study will be required to define best practice guidelines. As a general rule, however, identification of these co-occurring disorders and integration of specific pharmacological and psychosocial interventions for them within schizophrenia treatment programs will be essential if clinical outcomes for patients with schizophrenia are to be improved.

REFERENCES

Addington D, Addington J, Patten S: Gender and affect in schizophrenia. Can J Psychiatry 41:265–268, 1996

Addington D, Addington J, Patten S, et al: Double-blind, placebo-controlled comparison of the efficacy of sertraline as treatment for a major depressive episode in patients with remitted schizophrenia. J Clin Psychopharmacol 22:20–25, 2002

Addington J, Addington D: Effect of substance misuse in early psychosis. Br J Psychiatry Suppl 172:134–136, 1998

Addington J, Addington D: Impact of an early psychosis program on substance use. Psychiatr Rehabil J 25(1):60–67, 2001

Addington J, Leriger E, Addington D: Symptom outcome 1 year after admission to an early psychosis program. Can J Psychiatry 48:204–207, 2003

Albanese MJ: Safety and efficacy of risperidone in substance abusers with psychosis. Am J Addict 10:190–191, 2001

Albucher RC, Liberzon I: Psychopharmacological treatment in PTSD: a critical review. J Psychiatr Res 36:355–367, 2002

Alleback P, Varla A, Kristjansson E, et al: Risk factors for suicide among patients with schizophrenia. Acta Psychiatr Scand 76:414–419, 1987

Amador XF, Friedman JH, Kasapis C, et al: Suicidal behavior in schizophrenia and its relationship to awareness of illness. Am J Psychiatry 153:1185–1188, 1996

American Psychiatric Association: Diagnostic and Statistical Manual of Mental Disorders, 4th Edition, Text Revision. Washington, DC, American Psychiatric Association, 2000

Ananth J, Vandewater S, Kamal M, et al: Missed diagnosis of substance abuse in psychiatric patients. Hosp Community Psychiatry 40:297–299, 1989

Argyle N: Panic attacks in chronic schizophrenia. Br J Psychiatry 157:430–433, 1990

Arlow PB, Moran ME, Bermanzohn PC, et al: Cognitive-behavioral treatment of panic attacks in chronic schizophrenia. J Psychother Pract Res 6:145–150, 1997

Attiullah N, Eisen JL, Rasmussen SA: Clinical features of obsessive-compulsive disorder. Psychiatr Clin North Am 23:469–491, 2000

Azorin JM: Long term treatment of mood disorders in schizophrenia. Acta Psychiatr Scand 91 (suppl):20–23, 1995

Baker RW, Chengappa KN, Baird JW, et al: Emergence of obsessive compulsive symptoms during treatment with clozapine. J Clin Psychiatry 53:439–442, 1992

Baker RW, Ames D, Umbricht DS, et al: Obsessive-compulsive symptoms in schizophrenia: a comparison of olanzapine and placebo. Psychopharmacol Bull 32:89–93, 1996

Ballenger JC: Comorbidity of panic and depression: implications for clinical management. Int Clin Psychopharmacol 13 (suppl 4):S13–S17, 1998

Banov MD, Zarate CA, Tohen M, et al: Clozapine therapy in refractory affective disorders: polarity predicts response in long-term follow-up. J Clin Psychiatry 55:295–300, 1994

Barlow DH, Gorman JM, Shear MK, et al: Cognitive-behavioral therapy, imipramine, or their combination for panic disorder: a randomized controlled trial. JAMA 283:2529–2536, 2000

Barnes T, Curson DA, Liddle PF, et al: The nature and prevalence of depression in chronic schizophrenic in-patients. Br J Psychiatry 154:486–491, 1989

Barrowclough C, Haddock G, Tarrier N, et al: Randomized controlled trial of motivational interviewing, cognitive behavior therapy, and family intervention for patients with comorbid schizophrenia and substance use disorders. Am J Psychiatry 158:1706–1713, 2001

Bartels SJ, Drake RE: Depressive symptoms in schizophrenia: comprehensive differential diagnosis. Compr Psychiatry 29:467–483, 1988

Bartels SJ, Drake RE, McHugo GJ: Alcohol abuse, depression, and suicidal behavior in schizophrenia. Am J Psychiatry 149:394–395, 1992

Baxter D, Appleby L: Case register study of suicide risk in mental disorders. Br J Psychiatry 175:322–326, 1999

Bayle F, Krebs M, Epelbaum C, et al: Clinical features of panic attacks in schizophrenia. Eur Psychiatry 16:349–353, 2001

Baynes D, Mulholland C, Cooper SJ, et al: Depressive symptoms in stable chronic schizophrenia: prevalence and relationship to psychopathology and treatment. Schizophr Res 45:47–56, 2000

Becker RE: Implications of the efficacy of thiothixene and a chlorpromazine-imipramine combination for depression in schizophrenia. Am J Psychiatry 140:208–211, 1983

Berman I, Kalinowski A, Berman SM, et al: Obsessive and compulsive symptoms in chronic schizophrenia. Compr Psychiatry 36:6–10, 1995a

Berman I, Sapers BL, Chang HH, et al: Treatment of obsessive-compulsive symptoms in schizophrenic patients with clomipramine. J Clin Psychopharmacol 15:206–210, 1995b

Berman I, Merson A, Viegner B, et al: Obsessions and compulsions as a distinct cluster of symptoms: schizophrenia: a neuropsychological study. J Nerv Ment Dis 186:150–156, 1998

Berman I, Chang HH, Klegon DA: Obsessive-compulsive symptoms in schizophrenia: neuropsychological perspectives. Psychiatr Ann 29:525–528, 1999

Bermanzohn PC, Porto L, Arlow PB, et al: Obsessions and delusions: separate and distinct or overlapping? CNS Spectr 2:58–61, 1997

Bermanzohn PC, Porto L, Arlow PB, et al: Hierarchical diagnosis in chronic schizophrenia: a clinical study of co-occurring syndromes. Schizophr Bull 26:517–525, 2000

Bidaut-Russell M, Bradford SE, Smith EM: Prevalence of mental illnesses in adult offspring of alcoholic mothers. Drug Alcohol Depend 35:81–90, 1994

Birchwood M, Iqbal Z, Chadwick P, et al: Cognitive approach to depression and suicidal thinking in psychosis, 1: ontogeny of post-psychotic depression. Br J Psychiatry 177:516–521, 2000

Black DW, Warrack G, Winokur G: The Iowa record-linkage study, I: suicides and accidental deaths among psychiatric patients. Arch Gen Psychiatry 42:71–75, 1985

Blanco C, Schneier FR, Schmidt A, et al: Pharmacological treatment of social anxiety disorder: a meta-analysis. Depress Anxiety 18:29–40, 2003

Bland RC, Newman SC, Orn H: Schizophrenia: lifetime comorbidity in a community sample. Acta Psychiatr Scand 75:383–391, 1987

Blankertz LE, Cnaan RA: Assessing the impact of two residential programs for dually diagnosed homeless individuals. Soc Serv Rev 68:536–560, 1994

Bottlender R, Straub A, Moller HJ: Prevalence and background factors of depression in first admitted schizophrenic patients. Acta Psychiatr Scand 101:153–160, 2000

Boye B, Bentsen H, Ulstein I, et al: Relatives' distress and patients' symptoms and behaviours: a prospective study of patients with schizophrenia and their relatives. Acta Psychiatr Scand 104:42–50, 2001

Brady K, Anton R, Ballenger JC, et al: Cocaine abuse among schizophrenic patients. Am J Psychiatry 147:1164–1167, 1990

Brebion G, Smith M, Amador XF, et al: Clinical correlates of memory in schizophrenia: differential links between depression, positive and negative symptoms, and two types of memory impairment. Am J Psychiatry 154:1538–1543, 1997

Brebion G, Amador XF, Smith M, et al: Depression, psychomotor retardation, negative symptoms, and memory in schizophrenia. Neuropsychiatry Neuropsychol Behav Neurol 13:177–183, 2000

Breier A, Astrachan BM: Characterization of schizophrenic patients who commit suicide. Am J Psychiatry 141:206–209, 1984

Brown ES, Nejtek VA, Perantie DC, et al: Quetiapine in bipolar disorder and cocaine dependence. Bipolar Disord 4:406–411, 2002

Brunette M, Mueser KT, Drake RE, et al: Relationships between symptoms of schizophrenia and substance abuse. J Nerv Ment Dis 185:13–20, 1997

Brunette MF, Drake RE, Lynde D, et al: Toolkit for Integrated Dual Disorders Treatment. Rockville, MD, Substance Abuse and Mental Health Services Administration, 2002

Brunette M, Noordsy DL, Xie H, et al: Benzodiazepine use and abuse among patients with severe mental illness and co-occurring substance use disorders. Psychiatr Serv 54:1395–1401, 2003

Buchanan RW, Strauss ME, Breier A, et al: Attentional impairments in deficit and nondeficit forms of schizophrenia. Am J Psychiatry 154:363–370, 1997

Buckley P, Thompson P, Way L, et al: Substance abuse among patients with treatment-resistant schizophrenia: characteristics and implications for clozapine therapy. Am J Psychiatry 151:385–389, 1994

Buckley P, McCarthy M, Chapman P, et al: Clozapine treatment of comorbid substance abuse in patients with schizophrenia (abstract). Schizophr Res 36:272, 1999

Burgess P, Pirkis J, Morton J, et al: Lessons from a comprehensive clinical audit of users of psychiatric services who committed suicide. Psychiatr Serv 51:1555–1560, 2000

Carlsson A: The current status of the dopamine hypothesis of schizophrenia. Neuropsychopharmacology 1:179–186, 1988

Cassano GB, Pini S, Saettoni M, et al: Occurrence and clinical correlates of psychiatric comorbidity in patients with psychotic disorders. J Clin Psychiatry 59:60–68, 1998

Centers for Disease Control: Cigarette smoking among adults—United States, 2002. Morb Mortal Weekly Rep 53(20):428–431, 2004

Ceskova E, Cvesta J: Double-blind comparison of risperidone and haloperidol in schizophrenia and schizoaffective psychosis. Psychopharmacopsychiatry 26:121–124, 1993

Chambers RA, Self DW: Motivational responses to natural and drug rewards in rats with neonatal ventral hippocampal lesions: an animal model of dual diagnosis schizophrenia. Neuropsychopharmacology 2:889–905, 2002

Chambers RA, Krystal JH, Self DW: A neurobiological basis for substance abuse comorbidity in schizophrenia. Biol Psychiatry 50:71–83, 2001

Chang HH, Berman I: Treatment issues for patients with schizophrenia who have obsessive-compulsive symptoms. Psychiatr Ann 29:529–535, 1999

Clark RE, Xie H, Brunette MF: Benzodiazepine prescription practices and substance abuse in persons with severe mental illness. J Clin Psychiatry 65:151–155, 2004

Cohen LJ, Test MA, Brown RL: Suicide and schizophrenia: data from a prospective community treatment study [published erratum appears in Am J Psychiatry 147:1110]. Am J Psychiatry 147:602–607, 1990

Cosoff S, Hafner RJ: The prevalence of comorbid anxiety in schizophrenia, schizoaffective disorder and bipolar disorder. Aust N Z J Psychiatry 32:67–72, 1998

Craig T, Hwang MY, Bromet EJ: Obsessive-compulsive and panic symptoms in patients with first-admission psychosis. Am J Psychiatry 159:592–598, 2002

Craine L, Henson C, Colliver J, et al: Prevalence of a history of sexual abuse among female psychiatric patients in a state hospital system. Hosp Community Psychiatry 39:300–304, 1988

Cutler JL, Siris SG: "Panic-like" symptomatology in schizophrenic and schizoaffective patients with postpsychotic depression: observations and implications. Compr Psychiatry 32:465–473, 1991

Dalack GW, Healy DJ, Meador-Woodruff JH: Nicotine dependence in schizophrenia: clinical phenomena and laboratory findings. Am J Psychiatry 155:1490–1501, 1998

Darves-Bornoz J, Lemperiere T, Degiovanni A, et al: Sexual victimization in women with schizophrenia and bipolar disorder. Soc Psychiatry Psychiatr Epidemiol 30:78–84, 1995

Deganhardt L, Hall W, Lynskey M: Testing hypotheses about the relationship between cannabis use and psychosis. Drug Alcohol Depend 71:37–48, 2003

Delahanty J, Ram R, Postrado L, et al: Differences in rates of depression in schizophrenia by race. Schizophr Bull 27:29–38, 2001

Dervaux A, Bayle F, Laqueille X, et al: Is substance abuse in schizophrenia related to impulsivity, sensation seeking, or anhedonia? Am J Psychiatry 158:492–494, 2001

Dixon L, Green-Paden L, Delahanty J, et al: Variables associated with disparities in treatment of patients with schizophrenia and comorbid mood and anxiety disorders. Psychiatr Serv 52:1216–1222, 2001

Dougherty RJ: Naltrexone in the treatment of alcohol dependent dual diagnosed patients (abstract). J Addict Dis 16:107, 1997

Drake RE, Cotton PG: Depression, hopelessness and suicide in chronic schizophrenia. Br J Psychiatry 148:554–559, 1986

Drake RE, Mueser KT: Alcohol-use disorder and severe mental illness. Alcohol Health Res World 20:87–93, 1996

Drake RE, Wallach MA: Moderate drinking among people with severe mental illness. Hosp Community Psychiatry 44:780–782, 1993

Drake RE, Gates C, Whitaker A, et al: Suicide among schizophrenics: a review. Compr Psychiatry 26:90–100, 1985

Drake RE, Gates C, Cotton PG: Suicide among schizophrenics: a comparison of attempters and completed suicides. Br J Psychiatry 149:784–787, 1986

Drake RE, Osher FC, Wallach MA: Alcohol use and abuse in schizophrenia: a prospective community study. J Nerv Ment Dis 177:408–414, 1989

Drake RE, McHugo GJ, Clark RE, et al: Assertive community treatment for patients with co-occurring severe mental illness and substance use disorder: a clinical trial. Am J Orthopsychiatry 68:201–215, 1998

Drake RE, Xie H, McHugo GJ, et al: The effects of clozapine on alcohol and drug use disorders among schizophrenic patients. Schizophr Bull 26:441–449, 2000

Drake RE, Essock SM, Shaner A, et al: Implementing dual diagnosis services for clients with severe mental illness. Psychiatr Serv 52:469–472, 2001

Drake RE, Mueser KT, Brunette MF, et al: A review of treatments for people with severe mental illnesses and co-occurring substance use disorders. Psychiatr Rehabil J 27:360–374, 2004

Dufresne RL, Kass DJ, Becker RE: Bupropion and thiothixene versus placebo and thiothixene in the treatment of depression in schizophrenia. Drug Dev Res 12:259–266, 1988

Earle KA, Forquer SL, Volo AM, et al: Characteristics of outpatient suicides. Hosp Community Psychiatry 45:123–126, 1994

Egan MF, Goldberg TE, Kolachana BS, et al: Effect of COMT Val 108/158 Met genotype on frontal lobe function and risk for schizophrenia. Proc Natl Acad Sci U S A 98:6917–6922, 2001

Eisen JL, Beer DA, Pato MT, et al: Obsessive-compulsive disorder in patients with schizophrenia or schizoaffective disorder. Am J Psychiatry 154:271–273, 1997

Elk R, Dickman BJ, Teggin AF: Depression in schizophrenia: a study of prevalence and treatment. Br J Psychiatry 149:228–229, 1986

Emsley R, Oosthuizen P, Joubert A, et al: Depressive and anxiety symptoms in patients with schizophrenia and schizophreniform disorder. J Clin Psychiatry 60:747–751, 1999

Emsley R, Buckley P, Jones AM, et al: Differential effect of quetiapine on depressive symptoms in patients with partially responsive schizophrenia. J Psychopharmacol (Oxf) 17:210–215, 2003

Evins AE, Mays VK, Rigotti NA, et al: A pilot trial of bupropion added to cognitive behavioral therapy for smoking cessation in schizophrenia. Nicotine Tob Res 3:397–403, 2001

Fabisch K, Fabish H, Langs G, et al: Incidence of obsessive-compulsive phenomena in the course of acute schizophrenia and schizoaffective disorder. Eur Psychiatry 16:336–341, 2001

Fadda F, Mosca E, Colombo G, et al: Effects of spontaneous ingestion of ethanol on brain dopamine metabolism. Life Sci 44:281–287, 1989

Fenton WS: Comorbid conditions in schizophrenia. Curr Opin Psychiatry 14:17–23, 2001

Fenton WS, McGlashan TH: The prognostic significance of obsessive-compulsive symptoms in schizophrenia. Am J Psychiatry 143:437–441, 1986

Fenton WS, McGlashan TH, Victor BJ, et al: Symptoms, subtype, and suicidality in patients with schizophrenia spectrum disorders. Am J Psychiatry 154:199–204, 1997

Frame L, Morrison AP: Causes of posttraumatic stress disorder in psychotic patients. Arch Gen Psychiatry 58:305–306, 2001

Funahashi TM, Ibuki YM, Domon YM, et al: A clinical study on suicide among schizophrenics. Psychiatry Clin Neurosci 54:173–179, 2000

Gearon JS, Kaltman SI, Brown C, et al: Traumatic life events and PTSD among women with substance use disorders and schizophrenia. Psychiatr Serv 54:523–528, 2003

George TP, Sernyak MJ, Ziedonis D, et al: Effects of clozapine on smoking in chronic schizophrenic outpatients. J Clin Psychiatry 57:4–11, 1996

George TP, Ziedonis DM, Feingold A, et al: Nicotine transdermal patch and atypical antipsychotic medications for smoking cessation in schizophrenia. Am J Psychiatry 157:1835–1842, 2000

George TP, Vessicchio JC, Termine A, et al: A placebo controlled trial of bupropion for smoking cessation in schizophrenia. Biol Psychiatry 52:53–61, 2002

Glynn SH, Sussman S: Why patients smoke. Hosp Community Psychiatry 41:1027–1028, 1990

Goeders NE, Smith JE: Reinforcing properties of cocaine in the medial prefrontal cortex: primary action on presynaptic dopaminergic terminals. Pharmacol Biochem Behav 25:191–199, 1986

Goff DC: The comorbidity of obsessive-compulsive disorder and schizophrenia. Psychiatr Ann 29:533–536, 1999

Goff DC, Brotman AW, Kindlon D, et al: The delusion of possession in chronically psychotic patients. J Nerv Ment Dis 179:567–571, 1991

Goodman LA, Dutton MA: The relationship between victimization and cognitive schemata among episodically homeless, seriously mentally ill women. Violence Vict 11:159–174, 1996

Goodman WK, Price LH, Rasmussen SA, et al: The Yale-Brown Obsessive Compulsive Scale: development, use, and reliability. Arch Gen Psychiatry 46:1006–1011, 1989

Goodman LA, Dutton MA, Harris M: Episodically homeless women with serious mental illness: prevalence of physical and sexual assault. Am J Orthopsychiatry 65:468–478, 1995

Goodman LA, Dutton MA, Harris M: The relationship between violence dimensions and symptom severity among homeless, mentally ill women. J Trauma Stress 10:51–70, 1997

Goodman LA, Thompson KM, Weinfurt K, et al: Reliability of reports of violent victimization and posttraumatic stress disorder among men and women with serious mental illness. J Trauma Stress 12:587–599, 1999

Goodman LA, Salyers MP, Mueser KT, et al: Recent victimization in women and men with severe mental illness: prevalence and correlates. J Trauma Stress 14:615–632, 2001

Goodwin R, Lyons J, McNally R: Panic attacks in schizophrenia. Schizophr Res 58:213–220, 2002

Goodwin R, Fergusson DM, Horwood LJ: Panic attacks and psychoticism. Am J Psychiatry 161:88–92, 2004

Green AI, Zimmet SV, Strous RD, et al: Clozapine for comorbid substance use disorder and schizophrenia: do patients with schizophrenia have a reward-deficiency syndrome that can be ameliorated by clozapine? Harv Rev Psychiatry 6:287–296, 1999

Green AI, Salomon MS, Brenner MJ, et al: Treatment of schizophrenia and comorbid substance use disorder. Curr Drug Targets CNS Neurol Disord 1:129–139, 2002

Green AI, Burgess ES, Zimmet SV, et al: Alcohol and cannabis use in schizophrenia: effects of clozapine and risperidone. Schizophr Res 60:81–85, 2003

Green AI, Tohen M, Hamer RM, et al: First episode schizophrenia-related psychosis and substance use disorders: acute response to olanzapine and haloperidol. Schizophr Res 66:125–135, 2004

Greenfield SF, Strakowski SM, Tohen M, et al: Childhood abuse in first-episode psychosis. Br J Psychiatry 164:831–834, 1994

Grossman MH, Emanuel BS, Budarf ML: Chromosomal mapping of the human catechol-O-methyl transferase gene to 22q11.1-q112. Genomics 12:822–825, 1992

Gupta S, Black DW, Arndt S, et al: Factors associated with suicide attempts among patients with schizophrenia. Psychiatr Serv 49:1353–1355, 1998

Gut-Fayand A, Dervaux A, Olie J, et al: Substance abuse and suicidality in schizophrenia: a common risk factor linked to impulsivity. Psychiatry Res 102:65–72, 2001

Hafner H, Loffler W, Maurer K, et al: Depression, negative symptoms, social stagnation and social decline in the early course of schizophrenia. Acta Psychiatr Scand 100:105–118, 1999

Halperin S, Nathan P, Drummond P, et al: A cognitive-behavioural, group-based intervention for social anxiety in schizophrenia. Aust N Z J Psychiatry 34:809–813, 2000

Hamera E, Schneider JK, Stanley S: Alcohol, cannabis, nicotine, and caffeine use and symptoms distress in schizophrenia. J Nerv Ment Dis 183:559–565, 1995

Harkavy-Friedman JM, Nelson E: Management of the suicidal patient with schizophrenia. Psychiatr Clin North Am 20:625–640, 1997

Harris M: Modifications in service delivery and clinical treatment for women diagnosed with severe mental illness who are also the survivors of sexual abuse trauma. J Ment Health Adm 21:397–406, 2003

Harvey AG, Bryant RA, Tarrier N: Cognitive behaviour therapy for posttraumatic stress disorder. Clin Psychol Rev 23:501–522, 2003

Heila H, Isometsa ET, Henriksson MM, et al: Suicide and schizophrenia: a nationwide psychological autopsy study on age- and sex-specific clinical characteristics of 92 suicide victims with schizophrenia. Am J Psychiatry 154:1235–1242, 1997

Heila H, Isometsa ET, Henriksson MM, et al: Suicide victims with schizophrenia in different treatment phases and adequacy of antipsychotic medication. J Clin Psychiatry 60:200–208, 1999

Heinssen RKJ, Glass CR: Social skills, social anxiety, and cognitive factors in schizophrenia, in Handbook of Social and Evaluation Anxiety. Edited by Leitenberg H. New York, Plenum, 1990, pp 325–355

Herbener ES, Harrow M: The course of anhedonia during 10 years of schizophrenic illness. J Abnorm Psychol 111:237–248, 2002

Hoffmann H, Kupper Z, Kunz B: Hopelessness and its impact on rehabilitation outcome in schizophrenia: an exploratory study. Schizophr Res 43:147–158, 2000

Hofmann SG, Bufka LF, Brady KM, et al: Cognitive-behavioral treatment of panic in patients with schizophrenia: preliminary findings. Journal of Cognitive Psychotherapy 14:27–37, 2000

Hogarty GE, McEvoy JP, Ulrich RF, et al: Pharmacotherapy of impaired affect in recovering schizophrenic patients. Arch Gen Psychiatry 52:29–41, 1995

Holowka DW, King S, Saheb D, et al: Childhood abuse and dissociative symptoms in adult schizophrenia. Schizophr Res 60:87–90, 2003

Holthausen E, Wiersma D, Knegtering R, et al: Psychopathology and cognition in schizophrenia spectrum disorders: the role of depressive symptoms. Schizophr Res 39:65–71, 1999

Horwath E, Weissman M: The epidemiology and cross-national presentation of obsessive-compulsive disorder. Psychiatr Clin North Am 23:493–507, 2000

Hughes JR, Hatsukami DK, Mitchell JE, et al: Prevalence of smoking among schizophrenic outpatients. Am J Psychiatry 143:993–997, 1986

Hurlburt MS, Hough RL, Wood PA: Effects of substance abuse on housing stability of homeless mentally ill persons in supported housing. Psychiatr Serv 47:731–736, 1996

Hutchings PS, Dutton MA: Sexual assault history in a community mental health center clinical population. Community Ment Health J 29:59–63, 1993

Hwang MY, Opler LA: Management of schizophrenia with obsessive-compulsive disorder. Psychiatr Ann 30:23–28, 2000

Hwang MY, Morgan JE, Losconzey MF: Clinical and neuropsychological profiles of obsessive-compulsive schizophrenia: a pilot study. J Neuropsychiatry Clin Neurosci 12:91–94, 2000

Inskip HM, Harris EC, Barraclough B: Lifetime risk of suicide for affective disorder, alcoholism and schizophrenia. Br J Psychiatry 172:35–37, 1998

Iqbal Z, Birchwood M, Chadwick P, et al: Cognitive approach to depression and suicidal thinking in psychosis, 2: testing the validity of a social ranking model. Br J Psychiatry 177:522–528, 2000

Jacobson A, Richardson B: Assault experiences of 100 psychiatric inpatients: evidence of the need for routine inquiry. Am J Psychiatry 144:508–513, 1987

Jin H, Zisook S, Palmer BW, et al: Association of depressive symptoms with worse functioning in schizophrenia: a study in older outpatients. J Clin Psychiatry 62:797–803, 2001

Johnson DA: Depressions in schizophrenia: some observations on prevalence, etiology, and treatment. Acta Psychiatr Scand Suppl 291:137–144, 1981

Jones P, Cannon M: The new epidemiology of schizophrenia. Psychiatr Clin North Am 21:1–25, 1998

Kahn JP, Puertollano MA, Schane MD, et al: Adjunctive alprazolam for schizophrenia with panic anxiety: clinical observation and pathogenetic implications. Am J Psychiatry 145:742–744, 1988

Kaplan KJ, Harrow M: Positive and negative symptoms as risk factors for later suicidal activity in schizophrenics versus depressives. Suicide Life Threat Behav 26:105–121, 1996

Kavanagh DJ, Waghorn G, Jenner L, et al: Demographic and clinical correlates of comorbid substance use disorders in psychosis: multivariate analyses from an epidemiologic sample. Schizophr Res 66:115–124, 2004

Kendler KS: A twin study of individuals with both schizophrenia and alcoholism. Br J Psychiatry 147:48–53, 1985

Kendler KS, Masterson CC, Davis KL: Psychiatric illness in first-degree relatives of patients with paranoid psychosis, schizophrenia and medical illness. Br J Psychiatry 147:524–531, 1985

Kendler KS, Gallagher TJ, Abelson JM, et al: Lifetime prevalence, demographic risk factors, and diagnostic validity of nonaffective psychosis as assessed in a US community sample: the national comorbidity survey. Arch Gen Psychiatry 53:1022–1031, 1996a

Kendler KS, Karkowski-Shuman L, Walsh D: The risk for psychiatric illness in siblings of schizophrenics: the impact of psychotic and non-psychotic affective illness and alcoholism in parents. Acta Psychiatr Scand 94:49–55, 1996b

Kendler KS, O'Neill FA, Burke J, et al: Irish study on high-density schizophrenia families: field methods and power to detect linkage. Am J Med Genet 67:179–190, 1996c

Kessler RC, Sonnega A, Bromet EJ, et al: Posttraumatic stress disorder in the National Comorbidity Survey. Arch Gen Psychiatry 52:1048–1060, 1995

Khantzian EJ: The self-medication hypothesis of substance use disorders: a reconsideration and recent applications. Harv Rev Psychiatry 4:231–244, 1997

Kingsbury SJ, Salzman C: Disulfiram in the treatment of alcoholic patients with schizophrenia. Hosp Community Psychiatry 41:133–134, 1990

Kirli S, Caliskan M: A comparative study of sertraline versus imipramine in postpsychotic depressive disorder of schizophrenia. Schizophr Res 33:103–111, 1998

Kofoed LL, Kania J, Walsh T, et al: Outpatient treatment of patients with substance abuse and coexisting psychiatric disorders. Am J Psychiatry 143:867–872, 1986

Kopala L, Honer WG: Risperidone, serotonergic mechanisms, and obsessive-compulsive symptoms in schizophrenia. Am J Psychiatry 151:1714–1715, 1994

Koreen AR, Siris SG, Chakos M, et al: Depression in first-episode schizophrenia. Am J Psychiatry 150:1643–1648, 1993

Kramer MS, Vogel WH, DiJohnson C: Antidepressants in "depressed" schizophrenic inpatients: a controlled trial. Arch Gen Psychiatry 46:922–928, 1989

Krystal JH, D'Souza DC, Madonick S, et al: Toward a rational pharmacotherapy of comorbid substance abuse in schizophrenic patients. Schizophr Res 35:35–49, 1999

Kurland AA, Nagaraju A: Viloxazine and the depressed schizophrenic: methodological issues. J Clin Pharmacol 21:37–41, 1981

Labbate LA, Young PC, Arana GW: Panic disorder in schizophrenia. Can J Psychiatry 44:488–490, 1999

Lee ML: Clozapine and substance abuse in patients with schizophrenia. Can J Psychiatry 45:855–856, 1998

Lieberman J, Kane J, Alvir J: Provocative tests with psychostimulant drugs in schizophrenia. Psychopharmacology (Berl) 91:415–433, 1987

Littrell KH, Petty RG, Hilligoss NM, et al: Olanzapine treatment for patients with schizophrenia and substance abuse. J Subst Abuse Treat 21:217–221, 2001

Longo LP: Olanzapine for cocaine craving and relapse prevention in 2 patients. J Clin Psychiatry 63(7):595–596, 2002

Lysaker PH, Bell MD, Beam-Goulet J, et al: Relationship of positive and negative symptoms to cocaine abuse in schizophrenia. J Nerv Ment Dis 182:109–112, 1994

Lysaker PH, Bell MD, Bioty SM, et al: The frequency of associations between positive and negative symptoms and dysphoria in schizophrenia. Compr Psychiatry 36:113–117, 1995

Lysaker PH, Marks KA, Picone JB, et al: Obsessive and compulsive symptoms in schizophrenia: clinical and neurocognitive correlates. J Nerv Ment Dis 188:78–83, 2000

Lysaker PH, Meyer P, Evans JD, et al: Neurocognitive and symptom correlates of self-reported childhood sexual abuse in schizophrenia spectrum disorders. Ann Clin Psychiatry 13:89–92, 2001a

Lysaker PH, Meyer PS, Evans JD, et al: Childhood sexual trauma and psychosocial functioning in adults with schizophrenia. Psychiatr Serv 52:1485–1488, 2001b

Malla AK, Norman RMG: Prodromal symptoms in schizophrenia. Br J Psychiatry 164:287–293, 1994

Mandel MR, Severe JB, Schooler NR, et al: Development and prediction of postpsychotic depression in neuroleptic-treated schizophrenics. Arch Gen Psychiatry 39:197–203, 1982

Marazziti D, Dell'Osso L, Di Nasso E, et al: Insight in obsessive-compulsive disorder: a study of an Italian sample. Eur Psychiatry 17:407–410, 2002

Marder SR, Davis JM, Chouinard G: The effects of risperidone on the five dimensions of schizophrenia derived by factor analysis: combined results of the North American trials. J Clin Psychiatry 58:538–546, 1997

Marley J, Buila S: When violence happens to people with mental illness: disclosing victimization. Am J Orthopsychiatry 69:398–402, 1999

Martin RL, Cloninger CR, Guze SB, et al: Frequency and differential diagnosis of depressive syndromes in schizophrenia. J Clin Psychiatry 46:9–13, 1985

Maxwell S, Shinderman MS: Naltrexone in the treatment of dually diagnosed patients (abstract). J Addict Dis 16:125, 1997

Maxwell S, Shinderman MS: Use of naltrexone in the treatment of alcohol use disorders in patients with concomitant major mental illness. J Addict Dis 19:61–69, 2000

McDougle CJ, Epperson CN, Pelton GH, et al: A double-blind, placebo-controlled study of risperidone addition in serotonin reuptake inhibitor-refractory obsessive-compulsive disorder. Arch Gen Psychiatry 57:794–801, 2000

McEvoy J, Brown C: Smoking in first-episode patients with schizophrenia. Am J Psychiatry 156:1120–1121, 1999

McEvoy JP, Freudenreich O, McGee M, et al: Clozapine decreases smoking in patients with chronic schizophrenia. Biol Psychiatry 37:550–552, 1995

McEvoy J, Freudenreich O, McGee M, et al: Smoking and therapeutic response to clozapine in patients with schizophrenia. Biol Psychiatry 46:125–129, 1999

McGlashan TH, Bardenstein KK: Gender differences in affective, schizoaffective, and schizophrenic disorders. Schizophr Bull 16:319–329, 1990

McGlashan TH, Carpenter WT: Postpsychotic depression in schizophrenia. Arch Gen Psychiatry 33:231–239, 1976

Meltzer HY: Suicidality in schizophrenia: a review of the evidence for risk factors and treatment options. Curr Psychiatry Rep 4:279–283, 2002

Meltzer HY, Okayli G: Reduction of suicidality during clozapine treatment of neuroleptic-resistant schizophrenia: impact of risk-benefit assessment. Am J Psychiatry 152:183–190, 1995

Meltzer HY, Alphs L, Green AI, et al: Clozapine treatment for suicidality in schizophrenia: International Suicide Prevention Trial (InterSePT). Arch Gen Psychiatry 60:82–91, 2003

Messias E, Kirkpatrick B, Ram R, et al: Suspiciousness as a specific risk factor for major depressive episodes in schizophrenia. Schizophr Res 47:159–165, 2001

Miller WR, Rollnick S: Motivational Interviewing. New York, Guilford, 2002

Mohr N, Vythiulingum B, Emsley RA, et al: Quetiapine augmentation of serotonin reuptake inhibitors in obsessive-compulsive disorder. Int Clin Psychopharmacol 17:37–40, 2002

Moller HJ, Muller H, Borison R, et al: A path analytic approach to differentiate between direct and indirect drug effects on negative symptoms in schizophrenia patients: a re-evaluation of the North American risperidone study. Eur Arch Psychiatry Clin Neurosci 245:45–49, 1995

Moorey H, Soni SD: Anxiety symptoms in stable chronic schizophrenia. J Ment Health Adm 3:257–262, 1994

Morrison D, Clark D, Goldfarb E, et al: Worsening of obsessive-compulsive symptoms following treatment with olanzapine. Am J Psychiatry 155:855, 1998

Morrison RL, Bellack AS: Social functioning of schizophrenic patients: clinical and research issues. Schizophr Bull 13:715–725, 1987

Mueser KT, Yarnold PR, Levinson DF, et al: Prevalence of substance abuse in schizophrenia: demographic and clinical correlates. Schizophr Bull 16:31–56, 1990

Mueser KT, Drake RE, Clark RE, et al: Toolkit for Evaluating Substance Abuse in Persons With Severe Mental Illness. Cambridge, MA, Evaluation Center at Human Service Research Institute, 1995

Mueser KT, Goodman LA, Trumbetta SL, et al: Trauma and posttraumatic stress disorder in severe mental illness. J Consult Clin Psychol 66:493–499, 1998

Mueser KT, Noordsy DL, Drake RE, et al: Integrated Treatment for Dual Disorders: A Guide to Effective Practice. New York, Guilford, 2003a

Mueser KT, Noordsy DL, Fox M, et al: Disulfiram treatment for alcoholism in severe mental illness. Am J Addict 12:242–252, 2003b

Mueser KT, Salyers MP, Rosenberg SD, et al: Interpersonal trauma and posttraumatic stress disorder in patients with severe mental illness. Schizophr Bull 30:45–57, 2004

Muller-Siecheneder F, Muller MJ, Hillert A: Risperidone versus haloperidol and amitriptyline in the treatment of patients with a combined psychotic and depressive syndrome. J Clin Psychopharmacol 18:111–120, 1998

Mulholland C, Lynch G, King DJ, et al: A double-blind, placebo-controlled trial of sertraline for depressive symptoms in patients with stable, chronic schizophrenia. J Psychopharmacol 17(1):107–112, 2003

Murphy KC, Jones LA, Owen MJ: High rates of schizophrenia in adults with velo-cardio-facial syndrome. Arch Gen Psychiatry 56:940–945, 1999

Nechmad A, Ratzoni G, Poyurovsky M, et al: Obsessive-compulsive disorder in adolescent schizophrenia patients. Am J Psychiatry 160:1002–1004, 2003

Neria Y, Bromet EJ, Sievers S, et al: Trauma exposure and posttraumatic stress disorder in psychosis: findings from a first-admission cohort. J Consult Clin Psychol 70:246–251, 2002

Noordsy DL, Green AI: Pharmacotherapy for schizophrenia and co-occurring substance use disorders. Curr Psychiatry Rep 5:340–346, 2003

Noordsy DL, Drake RE, Biesanz JC, et al: Family history of alcoholism in schizophrenia. J Nerv Ment Dis 182:651–655, 1994

Noordsy DL, Torrey WC, Mead S, et al: Recovery-oriented pharmacology: redefining the goals of antipsychotic treatment. J Clin Psychiatry 61 (suppl 3):22–29, 2000

Noordsy DL, O'Keefe CD, Mueser KT, et al: Six-month outcomes for patients who switched to olanzapine treatment. Psychiatr Serv 52:501–507, 2001

Noordsy DL, Torrey WC, Mueser KT, et al: Recovery from severe mental illness: an intrapersonal and functional outcome definition. Int Rev Psychiatry 14:318–326, 2002

Nordentoft M, Jeppesen P, Abel M, et al: OPUS Study: suicidal behavior, suicidal ideation and hopelessness among patients with first-episode psychosis. Br J Psychiatry 181 (suppl 43): S98–S106, 2002

Norman RMG, Malla AK, Cortese L, et al: Aspects of dysphoria and symptoms of schizophrenia. Psychol Med 28:1433–1441, 1998

O'Malley SS, Jaffe AJ, Chang G, et al: Naltrexone and coping skills therapy for alcohol dependence: a controlled study. Arch Gen Psychiatry 49:881–887, 1992

Ohta M, Kokai M, Morita Y: Features of obsessive-compulsive disorder in patients primarily diagnosed with schizophrenia. Psychiatry Clin Neurosci 57:67–74, 2003

Oosthuizen P, Emsley RA, Roberts M, et al: Depressive symptoms at baseline predict fewer negative symptoms at follow-up in patients with first-episode schizophrenia. Schizophr Res 58:247–252, 2002

Osby U, Correia N, Brandt L, et al: Mortality and causes of death in schizophrenia in Stockholm County, Sweden. Schizophr Res 45:21–28, 2000

Owen RR, Fischer EP, Booth BM, et al: Medication noncompliance and substance abuse among patients with schizophrenia. Psychiatr Serv 47:853–858, 1996

Pallanti S, Quercioli L, Rossi A, et al: The emergence of social phobia during clozapine treatment and its response to fluoxetine augmentation. J Clin Psychiatry 60:819–823, 1999

Pallanti S, Quercioli L, Hollander E: Social anxiety in outpatients with schizophrenia: a relevant cause of disability. Am J Psychiatry 161:53–58, 2004

Patel JK, Salzman C, Green AI, et al: Chronic schizophrenia: response to clozapine, risperidone and paroxetine. Am J Psychiatry 154:543–546, 1997

Penn DL, Hope DA, Spaulding W, et al: Social anxiety in schizophrenia. Schizophr Res 11:277–284, 1994

Penn DL, Corrigan PW, Bentall RP, et al: Social cognition in schizophrenia. Psychol Bull 121:114–132, 1997

Petrakis IL, O'Malley SS, Rounsaville B, et al: Naltrexone augmentation of neuroleptic treatment in alcohol abusing patients with schizophrenia. Psychopharmacology (Berl) 172:291–297, 2004

Peuskens J: Risperidone in the treatment of patients with chronic schizophrenia: a multinational, multi-center, double-blind, parallel group study versus haloperidol. Br J Psychiatry 166:712–726, 1995

Pfanner C, Marazziti D, Dell'Osso L, et al: Risperidone augmentation in refractory obsessive-compulsive disorder: an open-label study. Int Clin Psychopharmacol 15:297–301, 2000

Poyurovsky M, Hermesh H, Weizman A: Fluvoxamine treatment in clozapine-induced obsessive-compulsive symptoms in schizophrenic patients. Clin Neuropharmacol 19:305–313, 1996

Poyurovsky M, Bergman Y, Shoshani D, et al: Emergence of obsessive-compulsive symptoms and tics during clozapine withdrawal. Clin Neuropharmacol 21:97–100, 1998

Poyurovsky M, Fuchs C, Weizman A: Obsessive-compulsive disorder in patients with first-episode schizophrenia. Am J Psychiatry 156:1998–2000, 1999a

Poyurovsky M, Isakov V, Hromnikov S, et al: Fluvoxamine treatment of obsessive-compulsive symptoms in schizophrenic patients: an add-on open study. Int Clin Psychopharmacol 14:95–100, 1999b

Poyurovsky M, Dorfman-Etrog P, Hermesh H, et al: Beneficial effects of olanzapine in schizophrenia patients with obsessive-compulsive symptoms. Int Clin Psychopharmacol 15:169–173, 2000

Poyurovsky M, Hramenkov S, Isakov V, et al: Obsessive-compulsive disorder in hospitalized patients with chronic schizophrenia. Psychiatry Res 102:49–57, 2001

Poyurovsky M, Kurs R, Weizman A: Olanzapine-sertraline combination in schizophrenia with obsessive-compulsive disorder. J Clin Psychiatry 64:611, 2003

Priebe S, Broker M, Gunkel S: Involuntary admission and posttraumatic stress disorder symptoms in schizophrenia patients. Compr Psychiatry 39:220–224, 1998

Provencher HL, Gregg R, Mead S, et al: The role of work in the recovery of persons with psychiatric disabilities. Psychiatr Rehabil J 26:132–144, 2002

Prusoff BA, Williams DH, Weissman MM, et al: Treatment of secondary depression in schizophrenia. Arch Gen Psychiatry 36:569–575, 1979

Read J, Argyle N: Hallucinations, delusions, and thought disorder among adult psychiatric inpatients with a history of child abuse. Psychiatr Serv 50:1467–1472, 1999

Regier DA, Farmer ME, Rae DS, et al: Comorbidity of mental disorders with alcohol and other drug abuse. JAMA 264:2511–2518, 1990

Reid WH, Mason M, Hogan T: Suicide prevention effects associated with clozapine therapy in schizophrenia and schizoaffective disorder. Psychiatr Serv 49:1029–1033, 1998

Resnick SG, Bond GR, Mueser KT: Trauma and posttraumatic stress disorder in people with schizophrenia. J Abnorm Psychol 112:415–423, 2003

Ridgely MS, Goldman HH, Willenbring M: Barriers to care of persons with dual diagnoses: organizational and financing issues. Schizophr Bull 16:123–132, 1990

Rolfe TJ, McGory P, Cooks J, et al: Cannabis use in first episode psychosis: incidence and short-term outcome (abstract). Schizophr Res 36:313, 1999

Rosenberg SD, Drake RE, Wolford GL, et al: Dartmouth Assessment of Lifestyle Instrument (DALI): a substance use disorder screen for people with severe mental illness. Am J Psychiatry 155:232–238, 1998

Rosenberg SD, Goodman LA, Osher FC, et al: Prevalence of HIV, hepatitis B, and hepatitis C in people with severe mental illness. Am J Public Health 91:31–37, 2001a

Rosenberg SD, Mueser KT, Friedman MJ, et al: Developing effective treatments for posttraumatic disorders among people with severe mental illness. Psychiatr Serv 52:1453–1461, 2001b

Ross CA, Anderson G, Clark P: Childhood abuse and the positive symptoms of schizophrenia. Hosp Community Psychiatry 45:489–491, 1994

Rossau CD, Mortensen PB: Risk factors for suicide in patients with schizophrenia: nested case-control study. Br J Psychiatry 171:355–359, 1997

Roy A: Risk factors for suicide in psychiatric patients. Arch Gen Psychiatry 39:1089–1095, 1982

Saarinen PI, Lehtonen J, Lonnqvist J: Suicide risk in schizophrenia: an analysis of 17 consecutive suicides. Schizophr Bull 25:533–542, 1999

Salyers MP, Mueser KT: Social functioning, psychopathology, and medication side effects in relation to substance use and abuse in schizophrenia. Schizophr Res 48:109–123, 2001

Sax KW, Strakowski SM, Keck PE, et al: Relationship among negative, positive, and depressive symptoms in schizophrenia and psychotic depression. Br J Psychiatry 168:68–71, 1996

Scheller-Gilkey G, Thomas SM, Woolwine BJ, et al: Increased early life stress and depressive symptoms in patients with comorbid substance abuse and schizophrenia. Schizophr Bull 28:223–231, 2002

Schmidtke L, Schorb A, Winkelmann G, et al: Cognitive frontal lobe dysfunction in obsessive-compulsive disorder. Biol Psychiatry 43:666–673, 1998

Schwartz CC, Myers JK: Life events and schizophrenia, I: comparison of schizophrenics with a community sample. Arch Gen Psychiatry 34:1238–1241, 1977

Schwartz RC, Cohen BN: Psychosocial correlates of suicidal intent among patients with schizophrenia. Compr Psychiatry 42:118–123, 2001

Selzer JA, Lieberman JA: Schizophrenia and substance abuse. Psychiatr Clin North Am 16:401–412, 1993

Shepherd M, Watt D, Falloon IR, et al: The natural history of schizophrenia: a five-year follow-up study of outcome and prediction in a representative sample of schizophrenics. Psychol Med 15:1–46, 1989

Singh AN, Saxena B, Nelson HL: A controlled clinical study of trazodone in chronic schizophrenic patients with pronounced depressive symptomatology. Curr Ther Res Clin Exp 23:485–501, 1978

Siris SG: Akinesia and postpsychotic depression: a difficult differential diagnosis. J Clin Psychiatry 38:240–243, 1987

Siris S: Pharmacological treatment of substance-abusing schizophrenic patients. Schizophr Bull 16:111–122, 1990

Siris SG: Diagnosis of secondary depression in schizophrenia: implications for DSM-IV. Schizophr Bull 17:75–98, 1991

Siris SG: Depression in schizophrenia: perspective in the era of "atypical" antipsychotics. Am J Psychiatry 157:1379–1389, 2000a

Siris SG: Management of depression in schizophrenia. Psychiatr Ann 30:13–19, 2000b

Siris S, Morgan V, Fagerstrom R, et al: Adjunctive imipramine in the treatment of post-psychotic depression: a controlled trial. Arch Gen Psychiatry 44:533–539, 1987

Siris SG, Adan F, Cohen M, et al: Postpsychotic depression and negative symptoms: an investigation of syndromal overlap. Am J Psychiatry 145:1532–1537, 1988

Siris S, Cutler J, Owen K: Adjunctive imipramine maintenance in schizophrenic patients with remitted post-psychotic depressions. Am J Psychiatry 146:1495–1497, 1989a

Siris SG, Aronson A, Sellew AP: Imipramine-responsive panic-like symptomatology in schizophrenia/schizoaffective disorder. Biol Psychiatry 25:485–488, 1989b

Siris SG, Bermanzohn PC, Mason SE, et al: Adjunctive imipramine for dysphoric schizophrenic patients with past histories of cannabis abuse. Prog Neuropsychopharmacol Biol Psychiatry 16:539–547, 1992

Siris SG, Mason SE, Bermanzohn PC, et al: Adjunctive imipramine in substance-abusing dysphoric schizophrenic patients. Psychopharmacol Bull 29:127–133, 1993

Smelson D, Losonczy M, Davis CW, et al: Risperidone decreases craving and relapses in individuals with schizophrenia and cocaine dependence. Can J Psychiatry 47:671–675, 2002

Soni S, Brownlee M: Alcohol abuse in chronic schizophrenics: implications for management in the community. Acta Psychiatr Scand 84:272–276, 1991

Stone WS, Faraone SV, Seidman LJ, et al: Concurrent validation of schizotaxia: a pilot study. Biol Psychiatry 50:434–440, 2001

Stratkowsky SM, Tohen M, Stoll AL, et al: Comorbidity in psychosis at first hospitalization. Am J Psychiatry 150:752–757, 1993

Strous RD, Patel JK, Zimmet S, et al: Clozapine/paroxetine in the treatment of schizophrenia with disabling obsessive compulsive features. Am J Psychiatry 156:973–974, 1999a

Strous RD, Patel JK, Zimmet SV, et al: Clozapine and paroxetine in the treatment of schizophrenia with obsessive-compulsive features. Am J Psychiatry 156:973–974, 1999b

Subotnik KL, Nuechterlein KH: Prodromal signs and symptoms of schizophrenic relapse. J Abnorm Psychol 97:405–412, 1988

Subotnik KL, Nuechterlein KH, Asarnow RF, et al: Depressive symptoms in the early course of schizophrenia: relationship to familial psychiatric illness. Am J Psychiatry 154:1551–1556, 1997

Swanson JW, Swartz MS, Essock SM, et al: The social-environmental context of violent behavior in persons treated for severe mental illness. Am J Public Health 92:1523–1531, 2002

Tamminga CA, Buchanan RW, Gold J: The role of negative symptoms and cognitive dysfunction in schizophrenia outcome. Int Clin Psychopharmacol 13:S21–S26, 1998

Taylor S: Meta-analysis of cognitive-behavioral treatments for social phobia. J Behav Ther Exp Psychiatry 27:1–9, 1996

Tibbo P, Kroetsch M, Chue P, et al: Obsessive-compulsive disorder in schizophrenia. J Psychiatr Res 34:139–146, 2000

Tibbo P, Swainson J, Chue P, et al: Prevalence and relationship to delusions and hallucinations of anxiety disorders in schizophrenia. Depress Anxiety 17:65–72, 2003

Tollefson G, Beasley CM, Tran PV, et al: Olanzapine versus haloperidol in the treatment of schizophrenia and schizoaffective disorders: results of an international collaborative trial. Am J Psychiatry 154:457–465, 1997

Tollefson GD, Sanger TM, Lu Y, et al: Depressive signs and symptoms in schizophrenia: a prospective blinded trial of olanzapine and haloperidol. Arch Gen Psychiatry 55:250–258, 1998

Tollefson GD, Andersen SW, Tran PV: The course of depressive symptoms in predicting relapse in schizophrenia: a double-blind, randomized comparison of olanzapine and risperidone. Biol Psychiatry 46:365–373, 1999

Treffert DA: Marijuana use in schizophrenia: a clear hazard. Am J Psychiatry 135:1213–1215, 1978

Tsuang MT, Fleming JA, Simpson JC: Suicide and schizophrenia, in The Harvard Medical School Guide to Suicide Assessment and Intervention. Edited by Jacobs DG. San Francisco, CA, Jossey-Bass, 1999, pp 287–299

Tsuang MT, Marder SR, Han A, et al: Olanzapine treatment for patients with schizophrenia and cocaine abuse. J Clin Psychiatry 63(12):1180–1181, 2002

van Balkom AJ, de Haan E, van Oppen P, et al: Cognitive and behavioral therapics alone versus in combination with fluvoxamine in the treatment of obsessive compulsive disorder. J Nerv Ment Dis 186:492–499, 1998

Veen ND, Selten J, van der Tweel I, et al: Cannabis use and age at onset of schizophrenia. Am J Psychiatry 161:501–506, 2004

Vlokh I, Mikhnyak S, Kachura O: Zoloft in management of depression in schizophrenia (abstract). Schizophr Res 41:209, 2000

Volpicelli JR, Alterman AI, Hayashida M, et al: Naltrexone in the treatment of alcohol dependence. Arch Gen Psychiatry 49:876–887, 1992

Waehrens J, Gerlach J: Antidepressant drugs in anergic schizophrenia: a double-blind cross-over study with maprotiline and placebo. Acta Psychiatr Scand 61:438–444, 1980

Walker A, Lanaza L, Arellano F, et al: Mortality in current and former users of clozapine. Epidemiology 8:671–677, 1997

Weiner E, Ball MP, Summerfelt A, et al: Effects of sustained-release bupropion and supportive group therapy on cigarette consumption in patients with schizophrenia. Am J Psychiatry 158:635–637, 2001

Weiss R, Hufford M: Substance abuse and suicide, in The Harvard Medical School Guide to Suicide Assessment and Intervention. Edited by Jacobs DG. San Francisco, CA, Jossey-Bass, 1999, pp 300–310

Westermeyer JF, Harrow M, Marengo JT: Risk for suicide in schizophrenia and other psychotic and nonpsychotic disorders. J Nerv Ment Dis 179:259–266, 1991

Wilkins JN: Pharmacotherapy of schizophrenia patients with comorbid substance abuse. Schizophr Bull 23:215–228, 1997

Yang YK, Nelson L, Kamaraju L, et al: Nicotine decreases bradykinesia-rigidity in haloperidol-treated patients with schizophrenia. Neuropsychopharmacology 27:684–686, 2002

Ziedonis D, Richardson T, Lee E, et al: Adjunctive desipramine in the treatment of cocaine abusing schizophrenics. Psychopharmacol Bull 28:309–314, 1992

Zimmet SV, Strous RD, Burgess ES, et al: Effects of clozapine on substance use in patients with schizophrenia and schizoaffective disorder: a retrospective survey. J Clin Psychopharmacol 20:94–98, 2000

Zisook S, McAdams LA, Kuck J, et al: Depressive symptoms in schizophrenia. Am J Psychiatry 156:1736–1743, 1999

NEUROCOGNITIVE IMPAIRMENTS

RICHARD S. E. KEEFE, PH.D.

CHARLES E. EESLEY, B.S.

COGNITIVE IMPAIRMENT IN SCHIZOPHRENIA

COGNITION AS A CORE FEATURE OF SCHIZOPHRENIA

Cognitive impairment associated with schizophrenia is now viewed as a potential psychopharmacological target for treatment (Hyman and Fenton 2003). Although cognition is not a formal part of the current diagnostic criteria for schizophrenia, DSM-IV-TR (American Psychiatric Association 2000) includes seven references to cognitive dysfunction in the description of the disorder. Diagnostic and scientific experts increasingly have expressed the idea that neurocognitive impairment is a core feature of the illness and not simply the result of the symptoms or the current treatments of schizophrenia.

PROFILE AND MAGNITUDE OF COGNITIVE IMPAIRMENT ASSOCIATED WITH SCHIZOPHRENIA

Severely impaired performance on cognitive tests is the strongest evidence for the importance of cognitive deficits in schizophrenia. In several cognitive domains, the aver-age impairment can reach 2 standard deviations below the healthy control mean (Harvey and Keefe 1997; Heinrichs and Zakzanis 1998; Saykin et al. 1991). Although approximately only 27% of patients with schizophrenia (and 85% of the general population) are not rated as "impaired" by clinical neuropsychological assessment (Palmer 1997), these patients tend to have the highest levels of premorbid functioning (Kremen et al. 2000) and demonstrate cognitive functioning that is considerably below what would be expected of them based on their premorbid levels and the education level of their parents. Recent analyses of data from 150 patients with schizophrenia suggest that up to 98% of patients perform more poorly on cognitive tests than would be predicted by their parents' education level (Keefe et al. 2005). In addition, comparisons of monozygotic twins discordant for schizophrenia suggest that almost all affected twins perform worse than their unaffected twin on cognitive tests (Goldberg et al. 1990). Therefore, it is likely that almost all patients with schizophrenia are functioning below the level that would be expected in the absence of the illness.

Neurocognitive tests often assess more than one domain of functioning, and many tests do not fit neatly into a single domain. Thus, descriptions of the profile of cognitive deficits in schizophrenia have varied across literature reviews. The domains that are most consistently cited as being severely impaired in schizophrenia are verbal memory, executive functions, attention or vigilance, verbal fluency, and motor speed (Harvey and Keefe 1997). Deficits in social cognition also appear to be severe, but this is a relatively new area of research with fewer studies to support this finding (Pinkham et al. 2003). The opinion of a group of experts who served on the Neurocognition Subcommittee for the CS project (www.matrics.ucla.edu) is that the most important domains of cognitive deficit in schizophrenia are working memory, attention/vigilance, verbal learning and memory, visual learning and memory, reasoning and problem solving, speed of processing, and social cognition (Nuechterlein et al. 2004).

The most striking aspect of the profile of cognitive deficits in patients with schizophrenia is that so few cognitive functions remain similar to those in healthy control subjects (Harvey and Keefe 1997; Saykin et al. 1994). In fact, as seen in Table 13–1, an estimate of the severity of neurocognitive impairment in patients with schizophrenia, based on an examination of the most methodologically sound studies completed, suggests that many important cognitive functions are in the severely impaired range (2–3 standard deviations below the normal mean) or moderately impaired range (1–2 standard deviations below the normal mean) (Harvey and Keefe 1997). A review and meta-analysis of 204 studies shows a consistent and stable difference between patients with schizophrenia ($n = 7,420$) and healthy control subjects ($n = 5,865$) in a wide range of domains of cognitive functioning (Heinrichs and Zakzanis 1998). Examples of tests that measure the most important components of cognitive impairment in schizophrenia are reviewed briefly here.

Vigilance and Attention

Many neurocognitive tests require vigilance functions, even if the test itself is not a measure of "pure" vigilance. *Vigilance* refers to the ability to maintain attention over time. A standard vigilance test used in many studies is the Continuous Performance Test (CPT). The "AX" version of the CPT (AX-CPT) requires that patients attend to a series of letters presented one at a time on a computer screen at a rate of one per second. Patients respond with a button press on the computer mouse or keyboard each time an "A" is followed by an "X." The AX-CPT has been shown to reveal severe vigilance impairments in patients with schizophrenia (Cornblatt and Keilp 1994).

Impairments in vigilance can result in difficulty following social conversations and an inability to follow important instructions regarding treatment, therapy, or work functions; simple activities such as reading or watch-

TABLE 13–1.   Cognitive impairments in schizophrenia and their severity[a]

Severe impairments (2–3 standard deviations [SD] below the mean[b])

- Serial learning
- Executive functioning
- Vigilance
- Motor speed
- Verbal fluency

Moderate impairments (1–2 SD below the mean)

- Distractibility
- Delayed recall
- Visuomotor skills
- Immediate memory span
- Working memory

Mild impairments (0.5–1 SD below the mean)

- Perceptual skills
- Delayed recognition memory
- Confrontation naming
- Verbal and full-scale IQ

No impairment

- Word recognition reading
- Long-term factual memory

[a]The estimated average severity scores are corrected on the basis of age and relative education level.
[b]The "mean" refers to the average level of performance of normal individuals who are similar in age and educational attainment.
Source.   Reprinted from Harvey PD, Keefe RSE: "Cognitive Impairment in Schizophrenia and Implications of Atypical Neuroleptic Treatment." *CNS Spectrums* 2:1–11, 1997. Used with permission.

ing television become labored or impossible. Reviews of the literature have suggested that vigilance deficits in patients with schizophrenia are related to various aspects of outcome, including social deficits, community functioning, and skills acquisition (Green 1996; Green et al. 2000).

Verbal Learning and Memory

The abilities involved in memory functioning include, but are not limited to, those associated with learning new information, retaining newly learned information over time, and recognizing previously presented material. In general, patients show larger deficits in learning than in retention. The findings for recognition are more equivocal, with most studies suggesting relatively mild deficits (Calev 1984; Saykin et al. 1991), yet large deficits also have been reported (Mohamed et al. 1999). The tests used to measure learning typically involve the ability to learn lists of words or written passages. Verbal list-learning tasks usually require the patient to listen to 12–16 words then immediately recall as many of the words as possible. Normal control subjects taking the California Verbal Learning Test can recall approximately 8 of 16 words after the first trial; patients with schizophrenia can recall only about 5 (Paulsen et al. 1995). After five consecutive trials of the same word list, most control subjects can recall at least 13 of the words, whereas patients with schizophrenia on average can recall only 9. Thus, patients are impaired both in their ability to immediately recall verbal material and in their ability to learn over time compared with control subjects. Patients are also impaired in recalling more interesting verbal material, such as stories (Hoff et al. 1992). Much empirical evidence points to the connection between verbal memory impairment and social deficits in patients with schizophrenia (Green 1996).

Visual Learning and Memory

Because visual information is not as easily expressed as verbal information, fewer tests sensitive to the deficits of schizophrenia have been developed, and this area of cognitive function has generally been found not to be as impaired as verbal memory (Heinrichs and Zaksanis 1998). Most tests require subjects to draw figures from memory or to indicate which among an array of figures was previously presented.

Studies of the relationship between poor visual memory and functional outcome have yielded mixed findings. Visual memory has been found to correlate modestly with employment status (J.M. Gold et al. 2003), job tenure (J.M. Gold et al. 2002), psychosocial rehabilitation success (Mueser et al. 1991), social functioning (Dickerson et al. 1999), quality of life ratings (Buchanan et al. 1994), and strongly with functional capacity (Twamley et al. 2003). Other studies have reported no significant correlations (Addington and Addington 2000; Addington et al. 1998; Ertugrul and Ulug 2002; Velligan et al. 2000).

Reasoning and Problem Solving

Although there are many tests of reasoning and problem solving, the most well known and most frequently used in schizophrenia research is the Wisconsin Card Sorting Test (WCST; Heaton 1981). In this test, patients are given a deck of cards with various numbers of colored shapes on them and are asked to match their cards to four "key" cards that have shapes on them that differ by color, form, and number. The first principle to which the subject needs to learn to sort the cards is *color*. After a patient demonstrates that he has learned that is the correct sorting principle, the principle changes to *form* without warning. Repeated sorting attempts by the previously correct principle are referred to as *perseverations*, and patients with schizophrenia, as with patients with frontal lobe damage, often make many of these errors. In fact, the very poor performance of patients with schizophrenia on the WCST (Goldberg et al. 1987) and the reduced activity of the dorsolateral prefrontal cortex during performance of this test (Weinberger et al. 1987) led to widespread pursuit of the hypothesis of frontal hypoactivation in schizophrenia. It is important to note, however, that the WCST measures a variety of cognitive functions and is not a pure measure of executive functions (Keefe 1995).

The rules of society and the workplace change regularly, and success in these arenas is often measured by one's ability to adapt to changes. Patients with schizophrenia who are impaired on measures of executive functions have difficulty adapting to the rapidly changing world around them.

Speed of Processing

Many neurocognitive tests require subjects to process information rapidly and can be compromised by impairments in processing speed. A standard example of this type of task is the Digit Symbol Test of the Wechsler Adult Intelligence Scale (Wechsler et al. 1997). Each numeral (1–9) is associated with a different simple symbol. Subjects are required to copy as many of the symbols associated with the numerals as possible in 90 seconds. This nonspecific cognitive impairment has been found to correlate with a variety of clinically important features of schizophrenia, such as daily life activities (Evans et al. 2003), job tenure (J.M. Gold et al. 2002), and independent living status (Brekke et al. 1997). It is also sensitive to medication side effects such as somnolence and extrapyramidal symptoms (Galletly et al. 2000).

Reduced processing speed can impair ability to keep in step with the task-oriented jobs that are frequently held by patients with schizophrenia. Increased response latency in social settings may hamper social relationships.

Verbal Fluency

Most cognitive assessments in treatment studies of schizophrenia have included measures of verbal fluency as a separate domain of functioning (Harvey and Keefe 2001; Keefe et al. 1999; Meltzer and McGurk 1999). Most of these tests measure either phonological fluency (also referred to as letter fluency) or semantic fluency. Phonological fluency refers to a patient's ability to produce as many words as possible beginning with a particular letter within, for instance, 60 seconds. Semantic fluency refers to the ability to produce words within a particular meaning-based category, such as "vegetables." Not only do schizophrenia patients produce fewer words than normal control subjects, but they often produce inappropriate examples, such as examples of fruits instead of vegetables. Impaired verbal fluency can damage functioning in social and vocational settings by making communication difficult and awkward.

Immediate/Working Memory

Immediate memory refers to the ability to hold a limited amount of information "on-line" for a brief period (usually a few seconds). Repeating a string of digits (*digits forwards*) is an example of immediate memory. The definition of working memory, on the other hand, is more complex and varies across studies. Some investigators consider working memory to be synonymous with immediate memory, whereas others believe it should require some manipulation of the information being held on-line. For example, repeating a series of digits in the reverse order than they were presented (*digits backward*) requires an active manipulation because the information needs to be both held on-line and then subsequently reordered. Patients typically show deficits on both tasks. These visual tasks involve keeping a visuospatial stimulus, such as a dot on a computer screen, or series of visual objects in mind while working on a related or unrelated task (reviewed in Keefe 2001).

Working memory has been described by various authors as a core component of the cognitive impairment in schizophrenia (Goldman-Rakic 1994; Keefe 2001; Silver et al. 2003) and is related to functional outcomes such as employment status (McGurk and Meltzer 2000) and job tenure (J.M. Gold et al. 2002). Much of the clinical relevance of working memory deficits in schizophrenia comes from strong correlations that working memory measures have with a variety of other cognitive domains impaired in schizophrenia, such as attention, planning, memory (reviewed in Keefe 2001), and intelligence (Baddeley 1992), as well as the advanced understanding of the neuroanatomy of working memory functions in human and nonhuman primates. This neuroanatomical work has suggested that neural circuitry that includes prefrontal cortical regions mediates aspects of working memory functions (Callicott et al. 1999; Goldman-Rakic 1987) and that this circuitry may be impaired in schizophrenia (Callicott et al. 1999).

Social Cognition

Theory-of-mind skills and social perception have been the general focus of the literature on social cognition in schizophrenia. *Theory of mind* is the ability to infer another's intentions and/or to represent the mental states of others. Individuals with schizophrenia perform poorly on measures of theory-of-mind abilities (Corcoran et al. 1995; Drury et al. 1998; Sarfati et al. 1997). The evidence regarding whether impairments in theory-of-mind skills are independent of a general cognitive deficit is mixed (Doody et al. 1998; Pinkham et al. 2003). Facial affect recognition and social cue perception are the two general areas into which studies of social perception in schizophrenia can be broken down. Reviews of the literature on facial affect recognition (Morrison et al. 1988; Penn et al. 1997) suggest that individuals with schizophrenia have stable deficits on tests of facial affect perception compared with healthy control subjects and psychiatric control subjects, and that perception of negative emotions and fear may be particularly impaired (Addington and Addington 1998; Edwards et al. 2001; Gaebel and Wolwer 1992). Tests of social cue perception use more dynamic stimuli that require multiple sensory modalities, such as watching videotapes of persons interacting. Patients with schizophrenia show consistent impairments on these tasks (Bell et al. 1997; Corrigan et al. 1990). In particular, they have more difficulty discerning other individuals' goals and intentions than what they are wearing or saying.

A variety of reports have described the strong relationship between cognitive function and social deficits in schizophrenia (reviewed by Trumbetta and Meuser 2000). Even so, there is growing evidence that social cognition is related to social impairments in schizophrenia, even after controlling for performance on neurocognitive tasks (Penn et al. 1996).

SUMMARY

Experts in cognition and schizophrenia have come to a clear consensus that cognitive impairment is a core feature of the illness. The profile of deficits is broad, severe, and is likely present in most if not all patients. Neurocognitive impairment has clear clinical relevance because cognitive impairment interferes with the everyday lives of patients in various important ways, from limiting social relationships to reducing the likelihood of employment.

NATURAL HISTORY OF NEUROCOGNITIVE IMPAIRMENT

Evidence shows that the time course of the development of cognitive deficits in schizophrenia patients appears to follow a predictable pattern (Figure 13–1). Some deficits may be present in childhood, followed by a decline in cog-

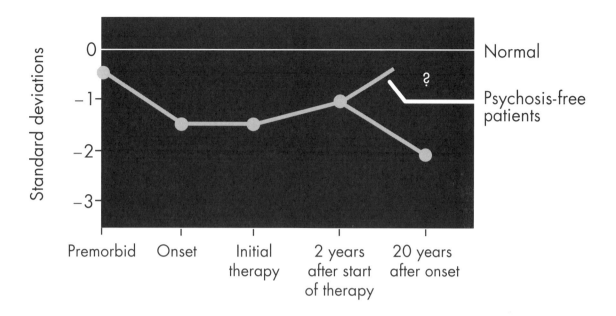

FIGURE 13–1. Course of cognitive impairment in patients with schizophrenia using first-generation antipsychotics.

Source. Reprinted from Keefe RSE: "Neurocognition," in *Current Issues in the Psychopharmacology of Schizophrenia.* Edited by Breier A, Tran PV, Herrera J, et al. Baltimore, MD, Lippincott Williams & Wilkins, 2001.

nitive function before the first episode. The severity of neurocognitive impairments becomes even more severe once psychosis develops. The long-term stability of neurocognitive impairment over time is not clear, but evidence for progression in nonelderly patients is lacking.

DEFICITS IN CHILDREN AT RISK FOR SCHIZOPHRENIA

Individuals who are genetically vulnerable to schizophrenia have notable cognitive impairments (Cornblatt and Keilp 1994), whereas individuals who are examined with cognitive assessments before they develop schizophrenia are found to have impairments in a variety of areas (Davidson et al. 1999). High-risk studies of children with one or two biological parents with schizophrenia (Cornblatt et al. 1999) have suggested that attention deficits can predict which children will develop schizophrenia in the future.

Follow-Back Studies

Several studies have used the follow-back method, in which adult patients with schizophrenia are identified and then linked with their records of cognitive assessments performed while they were children or adolescents (Davidson et al. 1999; Fuller et al. 2002; Jones et al. 1994). In the U.K. National Survey of Health and Development

study, data from 5,362 people indicated that children who went on to develop schizophrenia as adults differed significantly from the general population in a wide range of cognitive and behavioral domains (Jones et al. 1994). Low verbal, nonverbal, and mathematics/arithmetic educational test scores at all ages assessed were significant risk factors. Similar findings were generated from a population-based study that investigated the risk of schizophrenia in a sample of 50,000 18-year-old males conscripted into the Swedish Army between 1969 and 1970 (David et al. 1997). In the United States, scores from grades 4, 8, and 11 on the Iowa Tests for 70 children who later developed schizophrenia showed no significant differences from scores of control subjects at grades 4 and 8. However, for children who developed schizophrenia, test scores dropped significantly between grades 8 and 11, corresponding with the onset of puberty (Fuller et al. 2002). A small sample size and a nonrandom sample restrict the generalizability of these results.

Several studies have used a link between the Israeli Draft Board Registry and the National Psychiatric Hospitalization Case Registry. Israeli law requires that all adolescents between the ages of 16–17 years undergo preinduction assessment to determine their intellectual, medical, and psychiatric eligibility for military service. This assessment is compulsory and is administered to the entire unselected population of Israeli adolescents, including individuals who will be eligible for military service as well as those who will be excused from service based on medical, psychiatric, or social reasons. The results suggest that cognitive functions are significantly impaired in those adolescents who are later hospitalized for schizophrenia. These deficits thus precede the onset of psychosis in young people destined to develop schizophrenia, and, along with social isolation and organizational ability, cognitive deficits are a significant predictor of which young people will eventually develop a psychotic disorder (Davidson et al. 1999). One study from this series examined the cognitive performance of 44 patients with a first episode of schizophrenia and who had previously undergone cognitive assessment as part of their registration with the Israeli Draft Board. The stability of the deficits in these patients suggests that most of the cognitive impairment seen occurs prior to the first psychotic episode (Caspi et al. 2003).

These follow-back studies demonstrate consistently that cognitive impairment precedes the onset of illness in schizophrenia and schizoaffective illness.

Prodrome Studies

Cognitive deficits are also found in individuals who are identified as being at "ultra-high" risk (Yung and McGorry 1996) for schizophrenia by virtue of their family history of schizophrenia and/or the manifestation of mild signs and symptoms consistent with the prodromal symptoms of schizophrenia. Although several research groups are gathering data on this question, results have only recently begun to be reported (Brewer et al. 2003; Hawkins et al. 2004). Preliminary data also suggest that olfactory identification deficits predict which individuals at ultra-high risk will develop schizophrenia (Brewer et al. 2003).

FIRST-EPISODE PSYCHOSIS STUDIES

Once psychosis develops, cognitive deficits are severe (Bilder et al. 2000; DeLisi et al. 1995; Hoff et al. 1999; Mohamed et al. 1999; Stirling et al. 2003). Patients with a first episode of schizophrenia who have never taken antipsychotic medication already exhibit cognitive impairment (Brickman et al. 2004; Mohamed et al. 1999; Saykin et al. 1994). Motor functions and language functions may be more mildly impaired before medication treatment (Brickman et al. 2004). Initial treatment with first-generation antipsychotic medications does little to change these cognitive deficits (Bilder et al. 2000).

COGNITIVE CHANGES IN PATIENTS RECOVERING FROM ACUTE EXACERBATION

Several studies have investigated the longitudinal course of cognitive deficits in schizophrenia by repeatedly assessing cognition in samples that combine first-episode patients and those who have had an acute exacerbation of their symptoms. Patients recovering from an acute exacerbation of illness do not appear to demonstrate substantial changes in the severity of their cognitive impairment despite clear improvements in symptoms with treatment (S. Gold 1999; Hughes et al. 2003; Nopoulos et al. 1994; Sweeney et al. 1991).

LONGITUDINAL CHANGE IN COGNITIVE FUNCTION

There are many age-related changes in cognitive functioning in the normal population, especially in motor speed and memory functions (Moss and Albert 1988). The magnitude of change in long-term memory and ability to access and use previously learned material is more modest. Reading and vocabulary are tests of "old learning," therefore baseline functioning can be estimated from performance on these tests that show minimal aging-related changes. The possibility of detecting cognitive decline with aging is diminished because of floor effects on numerous tests. The types of cognitive functions that change with normal aging, such as new learning and recall, attention, and processing speed, are related to the deficits most commonly observed in schizophrenia patients early in life. Thus, aging-related changes are likely to affect those functions that are already severely impaired in adults with schizophrenia (Harvey 1999). The notion of neurodegeneration in schizophrenia has been controversial.

Evidence has been presented suggesting that schizophrenia is a neurodegenerative process, and some have concluded that schizophrenia is progressive (Lieberman 1999). Supportive evidence for this theory derives from the greater cognitive impairment reported in chronic patients compared with first-episode patients (Saykin et al. 1994). However, with a few notable exceptions (Bilder et al. 1992; Davidson et al. 1995; O'Donnell et al. 1995), cross-sectional studies generally have not found evidence of increased cognitive impairment in association with duration of illness, and older nonelderly patients do not manifest greater impairment than younger patients (Goldberg et al. 1993b; Heaton and Drexler 1987; Hyde et al. 1994; Zorrilla et al. 2000).

Definitive answers to questions regarding possible progression of cognitive impairment in schizophrenia must come from longitudinal studies. The available studies, however, have a variety of methodological limitations such as small or unrepresentative samples, no controls, limited assessment, or relatively short follow-up periods. One recent longitudinal study traced 111 first-episode schizophrenia patients over 10–12 years and found that visuospatial function, although spared in the first episode, may deteriorate over time, whereas executive deficits do not (Stirling et al. 2003). These longitudinal studies of neurocognitive impairment suggest that it is a stable, enduring feature of the illness, with very little change in chronic patients between assessment periods of up to 5 years (Heaton et al. 2001; Rund 1998).

Cognitive Functioning in Elderly Patients

There is some evidence that neurocognitive impairment in patients with schizophrenia may worsen over time in at least a subgroup of elderly patients with schizophrenia. Prominent cognitive impairments resembling dementia have been reported in older schizophrenic patients with a lifetime of poor functional outcome (Arnold et al. 1995; Davidson et al. 1995; Harvey et al. 1996).

On the basis of cross-sectional studies, elderly patients with schizophrenia appear to show some decline in cognitive function toward the end of life. However, this decline may be restricted to those patients who had an early onset of illness followed by a lifetime of poor functioning (Heaton et al. 1994; Hyde et al. 1994; Jeste et al. 1995; Zorrilla et al. 2000). Some of the inconsistency of these results may derive from the subject selection processes in these studies. Finally, cognitive decline in some elderly patients with schizophrenia has been found to be associated with tardive dyskinesia (Waddington and Youssef 1996) and neurological dysfunction (Goldstein and Zubin 1990).

Summary

Several studies have demonstrated that neurocognitive impairment is present in a mild form before the onset of psychosis in young people destined to develop schizophrenia. Neurocognitive impairment is severe in patients who have experienced their first psychotic episode, even before antipsychotic treatment is initiated. Although some early-phase patients may demonstrate a slight improvement in neurocognitive impairment with treatment, many patients do not improve at all. Following this early phase, neurocognitive impairment appears to be remarkably consistent, even in the presence of positive and negative symptom change, although few longitudinal studies have had follow-up periods of longer than 5 years. The course of neurocognitive impairment in elderly pa-

tients is uncertain, but some studies suggest that patients with the most chronic courses of illness may manifest a further, albeit gradual, cognitive decline in the latest years of life.

Early treatment with second-generation antipsychotics potentially could improve long-term cognitive and functional outcome and change the longitudinal course of illness described previously. (For further discussion, see subsection "Impact of Second-Generation Antipsychotics on Cognition" later in this chapter.)

RELATION OF NEUROCOGNITIVE IMPAIRMENT TO SCHIZOPHRENIA SYMPTOMS

In this section we address the relationship between neurocognitive impairment and symptoms. If neurocognitive deficits were the result of the symptoms of the illness, then the deficits would disappear when the symptoms do. However, this is usually not the case in patients with schizophrenia. Unlike patients with psychotic bipolar illness, whose performance on cognitive tests may improve when their psychotic symptoms remit, patients with schizophrenia do not show any change in performance when psychosis remits (Harvey et al. 1990).

Pseudospecificity

The impact of first-generation antipsychotics on cognition is very weak (Blyler and Gold 2000). The recalcitrance of neurocognitive impairment in the context of substantial symptom improvement is one of the most compelling lines of evidence of the independence of these symptom domains. However, recent studies investigating second-generation antipsychotics raise an important question about the potential "pseudospecificity" of cognitive improvement: If second-generation antipsychotics improve cognition and symptoms, is the cognitive improvement explained by the improvement in symptoms? Although substantial improvements in symptoms and mild improvements in cognition may be found with some second-generation drugs, the correlations between these two domains of improvement have largely been found not to be statistically significant (Bilder et al. 2002).

Cross-Sectional Studies of the Relation to Symptoms of Schizophrenia

Neurocognitive deficits are largely separate from both the positive and negative symptoms of the disorder. Cross-sectional relationships between neurocognition and positive symptoms, particularly for hallucinations and delusions, are usually quite weak (Addington and Addington 2000; Hughes et al. 2003; Strauss 1993). Generally, the variance shared by these variables is less than 10%. Relationships tend to be slightly stronger between neurocognition and negative or "deficit" symptoms (Addington and Addington 2000; Buchanan et al. 1997; Hughes et al. 2003; Tamlyn et al. 1992).

Positive Symptoms

It has been reported repeatedly that neurocognitive ability is not strongly correlated with severity of psychotic symptoms in patients with schizophrenia (Addington et al. 1991; Bilder et al. 1985; Strauss 1993). In acute exacerbation, the severity of positive symptoms has been found to be significantly correlated with *better* performance on select domains of cognitive function. Although some exceptions exist, such as isolated reports of significant correlations of positive symptoms with working memory (Bressi et al. 1996; Carter et al. 1996), source monitoring (Keefe et al. 2002), and auditory distractibility (Walker and Lewine 1988), the overall trend is for general neurocognitive impairment not to be correlated with positive symptoms. This low correlation across various patient samples, including first-episode (Mohamed et al. 1999), chronic (Addington et al. 1991; Tamlyn et al. 1992), and elderly (Davidson et al. 1995) patients, suggests that positive symptoms are clearly not the sole cause of the cognitive impairment found in patients with schizophrenia.

The low reliability of positive symptom assessment is a crucial factor (Strauss 1993). The subjective report of a psychotic patient may not reflect the true level of the patient's psychosis. Furthermore, the exclusion of patients who are too psychotic to be tested may serve to weaken any potential correlation between the severity of psychosis and neurocognitive impairment. Finally, those patients who have more intact cognitive abilities may be better able to recall and express their internal state including detailed delusions and hallucinations. These patients would thus receive higher scores on positive symptom rating scales, resulting in a reduction in any potential correlation between positive symptoms and neurocognitive impairment. Clearly, there are limitations to the assessment of positive symptoms, and the absence of cross-sectional correlations between positive symptoms severity and neurocognitive impairment is complex.

Negative Symptoms

Cognitive dysfunction is significantly correlated with various types of negative symptoms (Addington et al. 1991;

Cuesta et al. 1995; Morris et al. 1995; Strauss 1993; Summerfelt et al. 1991; Tamlyn et al. 1992). The greater variance shared between neurocognition and negative symptoms compared with positive symptoms may result from measurement overlap. For instance, the neurocognitive variable verbal fluency and the negative symptom variable poverty of speech both measure the speed at which a patient generates speech. A patient who generates speech at a slow rate will do so during a test of verbal fluency as well as in an interview during which he or she is being rated for poverty of speech.

Empirical studies suggest that motor functions are strongly correlated with negative symptoms (Cuesta et al. 1995; Manschreck et al. 1985), job success (McGurk et al. 2003), and outcome (Bilder et al. 1985). Deficient motor skills are represented in both the negative symptom and the cognitive dysfunction domain because symptoms such as blunted affect and motor retardation are observational measures of motor functioning (Alpert 1985; Andreasen 1989). Thus impaired motor skills in many ways lie at the core of negative symptoms in schizophrenia.

Whether the negative symptom of reduced motivation underlies the poor performance of patients with schizophrenia on cognitive tests is controversial. Although monetary reinforcement has been shown to improve performance on effortful cognitive tests such as the WCST in some studies (Summerfelt et al. 1991), especially in less difficult tasks, others have not shown these findings (Green et al. 1990). Increases in pupil size are associated with increased cognitive processing demands (Granholm et al. 1996). Therefore, pupillary response can measure engagement in a task. If the cognitive deficits of schizophrenic patients were caused by lack of interest or motivation, their pupillary response would be low throughout the period of cognitive assessment. Only during high-processing conditions do patients have abnormal pupillary responses, suggesting they put forth a normal amount of effort when being given cognitive tests, yet their decreased processing capacity leads them to be unable to engage in difficult tasks (Granholm et al. 1997).

On the contrary, cognitive deficits may cause reduced motivation. Individuals with cognitive deficits are less likely to be motivated to have goals and pursue them (reviewed by Deci and Flaste 1996). Patients with neurocognitive impairment are likely to be met with failure if they attempt to pursue employment, social, and even recreational avenues that require cognitive skill. Repeated failures are likely to cause discouragement and reduced motivation in people with schizophrenia.

In sum, a cross-sectional correlation of negative symptoms and neurocognitive impairment has been consistently reported, but the magnitude of this relation is modest.

Formal Thought Disorder

Deficits in semantic memory may lie at the heart of the cognition–thought disorder relation (Elvevag et al. 2002). This argument has recently been supported by empirical data suggesting that the difference between semantic fluency and phonological fluency, an indication of the severity of the impairment of the "semantic network" in schizophrenic patients, predicted the severity of their formal thought disorder (Goldberg et al. 1998). Thus, a patient's ability to have verbal information available (referred to as "semantic priming") may be the most important cognitive factor in formal thought disorder.

Affective Symptoms

Because many patients with schizophrenia also report depressed mood (Jin et al. 2001), if not a full depressive disorder, and because depression is associated with some cognitive impairment (Goldberg et al. 1993a), the role of depressed mood in neurocognitive impairment is important. Very few studies have examined this relationship directly. Further, the distinction between depressive symptoms and negative symptoms is sometimes difficult for raters and clinicians to make (Goldman et al. 1992; McKenna et al. 1989), yet factor analyses suggest that they are separate dimensions of schizophrenia (Lindenmayer et al. 1995; Willem Van der Does et al. 1995). Higher depression scores were significantly correlated with worse verbal memory task performance, which remained even after controlling for psychomotor retardation and processing speed performance (Brebion et al. 2001). Thus depression may influence the association between negative symptoms and cognitive impairments, and it also may have a direct deleterious effect on some aspects of neurocognitive impairment.

In conclusion, the cross-sectional correlations between neurocognitive impairment and symptoms are weaker than might be expected and vary depending on symptom domain. The consistency of this finding strongly supports the idea that neurocognitive impairment is not caused by psychosis.

LONGITUDINAL STUDIES

The relative independence of neurocognitive impairment and symptoms in cross-sectional studies appears to be supported by longitudinal studies. When patients with schizophrenia are successfully treated with first-generation antipsychotics, the severity of their symptoms is substantially reduced (Lieberman et al. 2003). However,

if neurocognitive function improves with first-generation antipsychotic treatment, the effects are small (Blyler and Gold 2000; DeLisi et al. 1995; S. Gold 1999; Hoff et al. 1999).

First, it is important to emphasize here that the stability of neurocognitive impairment occurs in the context of frequent variability of the symptoms of schizophrenia, especially the positive symptoms (Bilder et al. 2000). For example, in a study of patients tested during a psychotic exacerbation and then again, 1–2 years later, when symptoms had improved considerably, cognitive function was found to be very stable over time (Nopoulos et al. 1994). In a longitudinal study over a 1-year interval, cognitive and negative symptoms were correlated at each of the assessments, but there was no predictive relationship between these variables over time (Harvey et al. 1996). If negative symptoms were somehow causing poor performance on cognitive tests, a longitudinal relationship between these variables would have been expected. Second, when the differential relationship between cognitive and negative symptoms and adaptive functioning deficits has been examined, cognitive impairments have been found to be correlated more strongly with functional deficit than negative symptoms (Harvey et al. 1996, 1998). Third, in those patients whose functional status worsens over time, changes in cognitive impairment predict the level of change, whereas changes in negative symptoms do not (Harvey et al. 1998). These data suggesting a variable relationship of symptoms and neurocognitive impairment provide yet another line of support for the relative independence of these domains.

Another way to investigate the longitudinal relationship between neurocognitive impairment and symptoms is to calculate the correlation between change in neurocognitive impairment and symptom change. This approach addresses the issue of "pseudospecificity." Several studies have performed such analyses and although results are mixed, the findings have generally suggested that symptom change does not contribute substantially to cognitive change (Addington et al. 1991; Hoff et al. 1999).

IMPACT OF SECOND-GENERATION ANTIPSYCHOTICS ON COGNITION

Patients with schizophrenia have been treated with excessive doses of conventional antipsychotic medication for years. This treatment may have had direct adverse cognitive effects and led clinicians to use anticholinergic medications to control side effects. Lowering dosages of conventional antipsychotic medications has some modest cognitive benefit (Seidman et al. 1993), which suggests that use of excessive doses may have led to some of the failures of conventional medications to improve cognition (Harvey et al. 2004a).

Compared with first-generation antipsychotics, second-generation antipsychotics have some cognitive benefits (Harvey and Keefe 2001; Keefe et al. 1999). This issue is still controversial because many of the studies are methodologically limited. For instance, many comparisons of the cognitive benefit of second-generation and first-generation antipsychotics include excessive doses of first-generation antipsychotic medication, which may unfairly inflate the benefits attributable to second-generation antipsychotics by confusing them with dose effects. Further, there is evidence that unlike first-generation antipsychotics, second-generation medications may allow patients to benefit from practice-related improvements (Harvey et al. 2000). However, recent studies of first-episode patients on lower doses of first-generation antipsychotics suggest that second-generation antipsychotics have a greater cognitive enhancing effect (Harvey et al. 2004b; Keefe et al. 2004).

SUMMARY

The literature on neurocognitive impairment demonstrates consistently that cognitive impairment is not caused by the symptoms of schizophrenia. Most impressive is the zero-to-mild cross-sectional correlations between neurocognitive impairment and the positive symptoms of the illness. Whereas other aspects of schizophrenia, such as negative symptoms, appear to correlate with neurocognitive impairment, there is as much or more evidence supporting the idea that neurocognitive impairment causes negative symptoms as there is evidence that negative symptoms cause neurocognitive impairment. Although there is limited evidence of a relationship between changes in neurocognitive impairment and changes in symptoms over time, there is no clear evidence that improvements in neurocognitive impairment are caused by improvements in symptoms. In fact, most data point to the relative independence of these two targets of treatment in schizophrenia.

CLINICAL IMPORTANCE OF NEUROCOGNITIVE IMPAIRMENT

CROSS-SECTIONAL CORRELATIONS WITH FUNCTION

Although the literature suggests that neurocognitive impairment is not strongly correlated with symptoms, it has proven to be consistently related to a variety of other important aspects of the illness, such as social functioning (Liberman et al. 1986; Spaulding et al. 1986), functional impairments, unemployment (Brekke et al. 1997; Lysaker and Bell 1995; McGurk and Meltzer 2000; Velligan et al. 2000), quality of life (Fujii and Wylie 2003), relapse prevention (Fenton et al. 1997; Jarboe and Schwartz 1999), medical status, and economic cost (Knapp 1997; Sevy and Davidson 1995). Neurocognitive impairment also has considerable power to predict functional status years later.

Relation of Neurocognitive Impairment to Functioning

Functional outcome in schizophrenia is difficult to define and measure. The three types of functional outcome that most studies of neurocognitive deficits have examined are 1) community (social and occupational) outcome, 2) ability to solve simulations of interpersonal interactions, and 3) success in psychosocial rehabilitation programs. Strong support for associations between key areas of neurocognition and functional outcome are offered by two reviews of the literature (Green 1996; Green et al. 2000).

The connection between actual community functioning and cognition is weaker than the strong link between laboratory measures of community functioning or skills acquisition and cognition (Green 1996). In a 1-year follow-up study of patients with first-episode psychosis, the size of the correlations between the number and quality of actual social relations and various cognitive measures were found to be in the 0.25–0.35 range (Malla et al. 2002).

Across the studies reviewed by Green and colleagues (2000), all of the key neurocognitive constructs (secondary memory, immediate memory, vigilance, and executive functioning/card sorting) had significant relationships to functional outcome and effect sizes in the medium range. Cognitive impairments are also correlated with deficits in the performance of specific skills critical for independent living (Evans et al. 2003; Patterson et al. 2001).

Unemployment

Several studies of cognitive performance and vocational functioning have been conducted in rehabilitation settings (Bell and Bryson 2001; Lysaker and Bell 1995). Ratings of work behavior/performance are related to baseline scores on verbal memory tests and the WCST. Additionally, improvement in patient work performance in a 6-month work rehabilitation program was predicted by baseline performance on various cognitive tests.

A number of positive findings have been reported in studies examining correlates of competitive employment

(Beiser et al. 1994; Brekke et al. 1997; Velligan et al. 2000). Patients enrolled in school full-time or holding competitive employment show superior performance across measures of working memory, sustained attention, problem solving, and episodic memory when compared with unemployed patients (McGurk and Meltzer 2000), with scores of part-time workers falling between the other two groups. In addition, vocational functioning is significantly associated with performance on speed of processing tasks such as the Trail Making Parts A and B tests (McGurk et al. 2003).

McGurk and Meltzer (2000) evaluated the relationship of cognitive functioning and work status and concluded that neurocognitive performance plays a more important role than clinical symptoms in the ability of patients with schizophrenia to work. The implication is that patients with schizophrenia who have higher levels of cognitive impairment may require greater amounts of vocational support than those with lower levels of impairment (McGurk et al. 2003).

Quality of Life

Quality of life is often defined by the quality of social, occupational, and interpersonal aspects of life and is related to cognitive function. Some evidence suggests that reductions in quality of life are more strongly associated with cognitive deficits than other symptomatic features of the illness. Specifically, the relationship between subjective experience and social functioning has been shown to be mediated by executive functioning (Brekke et al. 2001). Patients have less realistic impressions of their social functioning if they also have more severe executive deficits.

The need for anticholinergic treatments is also associated with reductions in quality of life. Reductions in quality of life and anticholinergic medications may be related to the extrapyramidal side effect that triggers anticholinergic medication prescriptions. Nonetheless, anticholinergic medications reliably reduce cognitive functioning as well. In patients with schizophrenia, anticholinergic medications impair attention and memory functions (Spohn and Strauss 1989). These impairments can induce reductions in subjective quality of life. One study of patients with schizophrenia that examined the relationship between coping abilities and cognitive dysfunction suggested that more severe executive and memory deficits are related to decreased use of coping mechanisms (Wilder-Willis et al. 2002).

Fujii and Wylie (2003) studied the long-term effects of neurocognition on quality of life in patients with severe schizophrenia. They found that neurocognition does, in fact, have long-term predictive validity for quality of life and that therapeutics targeting neurocognition could improve quality of life in this population.

Relapse Prevention

Cognitive functions have been shown to be the strongest predictors of patients' ability to manage medications (Jeste et al. 2003). Cognitive deficits contribute to patterns of medication mismanagement that are associated with poor adherence and risk of relapse (Fenton et al. 1997; Jarboe and Schwartz 1999). In one study, memory impairment was the best predictor of partial compliance (Donohoe et al. 2001). Patients performing poorly in medication management tests also had poor global scores on a dementia inventory (Patterson et al. 2002). Decreased medication compliance in patients with schizophrenia has been shown to be related to poor performance on tests of attention and visual memory (Jarboe and Schwartz 1999).

Medical Comorbidity

Neurocognitive impairment is also related to medical comorbidities in schizophrenia. Deficits in organization (executive skills) directly affect patients' ability to seek treatment for medical problems. In elderly patients with schizophrenia, cognitive and functional impairments predicted the later incidence of new-onset medical problems, whereas medical problems did not predict the subsequent worsening of cognitive and self-care deficits (Friedman et al. 2002). Inability of patients with schizophrenia to reduce damaging habits such as smoking has been correlated with deficits in memory and attention (Buchanan et al. 1994; George et al. 2000). Thus, cognitive impairments were shown directly to effect new-onset medical problems in older patients.

Costs

A major factor in the costs (direct and indirect) associated with schizophrenia is cognitive impairment (Sevy and Davidson 1995). Factors leading to the increased cost include loss of ability for self-care, level of inpatient and outpatient care needed, and loss of productivity (for both patient and caretaker).

Although cognitive impairment by itself is rarely a reason for acute hospitalization of a patient with schizophrenia, it may contribute to the overall length of hospitalization. It may lead to early admission to nursing homes or long-term care facilities in the case of elderly patients.

CONCLUSION

A consensus has developed among experts in cognition and schizophrenia that cognitive impairment is a core feature of the illness. The course of neurocognitive impairment follows a characteristic pattern and following the early phase is consistent even when positive and negative symptoms change. Consistent with the demonstration that cognitive impairments are not a result of symptoms of schizophrenia, studies show on the whole the independence of these two targets for treatment. Long-term functional and cognitive outcome as well as the longitudinal course of the illness potentially could improve with early treatment using second-generation antipsychotics. Functional status years later can be predicted with considerable accuracy from the extent of neurocognitive impairments. The relationship has been established between cognition and many other facets of schizophrenia, from social functioning to unemployment to relapse prevention. Indeed, improved understanding and treatment of neurocognitive impairments in schizophrenia holds considerable promise for the field and for the lives of patients with schizophrenia.

REFERENCES

Addington J, Addington D: Facial affect recognition and information processing in schizophrenia and bipolar disorder. Schizophr Res 32:171–181, 1998

Addington J, Addington D: Neurocognitive and social functioning in schizophrenia: a 2.5 year follow-up study. Schizophr Res 44:47–56, 2000

Addington J, Addington D, Maticka-Tyndale E: Cognitive functioning and positive and negative symptoms in schizophrenia. Schizophr Res 5:123–134, 1991

Addington J, McCleary L, Munroe-Blum H: Relationship between cognitive and social dysfunction in schizophrenia. Schizophr Res 34:59–66, 1998

Alpert M: The signs and symptoms of schizophrenia. Compr Psychiatry 26:103–112, 1985

American Psychiatric Association: Diagnostic and Statistical Manual of Mental Disorders, 4th Edition, Text Revision. Washington, DC, American Psychiatric Association, 2000

Andreasen NC: Scale for the Assessment of Negative Symptoms (SANS). Br J Psychiatry 155 (suppl 7):53–58, 1989

Arnold SE, Gur RE, Shapiro RM, et al: Prospective clinico-pathologic studies of schizophrenia: accrual and assessment of patients. Am J Psychiatry 152:731–737, 1995

Baddeley A: Working memory. Science 255:556–559, 1992

Beiser M, Bean G, Erickson D, et al: Biological and psychosocial predictors of job performance following a first episode of psychosis. Am J Psychiatry 151:857–863, 1994

Bell M, Bryson G: Work rehabilitation in schizophrenia: does cognitive impairment limit improvement? Schizophr Bull 27:269–279, 2001

Bell M, Bryson G, Lysaker P: Positive and negative affect recognition in schizophrenia: a comparison with substance abuse and normal control subjects. Psychiatry Res 73:73–82, 1997

Bilder RM, Mukherjee S, Rieder RO, et al: Symptomatic and neuropsychological components of defect states. Schizophr Bull 11:409–419, 1985

Bilder RM, Lipschutz-Broch L, Reiter G, et al: Intellectual deficits in first-episode schizophrenia: evidence for progressive deterioration. Schizophr Bull 18:437–448, 1992

Bilder RM, Goldman RS, Robinson D, et al: Neuropsychology of first-episode schizophrenia: initial characterization and clinical correlates. Am J Psychiatry 157:549–559, 2000

Bilder RM, Goldman RS, Volavka J, et al: Neurocognitive effects of clozapine, olanzapine, risperidone, and haloperidol in patients with chronic schizophrenia or schizoaffective disorder. Am J Psychiatry 159:1018–1028, 2002

Blyer CR, Gold JM: Cognitive effects of conventional antipsychotics: another look, in Cognitive Functioning in Schizophrenia: Characteristics, Correlates, and Treatment. Edited by Sharma T, Harvey P. Oxford, England, Oxford University Press, 2000, pp 241–265

Brebion G, Gorman JM, Malaspina D, et al: Clinical and cognitive factors associated with verbal memory task performance in patients with schizophrenia. Am J Psychiatry 158:758–764, 2001

Brekke JS, Raine A, Ansel M, et al: Neuropsychological and psychophysiological correlates of psychosocial functioning in schizophrenia. Schizophr Bull 23:19–28, 1997

Brekke JS, Kohrt B, Green MF: Neuropsychological functioning as a moderator of the relationship between psychosocial functioning and the subjective experience of self and life in schizophrenia. Schizophr Bull 27:697–708, 2001

Bressi S, Miele L, Bressi C, et al: Deficit of central executive component of working memory in schizophrenia. New Trends in Experimental and Clinical Psychiatry 12:243–252, 1996

Brewer WJ, Wood SJ, McGorry PD, et al: Impairment of olfactory identification ability in individuals at ultra-high risk for psychosis who later develop schizophrenia. Am J Psychiatry 160:1790–1794, 2003

Brickman A, Buchsbaum M, Bloom R, et al: Neuropsychological functioning in first-break, never-medicated adolescents with psychosis. J Nerv Ment Dis 192:615–622, 2004

Buchanan RW, Holstein C, Breier A: The comparative efficacy and long-term effect of clozapine treatment on neuropsychological test performance. Biol Psychiatry 36:717–725, 1994

Buchanan RW, Strauss ME, Breier A, et al: Attentional impairments in deficit and nondeficit forms of schizophrenia. Am J Psychiatry 154:363–370, 1997

Calev A: Recall and recognition in chronic nondemented schizophrenics: use of matched tasks. J Abnorm Psychol 93:172–177, 1984

Callicott JH, Mattay VS, Bertolino A, et al: Physiological characteristics of capacity constraints in working memory as revealed by functional MRI. Cereb Cortex 9:20–26, 1999

Carter C, Robertson L, Nordahl T, et al: Spatial working memory deficits and their relationship to negative symptoms in unmedicated schizophrenia patients. Biol Psychiatry 40:930–932, 1996

Caspi A, Reichenberg A, Weiser M, et al: Cognitive performance in schizophrenia patients assessed before and following the first psychotic episode. Schizophr Res 65:87–94, 2003

Corcoran R, Mercer G, Frith CD: Schizophrenia, symptomatology and social influence: investigating "theory of mind" in people with schizophrenia. Schizophr Res 17:5–13, 1995

Cornblatt B, Keilp J: Impaired attention, genetics, and the pathophysiology of schizophrenia. Schizophr Bull 20:31–46, 1994

Cornblatt B, Obuchowski M, Roberts S, et al: Cognitive and behavioral precursors of schizophrenia. Dev Psychopathol 11:487–508, 1999

Corrigan PW, Davies-Farmer RM, Stolley MR: Social cue recognition in schizophrenia under variable levels of arousal. Cognit Ther Res 14:353–361, 1990

Cuesta MJ, Peralta V, Caro F, et al: Schizophrenic syndrome and Wisconsin Card Sorting Test dimensions. Psychiatry Res 58:45–51, 1995

David AS, Malmberg A, Brandt L, et al: IQ and risk for schizophrenia: a population-based cohort study. Psychol Med 27:1311–1323, 1997

Davidson M, Harvey PD, Powchik P, et al: Severity of symptoms in chronically institutionalized geriatric schizophrenic patients. Am J Psychiatry 152:197–207, 1995

Davidson M, Reichenberg A, Rabinowitz J, et al: Behavioral and intellectual markers for schizophrenia in apparently healthy male adolescents. Am J Psychiatry 156:1328–1335, 1999

Deci EL, Flaste R: Why We Do What We Do: Understanding Self-Motivation. New York, Penguin, 1996

DeLisi LE, Tew W, Xie S, et al: A prospective follow-up study of brain morphology and cognition in first-episode schizophrenic patients: preliminary findings. Biol Psychiatry 38:349–360, 1995

Dickerson F, Boronow JJ, Ringel N, et al: Social functioning and neurocognitive deficits in outpatients with schizophrenia: a 2-year follow-up. Schizophr Res 37:13–20, 1999

Donohoe G, Owens N, O'Donnell C, et al: Predictors of compliance with neuroleptic medication among inpatients with schizophrenia: a discriminant function analysis. Eur Psychiatry 16:293–298, 2001

Doody GA, Gotz M, Johnstone EC, et al: Theory of mind and psychoses. Psychol Med 28:397–405, 1998

Drury VM, Robinson EJ, Birchwood M: "Theory of mind" skills during an acute episode of psychosis and following recovery. Psychol Med 28:1101–1112, 1998

Edwards J, Pattison PE, Jackson HJ, et al: Facial affect and affective prosody recognition in first-episode schizophrenia. Schizophr Res 48:235–253, 2001

Elvevag B, Weickert T, Wechsler M, et al: An investigation of the integrity of semantic boundaries in schizophrenia. Schizophr Res 53:187–198, 2002

Ertugrul A, Ulug B: The influence of neurocognitive deficits and symptoms on disability in schizophrenia. Acta Psychiatr Scand 105:196–201, 2002

Evans JD, Heaton RK, Paulsen JS, et al: The relationship of neuropsychological abilities to specific domains of functional capacity in older schizophrenic patients. Biol Psychiatry 53:422–430, 2003

Fenton WS, Blyler CR, Heinssen RK: Determinants of medication compliance in schizophrenia: empirical and clinical findings. Schizophr Bull 23:637–651, 1997

Friedman JI, Harvey PD, McGurk SR, et al: Correlates of change in functional status of institutionalized geriatric schizophrenic patients: focus on medical comorbidity. Am J Psychiatry 159:1388–1394, 2002

Fujii DE, Wylie AM: Neurocognition and community outcome in schizophrenia: long-term predictive validity. Schizophr Res 59:219–223, 2003

Fuller R, Nopoulos P, Arndt S, et al: Longitudinal assessment of premorbid cognitive functioning in patients with schizophrenia through examination of standardized scholastic test performance. Am J Psychiatry 159:1183–1189, 2002

Gaebel W, Wolwer W: Facial expression and emotional face recognition in schizophrenia and depression. Eur Arch Psychiatry Clin Neurosci 242:46–52, 1992

Galletly CA, Clark CR, McFarlane AC, et al: The effect of clozapine on the speed and accuracy of information processing in schizophrenia. Prog Neuropsychopharmacol 24:1329–1338, 2000

George TP, Ziedonis DM, Feingold A, et al: Nicotine transdermal patch and atypical antipsychotic medications for smoking cessation in schizophrenia. Am J Psychiatry 157:1835–1842, 2000

Gold JM, Goldberg RW, McNary SW, et al: Cognitive correlates of job tenure among patients with severe mental illness. Am J Psychiatry 159:1395–1402, 2002

Gold JM, Wilk CM, McMahon RP, et al: Working memory for visual features and conjunctions in schizophrenia. J Abnorm Psychol 112:61–71, 2003

Gold S: Longitudinal study of cognitive function in first-episode and recent-onset schizophrenia. Am J Psychiatry 156:1342–1348, 1999

Goldberg TE, Weinberger DR, Berman KF, et al: Further evidence for dementia of the prefrontal type in schizophrenia? A controlled study of teaching the Wisconsin Card Sorting Test. Arch Gen Psychiatry 44:1008–1014, 1987

Goldberg TE, Ragland JD, Torrey EF, et al: Neuropsychological assessment of monozygotic twins discordant for schizophrenia. Arch Gen Psychiatry 47:1066–1072, 1990

Goldberg TE, Gold JM, Greenberg R, et al: Contrasts between patients with affective disorders and patients with schizophrenia on a neuropsychological test battery. Am J Psychiatry 150:1355–1362, 1993a

Goldberg TE, Hyde TM, Kleinman JE, et al: Course of schizophrenia: neuropsychological evidence for a static encephalopathy. Schizophr Bull 19:797–804, 1993b

Goldberg TE, Aloia MS, Gourovitch ML, et al: Cognitive substrates of thought disorder; I: the semantic system. Am J Psychiatry 155:1671–1676, 1998

Goldman RS, Tandon R, Liberzon I, et al: Measurement of depression and negative symptoms in schizophrenia. Psychopathology 25:49–56, 1992

Goldman-Rakic PS: Circuitry of the frontal association cortex and its relevance to dementia. Arch Gerontol Geriatr 6:299–309, 1987

Goldman-Rakic PS: Working memory dysfunction in schizophrenia. J Neuropsychiatry Clin Neurosci 6:348–357, 1994

Goldstein G, Zubin J: Neuropsychological differences between young and old schizophrenics with and without associated neurological dysfunction. Schizophr Res 3:117–126, 1990

Granholm E, Asarnow RF, Sarkin AJ, et al: Pupillary responses index cognitive resource limitations. Psychophysiology 33:457–461, 1996

Granholm E, Morris SK, Sarkin AJ, et al: Pupillary responses index overload of working memory resources in schizophrenia. J Abnorm Psychol 106:458–467, 1997

Green MF: What are the functional consequences of neurocognitive deficits in schizophrenia? Am J Psychiatry 153:321–330, 1996

Green MF, Ganzell S, Satz P, et al: Teaching the Wisconsin Card Sorting Test to schizophrenic patients. Arch Gen Psychiatry 47:91–92, 1990

Green MF, Kern RS, Braff DL, et al: Neurocognitive deficits and functional outcome in schizophrenia: are we measuring the "right stuff"? Schizophr Bull 26:119–136, 2000

Harvey PD: Treatment of cognitive deficits in elderly schizophrenic patients, in Improving Cognitive Function in the Schizophrenic Patient. Edited by Keefe RSE. Science Press, 1999, pp 32–43

Harvey PD, Keefe RSE: Cognitive impairment in schizophrenia and implications of atypical neuroleptic treatment. CNS Spectr 2:1–11, 1997

Harvey PD, Keefe RSE: Studies of cognitive change in patients with schizophrenia following novel antipsychotic treatment. Am J Psychiatry 158:176–184, 2001

Harvey PD, Keefe RS, Moskowitz J, et al: Attentional markers of vulnerability to schizophrenia: performance of medicated and unmedicated patients and normals. Psychiatry Res 33:179–188, 1990

Harvey PD, Lombardi J, Leibman M, et al: Cognitive impairment and negative symptoms in geriatric chronic schizophrenic patients: a follow-up study. Schizophr Res 22:223–231, 1996

Harvey PD, Howanitz E, Parrella M, et al: Symptoms, cognitive functioning, and adaptive skills in geriatric patients with lifelong schizophrenia: a comparison across treatment sites. Am J Psychiatry 155:1080–1086, 1998

Harvey PD, Moriarty PJ, Serper MR, et al: Practice-related improvement in information processing with novel antipsychotic treatment. Schizophr Res 46:139–148, 2000

Harvey PD, Green MF, Keefe RSE, et al: Cognitive functioning in schizophrenia: a consensus statement on its role in the definition and evaluation of effective treatments for the illness. J Clin Psychiatry 65:361–372, 2004a

Harvey PD, Meltzer H, Simpson GM, et al: Improvement in cognitive function following a switch to ziprasidone from conventional antipsychotics, olanzapine, or risperidone in outpatients with schizophrenia. Schizophr Res 66:101–113, 2004

Hawkins KA, Addington J, Keefe RS, et al: Neuropsychological status of subjects at high risk for a first episode of psychosis. Schizophr Res 67:115–122, 2004

Heaton RK: Wisconsin Card Sorting Test Manual. Odessa, FL, Psychological Assessment Resources, 1981

Heaton RK, Drexler M: Clinical neuropsychological findings in schizophrenia and aging, in Schizophrenia and Aging: Schizophrenia, Paranoia, and Schizophreniform Disorders in Later Life. Edited by Milner NE, Cohen GD. New York, Guilford, 1987, pp 145–161

Heaton RK, Paulsen JS, McAdams LA, et al: Neuropsychological deficits in schizophrenics: relationship to age, chronicity, and dementia. Arch Gen Psychiatry 51:469–476, 1994

Heaton RK, Gladsjo JA, Palmer BW, et al: Stability and course of neuropsychological deficits in schizophrenia. Arch Gen Psychiatry 58:24–32, 2001

Heinrichs RW, Zakzanis KK: Neurocognitive deficit in schizophrenia: a quantitative review of the evidence. Neuropsychology 12:426–444, 1998

Hoff AL, Riordan H, O'Donnell DW, et al: Neuropsychological functioning of first-episode schizophreniform patients. Am J Psychiatry 149:898–903, 1992

Hoff AL, Sakuma M, Wieneke M, et al: Longitudinal neuropsychological follow-up study of patients with first-episode schizophrenia. Am J Psychiatry 156:1336–1341, 1999

Hughes C, Kumari V, Soni W, et al: Longitudinal study of symptoms and cognitive function in chronic schizophrenia. Schizophr Res 59:137–146, 2003

Hyde TM, Nawroz S, Goldberg TE, et al: Is there cognitive decline in schizophrenia? A cross-sectional study. Br J Psychiatry 164:494–500, 1994

Hyman SE, Fenton WS: What are the right targets for psychopharmacology? Science 299:350–351, 2003

Jarboe KS, Schwartz SK: The relationship between medication noncompliance and cognitive function in patients with schizophrenia. J Am Psychiatr Nurses Assoc 5:S2–S8, 1999

Jeste DV, Harris MJ, Krull A, et al: Clinical and neuropsychological characteristics of patients with late-onset schizophrenia. Am J Psychiatry 152:722–730, 1995

Jeste SD, Patterson TL, Palmer BW, et al: Cognitive predictors of medication adherence among middle-aged and older outpatients with schizophrenia. Schizophr Res 63:49–58, 2003

Jin H, Zisook S, Palmer BW, et al: Association of depressive symptoms and functioning in schizophrenia: a study of older outpatients. J Clin Psychiatry 62:797–803, 2001

Jones P, Rodgers B, Murray R, et al: Child development risk factors for adult schizophrenia in the British 1946 birth cohort. Lancet 344:1398–1402, 1994

Keefe RSE: The contribution of neuropsychology to psychiatry. Am J Psychiatry 152:6–15, 1995

Keefe RSE: Neurocognition, in Current Issues in the Psychopharmacology of Schizophrenia. Edited by Breier A, Tran PV, Herrera J, et al. Baltimore, MD, Lippincott Williams & Wilkins, 2001, pp 192–208

Keefe RSE, Silva SG, Perkins DO, et al: The effects of atypical antipsychotic drugs on neurocognitive impairment in schizophrenia: a review and meta-analysis. Schizophr Bull 25:2201–222, 1999

Keefe RS, Arnold MC, Bayen UJ, et al: Source-monitoring deficits for self-generated stimuli in schizophrenia: multinomial modeling of data from three sources. Schizophr Res 57:51–67, 2002

Keefe RS, Seidman LJ, Christensen BK, et al: Comparative effect of atypical and conventional antipsychotic drugs on neurocognition in first-episode psychosis: a randomized, double-blind trial of olanzapine versus low doses of haloperidol. Am J Psychiatry 161:985–995, 2004

Keefe RS, Eesley CE, Poe MP: Defining a cognitive function decrement in schizophrenia. Biol Psychiatry 57:688–691, 2005

Knapp M: Costs of schizophrenia. Br J Psychiatry 171:509–518, 1997

Kremen WS, Seidman LJ, Faraone SV, et al: The paradox of normal neuropsychological function in schizophrenia. J Abnorm Psychol 109:743–752, 2000

Liberman RP, Mueser KT, Wallace CJ: Social skills training for schizophrenic individuals at risk for relapse. Am J Psychiatry 143:523–526, 1986

Lieberman JA: Is schizophrenia a neurodegenerative disorder? A clinical and neurobiological perspective. Biol Psychiatry 46:729–739, 1999

Lieberman JA, Tollefson G, Tohen M, et al: Comparative efficacy and safety of atypical and conventional antipsychotic drugs in first-episode psychosis: a randomized, double-blind trial of olanzapine versus haloperidol. Am J Psychiatry 160:1396–1404, 2003

Lindenmayer JP, Grochowski S, Hyman RB: Five factor model of schizophrenia: replication across samples. Schizophr Res 14:229–234, 1995

Lysaker P, Bell M: Work rehabilitation and improvements in insight in schizophrenia. J Nerv Ment Dis 183:103–106, 1995

Malla AK, Norman RMG, Manchanda LT: Symptoms, cognition, treatment adherence and functional outcome in first-episode psychosis. Psychol Med 32:1109–1119, 2002

Manschreck TC, Maher BA, Waller NG, et al: Deficient motor synchrony in schizophrenic disorders: clinical correlates. Biol Psychiatry 20:990–1002, 1985

McGurk SR, Meltzer HY: The role of cognition in vocational functioning in schizophrenia. Schizophr Res 45:175–184, 2000

McGurk SR, Mueser KT, Harvey PD, et al: Cognitive and symptom predictors of work outcomes for clients with schizophrenia in supported employment. Psychiatr Serv 54:1129–1135, 2003

McKenna PJ, Lund CE, Mortimer AM: Negative symptoms: relationship to other schizophrenic symptom classes. Br J Psychiatry 7:104–107, 1989

Meltzer HY, McGurk SR: The effects of clozapine, risperidone, and olanzapine on cognitive function in schizophrenia. Schizophr Bull 25:233–255, 1999

Mohamed S, Paulsen JS, O'Leary D, et al: Generalized cognitive deficits in schizophrenia: a study of first-episode patients. Arch Gen Psychiatry 56:749–754, 1999

Morris RG, Rushe T, Woodruffe PW, et al: Problem solving in schizophrenia: a specific deficit in planning ability. Schizophr Res 14:235–246, 1995

Morrison RL, Bellack AS, Mueser KT: Deficits in facial-affect recognition and schizophrenia. Schizophr Bull 14:67–83, 1988

Moss M, Albert M (eds): Geriatric Neuropsychology. New York, Guilford, 1988

Mueser KT, Bellack AS, Douglas MS, et al: Prediction of social skill acquisition in schizophrenic and major affective disorder patients from memory and symptomatology. Psychiatry Res 37:281–296, 1991

Nuechterlein KH, Barch DM, Gold JM, et al: Identification of separable cognitive factors in schizophrenia. Schizophr Res 72:29–39, 2004

Nopoulos P, Flashman L, Flaum M, et al: Stability of cognitive functioning early in the course of schizophrenia. Schizophr Res 14:29–37, 1994

O'Donnell BF, Faux SF, McCarley RW, et al: Increased rate of P300 latency prolongation with age in schizophrenia: electrophysiological evidence for a neurodegenerative process. Arch Gen Psychiatry 52:544–549, 1995

Palmer BW, Heaton RK, Paulsen JS, et al: Is it possible to be schizophrenic yet neuropsychologically normal? Neuropsychology 11:437–446, 1997

Patterson TL, Goldman S, McKibbin CL, et al: UCSD performance-based skills assessment: development of a new measure of everyday functioning for severely mentally ill adults. Schizophr Bull 27:235–245, 2001

Patterson TL, Lacro J, McKibbin CL, et al: Medication management ability assessment: results from a performance-based measure in older outpatients with schizophrenia. J Clin Psychopharmacol 22:11–19, 2002

Paulsen JS, Heaton RK, Sadek JR, et al: The nature of learning and memory impairments in schizophrenia. J Int Neuropsychol Soc 1:88–99, 1995

Penn DL, Spaulding W, Reed D, et al: The relationship of social cognition to ward behavior in chronic schizophrenia. Schizophr Res 20:327–335, 1996

Penn DL, Corrigan PW, Bentall RP, et al: Social cognition in schizophrenia. Psychol Bull 121:114–132, 1997

Pinkham AE, Penn DL, Perkins DO, et al: Implications for the neural basis of social cognition for the study of schizophrenia. Am J Psychiatry 160:815–824, 2003

Rund BR: A review of longitudinal studies of cognitive functions in schizophrenia patients. Schizophr Bull 24:425–435, 1998

Sarfati Y, Hardy-Bayle MC, Nadel J, et al: Attribution of mental states to others by schizophrenic patients. Cognitive Neuropsychiatry 2:1–17, 1997

Saykin AJ, Gur RC, Gur RE, et al: Neuropsychological function in schizophrenia: selective impairment in memory and learning. Arch Gen Psychiatry 48:618–624, 1991

Saykin AJ, Shtasel DL, Gur RE, et al: Neuropsychological deficits in neuroleptic naive patients with first-episode schizophrenia. Arch Gen Psychiatry 51:124–131, 1994

Seidman LJ, Pepple JR, Faraone SV: Neuropsychological performance in chronic schizophrenia in response to neuroleptic dose reduction. Biol Psychiatry 33:575–584, 1993

Sevy S, Davidson M: The cost of cognitive impairment in schizophrenia. Schizophr Res 17:1–3, 1995

Silver H, Feldman P, Bilker W, et al: Working memory deficit as a core neuropsychological dysfunction in schizophrenia. Am J Psychiatry 160:1809–1816, 2003

Spaulding WD, Storms L, Goodrich V, et al: Applications of experimental psychopathology in psychiatric rehabilitation. Schizophr Bull 12:560–577, 1986

Spohn HE, Strauss ME: Relation of neuroleptic and anticholinergic medication to cognitive functions in schizophrenia. J Abnorm Psychol 98:478–486, 1989

Stirling J, White C, Lewis S, et al: Neurocognitive function and outcome in first-episode schizophrenia: a 10-year follow-up of an epidemiological cohort. Schizophr Res 65:75–86, 2003

Strauss ME: Relations of symptoms to cognitive deficits in schizophrenia. Schizophr Bull 19:215–231, 1993

Summerfelt AT, Alphs LD, Funderburk FR, et al: Impaired Wisconsin Card Sort performance in schizophrenia may reflect motivational deficits. Arch Gen Psychiatry 48:282–283, 1991

Sweeney JA, Haas GL, Keilp JG, et al: Evaluation of the stability of neuropsychological functioning after acute episodes of schizophrenia: one-year follow-up study. Psychiatry Res 38:63–76, 1991

Tamlyn D, McKenna PJ, Mortimer AM, et al: Memory impairment in schizophrenia: its extent, affiliations and neuropsychological character. Psychol Med 22:101–115, 1992

Trumbetta, Susan L, Mueser, et al: Social functioning and its relationship to cognitive deficits over the course of schizophrenia, in Negative Symptom and Cognitive Deficit Treatment Response in Schizophrenia. Edited by Keefe RSE, McEvoy JP. Washington, DC, American Psychiatric Association, 2001, pp 33–67

Twamley EW, Doshi RR, Nayak GV, et al: Generalized cognitive impairments, ability to perform everyday tasks, and level of independence in community living situations of older patients with psychosis. Am J Psychiatry 159:2013–2020, 2003

Velligan DI, Bow-Thomas C, Mahurin RK, et al: Do specific neurocognitive deficits predict specific domains of community function in schizophrenia? J Nerv Ment Dis 188:518–524, 2000

Waddington JL, Youssef HA: Cognitive dysfunction in chronic schizophrenia followed prospectively over 10 years and its longitudinal relationship to the emergence of tardive dyskinesia. Psychol Med 26:681–688, 1996

Walker E, Lewine RJ: The positive/negative symptom distinction in schizophrenia: validity and etiological relevance. Schizophr Res 1:315–328, 1988

Wechsler D: Weschsler Adult Intelligence Scale—III. San Antonio, TX, Psychological Corporation, 1997

Weinberger DR: Implications of normal brain development for the pathogenesis of schizophrenia. Arch Gen Psychiatry 44:660–669, 1987

Wilder-Willis KE, Shear PK, Steffen JJ, et al: The relationship between cognitive dysfunction and coping abilities in schizophrenia. Schizophr Res 55:259–267, 2002

Willem Van der Does AJ, Dingemans PMAJ, Linszen DH, et al: Dimensions and subtypes of recent-onset schizophrenia: a longitudinal analysis. J Nerv Ment Dis 183:681–687, 1995

Yung AR, McGorry PD: The prodromal phase of first-episode psychosis: past and current conceptualizations. Schizophr Bull 22:353–370, 1996

Zorrilla LT, Eyler, Heaton RK, et al: Cross-sectional study of older outpatients with schizophrenia and healthy comparison subjects: no differences in age-related cognitive decline. Am J Psychiatry 157:1324–1326, 2000

SOCIAL COGNITIVE IMPAIRMENTS

DAVID L. PENN, PH.D.

JEAN ADDINGTON, PH.D.

AMY PINKHAM, M.A.

In this chapter, we provide an overview of social cognition in schizophrenia. Social cognition, which has been defined as "the human ability and capacity to perceive the intentions and dispositions of others" (Brothers 1990, p. 28), includes the cognitive processes involved in thoughts about the self, others, social situations, and social interactions (Penn et al. 1997). A related definition has been proposed by Adolphs (1999), who describes it as "the processes that subserve behavior in response to conspecifics, and, in particular, to those higher cognitive processes subserving the extreme, diverse, and flexible social behaviors that are seen in primates" (p. 469). These definitions characterize social cognition as being a key component of social behavior.

Unlike nonsocial cognition (or neurocognition), which has enjoyed a long history of investigation in schizophrenia, social cognition has only recently come to the forefront of interest, motivated in part by two factors. First, there is growing evidence of a neural network—composed of the prefrontal cortex, fusiform gyrus, superior temporal sulcus, and amygdala—specialized for the processing of social information (Adolphs 1999, 2001, 2002, 2003; Brothers 1990; Calder et al. 2001; Frith and Frith 1999;

Haxby et al. 2002; Phillips et al. 2003a, 2003b; Pinkham et al. 2003). Second, it is increasingly realized that nonsocial cognition, although significantly associated with social functioning, still cannot explain approximately 40%–80% in functioning (Penn et al. 1997, 2001; Pinkham et al. 2003; Silverstein 1997) and may in fact exert an influence on social functioning via social cognition (Green et al. 2000).

There is evidence, from work in clinical populations, for the relative independence of social cognition from other aspects of cognition. For example, individuals with either frontal or prefrontal cortex damage show impaired social behavior and functioning despite retaining intact cognitive skills (Anderson et al. 1999; Blair and Cipolotti 2000; Fine et al. 2001). A similar dissociation between social cognition and nonsocial cognitive skills often is observed in individuals with prosopagnosia, who show selective impairments in the perceptions of faces but preserved perception for nonsocial stimuli (Kanwisher 2000). Further evidence for the autonomy of social cognition is gleaned from studies on individuals with Williams syndrome and individuals with autism. Individuals with Williams syndrome tend to be outgoing and social despite

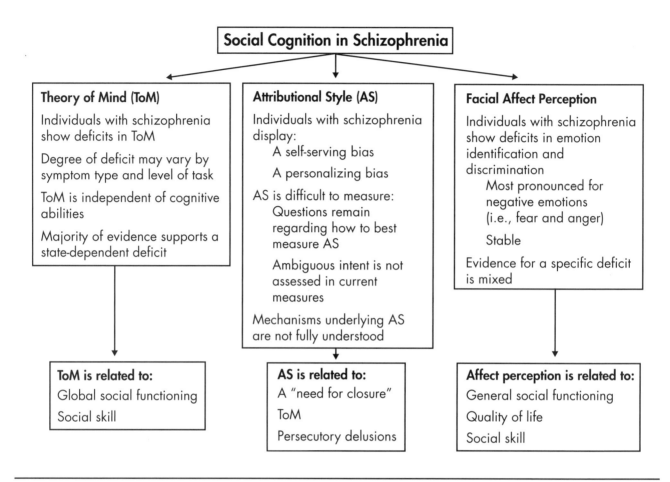

FIGURE 14–1. Major domains of social cognition in schizophrenia.

having below normal intelligence (Jones et al. 2000). Also, these individuals appear to have relatively preserved basic social cognitive skills despite having cognitive impairments (Tager-Flusberg et al. 1998). In contrast, individuals with high-functioning autism and Asperger's syndrome show impairments in social cognition and social behavior that are not related to general cognitive abilities (Heavey et al. 2000; Klin 2000). And even in nonclinical samples (e.g., scientists, mathematician) there is evidence for strengths in cognitive domains not translating into social cognitive domains (Baron-Cohen et al. 1999b). These findings lend support for the hypothesis that specific neural modules exist that are devoted to the processing of social information and that may have evolutionary significance (Fiddick et al. 2000).

In the ensuing sections, we review three major domains of social cognition in schizophrenia (Figure 14–1): 1) theory of mind, 2) attributional style, and 3) facial affect perception, with particular emphasis on the salient issues relevant to each domain (e.g., whether facial affect perception impairments in schizophrenia are caused by a specific or generalized performance deficit). We conclude

the chapter with a discussion of future research directions in this area.

THEORY OF MIND IN SCHIZOPHRENIA

Theory of mind (ToM) refers to the ability to represent the mental states of others and/or to make inferences about another's intentions. Skills that fall under the rubric of ToM include understanding false beliefs, hints, intentions, deception, metaphor, irony, and faux pas. A common way to conceptualize ToM skills is to place them in a hierarchical ordering of complexity. For example, false beliefs are often referred to as being of either first- or second-order ToM. *First-order ToM* involves the ability to understand that someone can hold a false belief about the state of the world, whereas *second-order ToM* is the more complex ability to understand that someone can have a false belief about the belief of another character (Frith and Corcoran 1996). One way of measuring first-order false belief is with the "Sally–Anne" task. In this task, the participant is read a scenario in which one character, Sally, places her ball in a basket and covers it with a cloth and then leaves the room. While she is gone, her friend Anne moves the ball to another location without Sally knowing. Sally then reenters the room, and the participant is asked where Sally thinks the ball is and where she will look for it. To answer correctly, the participant must understand that Sally still believes that the ball is in the basket where she left it and not in the new location. Likewise, a typical second-order task would involve a scenario that is read to the participants as is as follows:

> Sally and Ian are at the station because Sally has to catch a train home. Sally lives in Homesville, but the train does not stop at the Homesville station. Sally will have to get off at Neartown and walk. Sally goes to buy a magazine to read on her journey before she buys her ticket. While she is gone, there is an alteration to the timetable, and the train is now going to stop at Homesville. The guard tells Ian about this change, and Ian sets off to find Sally to tell her, but before Ian finds her, the guard meets Sally and tells her, "The train will now stop at Homesville." Ian eventually finds Sally who has just bought her ticket. (Frith and Corcoran 1996, p. 528)

After this story is read, the participant is asked which station Ian thinks Sally has bought her ticket for, and to answer correctly the participant must understand that Ian falsely believes that Sally still thinks the train is not stopping at Homesville. Thus, second-order false beliefs are higher in the hierarchy of complexity than first-order tasks. Accordingly, increasingly subtle ToM concepts such as hints, deception, metaphor, and irony are considered more difficult to understand than false beliefs.

The development of ToM abilities occurs over the course of infancy and childhood, with more difficult skills being learned as the child ages. Within the first year, infants begin to show joint attention, a sign of mentalizing, in which they will follow another person's gaze and seemingly attend to the focus of that person's attention (Frith 2001). Shortly thereafter, at approximately age 2 years, intentional gesturing and vocalization, abilities that are precursors of traditional ToM, emerge. At age 3 years children begin to incorporate mental state terms such as *know*, *think*, and *believe* into their vocabulary, and at age 4 years children acquire the ability to understand false beliefs, or first-order ToM (Leslie 1987). Second-order ToM abilities are thought to develop between the ages of 6 and 7 years, and from ages 8–11 years the more advanced ToM skills are obtained (Baron-Cohen et al. 1999a).

In the following section, ToM is reviewed specifically as it relates to schizophrenia. ToM deficits that are evident in individuals with schizophrenia are discussed as well as how these deficits relate to general cognitive abilities, phases of illness, and social functioning.

MIND DEFICITS

The finding that individuals with schizophrenia show impairments in ToM has been well established, and although these impairments are seen in other clinical disorders (i.e., autism), they appear to be most pronounced in schizophrenia (as compared with individuals with depression and mania) (Doody et al. 1998; Sarfati and Hardy-Bayle 1999). Some debate remains, however, about which symptom clusters are most related to this impairment. Corcoran and colleagues (1995) reported that individuals with predominantly negative symptoms performed worse on a hinting task than individuals with paranoia or delusions of control, a finding that was replicated in a subsequent study (Pickup and Frith 2001). Although these findings make sense given the similarities between negative symptoms in schizophrenia and behaviors observed in autism, other studies have contradicted these results. For example, Sarfati and colleagues have found that individuals with disorganization have more difficulty attributing intentions to social others than other subgroups of schizophrenia (Sarfati and Hardy-Bayle 1999; Sarfati et al. 1997, 1999). Similarly, Pilowsky and colleagues (2000) reported that the greatest degree of impairment is evident not only in individuals with disorganization but also in individuals with paranoia.

Corcoran (2001) noted that one possible explanation for the disparity in these findings could be differences in the categorization of symptoms across studies; however, a more comprehensive reconciliation is that the deficits may vary as a function of symptom and level of ToM task. Specifically, Corcoran and Frith (1996) proposed that individuals with both positive *and* negative symptoms show difficulty with both first- and second-order ToM tasks, whereas individuals with paranoid symptoms tend to pass first-order ToM tasks but fail second-order tasks. One study that drew on this hypothesis did not support the proposed pattern per se but did support the idea of an interaction between symptom and level of task. In this study, individuals with psychomotor poverty were more likely to fail both first- and second-order tasks, whereas individuals with disorganization passed first-order tasks but failed second-order ones, and individuals with reality distortion passed both first- and second-order tasks (Mazza et al. 2001). Thus, as of this writing, it appears that there is no clear-cut delineation between the symptoms of schizophrenia and impairments in ToM.

COGNITIVE ABILITIES

On the whole it appears that ToM deficits are independent of cognitive functioning (see Brune 2003 for an exception). For example, two studies that matched groups on IQ still found ToM impairments in individuals with schizophrenia compared with healthy and psychiatric control subjects (Frith and Corcoran 1996; Pickup and Frith 2001), and ability to correctly perform second-order ToM tasks was not correlated with any of the Weschler Adult Intelligence Scale subscale scores in a study by Drury and colleagues (1998). Additionally, Brunet and colleagues (2003b) have presented a very compelling argument for the specificity of ToM impairments. They compared the performance of individuals with schizophrenia and healthy participants on ToM tasks and two types of control stimuli: one that involved the determination of physical causality with human characters, and one that involved physical causality without human characters. The results indicated that individuals with schizophrenia could successfully complete sequences of physical causality, both with and without characters, but that they could not complete sequences involving the attribution of intentions or ToM. These results remained stable after controlling for verbal IQ.

In addition to these behavioral studies, neuroimaging research also supports the dissociation between ToM and cognitive abilities. Numerous neuroimaging studies of healthy individuals and individuals with autism suggest that there are specific neural structures that subserve ToM (reviewed in Pinkham et al. 2003). These structures, primarily the medial prefrontal cortex and to some extent the orbitofrontal cortex (Brodmann's areas 8 and 9), are activated in healthy individuals during ToM tasks but not during comparable non-ToM cognitive tasks. Moreover, for participants with autism who have shown deficits in ToM, these same areas do not activate during ToM tasks. At this time, only a few studies have attempted to identify the neural mechanisms of ToM in individuals with schizophrenia, and their results have been consistent with the previous research using other populations. In one such study, Russell and colleagues (2000) found that compared with healthy control participants, individuals with schizophrenia showed less activation of the middle frontal cortex, including portions of Brodmann's area 9, and made more errors on a mental state attribution task. A similar study also found no significant activation of the medial prefrontal cortex in individuals with schizophrenia during a nonverbal ToM task (Brunet et al. 2003a). Considered together, these studies make a convincing argument for the neural specificity of ToM in healthy populations as well as clinical populations such as patients with schizophrenia.

Lesion studies also provide evidence for a distinction between specific cognitive abilities and ToM. For example, in a study of individuals with damage to the prefrontal and frontal lobes, ToM was shown to be impaired, whereas executive function remained intact—a finding that is particularly interesting given that both ToM and executive function abilities have been localized to the prefrontal lobes (Rowe et al. 2001; Sylvester et al. 2003; Wagner et al. 2001). Likewise, a case study of an individual with amygdalar damage also demonstrated impaired ToM with intact executive functioning (Fine et al. 2001). Thus, a strong case can be made that ToM is generally independent from general cognitive functioning and that impairments in ToM are not caused by deficits in general intellectual abilities.

A STATE OR TRAIT DEFICIT?

An important question is whether ToM deficits are dependent on the individual's clinical state (i.e., stage of illness) or whether they are a trait characteristic. Several studies support the idea of a state-dependent relationship. One of the earliest studies to address this question found that individuals who had been diagnosed with schizophrenia but were in remission at the time of testing performed just as well as control subjects on a hinting ToM task (Corcoran et al. 1995)—a finding that has been replicated in multiple studies using a variety of ToM tasks including first-and second-order false belief tasks (Frith and Corcoran 1996; Pickup and Frith 2001), metaphor and irony tasks (Drury et al. 1998), and the hinting task (Corcoran 2003). One interesting addition to the "state argument" that deserves note is the idea that ToM deficits may get "turned on" during an acute episode and then "turned off" again when symptoms remit. Over time, the plasticity of this process may lessen such that individuals who have been ill for a long time show ToM deficits consistently across a range of symptoms (Brune 2003; Drury et al. 1998; Frith 1992; Sarfati et al. 2000).

Evidence supporting a trait hypothesis is not as readily available; however, a few studies do support this view. Herold and colleagues (2002) reported that individuals in remission were able to complete simple ToM tasks but that their performance was impaired on more complex ToM tasks compared with control subjects. Other studies have found that the first-degree relatives of individuals with schizophrenia performed worse than nonclinical control subjects but better than their relatives with schizophrenia on ToM tasks, which lends further support for a trait hypothesis (Janssen et al. 2003; Wykes et al. 2001).

SOCIAL FUNCTIONING

Thus far, the majority of research in this area has focused on identifying deficits in ToM and the nature of those deficits; however, a few recent studies have begun to look at how deficits in ToM may relate to social functioning and social outcome. Pollice and colleagues (2002) examined several domains of functioning in individuals with schizophrenia and found that ToM ability was related to global social functioning, even after controlling for IQ, and that it accounted for more variance in social functioning than cognitive factors such as verbal fluency, memory, and executive function.

Similarly, Pinkham and colleagues reported that performance on measures of ToM was correlated with both global and nonverbal social skill (A.E. Pinkham, D.L. Penn, E. Keifer, et al, unpublished data) . Thus, it appears that deficits in ToM may have an association with social functioning, which may have implications for targeting ToM in psychosocial treatment trials, as has been done in autism research (Hadwin et al. 1996, 1997; Ozonoff and Miller 1995; Swettenham 1996).

Overall, we may conclude that individuals with schizophrenia have impairments in ToM that appear to be independent from general cognitive abilities. Future work should elucidate further the relationship between specific symptoms and ToM deficits, and should continue to examine how deficits in ToM relate to the daily functioning of individuals with schizophrenia.

ATTRIBUTIONAL STYLE IN SCHIZOPHRENIA

Attributions refer to how one explains the causes for positive and negative outcomes. Much of the work on attributions, as applied to clinical populations, grew out of the groundbreaking research by Seligman and colleagues, who reported that individuals with depression make internal, stable, and global attributions for negative events (Abramson et al. 1978). Thus, a depressed individual who fails an exam will think that he or she is stupid (an internal attribution), that he or she will always fail exams (a stable attribution), and that he or she is a failure at everything (a global attribution). This type of attributional style does not appear to be a state-dependent characteristic of depression but is present in remitted states, leading to the hypothesis that for some individuals, it may be a vulnerability characteristic for depression (Just et al. 2001).

In this section, we discuss attributional style and schizophrenia. The bulk of the research in this area has focused on attributional style in individuals with paranoia or persecutory delusions; thus, this will be the focus of our review. We begin by providing an overview of the two most common attributional biases observed in individuals with persecutory delusions: a self-serving attributional style

and a personalizing bias. We conclude this section with a discussion of unanswered questions in this area.

SELF-SERVING AND PERSONALIZING BIASES

Attributional style in schizophrenia has received much attention over the past 15 years. Attributions are typically measured via questionnaires such as the Attributional Style Questionnaire (ASQ; Peterson et al. 1982), in which individuals are presented with hypothetical positive and negative outcomes. Such questionnaires are used to identify a reason for that outcome and then to rate it on dimensions corresponding to internal, stable, and global attributions. Unlike depression, however, the internal dimension has fostered the greatest interest in schizophrenia research.

The pioneer in attributional research in schizophrenia has been Richard Bentall at the Universities of Liverpool and Manchester (Bentall et al. 1994, 2001; Blackwood et al. 2001). Bentall and colleagues observed that individuals with paranoia or persecutory delusions (the former referring to diagnostic subtypes, the latter to symptom severity) tended to show a self-serving bias (i.e., taking credit for successful outcomes and denying responsibility for negative outcomes) that was, they argued, an exaggeration of the bias seen in nonclinical control subjects (and opposite to what is typically observed in depressed individuals) (Kaney and Bentall 1989).

However, as pointed out in a number of excellent reviews (Bentall et al. 2001; Garety and Freeman 1999), direct replication of the self-serving bias has been limited (Candido and Romney 1990), with studies either finding no evidence of a self-serving bias (Martin and Penn 2002; (A.E. Pinkham, D.L. Penn, E. Keifer, et al, unpublished data) or providing only partial support in the form of only an external attribution for negative outcomes (rather than the additional positive attribution for positive outcomes) (Fear et al. 1996; Kinderman and Bentall 1997; Krstev et al. 1999; Lyon et al. 1994; Sharp et al. 1997). On the basis of these findings, Garety and colleagues (1999) concluded that there is fairly strong evidence for people with persecutory delusions to attribute negative outcomes to external factors but less compelling evidence for a general self-serving bias.

The investigation of the tendency of individuals with persecutory delusions to attribute negative outcomes to external factors was refined with the development of the Internal, Personal, and Situational Attributions Questionnaire (IPSAQ; Kinderman and Bentall 1996a). Unlike the ASQ, which could only code attributions on the internality dimension as either internal or external, the IPSAQ allows for a distinction between external "personal" attributions (i.e., causes that are attributed to other people) and external "situational" attributions (i.e., causes that are attributed to situational factors). Specifically, participants are presented with 16 positive and 16 negative outcomes. The participant's task is to write down the reason for the outcome and then to classify that reason as being caused by him- or herself (internal), being caused by someone else (external-personal), or being caused by something else (external-situational). This distinction is in accord with the clinical experience of individuals with persecutory delusions, who often explain negative outcomes (e.g., someone not returning a phone call right away) as being due to malevolent intentions (e.g., that person is angry at them) rather than to a situational context (e.g., the person is out of town). Kinderman and Bentall (1996a) described this style of attributing negative outcomes to others, rather than to situations, as a "personalizing bias."

There is growing evidence in support of a personalizing bias for individuals with persecutory delusions (reviewed in Bentall et al. 2001; Garety and Freeman 1999). Specifically, a tendency toward a personalizing bias has been observed in people with persecutory delusions relative to individuals with depression (Kinderman and Bentall 1997) and nonclinical control subjects (Kinderman and Bentall 1997; Martin and Penn 2002) and may be most pronounced in individuals with acute, rather than remitted, symptoms (Randall et al. 2003). This tendency to blame others likely increases negative affect, defensiveness, avoidance, and possibly aggressive behaviors.

UNANSWERED QUESTIONS

The study of attributional style has yielded some interesting data about people with schizophrenia, namely, that attributions may be best understood within *symptom* rather than *diagnostic category* models and that people with persecutory delusions have a tendency to blame others, rather than situations, for negative outcomes. There remain, however, a number of unanswered questions that plague this area of research. First and foremost is how to measure attributions in this clinical population. Current measures of attributional style have been criticized as having poor psychometric properties (e.g., ASQ) or, because of being composed of hypothetical scenarios, as having questionable external validity (e.g., IPSAQ) (Bentall et al. 2001; Garety and Freeman 1999). These limitations have led some to argue that a more valid method of assessing attributions is to code them in the context of natural discourse rather than with paper-and-pencil questionnaires (Bentall et al. 2001).

In addition, extant measures of attributional style in schizophrenia research do not make a distinction among negative outcomes that vary in degree of intentionality.

For example, most people would agree that the following scenario involves a negative outcome in which the intent is clear: "A person jumps ahead of you on a grocery line and says, 'I'm in a rush.'" However, what would be the intent in the following situation? "You walk past a group of teenagers, and as you pass by you hear them laugh." One could argue that it is in the latter type of situation, in which the intent is ambiguous, that is particularly problematic for individuals with persecutory delusions, and research conducted with children with conduct disorders confirms this assertion. Aggressive children and adolescents are more likely to show a tendency to attribute negative outcomes to others (or what is also called a "hostile attribution bias") relative to control subjects in those situations that are most ambiguous with respect to intention (Crick and Dodge 1994; Dodge and Pettit 2003). Similar findings have linked a hostile attributional bias for ambiguous situations to aggressive behavior in adults (Epps and Kendall 1995), particularly with marital violence (Eckhardt et al. 1998), aggressive driving (Matthews and Norris 2002), and workplace aggression (Homant and Kennedy 2003). Thus, the current measures of attributional style in schizophrenia may be limited in their ability to evaluate attributions across situations that vary in intent (rather than just varying in outcome).

A final concern in the measurement of attributions in schizophrenia is *which* attributions to code: those that the participant generates or those that he or she subsequently rates? For example, the IPSAQ requires participants to generate causes to hypothetical outcomes and then to categorize that cause as internal, external-personal, or external-other. Early research using the IPSAQ focused on the responses that the participants categorized (Kinderman and Bentall 1996a, 1997). However, more recent work has found support for personalizing biases only when independent raters code participants' responses (Martin and Penn 2002; Randall et al. 2003), leading to the question of which response is the most valid index of attributions.

Perhaps the most pressing unanswered question in this area is the mechanism by which persecutory beliefs lead to attributional biases. An early model proposed by Bentall and colleagues (1994) argued that a self-serving attributional style had the function of protecting the individual with persecutory delusions from low self-esteem. Evidence in support of this model was garnered from research showing that individuals with persecutory delusions had an attributional style similar to that of depressed subjects when presented with an "opaque" attributional task (i.e., one that was presented as a memory task) (Lyon et al. 1994) but had an attributional style similar to nonclinical control subjects (i.e., a self-serving bias) on overt attributional tasks, suggesting the presence of an underlying negative self-concept, and a discrepancy between "covert" and "overt" self-esteem. This intriguing model has been challenged on two fronts, however. First, evidence in support of a "covert negative self-concept" was not replicated in subsequent studies (Krstev et al. 1999; Martin and Penn 2002; Peters et al. 1997). Second, the bulk of research has not found consistent patterns of discrepancies between overt and covert self-esteem in individuals with persecutory delusions, leading Garety and Freeman (1999) to conclude, "In view of this, one cannot conclude that there is yet strong empirical support for the persecutory delusions as defence theory" (p. 146).

Bentall and colleagues have subsequently revised the model in light of self-discrepancy theory (Higgins 1987). According to this theory, discrepancies may exist between one's actual self (i.e., attributes they believe they possess), one's ideal self (i.e., attributes they would like to possess), and one's "ought" self (i.e., attributes they believe they ought to have). In addition, Higgins posits that views of the self can be further broken down into two categories: 1) one's own view of the self and 2) one's view of how others view one. Discrepancies between aspects of the self (e.g., actual self vs. ought self) or from different views on the self (i.e., one's own view vs. how one thinks others view oneself) can have an impact on emotions. For example, depressive-type experiences may arise from discrepancies between actual versus ideal selves, whereas anxious type symptoms arise from discrepancies between actual versus ought selves.

Kinderman and Bentall (1996b) hypothesize that negative life events (e.g., negative evaluations by others) trigger a negative self-concept by creating discrepancies between an individual's perceptions of actual self and ideal self. Persecutory delusions function to reduce these discrepancies through an exaggeration of the self-serving bias found in normal populations (i.e., attributing negative outcomes to the actions of others and positive outcomes to one's own actions). Kinderman and Bentall (2000) point out that such a style reduces self-ideal discrepancies at the cost of increasing negative perceptions of others (i.e., a personalizing bias). Evidence in support of this model has been observed in nonclinical samples, whereby external attributions for negative events may reduce actual versus ideal-self discrepancies. And, in clinical samples, individuals with persecutory delusions relative to both clinical and nonclinical control subjects show consistent actual versus ideal-self views but discrepant actual versus ought views from others (namely, their parents) (Kinderman and Bentall 1996b). According to Bentall and colleagues (2001), this pattern is consistent with their model that predicts consistent actual versus ideal-self views at expense of attributing negative views to others.

This model is being further refined in light of Garety and Freeman's (1999) critique of the inconsistent findings regarding self-esteem and persecutory delusions, and the concern that attributions may be more of a state, than trait, characteristic (Bentall et al. 2001).

This concern has led Bentall and colleagues to consider why external-personal attributions are not corrected, even if they are made to reduce self-discrepancies. It has been demonstrated in nonclinical control subjects that when forming impressions of others, people automatically make dispositional judgments and only subsequently "correct" for situational factors (Gilbert et al. 1988; although see Penn et al. 2002 for a failure to replicate). For example, if you meet someone and they are not friendly, you might infer that they are a rude person. However, if you subsequently learn that that person had just received bad news (e.g., someone in their family had died), you would correct that impression in light of that social context.

Bentall and colleagues hypothesize that two factors may prevent people with persecutory delusions from correcting for situational information (or in considering social context). First, individuals with persecutory beliefs may have a greater need for "closure" (i.e., a desire to get a specific answer on a topic or issue, rather than dealing with ambiguity), a hypothesis with some preliminary support in samples with both nonclinical (Colbert and Peters 2002) and clinical levels of delusional ideation (Bentall and Swarbrick 2003). Second, individuals with persecutory delusions may be ignoring not only social context but also the "mental" context of others; in other words, impairments in theory of mind may contribute to personalizing biases. For example, if one of your co-workers does not return an e-mail, you might immediately infer that she is angry with you. However, if you have adequate theory of mind skills, you could use your knowledge of her character (based on previous experience) and conclude, "She has been complaining about how busy she is, so I wonder whether she is feeling overwhelmed and unable to get to all of her e-mail messages." This suggests that intact theory of mind skills will provide additional contextual information for the individual to consider when making attributions. Recent evidence from nonclinical (Kinderman et al. 1998; Taylor and Kinderman 2002) and clinical samples (Randall et al. 2003) supports the association between deficits in theory of mind and the tendency to make external-personal attributions. Thus, taken as a whole, these findings suggest that further examination of the relationship among need for closure, theory of mind, and attributions may yield insight into the mechanisms underlying attributional style and persecutory delusions.

FACIAL AFFECT RECOGNITION

One important component of social cognition that has been widely studied in schizophrenia is the ability to recognize affect in the faces of others. It has been relatively well established in the literature that individuals with schizophrenia generally show deficits in both identification and discrimination of facial affect. The many studies in this area have been reviewed previously (Edwards et al. 2002; Mandal et al. 1998; Pinkham et al. 2003). However, several questions have arisen that include the specificity of the deficit in terms of schizophrenia, the emotional valence of the deficit, the stability of the deficit, and the nature of the deficit, namely, whether the impairment is specific to emotions or due to generalized poor performance. Further, because social cognition has been implicated in the relationship between social and cognitive functioning, the relationship of facial affect recognition with both social and cognitive functioning needs to be addressed.

IS THE DEFICIT SPECIFIC TO SCHIZOPHRENIA?

Some studies have shown that individuals with schizophrenia perform more poorly than nonpatient and psychiatric control subjects on tests of facial affect recognition (Mandal 1986; Morrison et al. 1988; Muzekari and Bates 1977; Walker et al. 1980). However, the evidence is somewhat mixed. Some studies have demonstrated an advantage for those with depression compared with those with schizophrenia in facial affect recognition tasks (e.g., Gaebel and Wolwer 1992; Gessler et al. 1989); others have demonstrated that although schizophrenia subjects perform more poorly than nonpsychiatric control subjects, there is no difference between those with schizophrenia and those with depression (e.g., Schneider et al. 1995).

Addington and Addington (1998) reported that individuals with schizophrenia performed significantly worse on facial affect recognition tasks than individuals with bipolar disorder and nonclinical control subjects. In this study, even though individuals with bipolar disorder were impaired on a discrimination task as compared with control subjects, individuals with schizophrenia still performed significantly worse than the bipolar group. One study that has examined facial affect recognition in first-episode subjects found that schizophrenia spectrum–disordered patients performed more poorly than affective psychosis patients and normal control subjects on the fear and sadness subscales of two emotional labeling tasks (Edwards et al. 2001). Using both a videotaped test and still photographs, Bellack and colleagues (1996) did not find any differences between subjects with schizophrenia and

subjects with bipolar disorder on facial affect recognition. Differences between the schizophrenia group and control subjects were noted on the nonemotional perceptual tasks. Finally, in a recent study, Bolte and Poustka (2003) found that individuals with schizophrenia performed *better* than individuals with autism on a facial recognition test. Overall, these findings suggest that although individuals with schizophrenia are impaired in facial affect recognition relative to nonclinical control subjects, performance deficits compared with clinical control subjects are less consistently shown.

DOES THE DEFICIT OCCUR WITH ALL EMOTIONS?

Further research suggests that difficulties in affect recognition are a function of the kinds of emotions subjects are identifying. Subjects with schizophrenia appear to have more difficulty when the tasks involve the identification or discrimination of negative emotions (e.g., fear, anger) compared with more positive emotions such as happiness (Borod et al. 1993). In a study focusing on first-episode patients, Edwards and colleagues (2001) reported small but significant deficits in the recognition of fearful and sad emotions when compared with subjects with affective psychosis and healthy control subjects. In a recent study, individuals with schizophrenia showed an overall deficit in facial affect recognition when compared with control subjects, including increased impairment in the recognition of fear and disgust (Kohler et al. 2003). Further, of particular note in this study, the schizophrenia subjects tended to misattribute neutral features as negative. Thus, although studies are few, results are consistent that individuals with schizophrenia have more difficulty recognizing negative emotions, in particular fear and anger.

IS THE DEFICIT STABLE OVER TIME?

A number of cross-sectional studies have demonstrated a decrease in affect recognition deficits during remission (Gaebel and Wolwer 1992; Gessler et al. 1989). Penn and colleagues (2000) found that acutely ill individuals with schizophrenia perform worse than chronically ill yet stable inpatients on emotion perception tasks. The few longitudinal studies examining the stability of these deficits suggest that such deficits tend to remain. In the Addington and Addington (1998) study, despite a highly significant improvement in positive and negative symptoms from the time of hospitalization to the 3-month follow-up period, there was no improvement on either of the measures of facial affect recognition, suggesting that deficits on these facial affect recognition tasks are stable deficits that do not improve with an improvement in symptoms. This finding supports and improves on the results of Gaebel and Wolwer (1992) and Streit and colleagues (1997), whose followup periods were only 4 weeks. In a more recent study, the longitudinal stability (1 year) of deficits in facial affect recognition has been supported (Kee et al. 2003).

IS THE DEFICIT A RESULT OF A SPECIFIC OR GENERALIZED IMPAIRMENT?

One question that arises is whether these deficits in affect recognition are the result of a specific impairment in facial affect recognition or whether this deficit is related to a general impairment. Many of the studies we have reviewed did not involve the use of a differential design, which makes it unclear if the poor performance reflected a specific or a generalized impairment (Chapman and Chapman 1978). Implementation of a differential deficit design involves the inclusion of a control task that is matched for difficulty with the facial affect recognition task (Chapman and Chapman 1978). Results of using a differential design have been mixed.

A few studies have supported a differential deficit (Heimberg et al. 1992; Walker et al. 1984). Others have shown that, although schizophrenia subjects performed more poorly than control subjects on facial affect recognition tasks, they also performed more poorly on a control task, usually a facial recognition task (Addington and Addington 1998; Feinberg et al. 1986; Gessler et al. 1989; Kerr and Neale 1993; Mueser et al. 1996; Novic et al. 1984; Salem et al. 1996).

This finding suggests that facial affect impairment is more likely to be a generalized impairment rather than a specific impairment in facial affect recognition. Interestingly, a review by Penn and colleagues (1997) suggests otherwise. For example, in the Feinberg and colleagues (1986) and Novic and colleagues (1984) studies, support for the generalized deficit was weak. One contributing factor to this unclear picture of differential performance deficits is the nature of the "control" task, which typically is a face perception test. Thus, although this type of task controls for the affective quality of the stimulus, it is also a social stimulus, thus limiting the conclusions that can be made about a specific versus generalized deficit in social cognition proper. In an attempt to address this issue, Penn and colleagues (2000) reported contrasting results between patients experiencing an acute episode and patients with a more chronic course who were in extended care. The acutely ill group showed significant deficits in facial affect recognition after controlling for performance on social and nonsocial perception tasks. However, those in chronic care demonstrated deficits on control tasks as

well. Thus, facial affect recognition deficits might not necessarily result from generalized poor performance. Further work that uses a differential deficit design, which must include both social and nonsocial perception tasks, is clearly warranted to further our understanding of the deficit's specificity.

RELATIONSHIP AMONG FACIAL AFFECT RECOGNITION, NEUROCOGNITION, AND SOCIAL FUNCTIONING

In addition to impaired social cognition, it is well established that individuals with schizophrenia have impairments in social and neurocognitive functioning. Further, work has been conducted that attemps to establish a link between social and neurocognitive functioning (Addington and Addington 1999, 2000; Green 1996; Penn et al. 1996). Thus, social cognition may have direct relevance for social functioning, as it has been implicated in the relationship between social and cognitive functioning.

An important question is whether deficits on a facial affect recognition task are associated with deficits on tasks that demand selective attention, sustained attention, and perceptual load in relation to nonsocially relevant stimuli. Addington and Addington (1997) reported an association with impaired visual attention for those with schizophrenia, a partial association for those with bipolar disorder, and no association in the normal control group. It is likely that in the normal control group the facial perceptual tasks and the cognitive tasks are tapping distinct constructs, whereas in the schizophrenia group deficits may be revealing a unitary process of impairment rather than distinct impairments. This suggests that deficits in emotion recognition may be related to a more generalized impairment in processing complex visual stimuli that requires a high processing load. In other studies that addressed this issue, associations have been reported between facial affect recognition and memory, abstract thinking, language processing, and attention (Bryson et al. 1997; Kee et al. 1998; Sachs et al. 2004; Schneider et al. 1995; Silver and Shlomo 2001; Silver et al. 2002).

Several studies have demonstrated that facial affect recognition is significantly related to various aspects of social functioning, such as social skill, general social functioning, and quality of life (see Hooker and Park 2002; Ihnen et al. 1998; Kee et al. 2003; Mueser et al. 1996; Penn et al. 1996). This finding suggests that social cognition has *functional* significance for individuals with schizophrenia.

Only one study to date has attempted to examine the role of facial affect recognition as a potential mediator between cognitive and social functioning (Addington and Addington 2003). In this study, 50 first-episode subjects were compared with 59 subjects with a chronic course of schizophrenia and 55 nonpsychiatric control subjects over a 1-year period. On measures of facial affect recognition, a range of cognitive tasks, and social functioning measures, control subjects performed significantly better than the two patient groups. Further, there were significant associations among all three domains. However, using the mediational model of Baron and Kenny (1986), researchers found that facial affect recognition did not appear to mediate between cognitive and social functioning. Rather, it appeared to be a deficit that had a robust association with variables that predict poor outcome. Thus, this preliminary evidence suggests that facial affect recognition, although related to cognitive and social functioning, may be a distinct construct.

SUMMARY AND UNANSWERED QUESTIONS

Individuals with schizophrenia, both in the early and more chronic stages of the illness, show deficits in facial affect recognition. This impairment seems to be relatively stable over time, with most difficulty occurring with the recognition of negative emotions. Because of methodological problems and psychometric limitations, it has not been possible to draw conclusions about the specificity of these deficits to schizophrenia or about whether these impairments reflect generalized poor performance. Finally, it is clear that facial affect recognition is related to both neurocognition and social functioning, suggesting that it might have a role in the development of comprehensive psychosocial interventions.

A number of unanswered questions remain. First, given the heterogeneity of schizophrenia, it is important to determine whether specific symptoms relate, or contribute, to facial recognition deficits. For example, there is some evidence that individuals with persecutory delusions or paranoia perform better on facial recognition tasks relative to nonparanoid individuals with schizophrenia (Kline et al. 1992; Lewis and Garver 1995), particularly for naturalistic, rather than posed, emotions (Davis and Gibson 2000). Conversely, negative symptoms or the deficit syndrome may impair emotion perception (Bryson et al. 1998; Mueser et al. 1996; for exceptions, see Silver and Shlomo 2001; Streit et al. 1997). This finding suggests that a finer-grained analysis of facial affect recognition in schizophrenia may be obtained by forming symptom subgroups of individuals. Second, we still know little about the mechanisms underlying performance deficits in this social cognitive area, other than their association with neurocognition and illness phase. One promising area is

that of visual scanning, because individuals with schizophrenia show "restricted" scan paths relative to control subjects (Loughland et al. 2002; Streit et al. 1997), These restrictions may be most pronounced for individuals with persecutory delusions, who tend to look at nonthreatening and less essential features of scenes relative to control subjects (Phillips and David 1998; Phillips et al. 2000). Thus, how individuals acquire social information may lend insight into why they have difficulty in perceiving the emotions in others.

CONCLUSION

In this review, we have explored three key domains of social cognition in schizophrenia: theory of mind, attributional style, and facial affect recognition. Overall, it appears that individuals with schizophrenia display impairments in each of these domains and that these deficits in social cognition are in fact related to behavior. These findings, however, are just a start, and there is still a great deal of work that is needed before a more complete understanding of the role of social cognition in schizophrenia can be gained.

One question that needs to be addressed is the exact nature of the deficits presented here. The evidence provided in this review implies that there may be a generalized deficit in social cognition and that individuals with schizophrenia would perform poorly on any social cognitive task. This, however, may not be the case. Some of our own work suggests that individuals within the first 5 years of their illness can be impaired in one domain and not in another (i.e., social knowledge, but not theory of mind) and that deficits may be present on some measures of emotion perception but not others (i.e., the Bell Lysaker Emotion Recognition Task, but not the Facial Emotion Identification Task) (A. E. Pinkham, D. L. Penn, E. Keifer, et al, unpublished data). At this point, relatively few studies have simultaneously assessed multiple domains of social cognition to address this question.

Finally, there has been little direct work exploring the neural network that may subserve social cognition specifically in schizophrenia. A large body of literature addresses this issue in healthy individuals; however, this work has yet to be widely extended to schizophrenia despite compelling evidence that neural abnormalities in a specific social cognitive network may underlie social cognitive deficits (Pinkham et al. 2003). Such work may not only inform our understanding of abnormalities at the level of brain-behavior interactions but also shed light on the variability of social cognitive deficits between individuals and disorders.

REFERENCES

Abramson LY, Seligman MEP, Teasdale JD: Learned helplessness in humans: critique and reformulation. J Abnorm Psychol 78:40–74, 1978

Addington J, Addington D: Attentional vulnerability indicators in schizophrenia and bipolar disorder. Schizophr Res 23:197–204, 1997

Addington J, Addington D: Facial emotion recognition and information processing in schizophrenia and bipolar disorder. Schizophr Res 32:171–181, 1998

Addington J, Addington D: Neurocognitive and social functioning in schizophrenia. Schizophr Bull 25:173–182, 1999

Addington J, Addington D: Neurocognitive and social functioning in schizophrenia: a 2.5 year follow-up. Schizophr Res 44:47–56, 2000

Addington J, Addington D: Social cognition in first episode psychosis (abstract). Schizophr Res 60:63, 2003

Adolphs R: Social cognition and the human brain. Trends Cogn Sci 3:469–479, 1999

Adolphs R: The neurobiology of social cognition. Curr Opin Neurobiol 11:231–239, 2001

Adolphs R: Neural systems for recognizing emotion. Curr Opin Neurobiol 12:169–177, 2002

Adolphs R: Cognitive neuroscience of human social behavior. Nat Rev Neurosci 4:165–178, 2003

Anderson SW, Bechara A, Damasio H, et al: Impairment of social and moral behavior related to early damage in human prefrontal cortex. Nat Neurosci 2:1032–1037, 1999

Baron R, Kenny D: The moderator-mediator variable distinction in social psychological research: conceptual, strategic, and statistical considerations. J Pers Soc Psychol 51:1173–1182, 1986

Baron-Cohen S, O'Riordan M, Stone V, et al: Recognition of faux pas by normally developing children and children with Asperger syndrome or high-functioning autism. J Autism Dev Disord 29:407–418, 1999a

Baron-Cohen S, Wheelwright S, Stone V, et al: A mathematician, a physicist, and a computer scientist with Asperger syndrome: performance on folk psychology and folk physics tests. Neurocase 5:475–483, 1999b

Bellack AS, Blanchard JJ, Muser KT: Cue availability and affect perception in schizophrenia. Schizophr Bull 22:535–544, 1996

Bentall RP, Swarbrick R: The best laid schemas of paranoid patients: autonomy, sociotropy, and need for closure. Psychol Psychother 76:163–171, 2003

Bentall RP, Kinderman P, Kaney S: The self, attributional processes and abnormal beliefs: towards a model of persecutory delusions. Behav Res Ther 32:331–341, 1994

Bentall RP, Corcoran R, Howard R, et al: Persecutory delusions: a review and theoretical integration. Clin Psychol Rev 21:1143–1192, 2001

Blackwood NJ, Howard RJ, Bentall RP, et al: Cognitive neuropsychiatric models of persecutory delusions. Am J Psychiatry 158:527–539, 2001

Blair RJR, Cipolotti L: Impaired social response reversal: a case of "acquired sociopathy." Brain 123:1122–1141, 2000

Bolte S, Poustka F: The recognition of facial affect in autistic and schizophrenic subjects and their first-degree relatives. Psychol Med 33:907–915, 2003

Borod JC, Martin CC, Alpert M, et al: Perception of facial emotion in schizophrenic and right brain-damaged patients. J Nerv Ment Dis 181:494–501, 1993

Brothers L: The social brain: a project for integrating primate behavior and neurophysiology in a new domain. Concepts in Neuroscience 1:27–51, 1990

Brune M: Theory of mind and the role of IQ in chronic disorganized schizophrenia. Schizophr Res 60:57–64, 2003

Brunet E, Sarfati Y, Hardy-Bayle MC, et al: Abnormalities of brain function during a nonverbal theory of mind task in schizophrenia. Neuropsychologia 41:1574–1582, 2003a

Brunet E, Sarfati Y, Hardy-Bayle MC: Reasoning about physical causality and other's intentions in schizophrenia. Cognitive Neuropsychiatry 8:129–139, 2003b

Bryson G, Bell M, Lysaker P: Affect recognition in schizophrenia: a function of global impairment or a specific cognitive deficit. Psychiatry Res 71:105–113, 1997

Bryson G, Bell M, Kaplan E, et al: Affect recognition in deficit syndrome schizophrenia. Psychiatry Res 77:113–120, 1998

Calder AJ, Lawrence AD, Young AW: Neuropsychology of fear and loathing. Nat Rev Neurosci 2:352–363, 2001

Candido CL, Romney DM: Attributional style in paranoid versus depressed patients. Br J Med Psychol 63:355–363, 1990

Chapman L, Chapman J: The measurement of differential deficit. J Psychiatr Res 14:303–311, 1978

Colbert SM, Peters ER: Need for closure and jumping-to-conclusions in delusion-prone individuals. J Nerv Ment Dis 190:27–31, 2002

Corcoran R: Theory of mind and schizophrenia, in Social Cognition and Schizophrenia. Edited by Corrigan PW, Penn DL. Washington, DC, American Psychological Association, 2001, pp 149–174

Corcoran R: Inductive reasoning and the understanding of intention in schizophrenia. Cognitive Neuropsychiatry 8:223–235, 2003

Corcoran R, Frith CD: Conversational conduct and the symptoms of schizophrenia. Cognitive Neuropsychiatry 1:305–318, 1996

Corcoran R, Mercer G, Frith CD: Schizophrenia, symptomatology and social inference: investigating "theory of mind" in people with schizophrenia. Schizophr Res 17:5–13, 1995

Crick NR, Dodge KA: A review and reformulation of social information-processing mechanisms in children's social adjustment. Psychol Bull 115:74–101, 1994

Davis PJ, Gibson MG: Recognition of posed and genuine facial expressions of emotion in paranoid and non-paranoid schizophrenia. J Abnorm Psychol 109:445–450, 2000

Dodge KA, Pettit GS: A biopsychosocial model of the development of chronic conduct problems in adolescence. Dev Psychol 39:349–371, 2003

Doody GA, Gotz M, Johnstone EC, et al: Theory of mind and psychoses. Psychol Med 28:397–405, 1998

Drury VW, Robinson EJ, Birchwood M: "Theory of mind" skills during an acute episode of psychosis and following recovery. Psychol Med 28:1101–1112, 1998

Eckhardt CI, Barbour KA, Davison GC: Articulated thoughts of martially violent and nonviolent men during anger arousal. J Consult Clin Psychol 66:259–269, 1998

Edwards J, Jackson IIJ, Pattison PE, et al: Facial affect and affective prosody recognition in first-episode schizophrenia. Schizophr Res 48:235–253, 2001

Edwards J, Jackson, HJ, Pattitson PE: Emotion recognition via facial expression and affective prosody in schizophrenia: a methodological review. Clin Psychol Rev 22:789–832, 2002

Epps J, Kendall PC: Hostile attributional bias in adults. Cognit Ther Res 19:159–178, 1995

Fear CF, Sharp H, Healy D: Cognitive processes in delusional disorders. Br J Psychiatry 168:1–8, 1996

Feinberg TE, Rifkin A, Schaffer C, et al: Facial discrimination and emotional recognition in schizophrenia and affective disorders. Arch Gen Psychiatry 43:276–279, 1986

Fiddick L, Cosmides L, Tooby J: No interpretation without representation: the role of domain-specific representations and inferences in the Wason selection task. Cognition 77:1–79, 2000

Fine C, Lumsden J, Blair RJR: Dissociation between "theory of mind" and executive functions in a patient with early left amygdala damage. Brain 124:287–298, 2001

Frith CD: The Cognitive Neuropsychology of Schizophrenia. Hillsdale, NJ, Erlbaum, 1992

Frith CD, Corcoran R: Exploring "theory of mind" in people with schizophrenia. Psychol Med 26:521–530, 1996

Frith CD, Frith U: Interacting minds: a biological basis. Science 186:1692–1695, 1999

Frith U: Mind blindness and the brain in autism. Neuron 32:969–979, 2001

Gaebel W, Wolwer W: Facial expression and emotional face recognition in schizophrenia and depression. Eur Arch Psychiatry Clin Neurosci 242:46–52, 1992

Garety PA, Freeman D: Cognitive approaches to delusions: a critical review of theories and evidence. Br J Clin Psychol 38:113–154, 1999

Gessler S, Cutting J, Frith CD, et al: Schizophrenic inability to judge facial emotion: a controlled study. Br J Clin Psychol 28:19–29, 1989

Gilbert DT, Pelham BW, Krull DS: On cognitive busyness: when person perceivers meet persons perceived. J Pers Soc Psychol 54:733–740, 1988

Green MF: What are the functional consequences of neurocognitive deficits in schizophrenia? Am J Psychiatry 153:321–330, 1996

Green MF, Kern R, Braff DL, et al: Neurocognitive deficits and functional outcome in schizophrenia: are we measuring the right stuff? Schizophr Bull 26:119–136, 2000

Hadwin J, Baron-Cohen S, Howlin P, et al: Can we teach children with autism to understand emotions, belief, or pretense? Dev Psychopathol 8:345–365, 1996

Hadwin J, Baron-Cohen S, Howlin P, et al: Does teaching theory of mind have an effect on the ability to develop conversation in children? J Autism Dev Disord 27:519–535, 1997

Haxby JV, Hoffman EA, Gobbini MI: Human neural systems for face recognition and social communication. Biol Psychiatry 51:59–67, 2002

Heavey L, Phillips W, Baron-Cohen S, et al: The awkward moments test: a naturalistic measure of social understanding in autism. J Autism Dev Disord 30:225–236, 2000

Heimberg C, Gur RE, Erwin RJ, et al: Facial emotion discrimination, III: behavioral findings in schizophrenia. Psychiatry Res 42:253–265, 1992

Herold R, Tenyi T, Lenard K, et al: Theory of mind deficit in people with schizophrenia during remission. Psychol Med 32:1125–1129, 2002

Higgins ET: Self-discrepancy: a theory relating self and affect. Psychol Rev 94:319–340, 1987

Homant RJ, Kennedy DB: Hostile attribution in perceived justification of workplace aggression. Psychol Rep 92:185–194, 2003

Hooker C, Park S: Emotion processing and its relationship to social functioning in schizophrenia patients. Psychiatry Res 112:41–50, 2002

Ihnen GH, Penn DL, Corrigan PW, et al: Social perception and social skill in schizophrenia. Psychiatry Res 80:275–286, 1998

Janssen I, Krabbendam L, Jolles J, et al: Alterations in theory of mind in patients with schizophrenia and non-psychotic relatives. Acta Psychiatr Scand 108:110–117, 2003

Jones W, Bellugi U, Lai, et al: II: hypersociability in Williams syndrome. J Cogn Neurosci 12:30–46, 2000

Just N, Abramson LY, Alloy LB: Remitted depression studies as tests of the cognitive vulnerability hypotheses of depression onset: a critique and conceptual analysis. Clin Psychol Rev 21:63–83, 2001

Kaney S, Bentall RP: Persecutory delusions and attributional style. Br J Med Psychol 62:191–198, 1989

Kanwisher N: Domain specificity in face perception. Nat Neurosci 3:759–763, 2000

Kee KS, Kern RS, Green MF: Perception of emotion and neurocognitive functioning in schizophrenia: what's the link? Psychiatric Res 81:57–65, 1998

Kee KS, Green MF, Mintz J, et al: Is emotion processing a predictor of functional outcome in schizophrenia? Schizophr Bull 29:487–497, 2003

Kerr SL, Neale JM: Emotional perception in schizophrenia: specific deficit or further evidence of generalized poor performance? J Abnorm Psychol 102:312–318, 1993

Kinderman P, Bentall RP: A new measure of causal locus: the Internal, Personal, and Situational Attributions Questionnaire. Pers Individ Dif 20:261–264, 1996a

Kinderman P, Bentall RP: Self-discrepancies and persecutory delusions: evidence for a model of paranoid ideation. J Abnorm Psychol 105:106–113, 1996b

Kinderman P, Bentall RP: Causal attributions in paranoia and depression: internal, personal, and situational attributions for negative events. J Abnorm Psychol 106:341–345, 1997

Kinderman P, Bentall RP: Self-discrepancies and causal attributions: studies of hypothesized relationships. Br J Clin Psychol 39:255–273, 2000

Kinderman P, Dunbar R, Bentall RP: Theory of mind deficits and causal attributions. Br J Psychol 89:191–204, 1998

Klin A: Attributing social meaning to ambiguous visual stimuli in higher-functioning autism and Asperger syndrome: the social attribution task. J Child Psychol Psychiatry 41:831–846, 2000

Kline JS, Smith JE, Ellis HC: Paranoid and nonparanoid schizophrenic processing of facially displayed affect. J Psychiatr Res 26:169–182, 1992

Kohler CG, Turner TH, Bilker WB, et al: Facial emotion recognition in schizophrenia: intensity effects and error patterns. Am J Psychiatry 160:1768–1774, 2003

Krstev H, Jackson H, Maude D: An investigation of attributional style in first-episode psychosis. Br J Clin Psychol 38:181–194, 1999

Leslie AM: Pretense and representation: the origins of "theory of mind." Psychol Rev 94:412–426, 1987

Lewis SF, Garver DL: Treatment and diagnostic subtype in facial affect recognition in schizophrenia. J Psychiatr Res 29:5–11, 1995

Loughland CM, Williams LM, Gordon E: Visual scanpaths to positive and negative facial emotions in an outpatient schizophrenia sample. Schizophr Res 55:159–170, 2002

Lyon HM, Kaney S, Bentall RP: The defensive function of persecutory delusions: evidence from attributional tasks. Br J Psychiatry 164:637–646, 1994

Mandal MK: Judgment of facial affect among depressive and schizophrenics. Br J Clin Psychol 25:87–92, 1986

Mandal MK, Pandey R, Prasad AB: Facial expression of emotions and schizophrenia: a review. Schizophr Bull 24:399–412, 1998

Martin J, Penn DL: Attributional style among outpatients with schizophrenia with and without persecutory delusions. Schizophr Bull 28:131–141, 2002

Matthews BA, Norris FH: When is believing "seeing"? Hostile attribution bias as a function of self-reported aggression. J Appl Soc Psychol 32:1–32, 2002

Mazza M, De Riso A, Surian L, et al: Selective impairments of theory of mind in people with schizophrenia. Schizophr Res 47:299–308, 2001

Morrison RL, Bellack AS, Bashore TR: Perception of emotion among schizophrenic patients. Journal of Psychopathology and Behavioral Assessment 10:319–332, 1988

Mueser KT, Doonan R, Penn DL, et al: Emotional recognition and social competence in chronic schizophrenia. J Abnorm Psychol 105:271–275, 1996

Muzekari LH, Bates ME: Judgment of emotion among chronic schizophrenics. J Clin Psychol 33:662–666, 1977

Novic J, Luchins DJ, Perline R: Facial affect recognition in schizophrenia: is there a differential deficit? Br J Psychiatry 144:533–537, 1984

Ozonoff S, Miller JN: Teaching theory of minds: a new approach to social skills training for individuals with autism. J Autism Dev Disord 25:415–433, 1995

Penn DL, Spaulding W, Reed D, et al: The relationship of social cognition to ward behavior in chronic schizophrenia. Schizophr Res 20:327–335, 1996

Penn DL, Corrigan PW, Bentall RP, et al: Social cognition in schizophrenia. Psychol Bull 121:114–132, 1997

Penn DL, Combs DR, Ritchie M, et al: Emotion recognition in schizophrenia: further investigations of generalized versus specific deficit models. J Abnorm Psychol 109:512–516, 2000

Penn DL, Combs D, Mohamed S: Social cognition and social functioning in schizophrenia, in Social Cognition in Schizophrenia. Edited by Corrigan PW, Penn DL. Washington, DC, American Psychological Association, 2001, pp 97–121

Penn DL, Ritchie M, Francis, J, et al: Social perception in schizophrenia: the role of context. Psychiatry Res 109:149–159, 2002

Peters E, Day S, Garety P: From preconscious to conscious processing: where does the abnormality lie in delusions? Schizophr Res 24:120, 1997

Peterson C, Semmel A, Von Baeyer C, et al: The Attributional Style Questionnaire. Cognit Ther Res 3:287–300, 1982

Phillips ML, David AS: Abnormal visual scan paths: a psychophysiological marker of delusions in schizophrenia. Schizophr Res 29:235–245, 1998

Phillips ML, Senior C, David AS: Perception of threat in schizophrenics with persecutory delusions: an investigation using visual scan paths. Psychol Med 30:157–167, 2000

Phillips ML, Drevets WC, Rauch SL, et al: Neurobiology of emotion perception, I: the neural basis of normal emotion perception. Biol Psychiatry 54:504–514, 2003a

Phillips ML, Drevets WC, Rauch SL, et al: Neurobiology of emotion perception, II: implications for major psychiatric disorders. Biol Psychiatry 54:515–528, 2003b

Pickup GJ, Frith CD: Theory of mind impairments in schizophrenia: symptomatology, severity, and specificity. Psychol Med 31:207–220, 2001

Pilowsky T, Yirmiya N, Arbelle S, et al: Theory of mind abilities of children with schizophrenia, children with autism, and normally developing children. Schizophr Res 42:145–155, 2000

Pinkham AE, Penn DL, Perkins DO, et al: Implications for the neural basis of social cognition for the study of schizophrenia. Am J Psychiatry 160:815–824, 2003

Pollice R, Roncone R, Falloon IRH, et al: Is theory of mind in schizophrenia more strongly associated with clinical and social functioning than with neurocognitive deficits? Psychopathology 35:280–288, 2002

Randall F, Corcoran R, Day JC, et al: Attention, theory of mind, and causal attributions in people with persecutory delusions: a preliminary investigation. Cognitive Neuropsychiatry 8:287–294, 2003

Rowe AD, Bullock PR, Polkey CE, et al: "Theory of mind" impairments and their relationship to executive functioning following frontal lobe excisions. Brain 124:600–616, 2001

Russell TA, Rubia K, Bullmore ET, et al: Exploring the social brain in schizophrenia: left prefrontal underactivation during mental state attribution. Am J Psychiatry 157:2040–2042, 2000

Sachs G, Steger-Wuchese D, Krypsin-Exner I, et al: Facial recognition deficits and cognition in schizophrenia. Schizophr Res 68:27–35, 2004

Salem JE, Kring AM, Kerr SL: More evidence for generalized poor performance in facial emotion perception in schizophrenia. J Abnorm Psychol 105:480–483, 1996

Sarfati Y, Hardy-Bayle M: How do people with schizophrenia explain the behaviour of others? A study of theory of mind and its relationship to thought and speech disorganization in schizophrenia. Psychol Med 29:613–620, 1999

Sarfati Y, Hardy-Bayle M, Nadel J, et al: Attribution of mental states to others by schizophrenic patients. Cognitive Neuropsychiatry 2:1–17, 1997

Sarfati Y, Hardy-Bayle M, Brunet E, et al: Investigating theory of mind in schizophrenia: influence of verbalization in disorganized and non-disorganized patients. Schizophr Res 37:183–190, 1999

Sarfati Y, Passerieux C, Hardy-Bayle MC: Can verbalization remedy the theory of mind deficit in schizophrenia? Psychopathology 33:246–251, 2000

Schneider F, Gur RC, Gur RE, et al: Emotional processing in schizophrenia: neurobehavioral probes in relation to psychopathology. Schizophr Res 17:67–75, 1995

Sharp HM, Fear CF, Healy D: Attributional style and delusions: an investigation based on delusional content. Eur Psychiatry 12:1–7, 1997

Silver H, Shlomo N: Perception of facial emotions in chronic schizophrenia does not correlate with negative symptoms but correlates with cognitive and motor dysfunction. Schizophr Res 52:265–273, 2001

Silver H, Shlomo N, Turner T, et al: Perception of happy and sad facial expressions in chronic schizophrenia: evidence for two evaluative systems. Schizophr Res 55:171–177, 2002

Silverstein SM: Information processing, social cognition, and psychiatric rehabilitation in schizophrenia. Psychiatry 60:327–340, 1997

Streit M, Wolwer W, Gaebel W: Facial affect recognition and visual scanning behaviour in the course of schizophrenia. Schizophr Res 24:311–317, 1997

Swettenham J: Can children with autism be taught to understand false belief using computers? J Child Psychol Psychiatry 37:157–165, 1996

Sylvester CC, Wager TD, Lacey SC, et al: Switching attention and resolving interference: fMRI measures of executive functions. Neuropsychologia 41:357–370, 2003

Tager-Flusberg H, Boshart J, Baron-Cohen S: Reading the windows of the soul: evidence of domain-specific sparing in Williams syndrome. J Cogn Neurosci 10:631–639, 1998

Taylor JL, Kinderman P: An analogue study of attributional complexity, theory of mind deficits and paranoia. Br J Psychol 93:137–140, 2002

Wagner AD, Maril A, Bjork RA, et al: Prefrontal contributions to executive control: fMRI evidence for functional distinctions within lateral prefrontal cortex. Neuroimage 14:1337–1347, 2001

Walker E, Marwit S, Emory E: A cross-sectional study of emotion recognition in schizophrenics. J Abnorm Psychol 89:428–436, 1980

Walker E, McGuire M, Bettes B: Recognition and identification of facial stimuli by schizophrenics and patients with affective disorders. Br J Clin Psychol 23:37–44, 1984

Wykes T, Hamid S, Wagstaff K: Theory of mind and executive functions in the non-psychotic siblings of patients with schizophrenia (abstract). Schizophr Res 49 (suppl):148, 2001

SOCIAL AND VOCATIONAL IMPAIRMENTS

KIM T. MUESER, PH.D.

SHIRLEY M. GLYNN, PH.D.

SUSAN R. MCGURK, PH.D.

Problems with social relationships and role functioning, such as going to school or working, typically precede the onset of schizophrenia and continue throughout much of an affected person's life. In addition to psychotic symptoms that are hallmarks of schizophrenia, impaired social and vocational functioning are required for the diagnosis of schizophrenia according to both DSM-IV-TR (American Psychiatric Association 2000) and ICD-10 (World Health Organization 1992) classification systems. Thus, by definition, problems in social and vocational functioning are a critical feature of schizophrenia.

In this chapter, we summarize what is known about the nature of social and vocational impairment in schizophrenia and treatment strategies for improving functioning in these areas. We begin with a brief description of the onset and course of social and vocational dysfunction in schizophrenia. Although problems in social and vocational functioning are associated with each other, the strength of these associations is modest at best. In addition, rehabilitation strategies for addressing social and vocational functioning differ. Therefore, we describe the nature of social and vocational impairments and their treatment in separate sections of this chapter.

ONSET AND COURSE OF SOCIAL AND VOCATIONAL IMPAIRMENTS

Problems in the social functioning of patients with schizophrenia typically antedate the onset of the more obvious signs of the illness by many years. Although some people with schizophrenia have no social problems during childhood and adolescence before developing the early signs of schizophrenia, many others show a pattern of maladjustment (Baum and Walker 1995; Hans et al. 1992).

Two types of aberrant social functioning tend to occur in childhood and adolescence in people who later develop schizophrenia. First, some individuals are more shy, appear more awkward when interacting with peers, have fewer friends, and are generally more anxious and withdrawn than others around them (Zigler and Glick 1986). These individuals may seem peculiar to others or are viewed as loners with reduced social drive. They often fail to make close friends or develop romantic interests during adolescence. For these people, the onset of schizophrenia is often very gradual, even imperceptible, and the social impairments related to the illness appear to be mainly an exaggeration of problems in their premorbid social functioning.

A second pattern of maladjusted social behavior is reflected by individuals who appear to have impulse-control problems during childhood and adolescence and whose behavior may be marked by poor attention during school, fights, disregard for authority, and other problems commonly found in conduct disorder (Asarnow 1988; Cannon et al. 1993; Robins 1966; Rutter 1997). These individuals' social problems appear to stem more from their failure to recognize the rights and feelings of others than from their lack of understanding of basic social norms.

Although extensive research has documented problems in social functioning before the onset of schizophrenia, mounting evidence indicates that the prodromal period preceding the onset of psychotic symptoms in schizophrenia is longer than was once thought. Thus, at least some of the pervasive social impairments observed in people who later develop schizophrenia may actually be early signs of the illness and are not truly "premorbid." Work by Häfner and his colleagues (Häfner 2000; Häfner et al. 2003) has shown that the first signs of schizophrenia include depression and mild negative symptoms, followed by cognitive impairment and difficulties in role functioning. Problems in these areas tend to appear on average about 5 years before the emergence of psychotic symptoms, which is typically followed within a year by the first formal treatment (and often hospitalization).

In addition to reporting that the first signs of schizophrenia include both mood and social problems that precede the onset of psychotic symptoms by several years, Häfner and colleagues (1993, 1999) have shown that the age at which these difficulties first emerge is related to the person's subsequent social functioning over the course of his or her illness. Specifically, the older an individual is when he or she develops the first signs and symptoms of schizophrenia, the more social roles that person has been able to fulfill and the better that person's social functioning will be over the course of his or her illness. The frequently reported finding that women with schizophrenia tend to have better social functioning than men with schizophrenia (Haas and Garratt 1998), and experience a somewhat milder course of illness (Angermeyer et al. 1990), can be attributed to the later age at onset of schizophrenia for women (Häfner et al. 1993). Because women develop schizophrenia at a later age, they develop more social roles and thus enjoy a better level of functioning throughout the course of their psychiatric illness.

Over the long-term course of schizophrenia, social and vocational impairments tend to be relatively stable in the absence of concerted rehabilitation efforts. The consensus from long-term follow-up studies is that a signifi-

cant proportion of patients have partial or full symptom remissions and some improvement in their social functioning (Häfner and an der Heiden 2003; Harding and Keller 1998). The extent to which such gains occur has been the topic of much debate, but some degree of later life improvement is nevertheless quite common.

SOCIAL SKILLS AND SOCIAL FUNCTIONING

For too long, relapse prevention and symptom control were the exclusive goals of interventions for schizophrenia. However, with the advent of deinstitutionalization and community-based treatment, the importance of psychiatric patients being able to function competently in society has become increasingly recognized. More and more authors have begun to question the wisdom of constraining the definition of good outcome to few or no psychotic symptoms (Falloon 1984; Meltzer 1999). Consideration of the breadth of domains that most would consider integral to a successful life—work, intimacy, friendships, family, and avocations—has begun to influence the objectives of treatment interventions.

Psychiatric rehabilitation, a new field that reflects this broader conceptualization of outcome, has come to the forefront in schizophrenia treatment research (Bachrach 2000). The notion of recovery from schizophrenia is becoming more widespread, and it is not surprising that one of the most popular operationalizations of recovery includes independent functioning and peer relationships as core elements (Liberman et al. 2002). Both elements are well within the purview of the social functioning domain.

Any discussion of social functioning in schizophrenia commences with a need to define terms. When we discuss *social functioning*, we are typically describing domains of behavior that involve interactions with others; that is, the means by which individuals function in society. Social functioning in schizophrenia has been operationalized at both the microcomponent and macrocomponent level (Morrison and Bellack 1987). Many of the microcomponents of social functioning are subsumed under the rubric of *social skills*. These typically include the verbal, paralinguistic, and nonverbal components of interpersonal interactions—eye contact; facial expressions; length, frequency, and latency of speech utterances; proximity; use of hand gestures; and the like. A related variable involves social perception or cognition, including the accurate recognition of emotions in others (e.g., facial expressions), the ability to perceive relevant situational parameters, and understanding the possible motives of others (Penn et al. 1997). Some have conceptualized social skills as including "receiving" (social perception), "processing" (social cognition), and "sending" (social skills) skills (Donahoe et al. 1990; McFall 1982; Wallace et al. 1980) and have posited that deficits may occur in any of these domains. Many of the core symptoms of schizophrenia, especially those pertaining to cognitive deficits and negative symptoms, are reflected in the poor social skills often shown by persons with the disorder.

At a more macro level, social functioning can be seen as analogous to social adjustment. Here, the primary issue is role functioning in a variety of domains—worker, family member, friend, and parent. For adults, successful role functioning typically includes living independently, being financially self-sufficient through employment, having a strong social network of family and friends, and having satisfying avocations. In DSM-IV-TR, criterion B for schizophrenia reflects the poor and/or deteriorated role functioning inherent in the disorder.

SOCIAL SKILLS

Poor social skills have been understood as a core characteristic of schizophrenia from its first conceptualization as a disorder (Kraepelin 1919/1971). Among persons with schizophrenia, the predictors of better social skills include demographic characteristics such as being female (Mueser et al. 1990; Usall et al. 2002); cognitive factors such as high levels of verbal ability, verbal memory, and vigilance (Addington and Addington 2000); and psychopathological variables such as low levels of negative symptoms (Jackson et al. 1989; Patterson et al. 2001). Specific social skills are related to, but distinguishable from, global social competence (Appelo et al. 1992).

The negative outcomes accruing from poor social skills are apparent. For example, Nisenson et al. (2001) conducted a fascinating study in which research assistants were assigned to meet with inpatients with schizophrenia over a 2-week period. Across the 2 weeks, patients who had deficits in social skills, as reflected in unpleasant conversational topics or "strangeness," elicited increasingly more negative appraisals from the research assistants. In a similar vein, Penn et al. (2000) found, in ratings of the behavior of a group of individuals with schizophrenia, that poor social skills were associated with perceived "strangeness" and were then related to a desire for greater social distance.

Fortunately, antipsychotic medications can lead to improvements in social skills when an individual is acutely psychotic. For example, if a floridly psychotic person spends much of his or her time appearing to respond to internal stimuli (e.g., talking to self, looking off, not responding to questions), his or her social skills would be deemed poor. The administration of antipsychotic medications, which reduce the frequency of hallucinations, would be expected to decrease the patient's apparent response to the internal stimuli and thus improve his or her social skills. However, in individuals whose psychotic symptoms are under better control, either through medication or through their own adaptation, antipsychotic medications appear to have little effect on social skills (Bellack et al. 2004b). Here, targeted psychosocial interventions are necessary (Hogarty and Ulrich 1998).

Social skills training programs are among the most common of the psychosocial interventions for schizophrenia. Typically, these programs involve the use of cognitive-behavioral techniques grounded in learning theory (e.g., coaching, prompting, modeling, chaining, positive reinforcement) to improve specific components of social skills (Bellack et al. 2004a; Liberman et al. 1989). Sessions can be run individually or in a group and typically are offered in a time-limited fashion. Meetings are generally conducted in hospitals or clinics. Typical therapeutic goals might include improving assertiveness skills, affect recognition, family communication patterns, or conversational skills. Immediate outcome is usually assessed through role-plays and/or discussions of strategies that would be used to resolve interpersonal problems. Often, more global outcomes such as reduced relapse rates or improved role functioning are also evaluated. The steps of social skills training are summarized in Table 15–1.

Several reviews and meta-analyses indicated that social skills training programs can lead to improved outcomes (Benton and Schroeder 1990; Dilk and Bond 1996; Heinssen et al. 2000), although some have drawn more negative conclusions (Pilling et al. 2002; cf. Mueser and Penn 2004). One explanation for the negative findings may be that an obscure link often exists between the social skills intervention and more global outcomes evaluated in many studies. Social skills training would be expected to improve discrete behaviors and perhaps global adjustment or role functioning. However, some social skills trials have assessed more distal outcomes, such as treatment compliance and relapse, and these investigations have yielded mixed results. Even in studies in which benefits have been achieved in the clinic, there has been much debate about whether these benefits can be generalized to naturalistic settings (Liberman et al. 2001). For example, Dilk and Bond (1996) found that the estimated effects of social skills training programs were largest in studies in which the assessment setting and outcome measures were similar to those used in the training of skills and smallest in studies in which both differed. These results indicate that social skills training programs can affect specific behaviors, but it is often unclear when this modification of behavior will

TABLE 15–1. Steps of social skills training

1. Establish rationale for the skill.
   - Elicit reasons for learning the skill from group participants.
   - Acknowledge all contributions.
   - Provide additional reasons not mentioned by group members.
2. Discuss the steps of the skill.
   - Break down the skill into three or four steps.
   - Write the steps on a board or poster.
   - Discuss the reason for each step.
   - Check for understanding of each step.
3. Model the skill in a role-play.
   - Explain that you will demonstrate the skill in a role-play.
   - Plan out the role-play.
   - Use two leaders to model the skill.
   - Keep the role-play simple.
4. Review the role-play with the participants.
   - Discuss whether each step of the skill was used in the role-play.
   - Ask group members to evaluate the effectiveness of the role model.
   - Keep the review brief and to the point.
5. Engage a patient in a role-play of the same situation.
   - Request the patient to try the skill in a role-play with one of the leaders.
   - Ask the patient questions to make sure he or she understands their goal.
   - Instruct members to observe the patient.
   - Start with a patient who is more skilled or is likely to be compliant.
6. Provide positive feedback.
   - Elicit positive feedback from group members about the patient's skills.
   - Encourage feedback that is specific.
   - Cut off any negative feedback.
   - Praise effort and provide hints to group members about good performance.
7. Provide corrective feedback.
   - Elicit suggestions for how patient could do the skill better next time.
   - Limit the feedback to one or two suggestions.
   - Strive to communicate the suggestions in a positive, upbeat manner.

TABLE 15–1. Steps of social skills training (continued)

8. Engage the patient in another role-play of the same situation.
   - Request that the patient change one behavior in the role-play.
   - Check by asking questions to make sure the patient understands the suggestion.
   - Try to work on behaviors that are salient and changeable.
9. Provide additional feedback.
   - Focus first on the behavior that the patient was requested to change.
   - Engage patient in two to four role-plays with feedback after each one.
   - Use other behavior-shaping strategies to improve skills, such as coaching, prompting, supplemental modeling.
   - Be generous but specific when providing positive feedback.
10. Assign homework.
    - Give an assignment to practice the skill.
    - Ask group members to identify situations in which they could use the skill.
    - When possible, tailor the assignment to each patient's level of skill.

result in significant improvements in social adjustment. Better methods are necessary to generalize skills training in the clinic to the natural environment, such as in vivo practice of skills (Glynn et al. 2002) and the use of indigenous supporters to facilitate transfer of skills (Tauber et al. 2000).

SOCIAL FUNCTIONING

Social functioning occurs at the nexus between social skills and environmental opportunities to use these skills. In schizophrenia, both limited social skills and constrained environmental resources may lead to poor social functioning. Compared with those in the general population, persons with schizophrenia are less likely to marry and more likely to divorce if they do (Agerbo et al. 2004), less likely to have children (Nimgaonkar 1998), and less likely to be employed (Sturm et al. 1999). Predictors of poor social functioning include both individual and environmental variables. At the individual level, poorer social functioning has been related to being male (Usall et al. 2002) and psychophysiological variables (lower responsivity to environmental stressors and greater responses to skin conductance–orienting responses) (Brekke et al. 1997).

Interestingly, individuals with schizophrenia and concurrent substance use disorders tend to have better social functioning and greater social networks than do those without a substance use disorder (Carey et al. 2003; Salyers and Mueser 2001), possibly because of their better premorbid social functioning (Arndt et al. 1992). However, substance abuse in schizophrenia is also related to greater friction in family relationships (Kashner et al. 1991; Salyers and Mueser 2001) and at severe levels is associated with substantial social impairment and extrusion from social networks (Drake et al. 1998). At the environmental level, poorer social functioning is related to participation in less intensive rehabilitation programs (Brekke et al. 1997) and higher levels of ambient family stress (Miklowitz et al. 1983).

A variety of different strategies to improve social functioning in schizophrenia have been investigated, with some success. Three main strategies have been tried: 1) medication, 2) social skills training, and 3) environmental modifications. Although the findings are mixed, studies of long-term medication trials have reported greater benefits for second-generation over first-generation antipsychotic agents for improving social functioning, as measured by changes in outcomes such as global functioning, quality of life, and negative symptoms (Corrigan et al. 2003).

Several different skills-building approaches have been used. Participation in personal therapy, a multiyear individual therapy focusing on education about schizophrenia and development of stress tolerance, led to greater improvements in social functioning than did participation in supportive therapy or family therapy in a sample of 151 individuals with schizophrenia or schizoaffective disorder (Hogarty et al. 1997a, 1997b). In a sample of 528 individuals with a schizophrenia spectrum disorder, participation in family interventions, whether offered in monthly groups or in more intensive weekly sessions, was related to improvements in patient social leisure activity and self-care as rated by the family (Mueser et al. 2001c). Participation in a set of structured, manualized social and independent living skills groups was found to be related to increases in social adjustment in comparison to attending supportive group therapy (Marder et al. 1996). Extending this work, Glynn et al. (2002) found that using a community-based trainer to support practice of skills learned in the social and independent living skills groups led to greater improvements in social adjustment compared with attending the groups without the community-based trainer. In a unique study that compared the benefits of participating in a generic social skills training program like that described earlier with the benefits of participating in one targeting specific social areas (e.g., recreation, residence, vocational activity), Roder et al. (2002) found a trend for

improvement in all four groups for the targeted intervention.

The preceding discussion highlights both medication and skills training as ways to improve social functioning. The social and physical milieus are also susceptible to modification in the service of supporting better social functioning. In an innovative, environmentally focused study, Velligan et al. (2000) found that implementing a set of compensatory strategies (e.g., color coding, checklists, audible prompts) tailored to the participants' impediments in motivation, impulse control, and executive functioning led to greater improvements in functioning compared with a medication group or a medication group combined with an attention–placebo control intervention (i.e., equal time spent with a clinician engaged in supportive discussion and the provision of environmental adaptations such as posters and plants that were unrelated to the study goals).

The aforementioned studies suggest that profound changes in social functioning can occur as a result of medication, skills training, or environmental engineering. Most incorporated randomized designs, thus supporting the strength of the findings. Individuals with schizophrenia can experience improvements in social functioning over time, especially when exposed to well-considered, targeted treatments. Although control of symptoms is a laudable goal, improved social functioning is often the cornerstone of a successful community life.

The interventions described earlier yield important improvements in the social functioning of persons with schizophrenia; however, some of the greatest personal developmental tasks have yet to be adequately addressed by clinical researchers. Three important areas for consideration are living independently, establishing a romantic relationship, and raising children. Perhaps one explanation for why research and progress on interventions in these areas has lagged is that these are formidable life challenges, which can be daunting even for persons without psychiatric illnesses.

With regard to independent living, many have suggested that supported housing programs will lead to greater levels of self-sufficiency in schizophrenia (Rosenheck 2000). These programs typically provide persons with schizophrenia the opportunity to live in independent or quasi-independent settings with mental health staff available as resources and a planned, gradual transition to less supervision. In many programs, the ultimate goal is independent living. Unfortunately, the lack of randomized trials evaluating the benefits of supported housing program makes it impossible to discern whether they do, in fact, eventually lead to greater participant independence. A recent Cochrane review (Chilvers et al. 2002) found that although descriptions of 139 such programs were available in the scientific literature, none was conducted with the scientific rigor necessary to provide unbiased, useful information on whether supported housing really helps individuals move to greater independence.

A second compelling issue for many patients with schizophrenia today is their desire for a partner. Most individuals with the illness now spend most, if not all, of their lives outside of the hospital and long for a romantic relationship, just as their contemporaries without schizophrenia do. Unfortunately, this area has been little studied and is little understood. We do know that in Western societies (e.g., Finland and the United States), women with schizophrenia are more likely to marry than are their male counterparts (Bhatia et al. 2004; Salokangas et al. 2001). There are many posited reasons for this disparity (Haas and Garratt 1998; Riecher-Rössler and Häfner 2000), including the fact that 1) women tend to become ill later in life, so they may have already married before developing symptoms; 2) women may be more "marriageable" because it may be more acceptable for women to be out of the workforce and seen as homemakers, compared with men; and 3) more dependency is generally tolerated in women than in men in these societies. Similarly, cultural factors are thought to account for the absence of gender disparity in marriage rates among individuals with schizophrenia in India (Bhatia et al. 2004).

Nevertheless, we understand little at this point about how to help persons with the illness find and develop satisfactory, intimate partnerships with other individuals. Social stigma and poor self-esteem make this a very thorny road for many individuals with the illness. Most of the available textbooks on schizophrenia mention marriage little or not at all, and most family interventions for the illness highlight families of origin rather than partners (Schooler et al. 1997). Better ways to help persons with the illness develop satisfying social lives are sorely needed.

A final area of concern involves raising children (Brunette and Dean 2002). This issue has been studied primarily in women with schizophrenia, and the results are, not surprisingly, disturbing. In comparison to control subjects without schizophrenia, women with schizophrenia are less likely to have children (Haukka et al. 2003; Howard et al. 2002) but more likely to have difficulty raising their children if they do have them. Many lose custody (Miller and Finnerty 1996), and those who do raise their children may encounter difficulties resulting from their illness and poor social networks. Nevertheless, data suggest that being raised by a parent with schizophrenia is not necessarily equated with greater psychopathology in the offspring (Higgins et al. 1997), and many have called for professionals to provide more support to persons with

schizophrenia so that they will be able to rear their children successfully (Miller 1997).

Successful community functioning can be challenging for all persons. The experience of serious psychiatric illnesses such as schizophrenia often renders these challenges even more difficult. Mental health providers must take a broad view of their patients and take the time to understand and address social concerns in addition to symptom issues in order to provide optimal care and ensure the best possible outcomes.

VOCATIONAL FUNCTIONING

Poor occupational functioning is nearly a universal characteristic of schizophrenia, with competitive employment rates typically in the range of 10%–20% (Brekke et al. 1993; Marwaha and Johnson 2004; Mueser et al. 2001b) and invariably less than 50% (Priebe et al. 1998). Long-term outcome studies have reported occupational decline from premorbid levels in a significant proportion of persons with schizophrenia (Johnstone et al. 1990; Marneros et al. 1992). Moreover, this decline is evident as early as 6–18 months after the first episode (Beiser et al. 1994; Ho et al. 1998).

The high rate of unemployment among persons with schizophrenia has important implications for the effect of the disorder on the individual, the family, and society. From an individual perspective, high costs are associated with unemployment in schizophrenia, such as living in poverty with an increased vulnerability to victimization (Goodman et al. 2001; Walsh et al. 2003). In general, people with schizophrenia who are working function better across a range of different domains, and the attainment of work in previously unemployed persons is associated with increases in self-esteem, decreases in depression and psychotic symptoms, improved satisfaction with finances, and better overall functioning (Arns and Linney 1993; Bell et al. 1993, 1996; Bond et al. 2001b; Mueser et al. 1997; Torrey et al. 2000). The apparent clinical benefits of work for people with schizophrenia have led some to embrace the old adage that "work is good therapy" (Harding et al. 1987).

Low employment rates in schizophrenia also naturally lead to an increased dependence on the family for housing support and getting basic needs met. The high dependence of persons with schizophrenia on their family members, including cohabitation, contributes to significant objective and subjective burden on relatives (Baronet 1999; Maurin and Boyd 1990; Webb et al. 1998), which can culminate in high levels of anxiety and depression (Oldridge and Hughes 1992) and vulnerability to physical illness (Dyck et al. 1999) among caregivers. Even among people with schizophrenia who receive disability payments, family members still make significant financial and time contributions to the management of their illness and commonly associated disorders such as substance abuse and dependence (Clark 2001).

In addition, unemployment, resulting in lost productivity and the need for supplemental income, is a primary source of the high cost of schizophrenia, estimated to exceed $6 billion per year (Rice 1999). Indeed, the loss of productivity over most of the adult lifetime is a major reason that the combined economic and social costs of schizophrenia place it among the world's top 10 causes of disability-adjusted life-years (Murray and Lopez 1996), accounting for an estimated 2.3% of all burdens in developed countries and 0.8% in developing economies (U.S. Institute of Medicine 2001).

Finally, work is a critical component of how people in Western society define themselves, and the inability to work sets patients with mental illness, especially schizophrenia, apart from others and further contributes to their social marginalization (Crisp et al. 2000). Unfortunately, the stigma associated with schizophrenia may impede the ability of people with the illness to obtain jobs because of discrimination, which increases their stigmatization even more (Farina 1998; Wahl 1999). Increasing employment rates may decrease both stigmatizing public attitudes toward schizophrenia and self-stigmatizing beliefs among persons with the illness (Wahl 1997).

CORRELATES AND PREDICTORS OF WORK

A variety of sociodemographic, historical, and clinical correlates of work have been identified for persons with schizophrenia. As in the general population, level of education is related to work in schizophrenia (Mueser et al. 2001b). Given the evidence that educational attainment is more severely curtailed in schizophrenia compared with that in other disorders and the general population (Kessler et al. 1995), the association between education and work may partly account for the low work rates in people with this disorder. Similarly, history of competitive work, as well as current work status, is a potent predictor of future work in schizophrenia (Drake et al. 1996b; Mueser et al. 2001b).

Some research suggests that social skills are related to work performance in persons with schizophrenia (Arns and Linney 1995; Bellack et al. 1990; Furman et al. 1979; Mueser et al. 1986), and one study found that skills training improves employment outcomes (Tsang 2001). However, an even greater wealth of evidence points to the importance of symptoms and cognitive functioning as contributing factors to vocational functioning in schizo-

phrenia. Both psychotic and negative symptoms have been found to predict amount of employment in persons with schizophrenia not participating in vocational rehabilitation, both concurrently and prospectively (Beiser et al. 1994; Daradkeh and Karim 1994; Glynn et al. 1992; Mueser et al. 2001b; Racenstein et al. 2002).

Cognitive impairment is strongly related to a range of different domains of community functioning in schizophrenia (Green 1996; Green et al. 2000), including work (McGurk and Meltzer 2000). Specifically, cognitive functioning is related to work both in people not receiving vocational rehabilitation services (Bellack et al. 1999; J.M. Gold et al. 1999; McGurk and Mueser 2003; Mueser et al. 2001b) and in people receiving such services (Bell and Bryson 2001; Bryson et al. 1998; J.M. Gold et al. 2002; Lysaker et al. 1995; McGurk et al. 2003). A recent review of correlates and predictors of work in schizophrenia and other severe mental illnesses concluded that although symptoms and cognitive functioning predict work in schizophrenia, the associations tend to be stronger in patients not receiving employment services than among patients receiving such services (McGurk and Mueser 2004). A possible implication of these findings is that vocational rehabilitation may serve to compensate for the effects of illness-related impairments, both symptom and cognitive, on work.

VOCATIONAL REHABILITATION

The high rates of unemployment in patients with schizophrenia underscore the importance of improving employment outcomes in these individuals. Furthermore, most persons with schizophrenia express a desire for competitive work (Mueser et al. 2001b; Rogers et al. 1991). Various vocational rehabilitation models have been developed to address the poor work outcomes of persons with schizophrenia. Traditional approaches to vocational rehabilitation that use a "train-place" approach (i.e., in which patients engage in extensive preparation before getting a competitive job, such as vocational counseling, skills training, participating in job club, or sheltered work) found few beneficial effects on competitive work outcomes (Bond 1992). More recently, vocational rehabilitation models that emphasize rapid job search and attainment, and the provision of follow-along supports (most notably, supported employment), have been developed and empirically validated (Bond et al. 2001a).

Supported Employment

Purpose and scope. Supported employment is an approach to vocational rehabilitation for persons with schizophrenia and other severe mental illnesses that focuses on helping patients find competitive jobs in integrated community settings and on providing ongoing supports to facilitate good job performance or to help in the transition to another job. The supported employment model was first developed for persons with developmental disabilities (Wehman and Moon 1988) and was then adapted for individuals with schizophrenia and other severe mental illnesses (Becker and Drake 1994). The most widely studied approach to supported employment for severe mental illness is the Individual Placement and Support (IPS) model, which has been standardized in a manual (Becker and Drake 2003) and a fidelity scale (Bond et al. 1997).

First and foremost, supported employment emphasizes helping people with schizophrenia find competitive jobs in the community. The jobs that are most valued by individuals are those located in integrated community settings, thus providing contact with nondisabled persons and paying competitive wages (Bedell et al. 1998). Research, as described in the following subsection, suggests that many people with schizophrenia are capable of attaining competitive work in the community and that modest clinical benefits are associated with work (Arns and Linney 1993; Bell et al. 1996; Mueser et al. 1997). Furthermore, the focus of supported employment is on finding jobs with a minimum of prevocational activities, such as sheltered work or skills training. Some evidence indicates that delaying the job search in supported employment is associated with worse vocational outcomes (Bond and Dincin 1986; Bond et al. 1995), underscoring the importance of "striking while the iron is hot" and commencing the job search soon after the individual has expressed an interest in working.

The job search in supported employment is individualized for the patient and is informed by knowledge of the individual's job preferences, including type of work and extent of social contact. Matching patients' job preferences to the jobs obtained has implications for improving job tenure for persons receiving supported employment; people who obtain jobs that match their preferences report significantly higher levels of job satisfaction and remain in the job longer than do people whose jobs do not match their preferences (Becker et al. 1996; Mueser et al. 2001a).

Supported employment also differs from many other approaches to vocational rehabilitation in the provision of individual, time-unlimited support to maintain employment. The type of support provided by the supported employment specialist varies according to the needs and preferences of the individual. Some patients choose to disclose their psychiatric disability to prospective employers, whereas others do not. When patients prefer not to disclose their psychiatric disorder, the support provided is

"behind the scenes" and can involve activities such as planning the job search, practicing job interviewing, and problem solving to address conflicts and issues that arise on the job. When the person permits disclosure to a prospective employer, the employment specialist is also often directly involved in helping the patient acquire the job, liaising with the employer to ensure good job performance, and helping the person negotiate reasonable accommodations when needed.

Finally, supported employment services need to be closely integrated with the provision of clinical services to ensure the long-term retention of patients in vocational services (Mueser et al. 2004) and to address optimally clinical and treatment issues that may affect work (e.g., responding to the early warning signs of an impending relapse and managing medication side effects, such as sedation, that may interfere with work). One approach to integration of vocational and clinical services is to have the supported employment specialist function as a member of the patient's interdisciplinary treatment team and attend all team meetings, provide information about the patient's work-related activities, and obtain feedback and suggestions from other team members about how to help the individual attain his or her work goals. Having the employment specialist work alongside the clinical treatment team serves to highlight the importance of work in treatment planning and to ensure that all members of the team are supportive of improving the patient's vocational outcomes.

Research on supported employment. Over the past decade, a growing body of research has been conducted documenting the effectiveness of supported employment for persons with schizophrenia and other severe mental illnesses. Most of the research has examined the IPS model (Becker and Drake 2003), although research also has evaluated other models of supported employment. Five quasi-experimental studies have examined the effects of closing day treatment programs and initiating supported employment programs in their place (Bailey et al. 1998; Becker et al. 2001; Drake et al. 1994, 1996a; M. Gold and Marrone 1998). Across the studies, the conversion to a supported employment program was associated with significant increases in work, without any untoward effects observed, such as increases in relapses or rehospitalizations.

In addition to these quasi-experimental studies, 11 randomized controlled trials have reported the superiority of supported employment to a variety of other vocational rehabilitation approaches across the United States, as illustrated in Figure 15–1. These studies have shown that IPS or other approaches to supported employment result in significantly higher levels of competitive employment over

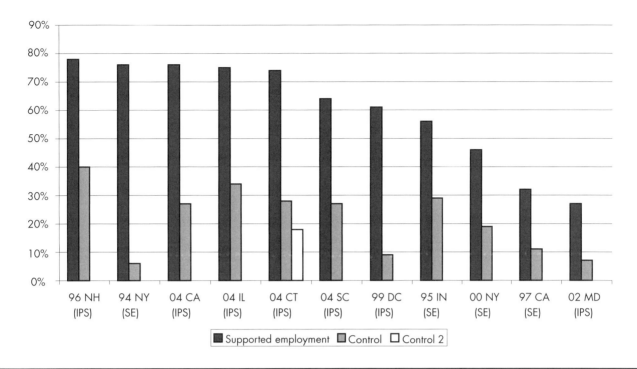

FIGURE 15–1. Cumulative rates of competitive employment over 1–2 years for persons with severe mental illness participating in 11 randomized controlled trials of supported employment programs.

IPS=Individual Placement and Support model of supported employment, SE=other supported employment model. Specific vocational programs used in comparisons with IPS and SE included sheltered work, brokered vocational rehabilitation services, prevocational preparation and skills training, psychosocial rehabilitation programs, and diversified vocational placement (i.e., access to multiple types of programs). See text for details.

1–2 years compared with other programs, including sheltered work in New York (Gervey and Bedell 1994); Washington, D.C. (Drake et al. 1999); and South Carolina (P.B. Gold et al., in press); brokered vocational rehabilitation services in California (Chandler et al. 1997; Twamley et al. 2004), New York (McFarlane et al. 2000), and Connecticut (Mueser et al. 2004); prevocational preparation and skills training in Indiana (Bond et al. 1995) and New Hampshire (Drake et al. 1996b); psychosocial rehabilitation programs in Connecticut (Mueser et al. 2004) and Maryland (Lehman et al. 2002); and diversified vocational placement (i.e., access to multiple types of programs) in Illinois (Bond 2004). Thus, significant research supports the effectiveness of supported employment for persons with severe mental illness.

CONCLUSION

Impairments in social and vocational functioning are a defining characteristic of schizophrenia and include poor quality of social relationships and difficulty with role functioning in areas such as school, work, and parenting.

Problems in social functioning appear to be at least partly related to symptoms of the illness, including psychotic, negative, and cognitive symptoms, but are not fully explained by those symptoms. Economic constraints and environmental factors such as stigma and discrimination also play a role in limiting social functioning.

Although impairments in functioning tend to be relatively stable and long term in schizophrenia, significant advances have been made in the development of interventions for improving functioning. Most notable among those interventions are social skills training to improve social functioning and supported employment to improve vocational outcomes.

REFERENCES

Addington J, Addington D: Neurocognitive and social functioning in schizophrenia: a 2.5 year follow-up study. Schizophr Res 7:47–56, 2000

Agerbo E, Byrne M, Eaton WW, et al: Marital and labor market status in the long run in schizophrenia. Arch Gen Psychiatry 61:28–33, 2004

American Psychiatric Association: Diagnostic and Statistical Manual of Mental Disorders, 4th Edition, Text Revision. Washington, DC, American Psychiatric Association, 2000

Angermeyer MC, Kuhn L, Goldstein JM: Gender and the course of schizophrenia: differences in treated outcome. Schizophr Bull 16:293–307, 1990

Appelo MT, Woonings FM, Van Nieuwenhuizen CJ, et al: Specific skills and social competence in schizophrenia. Acta Psychiatr Scand 85:419–422, 1992

Arndt S, Tyrrell G, Flaum M, et al: Comorbidity of substance abuse and schizophrenia: the role of pre-morbid adjustment. Psychol Med 22:379–388, 1992

Arns PG, Linney JA: Work, self, and life satisfaction for persons with severe and persistent mental disorders. Psychosocial Rehabilitation Journal 17:63–79, 1993

Arns PG, Linney JA: Relating functional skills of severely mentally ill clients to subjective and societal benefits. Psychiatr Serv 46:260–265, 1995

Asarnow JR: Children at risk for schizophrenia: converging lines of evidence. Schizophr Bull 14:613–631, 1988

Bachrach LL: Psychosocial rehabilitation and psychiatry in the treatment of schizophrenia—what are the boundaries? Acta Psychiatr Scand 102:6–10, 2000

Bailey EL, Ricketts SK, Becker DR, et al: Do long-term day treatment clients benefit from supported employment? Psychiatr Rehabil J 22:24–29, 1998

Baronet A-M: Factors associated with caregiver burden in mental illness: a critical review of the research literature. Clin Psychol Rev 19:819–841, 1999

Baum KM, Walker EF: Childhood behavioral precursors of adult symptom dimensions in schizophrenia. Schizophr Res 16:111–120, 1995

Becker DR, Drake RE: Individual placement and support: a community mental health center approach to vocational rehabilitation. Community Ment Health J 45:487–489, 1994

Becker DR, Drake RE: A Working Life for People With Severe Mental Illness. New York, Oxford University Press, 2003

Becker DR, Drake RE, Farabaugh A, et al: Job preferences of clients with severe psychiatric disorders participating in supported employment programs. Psychiatr Serv 47:1223–1226, 1996

Becker DR, Bond GR, McCarthy D, et al: Converting day treatment centers to supported employment programs in Rhode Island. Psychiatr Serv 52:351–357, 2001

Bedell JR, Draving D, Parrish A, et al: A description and comparison of experiences of people with mental disorders in supported employment and paid prevocational training. Psychiatr Rehabil J 21:279–283, 1998

Beiser M, Bean G, Erickson D, et al: Biological and psychosocial predictors of job performance following a first episode of psychosis. Am J Psychiatry 151:857–863, 1994

Bell MD, Bryson G: Work rehabilitation in schizophrenia: does cognitive impairment limit improvement? Schizophr Bull 27:269–279, 2001

Bell MD, Milstein RM, Lysaker PH: Pay and participation in work activity: clinical benefits for clients with schizophrenia. Psychosocial Rehabilitation Journal 17:173–177, 1993

Bell MD, Lysaker PH, Milstein RM: Clinical benefits of paid work activity in schizophrenia. Schizophr Bull 22:51–67, 1996

Bellack AS, Morrison RL, Wixted JT, et al: An analysis of social competence in schizophrenia. Br J Psychiatry 156:809–818, 1990

Bellack AS, Gold JM, Buchanan RW: Cognitive rehabilitation for schizophrenia: problems, prospects, and strategies. Schizophr Bull 25:257–274, 1999

Bellack AS, Mueser KT, Gingerich S, et al: Social Skills Training for Schizophrenia: A Step-By-Step Guide, 2nd Edition. New York, Guilford, 2004a

Bellack AS, Schooler NR, Marder SR, et al: Do clozapine and risperidone affect social competence and problem solving? Am J Psychiatry 161:364–367, 2004b

Benton MK, Schroeder HE: Social skills training with schizophrenics: a meta-analytic evaluation. J Consult Clin Psychol 58:741–747, 1990

Bhatia T, Franzos MA, Wood JA, et al: Gender and procreation among patients with schizophrenia. Schizophr Res 68:387–394, 2004

Bond GR: Vocational rehabilitation, in Handbook of Psychiatric Rehabilitation. Edited by Liberman RP. New York, MacMillan, 1992, pp 244–275

Bond GR: The Thresholds Study of Individual Placement and Support: progress report on a randomized controlled trial. Paper presented at the Research Seminar of New Hampshire-Dartmouth Psychiatric Research Center, Lebanon, NH, March 26, 2004

Bond G, Dincin J: Accelerating entry into transitional employment in a psychosocial rehabilitation agency. Rehabil Psychol 31:143–155, 1986

Bond G, Dietzen L, McGrew J, et al: Accelerating entry into supported employment for persons with severe psychiatric disabilities. Rehabil Psychol 40:91–111, 1995

Bond GR, Becker DR, Drake RE, et al: A fidelity scale for the Individual Placement and Support model of supported employment. Rehabil Couns Bull 40:265–284, 1997

Bond GR, Becker DR, Drake RE, et al: Implementing supported employment as an evidence-based practice. Psychiatr Serv 52:313–322, 2001a

Bond GR, Resnick SG, Drake RE, et al: Does competitive employment improve nonvocational outcomes for people with severe mental illness? J Consult Clin Psychol 69:489–501, 2001b

Brekke JS, Levin S, Wolkon GH, et al: Psychosocial functioning and subjective experience in schizophrenia. Schizophr Bull 19:600–608, 1993

Brekke JS, Raine A, Ansel M, et al: Neuropsychological and psychophysiological correlates of psychosocial functioning in schizophrenia. Schizophr Bull 23:19–28, 1997

Brunette MF, Dean W: Community mental health care of women with severe mental illness who are parents. Community Ment Health J 38:153–165, 2002

Bryson G, Bell MD, Kaplan E, et al: The functional consequences of memory impairments on initial work performance in people with schizophrenia. J Nerv Ment Dis 186:610–615, 1998

Cannon TD, Mednick SA, Parnas J, et al: Developmental brain abnormalities in the offspring of schizophrenic mothers. Arch Gen Psychiatry 50:551–564, 1993

Carey KB, Carey MP, Simons JS: Correlates of substance use disorder among psychiatric outpatients: focus on cognition, social role functioning, and psychiatric status. J Nerv Ment Dis 191:300–308, 2003

Chandler D, Meisel J, Hu T, et al: A capitated model for a cross-section of severely mentally ill clients: employment outcomes. Community Ment Health J 33:501–516, 1997

Chilvers R, Macdonald GM, Hayes AA: Supported housing for people with severe mental disorders. Cochrane Database Syst Rev (4):CD000453, 2002

Clark RE: Family support and substance use outcomes for persons with mental illness and substance use disorders. Schizophr Bull 27:93–101, 2001

Corrigan PW, Reinke RR, Landsberger SA, et al: The effects of atypical antipsychotic medications on psychosocial outcomes. Schizophr Res 63:97–101, 2003

Crisp AH, Gelder MG, Rix S, et al: Stigmatization of people with mental illnesses. Br J Psychiatry 177:4–7, 2000

Daradkeh TK, Karim L: Predictors of employment status of treated patients with DSM-III-R diagnoses: can logistic regression model find a solution? Int J Soc Psychiatry 40:141–149, 1994

Dilk MN, Bond GR: Meta-analytic evaluation of skills training research for individuals with severe mental illness. J Consult Clin Psychol 64:1337–1346, 1996

Donahoe CP, Carter MJ, Bloem WD, et al: Assessment of interpersonal problem-solving skills. Psychiatry 53:329–339, 1990

Drake RE, Becker DR, Biesanz JC, et al: Rehabilitative day treatment vs supported employment, I: vocational outcomes. Community Ment Health J 30:519–532, 1994

Drake RE, Becker DR, Biesanz BA, et al: Day treatment versus supported employment for persons with severe mental illness: a replication study. Psychiatr Serv 47:1125–1127, 1996a

Drake RE, McHugo GJ, Becker DR, et al: The New Hampshire Study of Supported Employment for people with severe mental illness: vocational outcomes. J Consult Clin Psychol 64:391–399, 1996b

Drake RE, Brunette MF, Mueser KT: Substance use disorder and social functioning in schizophrenia, in Handbook of Social Functioning in Schizophrenia. Edited by Mueser KT, Tarrier N. Boston, MA, Allyn & Bacon, 1998, pp 280–289

Drake RE, McHugo GJ, Bebout RR, et al: A randomized clinical trial of supported employment for inner-city patients with severe mental illness. Arch Gen Psychiatry 56:627–633, 1999

Dyck DG, Short R, Vitaliano PP: Predictors of burden and infectious illness in schizophrenia caregivers. Psychosom Med 61:411–419, 1999

Falloon IRH: Relapse: a reappraisal of assessment of outcome in schizophrenia. Schizophr Bull 10:293–299, 1984

Farina A: Stigma, in Handbook of Social Functioning in Schizophrenia. Edited by Mueser KT, Tarrier N. Boston, MA, Allyn & Bacon, 1998, pp 247–279

Furman W, Gleller M, Simon SJ, et al: The use of a behavioral rehearsal procedure for teaching job-interviewing skills to psychiatric patients. Behav Ther 10:157–167, 1979

Gervey R, Bedell JR: Supported employment in vocational rehabilitation, in Psychological Assessment and Treatment of Persons With Severe Mental Disorders. Edited by Bedell JR. Washington, DC, Taylor & Francis, 1994, pp 139–163

Glynn SM, Randolph ET, Eth S, et al: Schizophrenic symptoms, work adjustment, and behavioral family therapy. Rehabil Psychol 37:323–328, 1992

Glynn SM, Marder SR, Liberman RP, et al: Supplementing clinic-based skills training with manual-based community support sessions: effects on social adjustment of patients with schizophrenia. Am J Psychiatry 159:829–837, 2002

Gold JM, Queern C, Iannone VN, et al: Repeatable battery for the assessment of neuropsychological status as a screening test in schizophrenia, II: convergent/discriminant validity and diagnostic group comparisons. Am J Psychiatry 156:1944–1950, 1999

Gold JM, Goldberg RW, McNary SW, et al: Cognitive correlates of job tenure among patients with severe mental illness. Am J Psychiatry 159:1395–1402, 2002

Gold M, Marrone J: Mass Bay Employment Services (a service of Bay Cove Human Services, Inc.): a story of leadership and vision resulting in employment for people with mental illness. Roses and Thorns From the Grassroots: A Series Highlighting Organizational Change in Massachusetts, Vol 1, Spring 1998

Gold PB, Meisler N, Williams OH, et al: Randomized trial of supported employment integrated with Assertive Community Treatment for rural adults with severe mental illness. Schizophr Bull (in press)

Goodman LA, Salyers MP, Mueser KT, et al: Recent victimization in women and men with severe mental illness: prevalence and correlates. J Trauma Stress 14:615–632, 2001

Green MF: What are the functional consequences of neurocognitive deficits in schizophrenia? Am J Psychiatry 153:321–330, 1996

Green MF, Kern RS, Braff DL, et al: Neurocognitive deficits and functional outcome in schizophrenia: are we measuring the "right stuff"? Schizophr Bull 26:119–136, 2000

Haas GL, Garratt LS: Gender differences in social functioning, in Handbook of Social Functioning in Schizophrenia. Edited by Mueser KT, Tarrier N. Boston, MA, Allyn & Bacon, 1998, pp 149–180

Häfner H: Onset and early course as determinants of the further course of schizophrenia. Acta Psychiatr Scand 102 (suppl 407):44–48, 2000

Häfner H, an der Heiden W: Course and outcome of schizophrenia, in Schizophrenia, 2nd Edition. Edited by Hirsch SR, Weinberger DR. Oxford, England, Blackwell Scientific, 2003, pp 101–141

Häfner II, Maurer K, Löffler W, et al: The influence of age and sex on the onset and early course of schizophrenia. Br J Psychiatry 162:80–86, 1993

Häfner H, Löffler W, Maurer K, et al: Depression, negative symptoms, social stagnation and social decline in the early course of schizophrenia. Acta Psychiatr Scand 100:105–118, 1999

Häfner H, Maurer K, Löffler W, et al: Modeling the early course of schizophrenia. Schizophr Bull 29:325–340, 2003

Hans SL, Marcus J, Henson L, et al: Interpersonal behavior of children at risk for schizophrenia. Psychiatry 55:314–335, 1992

Harding C, Strauss J, Hafez H, et al: Work and mental illness, I: toward an integration of the rehabilitation process. J Nerv Ment Dis 175:317–326, 1987

Harding CM, Keller AB: Long-term outcome of social functioning, in Handbook of Social Functioning in Schizophrenia. Edited by Mueser KT, Tarrier N. Boston, MA, Allyn & Bacon, 1998, pp 134–148

Haukka J, Suvisaari J, Lonnqvist J: Fertility of patients with schizophrenia, their siblings, and the general population: a cohort study from 1950 to 1959 in Finland. Am J Psychiatry 160:460–463, 2003

Heinssen RK, Liberman RP, Kopelowicz A: Psychosocial skills training for schizophrenia: lessons from the laboratory. Schizophr Bull 26:21–46, 2000

Higgins J, Gore R, Gutkind D, et al: Effects of child-rearing by schizophrenic mothers: a 25-year follow-up. Acta Psychiatr Scand 96:402–404, 1997

Ho BC, Nopoulos PM, Flaum M, et al: Two-year outcome in first-episode schizophrenia: predictive value of symptoms for quality of life. Am J Psychiatry 155:1196–1201, 1998

Hogarty GE, Ulrich RF: The limitations of antipsychotic medication on schizophrenia relapse and adjustment and the contributions of psychosocial treatment. J Psychiatr Res 32:243–250, 1998

Hogarty GE, Greenwald D, Ulrich RF, et al: Three-year trials of personal therapy among schizophrenic patients living with or independent of family, II: effects of adjustment on patients. Am J Psychiatry 154:1514–1524, 1997a

Hogarty GE, Kornblith SJ, Greenwald D, et al: Three-year trials of personal therapy among schizophrenic patients living with or independent of family, I: description of study and effects on relapse rates. Am J Psychiatry 154:1504–1513, 1997b

Howard LM, Kumar C, Leese M, et al: The general fertility rate in women with psychotic disorders. Am J Psychiatry 159:991–997, 2002

Jackson HJ, Minas IH, Burgess PM, et al: Negative symptoms and social skills performance in schizophrenia. Schizophr Res 2:457–463, 1989

Johnstone EC, Macmillan JF, Frith CD, et al: Further investigation of the predictors of outcome following first schizophrenic episodes. Br J Psychiatry 157:182–189, 1990

Kashner M, Rader L, Rodell D, et al: Family characteristics, substance abuse, and hospitalization patterns of patients with schizophrenia. Hosp Community Psychiatry 42:195–197, 1991

Kessler RC, Foster CL, Saunders WB, et al: Social consequences of psychiatric disorders, I: educational attainment. Am J Psychiatry 152:1026–1032, 1995

Kraepelin E: Dementia Praecox and Paraphrenia (1919). Translated by Barclay RM. New York, Krieger, 1971

Lehman AF, Goldberg R, Dixon LB, et al: Improving employment outcomes for persons with severe mental illnesses. Arch Gen Psychiatry 59:165–172, 2002

Liberman RP, DeRisi WJ, Mueser KT: Social Skills Training for Psychiatric Patients. Needham Heights, MA, Allyn & Bacon, 1989

Liberman RP, Blair KE, Glynn SM, et al: Generalization of skills training to the natural environment, in The Treatment of Schizophrenia: Status and Emerging Trends. Edited by Brenner HD, Boker W, Genner R. Seattle, WA, Hogrefe & Huber, 2001, pp 104–120

Liberman RP, Kopelowicz A, Ventura J, et al: Operational criteria and factors related to recovery from schizophrenia. Int Rev Psychiatry 14:256–272, 2002

Lysaker PH, Bell MD, Zito WS, et al: Social skills at work: deficits and predictors of improvement in schizophrenia. J Nerv Ment Dis 183:688–692, 1995

Marder SR, Wirshing WC, Mintz J, et al: Two-year outcome for social skills training and group psychotherapy for outpatients with schizophrenia. Am J Psychiatry 153:1585–1592, 1996

Marneros A, Deister A, Rohde A: Comparison of long-term outcome of schizophrenic, affective and schizoaffective disorders [published erratum appears in Br J Psychiatry 161:868, 1992]. Br J Psychiatry Suppl (18):44–51, 1992

Marwaha S, Johnson S: Schizophrenia and employment: a review. Soc Psychiatry Psychiatr Epidemiol 39:337–349, 2004

Maurin JT, Boyd CB: Burden of mental illness on the family: a critical review. Arch Psychiatr Nurs 4:99–107, 1990

McFall RM: A review and reformulation of the concept of social skills. Behav Assess 4:1–33, 1982

McFarlane WR, Dushay RA, Deakins SM, et al: Employment outcomes in family aided assertive community treatment. Am J Orthopsychiatry 70:203–214, 2000

McGurk SR, Meltzer HY: The role of cognition in vocational functioning in schizophrenia. Schizophr Res 45:175–184, 2000

McGurk SR, Mueser KT: Cognitive functioning and employment in severe mental illness. J Nerv Ment Dis 191:789–798, 2003

McGurk SR, Mueser KT: Cognitive functioning, symptoms, and work in supported employment: a review and heuristic model. Schizophr Res 70:147–174, 2004

McGurk SR, Mueser KT, Harvey PD, et al: Cognitive and clinical predictors of work outcomes in clients with schizophrenia. Psychiatr Serv 54:1129–1135, 2003

Meltzer HY: Outcome in schizophrenia: beyond symptom reduction. J Clin Psychiatry 60:3–7, 1999

Miklowitz DJ, Goldstein MJ, Falloon IRH: Premorbid and symptomatic characteristics of schizophrenics from families with high and low levels of expressed emotion. J Abnorm Psychol 92:359–367, 1983

Miller LJ: Sexuality, reproduction, and family planning in women with schizophrenia. Schizophr Bull 23:623–635, 1997

Miller LJ, Finnerty M: Sexuality, pregnancy, and childrearing among women with schizophrenia-spectrum disorders. Psychiatr Serv 4:502–506, 1996

Morrison RL, Bellack AS: Social functioning of schizophrenic patients: clinical and research issues. Schizophr Bull 13: 715–725, 1987

Mueser KT, Penn DL: Meta-analysis examining the effects of social skills training on schizophrenia. Psychol Med 34: 1365–1367, 2004

Mueser KT, Foy DW, Carter MJ: Social skills training for job maintenance in a psychiatric patient. J Couns Psychol 33: 360–362, 1986

Mueser KT, Bellack AS, Morrison RL, et al: Gender, social competence, and symptomatology in schizophrenia: a longitudinal analysis. J Abnorm Psychol 99:138–147, 1990

Mueser KT, Becker DR, Torrey WC, et al: Work and nonvocational domains of functioning in persons with severe mental illness: a longitudinal analysis. J Nerv Ment Dis 185:419–426, 1997

Mueser KT, Becker DR, Wolfe R: Supported employment, job preferences, and job tenure and satisfaction. J Ment Health 10:411–417, 2001a

Mueser KT, Salyers MP, Mueser PR: A prospective analysis of work in schizophrenia. Schizophr Bull 27:281–296, 2001b

Mueser KT, Sengupta A, Schooler NR, et al: Family treatment and medication dosage reduction in schizophrenia: effects on patient social functioning, family attitudes, and burden. J Consult Clin Psychol 69:3–12, 2001c

Mueser KT, Clark RE, Haines M, et al: The Hartford study of supported employment for severe mental illness. J Consult Clin Psychol 72:479–490, 2004

Murray CJL, Lopez AD (eds): The Global Burden of Disease and Injury Series, Vol 1: A Comprehensive Assessment of Mortality and Disability From Diseases, Injuries, and Risk Factors in 1990 and Projected to 2020. Cambridge, MA, Harvard School of Public Health on behalf of the World Health Organization and the World Bank, Harvard University Press, 1996

Nimgaonkar VL: Reduced fertility in schizophrenia: here to stay? Acta Psychiatr Scand 98:348–353, 1998

Nisenson LG, Berenbaum H, Good TL: The development of interpersonal relationships in individuals with schizophrenia. Psychiatry 64:111–131, 2001

Oldridge ML, Hughes ICT: Psychological well-being in families with a member suffering from schizophrenia: an investigation into long-standing problems. Br J Psychiatry 161: 249–251, 1992

Patterson TL, Moscona S, McKibbin CL, et al: Social skills performance assessment among older patients with schizophrenia. Schizophr Res 30:351–360, 2001

Penn DL, Corrigan PW, Bentall RP, et al: Social cognition in schizophrenia. Psychol Bull 121:114–132, 1997

Penn DL, Kohlmaier JR, Corrigan PW: Interpersonal factors contributing to the stigma of schizophrenia: social skills, perceived attractiveness, and symptoms. Schizophr Res 45: 37–45, 2000

Pilling S, Bebbington P, Kuipers E, et al: Psychological treatments in schizophrenia, II: meta-analyses of randomized controlled trials of social skills training and cognitive remediation. Psychol Med 32:783–791, 2002

Priebe S, Warner R, Hubschmid T, et al: Employment, attitudes toward work, and quality of life among people with schizophrenia in three countries. Schizophr Bull 24:469–477, 1998

Racenstein JM, Harrow M, Reed R, et al: The relationship between positive symptoms and instrumental work functioning in schizophrenia: a 10-year follow-up study. Schizophr Res 56:95–103, 2002

Rice DP: Economic burden of mental disorders in the United States. Economics of Neuroscience 1:40–44, 1999

Riecher-Rössler A, Häfner H: Gender aspects in schizophrenia: bridging the border between social and biological psychiatry. Acta Psychiatr Scand Suppl 102:58–62, 2000

Robins LN: Deviant Children Grown Up. Huntington, NY, Robert E Krieger Publishing, 1966

Roder V, Brenner HD, Muller D, et al: Development of specific social skills training programmes for schizophrenia patients: results of multicentre study. Acta Psychiatr Scand 105:363–371, 2002

Rogers ES, Walsh D, Masotta L, et al: Massachusetts Survey of Client Preferences for Community Support Services (Final Report). Boston, MA, Center for Psychiatric Rehabilitation, 1991

Rosenheck R: Cost-effectiveness of services for mentally ill homeless people: the application of research to policy and practice. Am J Psychiatry 157:1563–1570, 2000

Rutter ML: Nature-nurture integration: the example of antisocial behavior. Am Psychol 52:390–398, 1997

Salokangas RK, Honkonen T, Stengard E, et al: To be or not to be married—that is the question of quality of life in men with schizophrenia. Soc Psychiatry Psychiatr Epidemiol 36:381–391, 2001

Salyers MP, Mueser KT: Social functioning, psychopathology, and medication side effects in relation to substance use and abuse in schizophrenia. Schizophr Res 48:109–123, 2001

Schooler NR, Keith SJ, Severe JB, et al: Relapse and rehospitalization during maintenance treatment of schizophrenia: the effects of dose reduction and family treatment. Arch Gen Psychiatry 54:453–463, 1997

Sturm R, Gresenz CR, Pacula RL, et al: Datapoints: labor force participation by persons with mental illness. Psychiatr Serv 50:1407, 1999

Tauber R, Wallace CJ, Lecomte T: Enlisting indigenous community supporters in skills training programs for persons with severe mental illness. Psychiatr Serv 51:1428–1432, 2000

Torrey WC, Mueser KT, Drake RE: Self-esteem as an outcome measure in vocational rehabilitation studies of adults with severe mental illness. Psychiatr Serv 51:229–233, 2000

Tsang HW: Applying social skills training in the context of vocational rehabilitation for people with schizophrenia. J Nerv Ment Dis 189:90–98, 2001

Twamley EW, Bartels SJ, Becker D, et al: Individual placement and support for middle-aged and older clients with schizophrenia. Paper presented at the International Association of Psychosocial Services, San Diego, CA, May 2004

U.S. Institute of Medicine: Neurological, Psychiatric, and Developmental Disorders: Meeting the Challenges in the Developing World. Washington, DC, National Academy of Sciences, 2001

Usall J, Haro JM, Ochoa S, et al: Influence of gender on social outcome in schizophrenia. Acta Psychiatr Scand 106:337–342, 2002

Velligan DI, Bow-Thomas CC, Huntzinger C, et al: Randomized controlled trial of the use of compensatory strategies to enhance adaptive functioning in outpatients with schizophrenia. Am J Psychiatry 157:1317–1323, 2000

Wahl O: Consumer Experience of Stigma. Fairfax, VA, George Mason University, Department of Psychology, 1997

Wahl OF: Telling Is Risky Business: Mental Health Consumers Confront Stigma. New Brunswick, NJ, Rutgers University Press, 1999

Wallace CJ, Nelson CJ, Liberman RP, et al: A review and critique of social skills training with schizophrenic patients. Schizophr Bull 6:42–63, 1980

Walsh E, Moran P, Scott C, et al: Prevalence of violent victimisation in severe mental illness. Br J Psychiatry 183:233–238, 2003

Webb C, Pfeiffer M, Mueser KT, et al: Burden and well-being of caregivers for the severely mentally ill: the role of coping style and social support. Schizophr Res 34:169–180, 1998

Wehman P, Moon MS: Vocational Rehabilitation and Supported Employment. Baltimore, MD, Paul Brookes, 1988

World Health Organization: The ICD-10 Classification of Mental and Behavioural Disorders: Clinical Descriptions and Diagnostic Guidelines. Geneva: World Health Organization, 1992

Zigler E, Glick M: A Developmental Approach to Adult Psychopathology. New York, Wiley, 1986

NATURAL HISTORY AND PREDICTORS OF CLINICAL COURSE

Diana O. Perkins, M.D., M.P.H.

Lydia Miller-Andersen, M.D.

Jeffrey A. Lieberman, M.D.

STAGES OF ILLNESS

The natural history of schizophrenia may be conceptualized in stages that include premorbid, prodromal, first-episode, early-course, and chronic phases, with the duration, course, and severity of symptoms in each phase highly variable. The *premorbid phase* includes the period before the emergence of any symptoms. Most individuals, however, have premorbid features that include subtle deficits in cognitive function (IQ, attention, verbal memory, executive function, motor skills) that negatively affect social and school function (Fuller et al. 2002; Niemi et al. 2003; Zammit et al. 2004). On average, the magnitude of these deficits is small, with the distribution overlapping substantially with that of the general population (Fuller et al. 2002). Thus, most individuals who will develop schizophrenia are not clearly distinguishable from their peers premorbidly.

Most individuals (about 75%–80%) experience a gradual emergence of symptoms before the onset of frank psycho-

sis—that is, a *prodrome* (Hafner et al. 1998) (see Chapter 19, "The Prodrome," this volume). Decline in cognitive, social, and vocational function may be one of the first symptoms to emerge as individuals move from the premorbid to the prodromal stage (Ang and Tan 2004; Fuller et al. 2002; Zammit et al. 2004). In a retrospective study of performance on standardized scholastic tests, individuals who later developed schizophrenia performed, on average, slightly lower than the norm in grade school and middle school (about the 45th percentile). By 11th grade, these individuals, on average, had experienced a decline in function, performing significantly below average on tests of reading (40th percentile), language (37th percentile), and sources of information (41st percentile) (Fuller et al. 2002).

Prodromal symptoms include frequent misperceptions: for example, seeing things out the corner of one's eye or hearing vague knocking or whistling noises. Prodromal symptoms also include subdelusional changes in thought content (e.g., becoming very suspicious of others) or ideas of reference. Individuals also complain of worsening problems with distractibility and attentional difficulties. These symptoms may impair ability to function at school, work, or socially, and the functional difficulties are often what brings the person to clinical attention (Addington et al. 2002). Much of the decline in social and occupational function associated with schizophrenia occurs during the prodrome, prior to the onset of frank psychosis (Hafner et al. 1999; Yung and McGorry 1996). Recent efforts have had some success at identifying individuals in the prodromal stage, prior to the onset of the full syndrome (Miller et al. 2003; Yung et al. 2004) (see Chapter 19, "The Prodrome," this volume).

Typically, schizophrenia spectrum disorders, including schizophrenia, schizoaffective disorder, and schizophreniform disorder, begin in adolescence or early adulthood. The average age at onset in women is about 29 years—somewhat older than the average age at onset in men (25 years) (Hafner et al. 1998; Jablensky and Cole 1997). Onset occurs for most individuals (about 75%) between ages 15 and 30 (Heiden and Hafner 2000). Age at onset may vary in specific populations. For example, among individuals who have a first-degree relative with a psychotic disorder, the age at onset may be similar for men and women (Gorwood et al. 1995). In addition, some evidence over the past century indicates later age at onset (Di Maggio et al. 2001; Stompe et al. 2000).

As the symptoms of schizophrenia emerge and the illness progresses, impairments in social and vocational function may occur. The diagnosis of schizophrenia requires hallucinations, delusions, or disorganization, but it is often the other associated impairments in cognitive function and the severity of negative symptoms that most contribute to social and vocational impairments (Green et al. 2000). The clinical progression of schizophrenia occurs during the initial decade of illness, followed by relative clinical stability (Hafner and an der Heiden 1997) or improvement (Harrison et al. 2001).

COURSE OF ILLNESS

Most individuals who develop a schizophrenic psychotic disorder will have a chronic illness. The severity of positive, negative, cognitive, and mood symptoms is highly variable, as is the severity of social and vocational disability. Long-term outcome varies from sustained recovery, to recurrent psychotic episodes with recovery between episodes, to varying severity of chronic, disabling, residual symptoms.

Two main strategies have been used to characterize outcome (Marengo 1994). One considers outcome in var-

ious domains, including symptomatic, social and work function, and activities of daily living. Although many studies have used their own descriptors, most modern studies have used standardized scales, especially the Disability Assessment Scale (DAS) to evaluate social and vocational function and the Global Assessment of Functioning (GAF) Scale or the Global Assessment Scale (GAS) to evaluate both symptoms and function. A second strategy emphasizes course patterns, characterizing onset (insidious or acute), symptom patterns (episodic or chronic), trajectory (stable or deteriorating), and summary evaluation of outcome (recovered or mild/moderate/severe end state) (Figure 16–1).

RECOVERY

Not all individuals who experience a psychotic illness meeting criteria for schizophrenia, schizoaffective disorder, or schizophreniform disorder develop chronic symptoms and functional impairment. Numerous prospective and follow-back outcome studies of individuals with first-episode schizophrenic psychotic disorders have been done. Definitions of *sustained recovery* are varied, but the studies shown in Figure 16–2 required both remission of symptoms and good social and vocational function. Note that definitions of *recovery* by and large do not require return to premorbid level of function, but instead emphasize resuming full participation in work and social life and absence of clinically significant psychopathology. These studies find that between 9% and 38% of the individuals meeting criteria for a schizophrenic psychotic disorder will enjoy a sustained symptomatic and functional recovery after one or more psychotic episodes. The sustained recovery may occur after multiple episodes and includes gradual improvement after a long period of illness (Harrison et al. 2001). Studies also find that 5%–22% of the patients recover from a first episode without subsequent recurrence of symptoms (see Figure 16–2) (Lee et al. 1998; Shepherd et al. 1989; Wiersma et al. 1998). At least one study did not find any patients who only had a single episode followed by recovery, however (Mason et al. 1996).

These studies, despite methodological limitations (Riecher-Rossler and Rossler 1998), paint a consistent picture: that as many as one of every five individuals who develop a schizophrenic psychotic disorder will have a sustained recovery and that a lower proportion completely recover from a first episode without subsequent relapse, even without maintenance antipsychotic medication.

The consistent finding that a substantial minority of individuals will recover from a first episode may be sur-

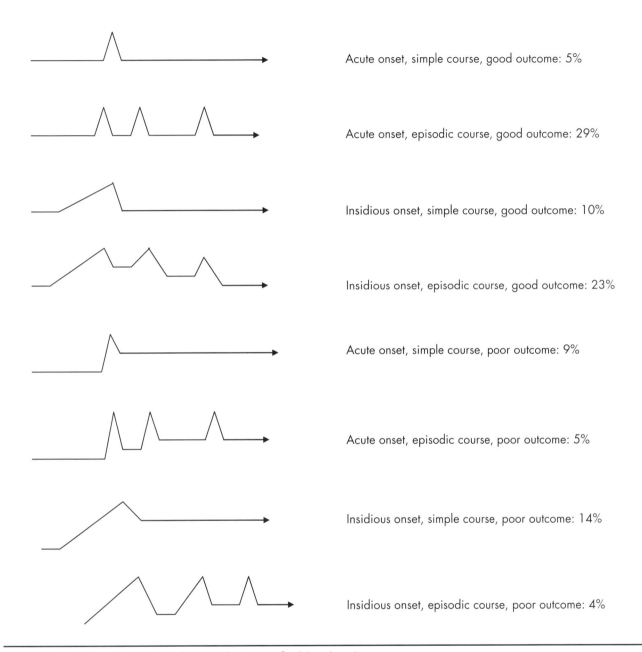

FIGURE 16–1. Long-term (15-year) course of schizophrenia.

Source. Reprinted from Harrison G, Hopper K, Craig T, et al.: "Recovery From Psychotic Illness: A 15- and 25-Year International Follow-up Study." *British Journal of Psychiatry* 178:506–517, 2001. Used with permission.

prising to clinicians who regularly treat schizophrenia. Functional disability and symptom chronicity occur in most patients who require chronic treatment, and recovery is rarely observed. The reason for the discrepancy between the observations of clinicians and the results of these epidemiological studies lies primarily in the fact that the recovered patients often do not seek ongoing treatment and thus are not part of the population of individuals who require chronic treatment.

CHRONIC SYMPTOMS AND DISABILITY

Long-term prospective and follow-back studies find a range of disability and symptom chronicity in individuals meeting criteria for a schizophrenic psychotic disorder. A significant minority—about 1 of every 10 patients—will have persistent, unremitting psychotic symptoms throughout the course of their illness (Thara et al. 1994; Wiersma et al. 1998). As is shown in Figure 16–3, by the chronic

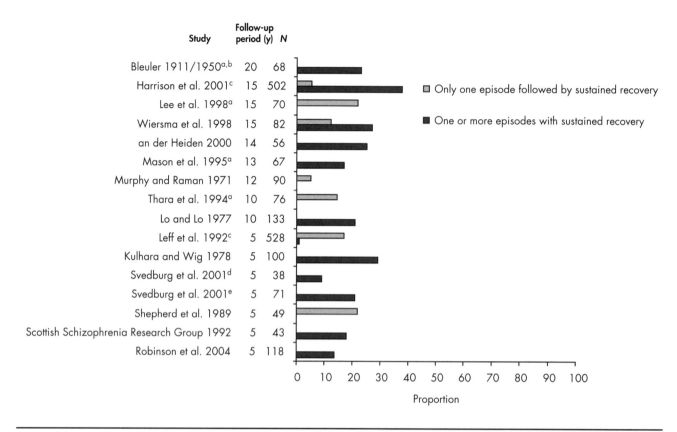

FIGURE 16–2.   Proportion of first-episode patients with sustained functional and symptomatic recovery.

[a]Reports from individual studies included in Harrison et al. 2001.

[b]Preantipsychotic era.

[c]International Pilot Study of Schizophrenia multisite study at 5- and 15-year follow-up; at 5-year follow-up, proportion with full remission and no further episode ranged from 5% to 42%.

[d]Subjects with schizophrenia only.

[e]Subjects with schizophrenia, schizophreniform disorder, or schizoaffective disorder.

stage of illness, a consistent prognostic picture emerges: about one-third of patients will have a relatively good outcome, with no more than mild symptoms and functional impairments; the remaining two-thirds will have moderate to severe symptoms and functional impairments. The same pattern of outcome is found when examining work and social function. For example, in a multicountry, 15-year follow-up study of first-episode patients, social and vocational function, as measured by the DAS, was good to excellent for 33%, fair for 23%, and poor for 44% (Harrison et al. 2001). When outcome is characterized in terms of disease course, about a third of patients also experience good outcomes with no or mild residual symptoms (Bleuler 1979; Harrison et al. 2001; Heiden and Hafner 2000).

DEATH

The most devastating outcome—premature death—occurs in a substantial minority of affected individuals. Long-term mortality is much higher for an individual

with schizophrenia than in the general population; as much as five times higher than the age-matched general population risk for men; and two times higher for women, with suicide accounting for about half of the excess mortality (Brown 1997; Brown et al. 2000; Mortensen and Juel 1993). About 1 of 10 individuals diagnosed with schizophrenia will die by suicide, with the highest risk occurring during the recovery period after initial diagnosis (Kua et al. 2003; Lee et al. 1998; Wiersma et al. 1998). Because the greatest risk of suicide appears to be during the recovery from a first episode, specialized treatment during this time may reduce death by suicide.

In addition, individuals with schizophrenia are at increased risk for death from cardiovascular disease, diabetes, lung disease, and accidents (Brown et al. 2000). The risk for these diseases may be in part genetically based; however, much of the risk may be related to lifestyle, social, and environmental factors and thus is potentially preventable.

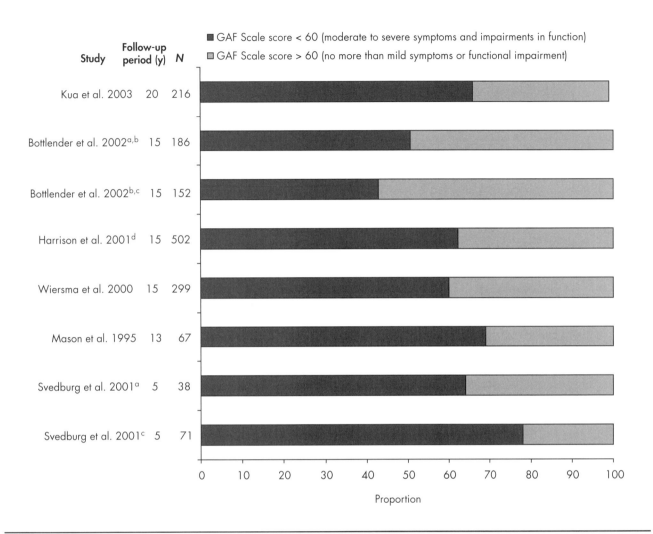

FIGURE 16–3.   Global outcomes as measured by Global Assessment of Functioning (GAF) Scale at follow-up.
[a]Subjects with schizophrenia only.
[b]GAF Scale score>61.
[c]Subjects with schizophrenia, schizophreniform disorder, or schizoaffective disorder.
[d]GAF Scale disability rating score>60 and Bleuler rating of "recovered."

TRENDS IN OUTCOME OVER TIME AND PLACE

The likelihood of a good symptomatic and functional outcome has varied over time and across place. The most likely explanation is that genetic and environmental factors that influence prognosis vary in a given population at a given time and thus affect disease outcome in that population. For example, some evidence suggests that outcome may have improved with the introduction of antipsychotics. In a meta-analysis of outcome studies conducted from 1895 to 1991, the proportion of individuals with schizophrenia who were "considered improved" after an average of 5.6 years (range=1–40 years) of follow-up differed between patients diagnosed in the first half of the century (35.4%) and those diagnosed in the second half

(48.5%) (Hegarty et al. 1994). The proportion "considered improved" declined over the decade from 1980 to 1990, to 36.4%, however. Because the meta-analysis was not limited to studies of individuals identified at a first episode, some of the results, especially the more recent reports, were likely to have excluded good-prognosis patients (e.g., single-episode recovered patients). Other methodological problems with the meta-analysis also limit conclusions that may be drawn (Dean 1995; Oken and McGeer 1995; Papezova and Czobor 1995; Warner 1995).

Nonetheless, when incidence studies are examined, a difference in outcome emerges between the first half of the century, during which, on average, 14% (range=0%–29%) experienced a good outcome, and the second half of

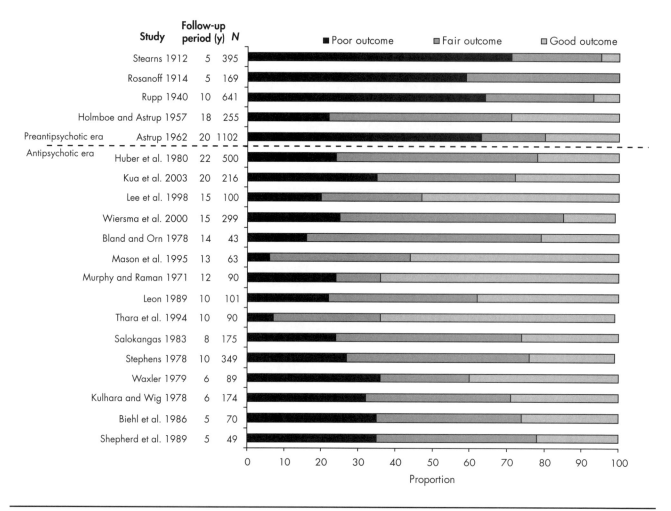

FIGURE 16–4.   Global outcome: before and after the introduction of antipsychotics.

the century, during which, on average, 29% (range=14%–64%) experienced a good outcome (Figure 16–4).

In addition, better outcome is consistently found in developing compared with developed countries. At 2-year follow-up of the well-designed and well-conducted World Health Organization International Pilot Study of Schizophrenia, about 63% of the individuals from developing country sites met criteria for remission compared with 37% of the subjects from developed country sites (Jablensky et al. 1992), and these difference persisted at 5-year follow-up (Leff et al. 1992). In addition, social function was rated as impaired at some point during follow-up for only 16% of the individuals from developing country sites compared with 42% of the individuals from developed country sites. These findings led to the idea that social-, cultural-, or biologically based differences between developing and developed countries may significantly affect the severity of schizophrenia (Jablensky 2000).

FACTORS ASSOCIATED WITH PROGNOSIS

The cause of the extreme heterogeneity in long-term outcome—from complete recovery to incapacitating symptoms and disability—is not known but is of obvious interest. Prognosis is very likely related in part to the extent and severity of the underlying disease pathology. Because of genetic and early environmental events that significantly affect brain development, some individuals may have a poor-prognosis disease that does not respond to available treatments. Disease course also may be related to environmental factors, including the extent that treatment is optimal, the support and demands of the patient's community, and the availability of resources to support recovery. Some individuals may have a neuroprogressive component to their disease that potentially could be prevented by optimal treatment and support (Lieberman et al. 2001).

To better predict prognosis and also to develop treatment strategies that could improve outcome, numerous studies have examined the relation between clinical, demographic, and treatment variables and outcome. Emerging results from molecular genetic studies are also beginning to shed light on biological factors that contribute to disease etiology and disease severity.

CLINICAL FEATURES

Clinical features associated with a poor prognosis include poor premorbid social and school function, insidious onset, earlier age at onset, prominent negative symptoms, more severe cognitive impairments, and male sex (Isohanni et al. 2004; Niemi et al. 2003). These features are intercorrelated, suggesting that together they characterize a poor-prognosis illness (Bottlender et al. 2002; Rund et al. 2004; Tiryaki et al. 2003). Some features, such as severe cognitive impairments and negative symptoms, may cause others, such as poor premorbid social and school function. As discussed earlier, individuals who develop schizophrenia have evidence of intellectual impairment in childhood, and these impairments may underlie the premorbid deficits in social and school function (Aylward et al. 1984; M. Cannon et al. 2002a; T.D. Cannon et al. 2000a; Ott et al. 1998; Zammit et al. 2004). Available studies suggest that lower IQ, poor school performance, and greater impairments in social function are associated with more severe illness course and greater functional deficits (Haas and Sweeney 1992; Munro et al. 2002; Roff 2001). Gradually emerging symptoms are also associated with poor prognosis (Harrison et al. 1996), and abrupt onset precipitated by stressful events is associated with a good prognosis (van Os et al. 1994). Progressive cognitive deficits during the premorbid stage and gradually emerging symptoms during the prodromal stage may contribute to functional decline and are in fact the earliest manifestations of a progressive component of the illness.

Recent evidence points to a high correlation between cognitive deficits and level of functional recovery (Verdoux et al. 2002). Cognitive deficits are not static through the course of illness but may improve, be stable, or decline over time. Declining neurocognitive function in particular may be a poor prognostic sign (Stirling et al. 2003).

The course and prognosis of schizophrenia differ for men and women. On average, women have a milder form of illness, with less severe psychopathology, better work and social function, greater likelihood of recovery, and less frequent and shorter hospitalizations (Lee et al. 1998; Leung and Chue 2000; Thara et al. 1994; Usall et al. 2002). Compared with men, women who develop schizophrenia are less likely to have poor prognostic clinical features, such as early age at onset, poor premorbid function, and obstetrical complications (Larsen et al. 1996). Speculations as to why women may have a more benign illness than men include the potential of estrogen to be neuroprotective and to have antipsychotic effects, the increased vulnerability to obstetrical complications in men, and the later age at onset in women allows development of social and vocational skills that are relatively preserved once the illness develops (Cyr et al. 2002; Hafner 2003; Leung and Chue 2000; Salem and Kring 1998).

DIAGNOSIS

Individuals meeting "narrow" criteria for schizophrenia, including the requirement of long duration of illness (e.g., greater than 6 months) and lack of prominent mood symptoms, consistently have a worse prognosis than do individuals with shorter duration of psychosis prior to treatment contact (e.g., schizophreniform, brief psychotic disorder) or those with prominent mood symptoms (e.g., schizoaffective disorder). For example, in one study, 9% of the persons meeting criteria for schizophrenia recovered compared with 21% meeting criteria for schizophrenia spectrum disorders (schizophrenia, schizophreniform disorder, and schizoaffective disorder) (Svedberg et al. 2001) (see Figure 16–2). The differences in prognosis related to diagnosis may be in part mediated by the other prognostic features, such as mode of onset and duration of illness, that are part of the diagnostic criteria.

ENVIRONMENTAL PROGNOSTIC FACTORS

Several environmental factors may affect brain development and thus influence risk of disease and ultimate disease severity (see Chapter 4, "Prenatal and Perinatal Factors"). Perinatal obstetric complications, especially maternal infectious disease, severe maternal malnutrition, maternal diabetes, and complications associated with fetal hypoxia, are environmental risk factors for schizophrenia (Alvir et al. 1999; M. Cannon et al. 2002b; Koponen et al. 2004; Kunugi et al. 2001). In addition, children who have a central nervous system viral infection may have a fivefold increase in risk for developing schizophrenia (Koponen et al. 2004). Obstetrical complications are associated with other poor prognostic features, such as poor premorbid function, male sex, and severe cognitive impairments (T.D. Cannon et al. 2002; Kotlicka-Antczak et al. 2001; Rosso et al. 2000). Perinatal complications may affect brain development at a critical period and, in a genetically vulnerable individual, increase risk, with more severe insults having more significant effect and thus resulting in a more severe illness (T.D. Cannon et al. 2000b).

Substance use disorders are about twice as common in individuals with schizophrenia as in those in the general population; about 40%–60% of patients meet criteria for a substance use disorder diagnosis (Cantor-Graae et al. 2001). Some evidence indicates that substance use may be associated with some good prognostic features, including better premorbid adjustment and less marked structural brain abnormalities, but on the whole, substance use is associated with greater psychopathology and a more severe illness course. Active use of alcohol or other drugs has been associated with more severe positive psychotic symptoms, more depressive symptoms, greater risk of suicide, and more frequent hospitalizations (Buhler et al. 2002; Farris et al. 2003; Margolese et al. 2004; Pencer and Addington 2003; Potkin et al. 2003). Substance use may influence prognosis, at least in part, by increasing the likelihood of treatment nonadherence (Coldham et al. 2002; Hunt et al. 2002). In addition, substance use disorders in themselves are associated with increased risk of suicide and functional impairments and so may be additive to the symptomatic and functional consequences of the psychotic disorder. Importantly, drugs of abuse have brain toxicity that may worsen the severity of the psychotic disorder (Farber and Olney 2003; McCann and Ricaurte 2004; Olney et al. 2002; Voruganti et al. 2001).

Evidence shows that cannabis use in particular may increase vulnerability to and severity of schizophrenia. Cannabis use is associated with an estimated twofold increase in risk for developing schizophrenia (Arseneault et al. 2004) and has been found to be associated with poor prognostic features, including early age at onset (Bersani et al. 2002; Veen et al. 2004). Cannabis use is associated with acute exacerbation of psychosis and may be associated with more frequent hospitalizations, poorer psychosocial functioning, and more severe psychopathology (Caspari 1999; van Os et al. 2002). Cannabis most likely increases risk of psychosis and worsens disease course directly, perhaps through effects on brain dopamine or other neurotransmitter systems (Voruganti et al. 2001), although (as is true with substance use generally) it is uncertain whether the association of cannabis use and outcome is causal or is mediated by other associated factors (Arseneault et al. 2004).

As discussed earlier, there is a consistent finding of substantially better prognosis for individuals with schizophrenic psychotic disorders in developing countries than in developed countries, perhaps because of some social or cultural factors that may improve prognosis (Jablensky 2000; Leff et al. 1992). Greater social support and less severe life stressors are proposed explanations. The availability of family support is associated with better long-term clinical and functional outcomes in first-episode patients (Salokangas 1997). Stressful life events may be associated with increased relapse risk in individuals with schizophrenia (Pallanti et al. 1997; Ventura et al. 1989), with effect of stress on dopamine and glutamate systems in the brain a theorized mechanism (Moghaddam 2002).

EFFECT OF TREATMENT ON PROGNOSIS

Although antipsychotic drugs are an effective treatment of psychosis, debate continues over whether the introduction of antipsychotics has affected the course and ultimate prognosis of schizophrenic psychotic disorders. The evidence that addresses this issue includes comparisons of outcomes before and after the availability of antipsychotics, clinical studies that examined the effect of maintenance antipsychotic treatment on outcome, and studies that examined the relation of duration of psychosis before first treatment initiation to outcome. This body of research provides indirect support for the notion that antipsychotic medications may positively influence prognosis.

Figure 16–4 shows the long-term outcome of first-episode (first treatment contact) patients from prospective or follow-back studies conducted prior to the introduction of antipsychotics and in the postantipsychotic era. Only studies of a first-episode cohort in which at least 75% of the subjects could be followed up are included. The included studies used different strategies and assessment measures, but all attempted to classify patients as having 1) "good" outcome, defined as minimal or no symptoms *and* reasonably productive social and vocational function; 2) "poor" outcome, defined as significant residual symptoms *and* poor social and vocational function; or 3) "fair" outcome, defined as intermediate between these two extremes.

The studies shown in Figure 16–4 point to a general improvement in long-term outcome since the introduction of antipsychotics. Before the availability of antipsychotics, the long-term prognosis of patients was poor for about half of all patients, whereas a quarter to a third of the patients in cohorts studied after the introduction of antipsychotics had poor outcome. The very early studies may not be comparable to studies done later for many reasons, including advancements in clinical assessment methodology, differences in diagnostic systems, and cultural and other health care system differences. These differences may well have biased the earlier studies toward cohorts of more severely ill patients, so this comparison is not conclusive. Supporting the observation of improved prognosis since the introduction of antipsychotics is an analysis of outcomes from a cohort of patients that bridged the introduction of antipsychotics. This study found that patients who received antipsychotics for their first psychotic episode 1) were more likely to have a complete remission than were those who had their first episode before antipsychotics were available (27.9% vs. 14.6%) and 2) generally had less severe psychopathology at long-term follow-up (mean=22 years) (Huber et al. 1980).

Epidemiological outcome studies generally do not report the relation of sustained recovery from a first psychotic episode and maintenance antipsychotic treatment (Harrison et al. 2001; Lee et al. 1998; Shepherd et al. 1989; Wiersma et al. 1998). Studies do report that antipsychotic use is associated with reduced likelihood of relapse after recovery from a first episode (Crow et al. 1986; Kane et al. 1982; Robinson et al. 1999). Recurrent episodes early in the course of illness are associated with increased likelihood of developing chronic residual positive and negative symptoms, suggesting that relapse may be related to risk of chronicity (Rabiner et al. 1986; Wiersma et al. 1998). In the 15-year follow-up of nine diverse sites from the World Health Organization International Pilot Study of Schizophrenia, the strongest predictor of long-term outcome was the amount of time the patient was psychotic in the first 2 years after illness onset (Harrison et al. 2001). Together, these findings support the notion that relapse prevention through maintenance antipsychotic use may improve long-term outcomes.

There is good evidence that the shorter the duration of the first episode of psychosis prior to initiating antipsychotics, the greater the level of symptomatic and functional recovery (Perkins et al. 2005). The relation of duration of initial untreated psychosis and outcome is independent of premorbid function or mode of onset. Thus, antipsychotic medication may affect a progressive pathological process.

As discussed earlier, available treatments, including antipsychotics, may positively affect prognosis. In addition to a general effect of antipsychotics on outcome, some medication treatments may offer greater clinical benefits. Clozapine clearly improves the outcome of a substantial proportion of very ill patients (Chakos et al. 2001) and also may reduce risk of suicide (Meltzer et al. 2003). A consensus is emerging that second-generation antipsychotics may offer greater benefits than the first-generation antipsychotics by reducing relapse risk (Csernansky et al. 2002; Dolder et al. 2003; Leucht et al. 2003), improving neurocognitive function (Keefe et al. 2004), and perhaps leading to greater reduction in psychopathology severity (Davis et al. 2003).

Finally, convincing evidence now suggests that specific psychotherapies, including family psychoeducation, other cognitive therapies directed at reducing severity of psychotic experiences, and therapies directed at improving antipsychotic treatment adherence, may improve symptomatic and functional outcome (Pilling et al. 2002).

GENETIC PROGNOSTIC FACTORS

The heterogeneity in outcome is theorized to be related to both environmental and genetic factors. Although the genetic basis of schizophrenia is not known, several genes have been associated with the disorder (see Chapter 3, "Genetics," in this volume). Some of these associated genes may in fact influence disease severity. For example, a polymorphism of the gene that codes for an enzyme involved in the metabolism of dopamine, catechol-O-methyltransferase, is associated with more severe symptoms in some (Herken and Erdal 2001; Inada et al. 2003; Strous et al. 2003) but not all (Tsai et al. 2004) studies. Similarly, a genetic alteration in the gene that codes for the N-methyl-D-aspartate receptor 2A subunit, involved in glutamate neurotransmission, has been associated with more severe symptoms (Itokawa et al. 2003). These associations are clearly speculative, but the hope is that future research will lead to an understanding of the genetic basis of schizophrenia, including genetic factors that affect prognosis.

CONCLUSION

The course of schizophrenia is highly heterogeneous, with outcomes ranging from complete recovery to chronic incapacity. Numerous factors are associated with outcome, and several treatment interventions may increase the likelihood of sustained recovery. First, antipsychotic treatment and other interventions should occur as close to psychosis onset as is possible. Second, long-term maintenance treatment is also associated with sustained recovery. Not every patient will require maintenance antipsychotic treatment to remain in recovery, but it is not currently possible to discern reliably those individuals who will have a benign course from those who will have a more severe course. Prevention of recurrent episodes is likely to be critical to preventing disease progression (Lieberman 1999). Finally, individual, group, and family interventions may enhance functional recovery, reduce the risk of suicide, and also reduce the severity of residual symptoms. Identification and treatment of comorbid substance use disorders also may reduce the risk of relapse and chronicity.

Although even more speculative, optimal prenatal care that includes appropriate vitamin supplementation and minimization of pre- and perinatal complications, including maternal infectious disease, gestational diabetes, and obstetrical complications, may influence disease risk as well as disease severity.

These strategies are not proven to ultimately affect disease course but are still clearly indicated in the optimal treatment of schizophrenia; however, such strategies may not be available because of limited resources and concerns over treatment costs. Treatment strategies that affect prognosis will likely prove to be cost-effective, given the tremendous economic and social burden posed by disabling symptoms.

REFERENCES

Addington J, van Mastrigt S, Hutchinson J, et al: Pathways to care: help seeking behaviour in first episode psychosis. Acta Psychiatr Scand 106:358–364, 2002

Alvir JM, Woerner MG, Gunduz H, et al: Obstetric complications predict treatment response in first-episode schizophrenia. Psychol Med 29:621–627, 1999

Ang YG, Tan HY: Academic deterioration prior to first episode schizophrenia in young Singaporean males. Psychiatry Res 121:303–307, 2004

Arseneault L, Cannon M, Witton J, et al: Causal association between cannabis and psychosis: examination of the evidence. Br J Psychiatry 184:110–117, 2004

Astrup C: Prognosis in Functional Psychoses: Clinical, Social, and Genetic Aspects. Springfield, IL, Charles C Thomas, 1962

Aylward E, Walker E, Bettes B: Intelligence in schizophrenia: meta-analysis of the research. Schizophr Bull 10:430–459, 1984

Bersani G, Orlandi V, Kotzalidis GD, et al: Cannabis and schizophrenia: impact on onset, course, psychopathology and outcomes. Eur Arch Psychiatry Clin Neurosci 252:86–92, 2002

Biehl H, Maurer K, Schubart C, et al: Prediction of outcome and utilization of medical services in a prospective study of first onset schizophrenics: results of a prospective 5-year follow-up study. Eur Arch Psychiatry Neurol Sci 236:139–147, 1986

Bland RC, Orn H: 14-Year outcome in early schizophrenia. Acta Psychiatr Scand 58:327–338, 1978

Bleuler M: On schizophrenic psychoses. Am J Psychiatry 136:1403–1409, 1979

Bottlender R, Sato T, Jager M, et al: The impact of duration of untreated psychosis and premorbid functioning on outcome of first inpatient treatment in schizophrenic and schizoaffective patients. Eur Arch Psychiatry Clin Neurosci 252:226–231, 2002

Brown S: Excess mortality of schizophrenia: a meta-analysis. Br J Psychiatry 171:502–508, 1997

Brown S, Inskip H, Barraclough B: Causes of the excess mortality of schizophrenia. Br J Psychiatry 177:212–217, 2000

Buhler B, Hambrecht M, Loffler W, et al: Precipitation and determination of the onset and course of schizophrenia by substance abuse—a retrospective and prospective study of 232 population-based first illness episodes. Schizophr Res 54:243–251, 2002

Cannon M, Caspi A, Moffitt TE, et al: Evidence for early childhood, pan-developmental impairment specific to schizophreniform disorder: results from a longitudinal birth cohort. Arch Gen Psychiatry 59:449–456, 2002a

Cannon M, Jones PB, Murray RM: Obstetric complications and schizophrenia: historical and meta-analytic review. Am J Psychiatry 159:1080–1092, 2002b

Cannon TD, Bearden CE, Hollister JM, et al: Childhood cognitive functioning in schizophrenia patients and their unaffected siblings: a prospective cohort study. Schizophr Bull 26:379–393, 2000a

Cannon TD, Rosso IM, Hollister JM, et al: A prospective cohort study of genetic and perinatal influences in the etiology of schizophrenia. Schizophr Bull 26:351–366, 2000b

Cannon TD, van Erp TG, Rosso IM, et al: Fetal hypoxia and structural brain abnormalities in schizophrenic patients, their siblings, and controls. Arch Gen Psychiatry 59:35–41, 2002

Cantor-Graae E, Nordstrom LG, McNeil TF: Substance abuse in schizophrenia: a review of the literature and a study of correlates in Sweden. Schizophr Res 48:69–82, 2001

Caspari D: Cannabis and schizophrenia: results of a follow-up study. Eur Arch Psychiatry Clin Neurosci 249:45–49, 1999

Chakos M, Lieberman J, Hoffman E, et al: Effectiveness of second-generation antipsychotics in patients with treatment-resistant schizophrenia: a review and meta-analysis of randomized trials. Am J Psychiatry 158:518–526, 2001

Coldham EL, Addington J, Addington D: Medication adherence of individuals with a first episode of psychosis. Acta Psychiatr Scand 106:286–290, 2002

Crow TJ, MacMillan JF, Johnson AL, et al: A randomised controlled trial of prophylactic neuroleptic treatment. Br J Psychiatry 148:120–127, 1986

Csernansky JG, Mahmoud R, Brenner R: A comparison of risperidone and haloperidol for the prevention of relapse in patients with schizophrenia. N Engl J Med 346:16–22, 2002

Cyr M, Calon F, Morissette M, et al: Estrogenic modulation of brain activity: implications for schizophrenia and Parkinson's disease. J Psychiatry Neurosci 27:12–27, 2002

Davis JM, Chen N, Glick ID: A meta-analysis of the efficacy of second-generation antipsychotics. Arch Gen Psychiatry 60:553–564, 2003

Dean CE: Schizophrenia: a 100-year retrospective. Am J Psychiatry 152:1694–1695, 1995

Di Maggio C, Martinez M, Menard JF, et al: Evidence of a cohort effect for age at onset of schizophrenia. Am J Psychiatry 158:489–492, 2001

Dolder CR, Lacro JP, Leckband S, et al: Interventions to improve antipsychotic medication adherence: review of recent literature. J Clin Psychopharmacol 23:389–399, 2003

Farber NB, Olney JW: Drugs of abuse that cause developing neurons to commit suicide. Brain Res Dev Brain Res 147:37–45, 2003

Farris C, Brems C, Johnson ME, et al: A comparison of schizophrenic patients with or without coexisting substance use disorder. Psychiatr Q 74:205–222, 2003

Fuller R, Nopoulos P, Arndt S, et al: Longitudinal assessment of premorbid cognitive functioning in patients with schizophrenia through examination of standardized scholastic test performance. Am J Psychiatry 159:1183–1189, 2002

Gorwood P, Leboyer M, Jay M, et al: Gender and age at onset in schizophrenia: impact of family history. Am J Psychiatry 152:208–212, 1995

Green MF, Kern RS, Braff DL, et al: Neurocognitive deficits and functional outcome in schizophrenia: are we measuring the "right stuff"? Schizophr Bull 26:119–136, 2000

Haas GL, Sweeney JA: Premorbid and onset features of first-episode schizophrenia. Schizophr Bull 18:373–386, 1992

Hafner H: Gender differences in schizophrenia. Psychoneuroendocrinology 28 (suppl 2):17–54, 2003

Hafner H, an der Heiden W: Epidemiology of schizophrenia. Can J Psychiatry 42:139–151, 1997

Hafner H, an der Heiden W, Behrens S, et al: Causes and consequences of the gender difference in age at onset of schizophrenia. Schizophr Bull 24:99–113, 1998

Hafner H, Loffler W, Maurer K, et al: Depression, negative symptoms, social stagnation and social decline in the early course of schizophrenia. Acta Psychiatr Scand 100:105–118, 1999

Harrison G, Croudace T, Mason P, et al: Predicting the long-term outcome of schizophrenia. Psychol Med 26:697–705, 1996

Harrison G, Hopper K, Craig T, et al: Recovery from psychotic illness: a 15- and 25-year international follow-up study. Br J Psychiatry 178:506–517, 2001

Hegarty JD, Baldessarini RJ, Tohen M, et al: One hundred years of schizophrenia: a meta-analysis of the outcome literature. Am J Psychiatry 151:1409–1416, 1994

an der Heiden W, Hafner H: The epidemiology of onset and course of schizophrenia. Eur Arch Psychiatry Clin Neurosci 250:292–303, 2000

Herken H, Erdal ME: Catechol-O-methyltransferase gene polymorphism in schizophrenia: evidence for association between symptomatology and prognosis. Psychiatr Genet 11 (2):105–109, 2001

Holmboe R, Astrup C: A follow-up study of 255 patients with acute schizophrenia and schizophreniform psychoses. Acta Psychiatr Neurol Scand 32:9–61, 1957

Huber G, Gross G, Schuttler R, et al: Longitudinal studies of schizophrenic patients. Schizophr Bull 6:592–605, 1980

Hunt GE, Bergen J, Bashir M: Medication compliance and comorbid substance abuse in schizophrenia: impact on community survival 4 years after a relapse. Schizophr Res 54:253–264, 2002

Inada T, Nakamura A, Iijima Y: Relationship between catechol-O-methyltransferase polymorphism and treatment-resistant schizophrenia. Am J Med Genet B Neuropsychiatr Genet 120(1):35–39, 2003

Isohanni M, Isohanni I, Koponen H, et al: Developmental precursors of psychosis. Curr Psychiatry Rep 6:168–175, 2004

Itokawa M, Yamada K, Yoshitsugu K, et al: A microsatellite repeat in the promoter of the N-methyl-D-aspartate receptor 2A subunit (GRIN2A) gene suppresses transcriptional activity and correlates with chronic outcome in schizophrenia. Pharmacogenetics 13:271–278, 2003

Jablensky A: Epidemiology of schizophrenia: the global burden of disease and disability. Eur Arch Psychiatry Clin Neurosci 250:274–285, 2000

Jablensky A, Cole SW: Is the earlier age at onset of schizophrenia in males a confounded finding? Results from a cross-cultural investigation. Br J Psychiatry 170:234–240, 1997

Jablensky A, Sartorius N, Ernberg G, et al: Schizophrenia: manifestations, incidence and course in different cultures: a World Health Organization ten-country study [published erratum appears in Psychol Med Monogr Suppl 22(4):following 1092, 1992]. Psychol Med Monogr Suppl 20:1–97, 1992

Kane JM, Rifkin A, Quitkin F, et al: Fluphenazine vs placebo in patients with remitted, acute first-episode schizophrenia. Arch Gen Psychiatry 39:70–73, 1982

Keefe RS, Seidman LJ, Christensen BK, et al: Comparative effect of atypical and conventional antipsychotic drugs on neurocognition in first-episode psychosis: a randomized, double-blind trial of olanzapine versus low doses of haloperidol. Am J Psychiatry 161:985–995, 2004

Koponen H, Rantakallio P, Veijola J, et al: Childhood central nervous system infections and risk for schizophrenia. Eur Arch Psychiatry Clin Neurosci 254:9–13, 2004

Kotlicka-Antczak M, Gmitrowicz A, Sobow TM, et al: Obstetric complications and Apgar score in early onset schizophrenic patients with prominent positive and prominent negative symptoms. J Psychiatr Res 35:249–257, 2001

Kua J, Wong KE, Kua EH, et al: A 20-year follow-up study on schizophrenia in Singapore. Acta Psychiatr Scand 108:118–125, 2003

Kulhara P, Wig NN: The chronicity of schizophrenia in North West India: results of a follow-up study. Br J Psychiatry 132:186–190, 1978

Kunugi H, Nanko S, Murray RM: Obstetric complications and schizophrenia: prenatal underdevelopment and subsequent neurodevelopmental impairment. Br J Psychiatry Suppl 40:S25–S29, 2001

Larsen TK, McGlashan TH, Johannessen JO, et al: First-episode schizophrenia, II: premorbid patterns by gender. Schizophr Bull 22:257–269, 1996

Lee PW, Lieh-Mak F, Wong MC, et al: The 15-year outcome of Chinese patients with schizophrenia in Hong Kong. Can J Psychiatry 43:706–713, 1998

Leff J, Sartorius N, Jablensky A, et al: The International Pilot Study of Schizophrenia: five-year follow-up findings. Psychol Med 22:131–145, 1992

Leon CA: Clinical course and outcome of schizophrenia in Cali, Colombia: a 10-year follow-up study. J Nerv Ment Dis 177:593–606, 1989

Leucht S, Barnes TR, Kissling W, et al: Relapse prevention in schizophrenia with new-generation antipsychotics: a systematic review and exploratory meta-analysis of randomized, controlled trials. Am J Psychiatry 160:1209–1222, 2003

Leung A, Chue P: Sex differences in schizophrenia, a review of the literature. Acta Psychiatr Scand Suppl 401:3–38, 2000

Lieberman JA: Is schizophrenia a neurodegenerative disorder? A clinical and neurobiological perspective. Biol Psychiatry 46:729–739, 1999

Lieberman JA, Perkins D, Belger A, et al: The early stages of schizophrenia: speculations on pathogenesis, pathophysiology, and therapeutic approaches. Biol Psychiatry 50:884–897, 2001

Lo WH, Lo T: A ten-year follow-up study of Chinese schizophrenics in Hong Kong. Br J Psychiatry 131:63–66, 1977

Marengo J: Classifying the courses of schizophrenia. Schizophr Bull 20:519–536, 1994

Margolese HC, Malchy L, Negrete JC, et al: Drug and alcohol use among patients with schizophrenia and related psychoses: levels and consequences. Schizophr Res 67:157–166, 2004

Mason P, Harrison G, Glazebrook C, et al: Characteristics of outcome in schizophrenia at 13 years. Br J Psychiatry 167(5):596–603, 1995

Mason P, Harrison G, Glazebrook C, et al: The course of schizophrenia over 13 years: a report from the International Study on Schizophrenia (ISoS) coordinated by the World Health Organization. Br J Psychiatry 169:580–586, 1996

McCann UD, Ricaurte GA: Amphetamine neurotoxicity: accomplishments and remaining challenges. Neurosci Biobehav Rev 27:821–826, 2004

Meltzer HY, Alphs L, Green AI, et al: Clozapine treatment for suicidality in schizophrenia: International Suicide Prevention Trial (InterSePT). Arch Gen Psychiatry 60:82–91, 2003

Miller TJ, McGlashan TH, Rosen JL, et al: Prodromal assessment with the structured interview for prodromal syndromes and the scale of prodromal symptoms: predictive validity, interrater reliability, and training to reliability. Schizophr Bull 29:703–715, 2003

Moghaddam B: Stress activation of glutamate neurotransmission in the prefrontal cortex: implications for dopamine-associated psychiatric disorders. Biol Psychiatry 51:775–787, 2002

Mortensen PB, Juel K: Mortality and causes of death in first admitted schizophrenic patients. Br J Psychiatry 163:183–189, 1993

Munro JC, Russell AJ, Murray RM, et al: IQ in childhood psychiatric attendees predicts outcome of later schizophrenia at 21 year follow-up. Acta Psychiatr Scand 106:139–142, 2002

Murphy HB, Raman AC: The chronicity of schizophrenia in indigenous tropical peoples: results of a twelve-year follow-up survey in Mauritius. Br J Psychiatry 118:489–497, 1971

Niemi LT, Suvisaari JM, Tuulio-Henriksson A, et al: Childhood developmental abnormalities in schizophrenia: evidence from high-risk studies. Schizophr Res 60:239–258, 2003

Oken RJ, McGeer PL: Schizophrenia: a 100-year retrospective. Am J Psychiatry 152:1692–1693, 1995

Olney JW, Wozniak DF, Jevtovic-Todorovic V, et al: Drug-induced apoptotic neurodegeneration in the developing brain. Brain Pathol 12:488–498, 2002

Ott SL, Spinelli S, Rock D, et al: The New York High-Risk Project: social and general intelligence in children at risk for schizophrenia. Schizophr Res 31:1–11, 1998

Pallanti S, Quercioli L, Pazzagli A: Relapse in young paranoid schizophrenic patients: a prospective study of stressful life events, P300 measures, and coping. Am J Psychiatry 154:792–798, 1997

Papezova H, Czobor P: Schizophrenia: a 100-year retrospective. Am J Psychiatry 152:1693–1694, 1995

Pencer A, Addington J: Substance use and cognition in early psychosis. J Psychiatry Neurosci 28:48–54, 2003

Pilling S, Bebbington P, Kuipers E, et al: Psychological treatments in schizophrenia, I: meta-analysis of family intervention and cognitive behaviour therapy. Psychol Med 32:763–782, 2002

Potkin SG, Alphs L, Hsu C, et al: Predicting suicidal risk in schizophrenic and schizoaffective patients in a prospective two-year trial. Biol Psychiatry 54:444–452, 2003

Rabiner CJ, Wegner JT, Kane JM: Outcome study of first-episode psychosis, I: relapse rates after 1 year. Am J Psychiatry 143:1155–1158, 1986

Riecher-Rossler A, Rossler W: The course of schizophrenic psychoses: what do we really know? A selective review from an epidemiological perspective. Eur Arch Psychiatry Clin Neurosci 248(4):189–202, 1998

Robinson D, Woerner MG, Alvir JM, et al: Predictors of relapse following response from a first episode of schizophrenia or schizoaffective disorder. Arch Gen Psychiatry 56:241–247, 1999

Robinson DG, Woerner MG, McMeniman M, et al: Symptomatic and functional recovery from a first episode of schizophrenia or schizoaffective disorder. Am J Psychiatry 161:473–479, 2004

Roff JD: Comparison of childhood problem behaviors in boys with subsequent schizophrenic, antisocial, and good adult outcomes. Psychol Rep 89:633–640, 2001

Rosanoff AJ: A statistical study of prognosis in insanity. J Am Med Assoc 62:3–6, 1914

Rosso IM, Cannon TD, Huttunen T, et al: Obstetric risk factors for early onset schizophrenia in a Finnish birth cohort. Am J Psychiatry 157:801–807, 2000

Rund BR, Melle I, Friis S, et al: Neurocognitive dysfunction in first-episode psychosis: correlates with symptoms, premorbid adjustment, and duration of untreated psychosis. Am J Psychiatry 161:466–472, 2004

Rupp CFEK: A five to ten year follow-up study of 641 schizophrenic cases. Am J Psychiatry 96:877–888, 1940

Salem JE, Kring AM: The role of gender differences in the re-duction of etiologic heterogeneity in schizophrenia. Clin Psychol Rev 18:795–819, 1998

Salokangas RK: Prognostic implications of the sex of schizo-phrenic patients. Br J Psychiatry 142:145–151, 1983

Salokangas RK: Living situation, social network and outcome in schizophrenia: a five-year prospective follow-up study. Acta Psychiatr Scand 96:459–468, 1997

Shepherd M, Watt D, Falloon I, et al: The natural history of schizophrenia: a five-year follow-up study of outcome and prediction in a representative sample of schizophrenics. Psychol Med Monogr Suppl 15:1–46, 1989

Stearns AW: The prognosis in dementia praecox. Boston Medi-cal and Surgical Journal 167:158–160, 1912

Stephens JH: Long-term prognosis and followup in schizophre-nia. Schizophr Bull 4:25–47, 1978

Stirling J, White C, Lewis S, et al: Neurocognitive function and outcome in first-episode schizophrenia: a 10-year follow-up of an epidemiological cohort. Schizophr Res 65:75–86, 2003

Stompe T, Ortwein-Swoboda G, Strobl R, et al: The age of on-set of schizophrenia and the theory of anticipation. Psychi-atry Res 93:125–134, 2000

Strous RD, Nolan KA, Lapidus R, et al: Aggressive behavior in schizophrenia is associated with the low enzyme activity COMT polymorphism: a replication study. Am J Med Genet 120B:29–34, 2003

Svedberg B, Mesterton A, Cullberg J: First-episode non-affective psychosis in a total urban population: a 5-year follow-up. Soc Psychiatry Psychiatr Epidemiol 36:332–337, 2001

Thara R, Henrietta M, Joseph A, et al: Ten-year course of schizophrenia—the Madras longitudinal study. Acta Psy-chiatr Scand 90:329–336, 1994

The Scottish First Episode Schizophrenia Study, VIII: five-year follow-up: clinical and psychosocial findings. The Scottish Schizophrenia Research Group. Br J Psychiatry 161:496–500, 1992

Tiryaki A, Yazici MK, Anil AE, et al: Reexamination of the char-acteristics of the deficit schizophrenia patients. Eur Arch Psychiatry Clin Neurosci 253:221–227, 2003

Tsai SJ, Hong CJ, Liao DL, et al: Association study of a functional catechol-O-methyltransferase genetic polymorphism with age of onset, cognitive function, symptomatology and prognosis in chronic schizophrenia. Neuropsychobiology 49:196–200, 2004

Usall J, Haro JM, Ochoa S, et al: Influence of gender on social outcome in schizophrenia. Acta Psychiatr Scand 106:337–342, 2002

van Os J, Fahy TA, Bebbington P, et al: The influence of life events on the subsequent course of psychotic illness: a pro-spective follow-up of the Camberwell Collaborative Psy-chosis Study. Psychol Med 24:503–513, 1994

van Os J, Bak M, Hanssen M, et al: Cannabis use and psycho-sis: a longitudinal population-based study. Am J Epidemiol 156:319–327, 2002

Veen ND, Selten JP, van der Tweel I, et al: Cannabis use and age at onset of schizophrenia. Am J Psychiatry 161:501–506, 2004

Ventura J, Nuechterlein KH, Lukoff D, et al: A prospective study of stressful life events and schizophrenic relapse. J Abnorm Psychol 98:407–411, 1989

Verdoux H, Liraud F, Assens F, et al: Social and clinical conse-quences of cognitive deficits in early psychosis: a two-year follow-up study of first-admitted patients. Schizophr Res 56:149–159, 2002

Voruganti LN, Slomka P, Zabel P, et al: Cannabis induced dopamine release: an in-vivo SPECT study. Psychiatry Res 107:173–177, 2001

Warner R: Schizophrenia: a 100-year retrospective. Am J Psy-chiatry 152:1693–1695, 1995

Waxler NE: Is outcome for schizophrenia better in nonindustri-al societies? The case of Sri Lanka. J Nerv Ment Dis 167:144–158, 1979

Wiersma D, Nienhuis FJ, Slooff CJ, et al: Natural course of schizophrenic disorders: a 15-year followup of a Dutch in-cidence cohort. Schizophr Bull 24:75–85, 1998

Yung AR, McGorry PD: The prodromal phase of first-episode psychosis: past and current conceptualizations. Schizophr Bull 22:353–370, 1996

Yung AR, Phillips LJ, Yuen HP, et al: Risk factors for psychosis in an ultra high-risk group: psychopathology and clinical features. Schizophr Res 67:131–142, 2004

Zammit S, Allebeck P, David AS, et al: A longitudinal study of premorbid IQ score and risk of developing schizophre-nia, bipolar disorder, severe depression, and other nonaf-fective psychoses. Arch Gen Psychiatry 61:354–360, 2004

CHAPTER 17

PHARMACOTHERAPIES

T. Scott Stroup, M.D., M.P.H.

John E. Kraus, M.D., Ph.D.

Stephen R. Marder, M.D.

Pharmacological treatments are an essential component of a comprehensive approach to the treatment of schizophrenia. Rational pharmacotherapies can contribute greatly to symptom relief and to a broader psychosocial recovery for affected individuals. However, antipsychotic drugs do not cure schizophrenia. Moreover, if not used judiciously, drug therapies can create significant financial, side-effect, and medical morbidity burdens that may hinder progress toward personal and treatment goals. Importantly, evidence-based plans of care should be individualized and should integrate both appropriate pharmacotherapies and psychosocial interventions (Lehman et al. 2004a).

In this chapter, we discuss drugs commonly used in the treatment of schizophrenia. The goal of pharmacological treatment of schizophrenia is to minimize symptoms and functional impairments to allow individuals to pursue personal goals as best as possible. Antipsychotic drugs are commonly used to treat positive symptoms, such as hallucinations, delusions, and disorganized speech and behavior, and negative symptoms, including anhedonia, avolition, alogia, affective flattening, and social withdrawal. Antipsychotic drugs are also to treat behavioral disturbances such as aggression and hostility and to reduce anxiety and suicidal behaviors. Anxiolytics, antidepressants,

and mood-stabilizing drugs are often used as adjunctive treatments for mood symptoms. Because cognitive impairments are common in schizophrenia and are related to functional outcomes, cognitive functioning is now an important focus of research and a possible target of pharmacotherapies; however, there are neither U.S. Food and Drug Administration (FDA)–approved nor commonly used drugs available for this purpose in schizophrenia.

In the following sections, we describe common features of all antipsychotic drugs, then features of first- and second-generation drugs, and finally specific information about distinguishing features of the drugs. Contentious views of the drugs' features are driven by fierce market competition among pharmaceutical companies for a global market for antipsychotic drugs valued at $12.2 billion in 2003 (IMS Health Inc. 2004). Common side effects of antipsychotic drugs are discussed in more detail in a later section of this chapter (see subsection "Common Side Effects").

ANTIPSYCHOTIC DRUGS

Modern drug treatment for schizophrenia dates to the early 1950s, when Deniker and Delay reported the antipsychotic effects of chlorpromazine (Healy 2002). Chlorpromazine was introduced in the United States in 1954, followed over the next three decades by several drugs, including fluphenazine, haloperidol, perphenazine, and thioridazine, with similar therapeutic effects. All of these so-called first-generation antipsychotics block postsynaptic dopamine receptors in the brain, with the dopamine blockade in frontal cortical and limbic regions thought to account for the antipsychotic effect. The first-generation antipsychotics also interact with other neurotransmitter systems that are thought primarily to cause side effects rather than the desired antipsychotic effect.

Antipsychotic medicines ameliorate psychotic symptoms such as hallucinations, delusions, and disorganized speech or behavior. The drugs reduce the intensity of the symptoms, shorten exacerbations of illness, and reduce the risk of relapse. An early landmark study led by the U.S. National Institute of Mental Health (NIMH) found that approximately 60% of the subjects who received first-generation antipsychotic drugs, as compared with 20% of placebo-treated subjects, had a nearly complete resolution of acute positive symptoms during a 6-week trial (Guttmacher 1964). Only 8% of the medication-treated subjects showed no improvement or worsening, whereas almost half of the placebo-treated subjects did not improve or worsened. Positive and negative symptoms improved with antipsychotic treatment, but positive symptoms responded to a greater degree and more consistently than did negative symptoms. Subsequent research showed that patients with schizophrenia who achieve remission and then consistently take antipsychotic drugs are about three times less likely to relapse than patients who do not take the medicines consistently (Hogarty et al. 1976).

The introduction of a second generation of antipsychotic drugs began with clozapine in 1990. Clozapine was approved by the FDA after it was shown to have greater efficacy than chlorpromazine in patients with refractory symptoms. In the critical study of clozapine in treatment-resistant patients, 30% of the clozapine-treated patients met positive symptom response criteria compared with only 4% of the chlorpromazine-treated patients (Kane et al. 1988a). However, clozapine's significant risk of agranulocytosis and other life-threatening side effects greatly limited its use.

Clozapine's unique pharmacological profile, with prominent effects on neurotransmitter receptors other than dopamine and a different side-effect profile from that of the chlorpromazine-like drugs, led to the development and introduction of a second generation of drugs with pharmacological similarities to clozapine. These drugs, including risperidone, olanzapine, quetiapine, ziprasidone, and aripiprazole, attempted to mimic clozapine's superior

effectiveness without its risk of agranulocytosis. Like the first generation of drugs, second-generation antipsychotics also affect postsynaptic dopamine receptors, but other pharmacological actions are thought to influence significantly their therapeutic effects as well as their side effects. There is no consensus definition of second-generation or atypical antipsychotic drugs, but antagonism of central serotoninergic receptors and perhaps relatively loose binding to dopamine$_2$ (D$_2$) receptors are thought to be key features in their actions. A purported distinguishing feature of second-generation antipsychotics is that they produce fewer extrapyramidal side effects (EPS) (e.g., akathisia, parkinsonian symptoms, dystonia) than the first-generation or typical drugs at recommended antipsychotic doses.

FIRST-GENERATION OR TYPICAL ANTIPSYCHOTICS

First-generation antipsychotic drugs share the same presumed mechanism of action (blockade of dopamine receptors) and do not appear to differ in efficacy. Their side effects tend to vary according to drug potency. High-potency drugs have a stronger affinity for dopamine receptors than low-potency drugs; lower dosages of the high-potency drugs achieve the same antipsychotic effect as higher dosages of low-potency drugs (Table 17–1). The drugs' different effects on dopamine receptors and on other neurotransmitter systems determine their pharmacological actions and side effects. High-potency drugs (e.g., haloperidol and fluphenazine) have a high risk of EPS, moderate risk of sedation, and low risk of anticholinergic (e.g., dry mouth, constipation, blurred vision) and antiadrenergic (e.g., orthostatic hypotension) effects. Low-potency drugs (e.g., chlorpromazine and thioridazine) have a lower risk of EPS, high risk of sedation, and high risk of anticholinergic and antiadrenergic side effects. Medium-potency drugs (e.g., loxapine, molindone, perphenazine, and thiothixine) tend to have a moderate risk of these common side effects. Side-effect profiles of commonly used antipsychotic medications are summarized in Table 17–2.

Chlorpromazine, a low-potency first-generation antipsychotic, has been available since 1954. It is effective in treating schizophrenic psychopathology but is associated with substantial weight gain, sedation, orthostatic hypotension, anticholinergic side effects, and modest EPS when used at currently recommended doses. Perphenazine, a mid-potency first-generation antipsychotic, has been available since 1958. It is effective in treating schizophrenic psychopathology but is associated with moderate hypotension and EPS when used at currently recommended doses. Haloperidol, a high-potency first-generation antipsychotic, has been available since 1967. Widely used,

TABLE 17–1. Oral antipsychotic medications in common use

Antipsychotic medication	Recommended dosage range (mg/day)[a]	Chlorpromazine equivalents (mg/day)[b]	Half-life (hours)[c]	Potency[d]
First-generation agents				
Chlorpromazine	300–1,000	100	6	L
Mesoridazine	150–400	50	36	L
Thioridazine	300–800	100	24	L
Loxapine	30–100	10	4	M
Molindone	30–100	10	24	M
Thiothixene	15–50	5	34	M
Perphenazine	16–64	10	10	M
Trifluoperazine	15–50	5	24	M
Fluphenazine	5–20	2	33	H
Haloperidol	5–20	2	21	H
Second-generation agents				
Clozapine	150–600		12	
Risperidone	2–8		24	
Olanzapine	10–30		33	
Quetiapine	300–750		6	
Ziprasidone	120–160		7	
Aripiprazole	10–30		75	

Note. L=low potency; M=medium potency; H=high potency.

[a]Dose range recommendations are adapted from the 2003 Schizophrenia Patient Outcomes Research Team recommendations (Lehman et al. 2004a). In persons experiencing a first episode of psychosis, lower doses may be adequate. The upper dose recommendations for quetiapine and ziprasidone may not incorporate these drugs' full therapeutic range.

[b]Chlorpromazine equivalents represent the approximate dose equivalent to 100 mg of chlorpromazine (relative potency). Chlorpromazine equivalents are used only with first-generation antipsychotics.

[c]The half-life of a drug is the amount of time required for the plasma drug concentration to decrease by one-half. The half-life of a drug does not include the half-life of its active metabolites.

[d]Relative potency classifications are used only with first-generation antipsychotics.

Source. Adapted from Lehman et al. 2004b.

haloperidol is effective in reducing schizophrenic psychopathology and in reducing acutely agitated behaviors. It is associated with severe EPS but with little sedation, orthostatic hypotension, and weight gain and few anticholinergic side effects. Haloperidol's short-acting injections are commonly used in emergency situations when rapid effects are needed, whereas a long-acting haloperidol formulation is used when patients have trouble regularly taking oral antipsychotic medications.

SECOND-GENERATION OR ATYPICAL ANTIPSYCHOTICS

Second-generation antipsychotics available in the United States as of 2004, listed in order of their approval by the

FDA, are clozapine, risperidone, olanzapine, quetiapine, ziprasidone, and aripiprazole. Summary information about each of the second-generation antipsychotics follows. As would be expected, drugs that have been available for clinical use for a longer time have been the subject of more research studies and have better-known patterns of side effects, both short- and long-term.

Clozapine

Clozapine was approved for use in the United States in 1990, despite a significant risk of the potentially lethal side effect agranulocytosis, because of its unique efficacy in patients with symptoms that were resistant to treatment. The key study in its approval by the FDA, conducted by

TABLE 17–2. Selected side effects of commonly used antipsychotic medications

Medication	EPS	Prolactin elevation	Weight gain	Glucose abnormalities	Lipid abnormalities	QTc prolongation	Sedation	Hypotension	Anticholinergic side effects
Chlorpromazine	+	+?	+++	+?	+?	+?	+++	+++	+++
Perphenazine	++	+	+?	+?	+?	0	+	+	0
Haloperidol	+++	++	+	0	0	0	++	0	0
Clozapine[a]	0[b]	0	+++	+++	+++	0	+++	+++	+++
Risperidone[c]	+	+++	++	++	++	+	+	+	0
Olanzapine	+	0	+++	+++	+++	0	+++	+	+
Quetiapine[c,d]	+	0	++	++	++	0	+++	++	++
Ziprasidone[e]	+	+	0	0	0	+	0	0	0
Aripiprazole[e,f]	+	0	0	0	0	0	+	0	0

Note. EPS=extrapyramidal side effects (includes akathisia, dystonias, and implied risk of tardive dyskinesia; TD=tardive dyskinesia; 0=no risk or rarely causes side effects at therapeutic dose; +=mild or occasionally causes side effects at therapeutic dose; ++=sometimes causes side effects at therapeutic dose; +++=frequently causes side effects at therapeutic dose; ?=data too limited to rate with confidence.

[a]Clozapine also causes agranulocytosis, seizures, and myocarditis.

[b]Possible exception of akathisia.

[c]Discrepant results for risperidone and quetiapine regarding glucose and lipid abnormalities.

[d]Quetiapine also carries warning about potential development of cataracts.

[e]Because ziprasidone and aripiprazole are relatively new drugs, there are limited long-term data on side effects.

[f]Aripiprazole also causes nausea and headache.

Source.   Adapted from Lehman et al. 2004b and American Diabetes Association, American Psychiatric Association, American Association of Clinical Endocrinologists, et al. 2004.

Kane and colleagues (1988b), entered 268 patients with treatment-resistant schizophrenia into a trial comparing clozapine and chlorpromazine. Treatment resistance was defined as having failed to respond to at least three prior antipsychotics, with no period of good functioning in the past 5 years, then having no response to haloperidol in a 6-week lead-in trial. After 6 weeks of double-blind treatment, 30% of the clozapine-treated group but only 4% of the chlorpromazine-treated group met a priori response criteria. Response was defined as a reduction greater than 20% from baseline in the Brief Psychiatric Rating Scale (BPRS) total score plus either a posttreatment Clinical Global Impression (CGI) score of 3 (mild) or less or a posttreatment BPRS total score of 35 or lower (also representing a mild level of psychiatric symptoms).

A later meta-analysis of randomized, double-blind trials comparing clozapine with a typical antipsychotic drug in patients with treatment-refractory schizophrenia showed an advantage for clozapine with regard to total psychopathology, categorical response to treatment (the number of patients who met a cutoff point for response), extrapyramidal symptoms, tardive dyskinesia (TD), and study completion rates (Chakos et al. 2001). Clozapine-treated patients were 2.5 times more likely to respond than were those receiving first-generation drugs (Chakos et al. 2001). Furthermore, clozapine has been found effective in reducing suicidal behaviors in patients with schizophrenia or schizoaffective disorder at high risk for suicide (Meltzer et al. 2003) and in reducing hostility and aggression among patients with treatment-resistant symptoms (Chengappa et al. 2002; Citrome et al. 2001).

Unfortunately, 0.5%–1% of patients develop clozapine-induced agranulocytosis (Alvir et al. 1993), and this risk has limited clozapine's use. In addition to agranulocytosis, seizures occur in up to 2% of patients, and a small but increased risk of myocarditis or cardiomyopathy is seen. Common side effects of clozapine include sedation, hypotension, and tachycardia (Table 17–2). Furthermore, clozapine is associated with substantial weight gain and a higher risk of glucose and lipid abnormalities compared with most other antipsychotic drugs (American Diabetes Association et al. 2004). Nevertheless, because of its efficacy in reducing refractory positive symptoms, with virtually no acute EPS or TD, clozapine represents a unique and important treatment option for severely ill patients for whom adequate medical supervision is available. Furthermore, the success of clozapine provided the impetus for the development of other antipsychotic drugs and hope for better outcomes.

Risperidone

Risperidone was approved for use in the United States in 1994. Existing evidence suggests that risperidone is at least equal in efficacy to first-generation antipsychotics in the treatment of schizophrenic symptoms, with a lower incidence rate of EPS at recommended dosages (2–8 mg/day). A meta-analysis of 12 short-term and 2 long-term trials of risperidone compared with a first-generation antipsychotic in the treatment of schizophrenia found no advantage for risperidone in reducing positive or negative symptoms but found that risperidone caused fewer EPS (Kennedy et al. 2000). In a trial that compared relapse rates of stable outpatients randomly assigned to risperidone or haloperidol over a period of more than a year, patients taking risperidone were significantly less likely to relapse than were patients taking haloperidol (34% vs. 60% in a Kaplan-Meier analysis) (Csernansky et al. 2002). Risperidone may also have advantages over haloperidol in improving neurocognitive functioning (Bilder et al. 2002). In comparison to other second-generation antipsychotics in the treatment of global schizophrenic psychopathology, risperidone is similarly effective (Conley and Mahmoud 2001; Mullen et al. 2001; Tran et al. 1997b).

Common side effects of risperidone are summarized in Table 17–2. At typical dosages (2–8 mg/day), risperidone has a low risk of EPS, but this risk increases at higher doses. Risperidone frequently causes serum prolactin elevation and sometimes causes weight gain, glucose abnormalities, and lipid abnormalities. Risperidone occasionally causes orthostatic hypotension. A long-acting, injectable microsphere formulation of risperidone for injection became available in 2003 to help enhance treatment adherence.

Olanzapine

The FDA approved olanzapine in 1996 for the treatment of schizophrenia. In acute treatment studies, olanzapine is effective in reducing positive and negative symptoms. Olanzapine is at least as effective as first-generation antipsychotics and other second-generation antipsychotics other than clozapine in reducing global psychopathology, positive symptoms, and negative symptoms and in improving neurocognitive functioning. In some but not all studies, olanzapine had advantages over other treatments (Conley and Mahmoud 2001; Tollefson et al. 1997, 2001; Tran et al. 1997a, 1997b).

Common side effects of olanzapine are summarized in Table 17–2. Olanzapine frequently causes sedation and weight gain at therapeutic doses and is thought to cause more glucose and lipid abnormalities than do first-generation antipsychotics and other second-generation antipsychotics except clozapine (American Diabetes Association et al. 2004). Olanzapine does not increase prolactin levels. Compared with first-generation antipsychotics, olanzapine is less likely to cause EPS.

Quetiapine

Quetiapine was approved for the treatment of schizophrenia in the United States in 1998. Two meta-analyses have shown quetiapine to have efficacy similar to that of haloperidol in treating symptoms of schizophrenia (Davis et al. 2003; Leucht et al. 1999). Because of a half-life of only 6 hours, doses of quetiapine should be given two or three times daily, although a small study suggested that once-daily dosing may be feasible (Chengappa et al. 2003). At recommended dosages, quetiapine causes no elevation in prolactin levels and little or no EPS (Table 17–2). It often causes sedation and sometimes causes hypotension, weight gain, and lipid and glucose abnormalities. Because of its sedative properties, quetiapine is sometimes selected for patients with prominent insomnia.

Ziprasidone

The FDA approved ziprasidone in 2001 for the treatment of schizophrenia. With a half-life of 7 hours, it is recommended as a twice-daily drug. Administration with food enhances absorption. Ziprasidone causes little or no weight gain, a feature that distinguishes it from most other antipsychotics. Unlike other first- and second-generation antipsychotics, it very rarely causes sedation. Ziprasidone rarely causes EPS (except possibly akathisia). It is rarely associated with glucose or lipid abnormalities but sometimes causes prolactin elevations (Table 17–2).

Approval of ziprasidone was delayed by the FDA in 1998 because of clinical trial data that showed that it delayed cardiac repolarization, as measured by the QTc interval on electrocardiograms (ECGs). Because QTc prolongation is associated with torsades de pointes, a potentially fatal ventricular arrhythmia, additional safety data were required. Ziprasidone was approved when it was shown that 4,000 patients had been treated in clinical trials with ziprasidone without evidence of torsades de pointes or sudden death. The FDA issued a warning about QTc prolongation and instructed prescribers to avoid coadministration with other QTc-prolonging drugs and to avoid prescribing ziprasidone to other patients with histories of or at significant risk for cardiac arrhythmias. The FDA did not, however, require pretreatment ECGs. Clinical use over several years now indicates that ziprasidone can be safely used with current labeling related to QTc prolongation and that metabolic inhibitors of ziprasidone do not further increase QTc (Harrigan et al. 2004).

Aripiprazole

Aripiprazole was approved by the FDA for treatment of schizophrenia in 2002. Unlike all other approved antipsychotics, aripiprazole has partial agonist activity at dopamine D_2 receptors. This has the theoretical advantage of agonist activity when dopamine levels are relatively low and antagonist activity when dopamine levels are high (Lieberman 2004).

Of the common antipsychotic side effects (Table 17–2), aripiprazole is associated with only occasional or mild sedation. It is very rarely associated with weight gain, glucose or lipid abnormalities, or hypotension. Aripiprazole sometimes causes an akathisia-like syndrome, but it rarely causes other forms of EPS. Headache, insomnia, and nausea early in treatment are relatively more common for aripiprazole than for other antipsychotics.

COMMON SIDE EFFECTS: MONITORING AND MANAGEMENT RECOMMENDATIONS

Extrapyramidal Side Effects

Antipsychotic-induced EPS may occur acutely or after long-term treatment. First-generation antipsychotics, in particular high-potency neuroleptics, are more likely than second-generation antipsychotics to cause EPS when the drugs are used at usual therapeutic doses. However, as can be noted in Table 17–2, considerable variation in the incidence of EPS is seen among both the first-generation antipsychotics and the second-generation antipsychotics. Common acute EPS include akathisia, parkinsonism, and dystonia. Importantly, each of these side effects often responds to medication treatment (Table 17–3). Each type of acute EPS has a characteristic time of onset. Akathisia typically occurs a few hours to days after medication administration, dystonia within the first few days, and parkinsonism within a few days to weeks after starting a new drug or after a dosage increase (Casey 1993).

Akathisia. *Akathisia*, a subjective feeling of restlessness accompanied by restless movements, usually in the legs or feet, is the most common form of EPS. Severe akathisia can be diagnosed when frequent pacing, restless foot movements, or an inability of patients to sit still is present. This condition must be differentiated from psychotic agitation, which is often a response to disturbing hallucinations or delusions, but also may represent hostility related to acute psychosis or increased motor activity associated with excited catatonia. Patients who experience milder akathisia may not have any evidence of increased motor activity but may experience an unpleasant sensation of restlessness subjectively similar to anxiety. Patients should

TABLE 17–3. Selected medications for treating extrapyramidal side effects

Generic name	Dosage (mg/day)	Elimination half-life (hours)	Targeted EPS
Benztropine mesylate[a]	0.5–6.0	24	Akathisia, dystonia, parkinsonism
Trihexyphenidyl hydrochloride	1–15	4	Akathisia, dystonia, parkinsonism
Amantadine	100–300	10–14	Akathisia, parkinsonism
Propranolol	30–90	3–4	Akathisia
Lorazepam[a]	1–6	12	Akathisia
Clonazepam	1–3	20–50	Akathisia
Diphenhydramine[a]	25–50	4–8	Akathisia, dystonia, parkinsonism

[a]Available in oral and parenteral forms.
Source. Adapted from Lehman et al. 2004b.

be closely monitored for akathisia when starting a new antipsychotic drug or when the dosage is increased. Severe, unrelenting akathisia has been associated with an increased risk of suicidal behaviors. If symptoms of schizophrenia are adequately treated, lowering the antipsychotic dose is a feasible first approach to reduce akathisia. Another common approach is to change to an antipsychotic less likely to cause akathisia (e.g., a second-generation antipsychotic). Drug treatments for akathisia include β-blockers, anticholinergic agents, or benzodiazepines (Table 17–3). Evidence from controlled trials is inadequate to compare the efficacy of the various treatments for akathisia.

Drug-induced parkinsonism (pseudoparkinsonism). *Drug-induced parkinsonism* (pseudoparkinsonism) may include the classic Parkinson's disease symptoms of tremor, muscular rigidity, and a decrease in spontaneous movements (bradykinesia), as well as cognitive slowing and apathy. Milder forms of parkinsonism may include decreased expressive gestures, decreased facial expressiveness, or diminished arm swing. Recognition and management of parkinsonism are important because it is frequently associated with poor adherence to antipsychotic medication regimens (Perkins 2002; Robinson et al. 2002). The initial approach to parkinsonian side effects is to lower the dose of antipsychotic if feasible. Common drug treatments for parkinsonism include anticholinergic medications, as seen in Table 17–3. Another common approach is to change to an antipsychotic less likely to cause parkinsonism (e.g., a second-generation antipsychotic).

Dystonias. *Dystonias* are intermittent or sustained muscular spasms and abnormal postures affecting mainly the musculature of the head and neck but sometimes the trunk

and lower extremities. Common forms of dystonia include abnormal positioning of the neck (torticollis), impaired swallowing (dysphagia), hypertonic or enlarged tongue, and deviations of the eyes (oculogyric crisis). These reactions usually appear within the first few days of treatment with antipsychotic drugs and sometimes occur within minutes to hours. These reactions can be painful and dramatic. They occur most commonly with high-potency first-generation antipsychotics, particularly when they are given in substantial doses (e.g., haloperidol 5–10 mg) to drug-naïve patients. For this reason, prophylactic treatment with benztropine 1–2 mg is recommended if starting high-potency first-generation antipsychotics at these substantial doses, which may be required in emergency situations. Acute dystonic reactions are treated with diphenhydramine 25–50 mg or benztropine 1–2 mg. Usually, these treatments are given intramuscularly to provide rapid relief for the considerable discomfort of dystonias.

Neuroleptic malignant syndrome. *Neuroleptic malignant syndrome* (NMS), another neurological side effect, is characterized by rigidity, hyperthermia, mental status changes, and autonomic instability. NMS has a lifetime incidence of approximately 0.2% among antipsychotic users (Caroff 2003). Hyperthermia and severe muscle rigidity may lead to rhabdomyolysis and renal failure. Serum levels of creatine kinase may rise dramatically. Risk factors for NMS include rapid dose escalation of high-potency first-generation antipsychotics, parenteral administration, and underlying neurological impairment. NMS is probably less common with second- than with first-generation drugs, but the incidence with first-generation antipsychotics may be decreasing because lower doses than in the past are now commonly used.

NMS may be fatal if untreated. Treatment includes discontinuation of the antipsychotic and supportive care. Temperature reduction by cooling blankets if necessary and correction of fluid imbalances are crucial. The dopamine agonist bromocriptine (2.5 mg every 8 hours) has been shown to reduce NMS duration and mortality. The muscle relaxant dantrolene (1–2.5 mg/kg intravenously every 6 hours) is also commonly used, although there is no strong evidence of its effectiveness. Electroconvulsive therapy is indicated if catatonia related to NMS persists or response is otherwise inadequate with drugs and supportive care. If NMS occurs, need for an antipsychotic medication should be carefully assessed before antipsychotic treatment is resumed. When another trial of an antipsychotic drug is attempted, second-generation antipsychotics (in particular, clozapine) are preferred. A rechallenge should begin with low doses and slow titration.

Tardive dyskinesia and other tardive syndromes.
Tardive dyskinesia and other tardive (late-onset) syndromes are involuntary, repetitive, purposeless, hyperkinetic, abnormal movements of the mouth, face and tongue, trunk, and extremities that occur during or following the cessation of long-term antipsychotic drug therapy. According to DSM-IV-TR (American Psychiatric Association 2000) diagnostic criteria, the abnormal movements should be present for at least 4 weeks, and patients should have been exposed to an antipsychotic for at least 3 months. The onset of the abnormal movements should occur either while the patient is receiving an antipsychotic or within 4 weeks of discontinuing an oral or 8 weeks after the withdrawal of a long-acting injectable antipsychotic. Oral-facial movements occur in about three-fourths of TD patients and can include lip smacking, sucking, puckering, and grimacing. Other movements include irregular movements of the limbs, particularly choreoathetoid-like movements of the fingers and toes and slow, writhing movements of the trunk. When severe, TD is disfiguring. In addition to TD, tardive dystonias and tardive akathisia have been described.

Tardive dyskinesia occurs at the rate of 4%–5% per year in the adult, nongeriatric population taking a first-generation antipsychotic (Glazer et al. 1993; Kane et al. 1985; Morgenstern and Glazer 1993). The risk may be five to six times higher in the elderly, with some data suggesting that as many as 29% of elderly patients will develop TD each year (Jeste et al. 1999). A systematic review of 1-year studies involving second-generation antipsychotics found a lower risk of TD in patients taking second-generation antipsychotics (annual risk=2.1%) than in patients taking the high-potency first-generation antipsychotic haloperidol (annual risk=5.2%) (Correll et al. 2004). This review did

not include clozapine, but clozapine-induced TD is thought to be extremely rare. Nor did the review include low- or medium-potency antipsychotics, which cause fewer acute EPS than haloperidol and may thus have a lower risk of TD. Risk factors for TD include increased age, female gender, higher dosages of antipsychotics, and longer periods of treatment.

Treatment of TD has largely been unsuccessful, but some data from controlled trials (Adler et al. 1993) suggest that the antioxidant vitamin E may be useful in less chronic cases. Second-generation antipsychotics (in particular, clozapine) have been used to treat TD, but there have been no methodologically rigorous trials to support this practice. The recommended clinical approach is to use the lowest possible dose of antipsychotic that is effective and to consider changing to a medication with lower risk of TD (i.e., a second-generation antipsychotic) if TD is an important concern.

Monitoring for EPS. Guidelines from the Mount Sinai Conference on Medical Monitoring (Marder et al. 2004) recommend an assessment of EPS prior to starting an antipsychotic and at weekly intervals until the dose has been stabilized for at least 2 weeks. Although the second-generation antipsychotics are associated with a reduced risk of EPS, it is not uncommon for patients receiving these drugs—with the possible exception of clozapine—to experience mild akathisia or rigidity.

The examination for EPS includes observing patients for restlessness movements and inquiring if the patient feels restless. Asking patients if they are having difficulty sitting still can be helpful. Parkinsonism is evaluated by observing the patient's gait and examining for rigidity in the elbow and wrist. Dystonias usually present as urgent events reported by patients.

Regular monitoring for TD should be a component of management strategies with antipsychotics. The Mount Sinai guidelines (Marder et al. 2004) recommend examining patients for TD before starting an antipsychotic and at 6-month intervals for first-generation antipsychotics and yearly for second-generation antipsychotics. Patients who are at high risk, including the elderly and those who are sensitive to EPS, should be examined every 6 months. The Abnormal Involuntary Movement Scale (AIMS; 1988) provides instructions for examining patients as well as means for recording the results of the examination.

Metabolic Effects

In 2004, a joint panel of the American Diabetes Association, American Psychiatric Association, American Association of Clinical Endocrinologists, and the North Amer-

TABLE 17–4. Suggested monitoring protocol for patients taking second-generation antipsychotics

	Baseline	4 weeks	8 weeks	12 weeks	Quarterly	Annually	Every 5 years
Personal or family history	X					X	
Weight (body mass index)	X	X	X	X	X		
Waist circumference	X			X		X	
Blood pressure	X			X		X	
Fasting plasma glucose	X			X		X	
Fasting lipid profile	X			X			X

Note. More frequent assessments may be warranted based on clinical status.
Source. American Diabetes Association, American Psychiatric Association, American Association of Clinical Endocrinologists, et al. 2004.

ican Association for the Study of Obesity (2004) issued a consensus statement asking physicians to screen carefully and monitor patients who take antipsychotic drugs for signs of rapid weight gain or other problems that could lead to diabetes, obesity, and heart disease. Table 17–4 shows the panel's recommendation for baseline and follow-up monitoring of factors relevant to these issues. Similarly, at the Mount Sinai Conference on Medical Monitoring, a group of mental health clinicians and researchers and medical experts who convened to review data on the metabolic effects of antipsychotics developed detailed consensus recommendations for approaching metabolic side effects, which are described in the following subsections (Marder et al. 2004).

Weight gain. Individuals with schizophrenia are more likely than the population at large to be overweight or obese (Allison et al. 1999a). Antipsychotics vary in their association with weight gain. A meta-analysis by Allison et al. (1999b) estimated the amount of weight gain associated with moderate doses of several antipsychotics over 10 weeks. Among the drugs studied, the mean increases were 0.04 kg with ziprasidone, 0.39 kg with molindone, 0.43 kg with fluphenazine, 1.13 kg with haloperidol, 2.10 kg with risperidone, 2.58 kg with chlorpromazine, 3.19 kg with thioridazine, 4.15 kg with olanzapine, and 4.45 kg with clozapine. These differences in weight gain liabilities have been confirmed by other studies (Wirshing et al. 1999). Quetiapine was not included in the study above but is associated with modest weight gain (American Diabetes Association et al. 2004). Aripiprazole, also not included in the study above and for which there are few long-term data, is associated with little or no weight gain (American Diabetes Association et al. 2004).

The Mount Sinai consensus recommendation is that mental health providers should monitor and chart the body mass index (BMI: weight in kg/height in m^2) of every

patient with schizophrenia, regardless of the antipsychotic medication prescribed (Marder et al. 2004). Individuals with a BMI greater than 25 are at increased risk for diabetes, heart disease, certain cancers, and other weight-associated disorders. Patients should be weighed at every visit for the first 6 months following a medication change. BMI monitoring should be supplemented by measurement and recording of the patient's waist circumference. A waist circumference greater than 40 inches for men or greater than 35 inches for women is a criterion of the metabolic syndrome and places a person at elevated risk for diabetes. The relative risk of weight gain for the different antipsychotic medications should be a consideration in drug selection for patients who have a BMI greater than 25. Interventions for patients who gain weight may include closer monitoring of weight, engagement in a weight management program, or a change in antipsychotic medication. If a patient is taking a medication that is associated with a high risk for weight gain, the clinician should consider switching to medication with less weight gain liability.

Diabetes. Diabetes is more prevalent in individuals with schizophrenia than in the general population (Dixon et al. 2000). This may be related to the high rates of obesity associated with schizophrenia or to a possible association of schizophrenia with insulin resistance (American Diabetes Association et al. 2004). Other evidence suggests that antipsychotics have the potential for increasing the risk of diabetes. This could be either a result of antipsychotic-associated weight gain or a direct effect of antipsychotic drugs on insulin resistance. Most attention has focused on the second-generation antipsychotics, although it is likely that the first-generation antipsychotics also differ in their tendencies to cause weight gain and diabetes. As indicated in Table 17–2, the second-generation antipsychotics that are most associated with weight gain—clozapine and olanzapine—are also most associated with glucose abnormalities. The FDA, however, issued a warning that all second-generation antipsychotics increase the risk of hyperglycemia and diabetes (U.S. Food and Drug Administration 2004).

Mental health practitioners should be aware of risk factors for diabetes and the symptoms of new-onset diabetes (including weight change, polyuria, and polydipsia) and should inform patients about these symptoms and monitor for their presence at regular intervals. Furthermore, a baseline measure of glucose should be collected for all patients before starting a new antipsychotic. A fasting glucose level is preferred, but a hemoglobin A_{1C} level is sufficient if fasting glucose is not feasible. Patients who have significant risk factors for diabetes (family history, BMI>25, waist circumference>35 inches for women and 40 inches for men) should have fasting glucose or hemoglobin A_{1C} levels monitored 4 months after starting an antipsychotic and then yearly. Patients who are gaining weight should have fasting glucose or hemoglobin A_{1C} levels monitored every 4 months. Both the Mount Sinai guidelines (Marder et al. 2004) and the American Diabetes Association, American Psychiatric Association, American Association of Clinical Endocrinologists, et al. (2004) recommend measuring fasting blood glucose level before starting an antipsychotic, 4 months later, and then annually.

Mental health providers should ensure that patients with diagnosed diabetes are followed up by an appropriate medical provider. The patient's psychiatrist and medical care provider should communicate when medication changes are instituted that may affect the control of the patient's diabetes. If symptoms of diabetes are reported, a random blood glucose level should be collected, and if the level is elevated (≥126 if fasting or ≥200 if nonfasting), the patient should be referred to a medical care provider.

Dyslipidemia. Elevated levels of total cholesterol, low-density lipoprotein (LDL) cholesterol, and triglycerides may, in part, account for the high risk of coronary heart disease in schizophrenia. Studies of second-generation antipsychotics indicate that the tendency of these agents to cause weight gain is also associated with their risk for worsening serum lipid levels. Table 17–2 summarizes the associations between antipsychotics and dyslipidemias.

Mental health providers should be aware of the lipid profiles for all patients with schizophrenia. The National Cholesterol Education Program (Grundy et al. 2004) and the U.S. Preventive Services Task Force (2001) guidelines provide direction for screening and treating patients who are at high risk for cardiovascular disease. If a lipid panel is not available, one should be obtained and reviewed. As noted in Table 17–4, the American Diabetes Association,

American Psychiatric Association, American Association of Clinical Endocrinologists, et al. (2004) recommend monitoring lipid levels before medication changes, after 12 weeks, and then every 5 years. Patients who fulfill criteria for the metabolic syndrome should be carefully monitored by a medical care provider.

Prolactin. First-generation antipsychotics and risperidone (as well as sulpiride and amisulpiride) elevate serum prolactin levels through blockade of dopamine receptors in the anterior pituitary. Consequences may include decreased libido, anorgasmia, amenorrhea, galactorrhea, and gynecomastia. Dopamine receptor antagonists, such as first-generation antipsychotics, have been associated with an increased risk of breast cancer, possibly related to elevated prolactin (Wang et al. 2002). Growing evidence suggests that high levels of prolactin increase the risk of osteoporosis by reducing estrogen levels (Abraham et al. 2003; Becker et al. 2003; Meaney et al. 2004). Aripiprazole, which has agonist effects on pituitary dopamine receptors, can be associated with decreases in serum prolactin levels that are not thought to have clinical significance.

The Mount Sinai guidelines recommend yearly monitoring of patients taking antipsychotics for symptoms of prolactin elevation, including galactorrhea, decreased libido, or menstrual disturbances in women and decreased libido or erectile or ejaculatory disturbances in men (Marder et al. 2004). Patients who are receiving an agent that is associated with prolactin elevation (e.g., first-generation antipsychotics or risperidone) should be asked about symptoms of prolactin elevation at each visit after starting the agent until they are receiving a stable dose. If any symptoms of prolactin elevation are present, prolactin should be measured and, if possible, other medical causes ruled out. Consideration also should be given to a medication change to a prolactin-sparing antipsychotic. If, after a change in antipsychotic, the signs and symptoms disappear and the prolactin level declines to normal, an endocrine workup is not needed. For patients with symptomatic antipsychotic-induced hyperprolactinemia, hormone replacement therapy (estrogen/progestogen for women and testosterone in men) is considered the first choice for medication treatment (Miller 2004). As a last resort, treatment with a dopamine agonist (e.g., cabergoline or bromocriptine) may effectively lower prolactin levels, but psychotic exacerbation is a risk warranting careful monitoring.

Other Side Effects

Antipsychotics can also cause varying amounts of sedation and postural hypotension, as noted in Table 17–2. Patients should be asked about these side effects at each visit after starting an antipsychotic until tolerance develops. If the side effects do not resolve, a change to an antipsychotic with a lower risk of sedation or hypotension is indicated.

Tachycardia may be a side effect of certain agents, particularly clozapine. In addition, mental health providers are often in the best position to diagnose hypertension. Blood pressure and pulse also should be monitored at each visit after starting an antipsychotic until the dosage is stable. Thereafter, pulse and blood pressure should be measured at least every 6 months.

Neuroleptic dysphoria, an unpleasant subjective response to antipsychotic medicines, is associated with poor adherence to antipsychotic medication regimens (Perkins 2002; Van Putten et al. 1984; Weiden et al. 1989). Because neuroleptic dysphoria has been associated with akathisia and parkinsonism, it may be more common with first-generation antipsychotics than with second-generation antipsychotics (Perkins 2002).

MAINTENANCE TREATMENT EFFECTS AND RELAPSE PREVENTION

Many studies have reported that maintenance antipsychotic treatment for schizophrenia that has responded to antipsychotic medication reduces symptom relapse and rehospitalization (Davis 1975; Kane and Lieberman 1987). A reasonable estimate, based on controlled clinical trials of drug discontinuation, is that stopping antipsychotics after 1 year of maintenance treatment will result in relapse in about two-thirds of patients, whereas only one-third of the patients who continue to take antipsychotic medicines will relapse. Hogarty and colleagues (1976) found a relapse rate of 66% within 1 year of treatment discontinuation even among patients who had been successfully maintained in the community for 2–3 years with antipsychotic drugs. First-episode patients who meet symptom response criteria may have lower relapse rates. During the year following initial recovery, a relapse rate of 40% has been reported for patients taking placebo as compared with 0% for patients taking medication (Kane et al. 1982). Furthermore, Robinson and colleagues (1999a) showed that discontinuing drug therapy increased the risk of relapse almost five times in a sample of patients with first-episode schizophrenia or schizoaffective disorder over several years of follow-up.

The benefits of maintenance antipsychotic drug treatment are tempered by the risk of long-term side effects, such as the development of TD as well as obesity, diabetes, hyperlipidemias, and other factors associated with heart disease. Use of low doses of antipsychotic drugs has

intuitive appeal for minimizing side-effect risk. However, maintenance studies of the dose–response relation for up to 1 year of continuous antipsychotic drug treatment indicated that standard drug doses (fluphenazine decanoate, 12.5–50 mg biweekly; haloperidol decanoate, 50–200 mg monthly) provide significantly greater prophylaxis against relapse than do doses of one-half to one-tenth as much (Hogarty et al. 1988; Johnson et al. 1987; Kane et al. 1983, 1986; Marder et al. 1987; Schooler 1993). A targeted approach that involves slowly titrating stabilized patients off medication with reintroduction of the medication when signs or symptoms of imminent relapse occur has not been found to reduce the risk of TD and is associated with risks of symptom exacerbation and relapse (Carpenter et al. 1990; Gaebel et al. 1993; Herz et al. 1991; Jolley et al. 1990; Schooler 1993). The Schizophrenia Patient Outcomes Research Team (Lehman et al. 2004a) and the American Psychiatric Association "Practice Guideline for the Treatment of Patients With Schizophrenia" (Lehman et al. 2004b) recommend continuous maintenance treatment for all patients with chronic schizophrenia. Targeted, intermittent therapy is acceptable only for patients who cannot tolerate or will not accept continuous antipsychotic treatment.

COMPARATIVE EFFECTIVENESS OF FIRST- AND SECOND-GENERATION ANTIPSYCHOTICS

The second-generation antipsychotics were developed with the hope that they would lead to improved outcomes for individuals with schizophrenia, in part by reducing negative symptoms and the burden of extrapyramidal side effects. Although advantages for clozapine have been shown in many studies, it remains unclear whether the newer second-generation drugs have significant advantages in effectiveness and side-effect profiles over first-generation antipsychotics when they are prescribed at appropriate doses. A meta-analysis by Geddes and colleagues (2000) showed a modest advantage for second-generation antipsychotics in efficacy and EPS as compared with typical antipsychotics. However, in trials in which the mean dose of the drug compared with the second-generation antipsychotic drug was less than the equivalent of 12 mg of haloperidol, an advantage for second-generation drugs with regard to extrapyramidal symptoms remained, but no difference in overall efficacy was found between first- and second-generation antipsychotic drugs. Other meta-analyses (Davis et al. 2003; Leucht et al. 1999, 2003) support the notion that some second-generation antipsychotics may have advantages in short-term efficacy and relapse prevention over 1 year.

TABLE 17–5.   Long-acting antipsychotic drugs

	How supplied	Half-life (days)	Starting dose (mg)	Second dose (mg)	Maintenance dose (mg)
Fluphenazine decanoate	25 mg/mL or 100 mg/mL		12.5 im	12.5–25 (6–14 days later)	12.5–50 im every 2–3 weeks
Haloperidol decanoate	50 mg/mL or 100 mg/mL	21	50 im	50–100 (3–28 days later)	50–200 im every 3–4 weeks
Risperidone microspheres	Prepared packages of 25, 37.5, and 50 mg	3–6	25 im	25–50 (2 weeks later)	25–50 im every 2 weeks

Note.   im=intramuscularly.

According to exhaustive reviews conducted by the Schizophrenia Patient Outcomes Research Team (PORT) on evidence available through 2003, there is no clear evidence that supports the use of SGAs over FGAs for either acute or maintenance treatment of schizophrenia when considering positive and negative symptom efficacy alone (Lehman et al. 2004a).

Long-term trials with SGAs may yet demonstrate greater effectiveness in the maintenance treatment of schizophrenia compared with FGAs, as measured by reduced rates of relapse, improved social reintegration, and decreased risk of tardive dyskinesia. However, a multicenter, NIMH-funded trial (the Clinical Antipsychotic Trials of Intervention Effectiveness: Schizophrenia Trial) designed to determine the longer-term (18-month) effectiveness and tolerability of the SGAs relative to each other and to a representative FGA in chronic schizophrenia found no substantial advantages of the newer agents as compared with perphenazine with regard to symptom reduction or EPS (Lieberman et al. 2005). It is unclear at present whether advantages of SGAs in other symptom domains, such as cognitive functioning, will emerge.

LONG-ACTING INJECTABLE (DEPOT) ANTIPSYCHOTIC MEDICATIONS

Long-acting injectable antipsychotics, also known as *depot antipsychotics*, are commonly thought to have important advantages over oral medications in some situations. The primary reason long-acting formulations are used is to improve adherence with treatment regimens; thus, they are recommended for individuals who do not regularly take medications or who are expected not to do so. Another purported advantage is less fluctuation in drug levels than with oral medications, which is thought to lower the incidence of side effects (Ereshefsky et al. 1990). Other advantages are a clear knowledge of an individual's treatment adherence because of the need for injections and improved surveillance for missed medicine doses. An-

other possible advantage is increased contact with caregivers because injections are needed every 2–4 weeks instead of the typical monthly or less frequent appointment schedules. Disadvantages are that some patients do not like regular injections, the injections can be painful, and the requirement for regular injections can be inconvenient for clinicians as well as patients. Table 17–5 contains summary information on the long-acting injectable antipsychotics available in the United States.

The evidence to support any advantages of depot antipsychotics over oral antipsychotics is limited. Randomized controlled trials comparing oral with depot neuroleptics have been extremely rare. One well-designed study was a random-assignment, double-blind study that compared oral and depot fluphenazine for schizophrenia over 1 year (Schooler et al. 1980). Eligible participants were recruited from among newly hospitalized patients intended to represent "the broad range of schizophrenic patients." Eligibility for the study was explicitly "not based on prior illness, presumed prognosis, or prior medication-taking behavior." There was no fixed dosage ratio of oral fluphenazine and fluphenazine decanoate; oral and depot forms of fluphenazine were allowed to vary according to clinical judgment. No reports from this study identified significant differences between the two treatments on relapse, symptoms, or social adjustment.

Rifkin et al. (1977) compared oral fluphenazine, depot fluphenazine, and placebo in a 1-year study of 175 remitted patients with schizophrenia. They found that both active medicines were more effective than placebo in preventing relapse, but they found no differences between the depot and the oral agents. With regard to side effects, they found markedly more side effects with fluphenazine decanoate than with oral fluphenazine. The authors speculated that this was in part a result of overly high doses of fluphenazine decanoate relative to oral fluphenazine.

Hogarty and others (1979) compared randomly assigned oral fluphenazine and fluphenazine decanoate to 105 persons with schizophrenia in the context of high and low degrees of social therapy over 2 years. In the first year, they found no differences in relapse rates (oral fluphenazine = 39.5%, fluphenazine decanoate=35.1%) and no effect of social therapy. When they examined relapse rates from month 2 to 24, the difference in relapse rates was large (oral fluphenazine=60.8%, fluphenazine decanoate = 35.6%) but not statistically significant.

A randomized study of the effect of various dosages of haloperidol found that the highest dosage studied, 200 mg intramuscularly every 4 weeks, was associated with a lower rate of symptom exacerbations (15%) over 1 year than were lower dosages (Kane et al. 2002). Surprisingly, this study found little increase in side effects or subjective discomfort for persons taking 100 mg or 50 mg monthly.

The long-acting injectable formulation of risperidone was approved by the FDA in 2003 and is efficacious in reducing psychotic symptoms (Kane et al. 2003). In the Kane et al. study, patients taking the highest recommended dosage (50 mg every 2 weeks) were significantly more likely to require anticholinergic medicines for EPS than were patients taking 25 mg every 2 weeks or placebo. To date, no published data have compared this first depot second-generation antipsychotic with any depot first-generation antipsychotic.

IMPLEMENTING AND MONITORING ANTIPSYCHOTIC DRUG TREATMENT

DOSING

Recommended dose ranges for commonly used oral antipsychotics appear in Table 17–1. Few data support the usefulness of doses beyond the range of 300–1,000 mg/day of chlorpromazine or the equivalent dose of other antipsychotics. Large doses of chlorpromazine daily (e.g., 2,000 mg or more) or equivalent doses of other first-generation antipsychotics are not associated with greater efficacy (Bjorndal et al. 1980; Ericksen et al. 1978; McCreadie and MacDonald 1977; Neborsky et al. 1981; Quitkin et al. 1975) but can lead to a greater incidence of side effects. Some reports of positive results with high doses of olanzapine have not been confirmed in rigorous studies (Conley et al. 2003; Sheitman et al. 1997). The administration of large parenteral doses of antipsychotics within a 24-hour period ("rapid neuroleptization") has not shown any gains in efficacy over standard treatment and is not a recommended strategy (Lehman et al. 2004a).

During the treatment of an acute episode of schizophrenia, antipsychotic drugs usually have a therapeutic effect within 1–3 weeks, with most gains in the first 6–8 weeks (Davis et al. 1989). Some patients, however, may require several months to achieve a full clinical response and symptom remission. This also applies to first-episode patients, whose symptoms typically respond relatively rapidly to modest doses of antipsychotic medications (Lieberman 1993). When patients' symptoms do not respond to a standard course of treatment, clinicians generally increase the dose, switch to another antipsychotic drug, or maintain the initial treatment for an extended period. Little evidence from controlled clinical trials supports the efficacy of any of these strategies (Kinon et al. 1993; Levinson et al. 1990; Rifkin et al. 1991; Van Putten et al. 1990; Volavka et al. 1992), although an individual patient may show a better response to one particular drug than to another (Gardos 1974). Another common approach, also without strong evidence for effectiveness, is simultaneous use of more than one antipsychotic. This strategy, known as *antipsychotic polypharmacy*, is discussed later in this chapter (see section "Antipsychotic Polypharmacy" later in this chapter).

ROUTE OF ADMINISTRATION

Oral pills are the most commonly used form of antipsychotic medication and are suitable for most patients in most situations. Liquids and dissolvable tablets are useful for patients who cannot or will not swallow pills or who prefer this form. Short-acting injections that are rapidly active are available for emergency treatment of agitated, psychotic patients or others in need of rapid decreases in symptoms or dangerous behavior.

Long-acting injections are recommended for patients with frequent relapses on oral medications, poor adherence to oral medication regimens, or a preference for injections (Lehman et al. 2004a). Despite limited evidence from well-conducted clinical trials, this recommendation is supported by the experience of clinicians who believe that long-acting injections work well for patients who cannot or will not consistently take oral medications and that adherence with injectable regimens is easier to monitor than with oral regimens.

IMPLEMENTING CLOZAPINE TREATMENT

A complete blood count with differential should be obtained before starting clozapine to make sure the patient is not granulocytopenic (white blood cell count<3,000/mm^3). General and cardiovascular health should be assessed because of the side effects of orthostatic hypotension and tachycardia and the rare occurrence of life-threatening cardiovascular side effects. The initial dosage should be 12.5–25 mg once or twice daily. Increases should be made gradually (increase by 25–50 mg/day) because risks of sedation, hypotension, and seizures are higher with rapid dose escalation. The target dosage is 300–800 mg/day. The minimum effective dose should be used. If response is inadequate once 600 mg/day is reached, a blood level should be obtained because there appears to be a therapeutic threshold of about 350 ng/mL. If this level has not been obtained, slow upward titration of the clozapine dosage to 800 mg/day is recommended. One important drug interaction is with selective serotonin reuptake inhibitors and other drugs that are metabolized by the cytochrome P450 2D6 isozyme (e.g., fluoxetine, fluvoxamine), which can lead to significant increases in clozapine plasma levels.

To limit the risk of agranulocytosis, a complete blood count must be repeated weekly for the first 6 months and biweekly after that. Clozapine should not be given if the white blood cell count declines below 2,000/mm^3 or the absolute neutrophil count declines below 1,000/mm^3. Drugs known to suppress bone marrow function (e.g., carbamazepine) should not be used with clozapine.

There is no clear consensus on how to monitor for myocarditis. However, because the risk appears greatest in the first 2 months of clozapine therapy, at some centers, serum creatine kinase levels and ECGs are obtained before treatment and every 2 weeks during these first 2 months. Patients should be monitored carefully for chest discomfort, shortness of breath, or unusual fatigue during this time. A conservative approach is to discontinue clozapine if any signs or symptoms of myocarditis develop early in treatment. Clozapine should be stopped if substantial evidence of a new cardiac problem is found early in treatment, but if signs and symptoms are nonspecific, then a cardiology consultation may be helpful in determining the diagnosis and may prevent unnecessary discontinuation of this very useful medication.

Because clozapine is the best available drug treatment for refractory symptoms, a trial should last 8–12 weeks at an effective dosage. Clinical benefits may continue to accrue for up to 12 months. If effective, clozapine should be continued as a maintenance treatment. But because of its side effects and the need for continued white blood cell monitoring, if clozapine does not offer advantages over previous treatments, then it should be slowly discontinued after 6 months of treatment and replaced with a new or previously helpful treatment.

TREATMENT TARGETS: RESPONSE CRITERIA

Although drugs classified as antipsychotics may have a wide range of therapeutic effects, the primary standard of efficacy has been the reduction of positive psychotic symptoms such as delusions, hallucinations, and disorganization. Antipsychotic drugs that have been approved by regulatory agencies are all superior to placebo in reducing positive psychotic symptoms. Antipsychotic drugs also reduce negative symptoms (i.e., affective flattening, alogia, and avolition), but the magnitude of the effect is smaller than the effect on positive symptoms (Leucht et al. 1999), and any effect on residual negative symptoms or the deficit syndrome is small (Carpenter 1996; Kirkpatrick et al. 2000). The clearest types of negative symptoms that can be reduced with antipsychotic medicines are those secondary to positive symptoms, such as social withdrawal and avoidance due to delusions or paranoia (Carpenter et al. 1988). As positive symptoms decrease in response to antipsychotic drugs, the secondary negative symptoms also diminish.

Because cognitive impairments are common in schizophrenia and have been shown to relate more strongly to functional outcomes than to positive symptom severity, cognitive functioning is now an important focus of research and a possible target of pharmacotherapies (Green 1996; Harvey et al. 1998). The cognitive domains under study include learning and secondary memory, motor function, verbal fluency, attention, and executive functioning. Second-generation antipsychotic drugs may have advantages over first-generation antipsychotics in terms of neurocognitive functioning as a result of either fewer neurocognitive adverse effects or direct, positive therapeutic effects (Kinon and Lieberman 1996). Evidence for this remains inconclusive.

FACTORS INFLUENCING ANTIPSYCHOTIC RESPONSE

Significant efforts are under way to identify factors that may be associated with antipsychotic treatment refractoriness because preventive measures may offer more hope than new drugs. For example, a delay in treatment of the first episode of schizophrenia (Addington et al. 2004; Loebel et al. 1992) and in the treatment of acute exacerbations (May et al. 1976; Wyatt 1995) is associated with poorer clinical outcomes. Robinson and colleagues (1999b) reported that 87% of their sample of first-episode patients with schizophrenia or schizoaffective disorder responded to treatment within 1 year. Male gender, a history of obstetric complications, poorer attention at baseline, more severe hallucinations and delusions, and the development of EPS during antipsychotic treatment were associated with a significantly lower likelihood of response.

OTHER PHARMACOLOGICAL TREATMENTS

Because antipsychotic medications often fail to resolve the full range of schizophrenic psychopathology and other common symptoms (e.g., anxiety, depression, mood instability, motor unrest), adjunctive treatments are commonly tried. Adjunctive pharmacological treatments in patients with schizophrenia have been the subject of numerous reviews (Christison et al. 1991; Donaldson et al. 1983; Farmer and Blewett 1993; Johns and Thompson 1995; Lehman et al. 2004b; Lindenmayer 1995; Meltzer 1992; Rifkin 1993; Siris 1993). In addition, some psychotropic medications other than antipsychotics have been used alone to treat schizophrenia. Below we summarize information on the use of anxiolytics/hypnotics, antidepressants, mood stabilizers, and dopamine agonists to treat either symptoms of schizophrenia or common comorbid conditions.

ANTIANXIETY OR HYPNOTIC DRUGS

Benzodiazepines have been prescribed for patients with schizophrenia since the early 1960s, but there has been little recent systematic research in this area. This lack of research may be due to the potential for dependency and reluctance to prescribe these agents to patients with comorbid substance abuse or substance use disorders. In addition, reports indicate that benzodiazepines may result in a "disinhibiting" (Karson et al. 1982) or worsening of psychopathology in some patients (Wolkowitz and Pickar 1991).

Carpenter and colleagues (1999) studied whether diazepam could help to prevent a psychotic relapse when given for symptoms thought to be prodromal of an impending psychotic exacerbation. In their double-blind, randomized clinical trial of 53 patients with schizophrenia, they compared diazepam with placebo and with fluphenazine and found that diazepam was superior to placebo and comparable to fluphenazine in preventing a psychotic relapse.

Few studies in the literature have rigorously tested the use of benzodiazepines to treat nonpsychotic symptoms common in people with schizophrenia. Nevertheless, some evidence suggests that schizophrenia patients with anxiety, depression, hostility, irritability, and motor unrest may benefit from benzodiazepines (Wolkowitz and Pickar 1991). A very small study that examined benzodiazepine response among six anxious schizophrenia patients under double-blind conditions over 12 weeks concluded that some patients from this subgroup may experience reduced anxiety with a benzodiazepine used adjunctively to antipsychotics (Kellner et al. 1975). Although benzodiazepines are frequently used as hypnotic agents in clinical practice, no controlled studies have established their efficacy in patients with schizophrenia. At a minimum, the benzodiazepines appear to be a useful adjunct to antipsychotics in the treatment of agitation or anxiety in patients with schizophrenia.

ANTIDEPRESSANTS

Antidepressants do not appear to be effective as an adjunctive treatment for positive psychotic symptoms (Siris et al. 1978) and may worsen symptoms in persons who are acutely psychotic (Plasky 1991). The efficacy of antidepressants for negative symptoms of schizophrenia has been examined in several studies but the effect, if any, is modest (Berk et al. 2001; Lee et al. 1998; Silver and Nassar 1992; Silver et al. 2000).

Because secondary or postpsychotic depression among patients with schizophrenia is common, antidepressants are widely used to treat depression among persons with schizophrenia, although the evidence for the effectiveness of this strategy is modest. In a review of six double-blind, placebo-controlled studies that used tricyclic antidepressants in addition to an antipsychotic, two reported a significant reduction in depression (Plasky 1991). These two studies involved patients whose acute psychosis was under control, suggesting that adjunctive antidepressant treatment may be most successful for the treatment of depression when an acute psychotic episode has stabilized. However, in two studies of acutely psychotic patients, the antidepressants appeared to have resulted in a worsening of the psychosis (Plasky 1991). Subsequent research has supported the use of antidepressants for schizophrenic patients with depression whose psychotic symptoms have stabilized (Hogarty et al. 1995; Siris et al. 1994). Definitive conclusions cannot be drawn about antidepressant use for schizophrenia patients with depression, however, because few methodologically rigorous studies are available. Nevertheless, adjunctive antidepressant treatment is warranted when a patient reports persistent symptoms of depression when he or she is not in an acute episode of illness.

Important practical issues must be considered when antidepressants are used in combination with clozapine. Selective serotonin reuptake inhibitors—in particular, fluvoxamine, fluoxetine, and sertraline—inhibit the metabolism of clozapine and can cause large increases in clozapine levels that are potentially toxic. Serum clozapine levels and side effects, particularly anticholinergic side effects, should be monitored when using the combination of selective serotonin reuptake inhibitors and clozapine. Because bupropion and clozapine both increase the risk of seizures, this combination is not recommended.

LITHIUM

Lithium has been used as monotherapy and as an adjunct to antipsychotics in the treatment of schizophrenia (Atre-Vaidya and Taylor 1989; Christison et al. 1991). Antipsychotics are superior to lithium as a treatment for acute psychosis in schizophrenic patients, although some patients may improve while taking lithium alone (Atre-Vaidya and Taylor 1989). There is no convincing evidence of the efficacy of lithium as an adjunctive agent to antipsychotics for schizophrenia. However, because of reports of benefit in some treatment-refractory patients, a trial of lithium should be considered if a patient has not adequately responded or was unable to tolerate a second-generation agent (e.g., clozapine). When concern about potentially toxic interactions between an antipsychotic and lithium was investigated (Cohen and Cohen 1974), little evidence supporting this association was found (Rifkin 1993).

ANTICONVULSANTS

Carbamazepine

Leucht and colleagues (2002) reviewed eight studies that compared carbamazepine plus antipsychotics with placebo plus antipsychotics in the treatment of schizophrenia. They concluded that carbamazepine should not be recommended for routine clinical use for treatment of schizophrenia or augmentation of antipsychotic treatment of schizophrenia. The review qualified that conclusion by indicating that a trial of carbamazepine may be warranted for those with a history of response to carbamazepine or for patients with associated electroencephalogram abnormalities.

For the subpopulation of aggressive, agitated patients, some evidence supports carbamazepine as an adjunctive agent to antipsychotics in the treatment of schizophrenia. Because of carbamazepine's ability to upregulate hepatic enzymes, plasma antipsychotic levels may be lowered when carbamazepine is used. If antipsychotic efficacy is lost, antipsychotic levels can be checked, or the dosage can be increased (Christison et al. 1991). Because of carbamazepine's risk of bone marrow toxicity, including agranulocytosis, it should not be used in combination with clozapine.

Valproate

Valproate (the active component of valproic acid and divalproex) is widely used as an adjunctive treatment for schizophrenia, but evidence supporting its use as a maintenance treatment is limited (Citrome 2003). Linnoila

and colleagues (1976) found that the combination of valproate with an antipsychotic was superior to an antipsychotic alone in reducing global psychopathology in a double-blind, crossover study of 32 patients with dyskinesias. In a small 21-day double-blind, randomized, placebo-controlled study of valproate as adjunctive treatment to haloperidol in 12 hospitalized patients with acute exacerbations of chronic schizophrenia, Wassef et al. (2000) found that the valproate group showed greater improvements than the placebo group on measures of psychopathology. Casey et al. (2003) conducted a 28-day double-blind, randomized controlled trial of 249 patients with schizophrenia that compared combination therapy of divalproex and risperidone or olanzapine with risperidone or olanzapine monotherapy and found faster improvement in psychopathology with combination therapy. Although the differences in psychopathology were not significant at the end of the 28 days, fewer combination therapy patients dropped out of the study compared with monotherapy patients (10% vs. 20%). Definitive conclusions on the efficacy of valproate for the long-term treatment of schizophrenia are premature, however. Although valproate is sometimes used as an adjunctive treatment for treatment-refractory patients, no strong evidence supports this use (Conley et al. 2003).

DOPAMINE AGONISTS

Dopamine agonists have been associated with an exacerbation of psychotic symptoms in schizophrenic patients, but they also have been used as a treatment for negative symptoms. The strategy of using dopamine agonists for negative symptoms is consistent with the hypothesis that a hypodopaminergic state may be their cause (Carpenter 1995; Lynch 1992). L-Dopa, bromocriptine, and dextroamphetamine all have been studied in relatively small trials with only inconsistent and modest effects (Brambilla et al. 1979; Christison et al. 1991; Gattaz et al. 1989; Gerlach and Luhdorf 1975; Inanaga et al. 1975).

Dopamine agonists have been insufficiently studied to draw definitive conclusions, but they may represent an underused class of medication for the treatment of negative symptoms. Clinicians are understandably hesitant to use these agents because of the risk of exacerbating symptoms, even though this risk may be small if patients are given maintenance antipsychotics (Perovich et al. 1989).

GLUTAMATERGIC AGENTS

Because phencyclidine inhibits the neurotransmission of glutamate through N-methyl-D-aspartate (NMDA) receptors (i.e., is an NMDA antagonist) and has been shown to produce a syndrome similar to schizophrenic psychosis, it was hypothesized that reduced glutamate activity (possibly through NMDA receptor hypofunction) caused the symptoms of schizophrenia (Anis et al. 1983; Javitt and Zukin 1991; Luby et al. 1959). The potential therapeutic effects of three glutamatergic agents on schizophrenia have been studied to date: glycine (Heresco-Levy et al. 1996; Javitt et al. 1994), D-cycloserine (Goff et al. 1995, 1999a, 1999b; Rosse et al. 1996), and D-serine (Tsai et al. 1998, 1999).

Each of the three agents showed some benefit as an adjunctive treatment for psychotic symptoms when dosed appropriately, except when used with clozapine. Although dosing challenges with glycine and D-cycloserine may make them impractical for clinical use, studies of these compounds provide strong support for a role of glutamate in the pathophysiology of schizophrenia and further the understanding of the pharmacological mechanism of clozapine. D-Serine is the most promising agent in this group according to current findings. Investigators hope that this line of research will lead to improved symptom reduction for patients with schizophrenia and clues for the development of other novel therapeutic agents.

ANTIPSYCHOTIC POLYPHARMACY

Although antipsychotic polypharmacy is a common treatment strategy, little evidence supports its use (Covell et al. 2002; Freudenreich and Goff 2002; A.L. Miller and Craig 2002; Weissman 2002). However, augmenting clozapine with other antipsychotics has some support in the literature. Part of the rationale for combined therapy is the use of agents with higher D_2 receptor potency than that of clozapine, which has a relatively low affinity for and fast dissociation constant at this receptor type (Chong et al. 2000; Kapur and Seeman 2000, 2001; Shiloh et al. 1997). Shiloh and colleagues, in a double-blind, placebo-controlled study, evaluated the effectiveness of sulpiride, a selective D_2 antagonist, as an add-on to clozapine. They found that clozapine-treated patients who received concomitant sulpiride (600 mg) had significant improvement in both positive and negative symptoms as compared with those who received placebo (Shiloh et al. 1997). This finding has had further support from case reports of sulpiride combined with clozapine (Stubbs et al. 2000) and sulpiride combined with other atypical antipsychotics (Raskin et al. 2000).

Similarly, risperidone, an atypical antipsychotic with relatively high D_2 receptor potency, has been found to improve symptoms in clozapine-treated patients. An investigation of the effect of risperidone as an add-on to clo-

zapine in an open 4-week trial involving 12 patients found that 10 of the 12 patients had a 20% or greater reduction in the BPRS score (Henderson and Goff 1996). A placebo-controlled trial involving 40 patients has added evidence to support the addition of risperidone to clozapine in patients who are nonresponsive or only partially responsive to clozapine alone (Josiassen et al. 2005). This study found greater reduction in overall symptoms and in positive and negative symptoms in patients taking risperidone and clozapine compared with those taking placebo and clozapine.

Case reports and case series have used clozapine with loxapine (Mowerman and Siris 1996), pimozide (Friedman et al. 1997), and olanzapine (Gupta et al. 1998), but, again, controlled trials are lacking. Case series also have investigated the combination of clozapine with quetiapine (Reinstein et al. 1999) or with ziprasidone (Kaye 2003) and have shown a reduced need for clozapine (as reflected by lower clozapine dose following addition of the second antipsychotic) and a reduced clozapine side-effect burden, but these findings must be considered preliminary.

In summary, concomitant use of another antipsychotic, particularly one with relatively higher D_2 receptor potency, with clozapine in patients with persistent symptoms may offer some benefit, but controlled trials are needed to verify the observations of open trials (Freudenreich and Goff 2002). This verification is important given the potential adverse effects of antipsychotic polypharmacy, as has been reported for risperidone combined with clozapine (Chong et al. 1997; Henderson et al. 2001; Kontaxakis et al. 2002).

Aside from the clozapine literature, no controlled studies have examined the use of two or more antipsychotics in the treatment of refractory schizophrenia. Still, antipsychotic polypharmacy is common, and anecdotal evidence suggests that in some patients, combined use of antipsychotics may improve symptoms as compared with antipsychotic monotherapy. A small case series has been published suggesting that combined treatment with risperidone and olanzapine shows benefit in treatment-refractory patients (Lerner et al. 2000). Similarly, a case series found clinical improvement in olanzapine-treated patients after the addition of sulpiride (Raskin et al. 2000), an observation congruent with the clozapine literature. We recommend clozapine monotherapy prior to any adjunctive pharmacotherapy or antipsychotic polypharmacy for the treatment of schizophrenia. Unfortunately, in the event of clozapine refusal or intolerance, few data are available to guide the use of specific antipsychotic combinations.

REFERENCES

Abnormal Involuntary Movement Scale (AIMS). Psychopharmacol Bull 24:781–783, 1988

Abraham G, Paing WW, Kaminski J, et al: Effects of elevated serum prolactin on bone mineral density and bone metabolism in female patients with schizophrenia: a prospective study. Am J Psychiatry 160:1618–1620, 2003

Addington J, Van Mastrigt S, Addington D: Duration of untreated psychosis: impact on 2-year outcome. Psychol Med 34: 277–284, 2004

Adler LA, Peselow E, Rotrosen J, et al: Vitamin E treatment of tardive dyskinesia. Am J Psychiatry 150:1405–1407, 1993

Allison DB, Fontaine KR, Heo M, et al: The distribution of body mass index among individuals with and without schizophrenia. J Clin Psychiatry 60:215–220, 1999a

Allison DB, Mentore JL, Heo M, et al: Antipsychotic-induced weight gain: a comprehensive research synthesis. Am J Psychiatry 156:1686–1696, 1999b

Alvir JM, Lieberman JA, Safferman AZ, et al: Clozapine-induced agranulocytosis: incidence and risk factors in the United States. N Engl J Med 329:162–167, 1993

American Diabetes Association, American Psychiatric Association, American Association of Clinical Endocrinologists, et al: Consensus development conference on antipsychotic drugs and obesity and diabetes. J Clin Psychiatry 65:267–272, 2004

American Psychiatric Association: Diagnostic and Statistical Manual of Mental Disorders, 4th Edition, Text Revision. Washington, DC, American Psychiatric Association, 2000

Anis N, Berry SC, Burton NR, et al: The dissociative anesthetics, ketamine and phencyclidine, selectively reduce excitation of central mammalian neurons by N-methyl-aspartate. Br J Pharmacol 79:565–575, 1983

Atre-Vaidya N, Taylor MA: Effectiveness of lithium in schizophrenia: do we really have an answer? J Clin Psychiatry 50:170–173, 1989

Becker D, Liver O, Mester R, et al: Risperidone, but not olanzapine, decreases bone mineral density in female premenopausal schizophrenia patients. J Clin Psychiatry 64:761–766, 2003

Berk M, Ichim C, Brook S: Efficacy of mirtazapine add on therapy to haloperidol in the treatment of the negative symptoms of schizophrenia: a double-blind randomized placebo-controlled study. Int Clin Psychopharmacol 16:87–92, 2001

Bilder RM, Goldman RS, Volavka J, et al: Neurocognitive effects of clozapine, olanzapine, risperidone, and haloperidol in patients with chronic schizophrenia or schizoaffective disorder. Am J Psychiatry 159:1018–1028, 2002

Bjorndal N, Bjerre M, Gerlach J, et al: High dosage haloperidol therapy in chronic schizophrenic patients: a double-blind study of clinical response, side effects, serum haloperidol, and serum prolactin. Psychopharmacology (Berl) 67:17–23, 1980

Brambilla F, Bellodi L, Negri F, et al: Dopamine receptor sensitivity in the hypothalamus of chronic schizophrenics after haloperidol therapy: growth hormone and prolactin response to stimuli. Psychoneuroendocrinology 4:329–339, 1979

Caroff S: Neuroleptic malignant syndrome: still a risk, but which patients may be in danger? Current Psychiatry 2:36–42, 2003

Carpenter WT Jr: Serotonin-dopamine antagonists and treatment of negative symptoms. J Clin Psychopharmacol 15: 30S–35S, 1995

Carpenter WT Jr: The treatment of negative symptoms: pharmacological and methodological issues. Br J Psychiatry Suppl (29):17–22, 1996

Carpenter WT Jr, Heinrichs DW, Wagman AM: Deficit and nondeficit forms of schizophrenia: the concept. Am J Psychiatry 145:578–583, 1988

Carpenter WT Jr, Hanlon TE, Heinrichs DW, et al: Continuous versus targeted medication in schizophrenic outpatients: outcome results. Am J Psychiatry 147:1138–1148, 1990

Carpenter WT Jr, Buchanan RW, Kirkpatrick B, et al: Diazepam treatment of early signs of exacerbation in schizophrenia. Am J Psychiatry 156:299–303, 1999

Casey DE: Neuroleptic-induced acute extrapyramidal syndromes and tardive dyskinesia. Psychiatr Clin North Am 16:589–610, 1993

Casey DE, Daniel DG, Wassef AA, et al: Effect of divalproex combined with olanzapine or risperidone in patients with an acute exacerbation of schizophrenia. Neuropsychopharmacology 28:182–192, 2003

Chakos M, Lieberman J, Hoffman E, et al: Effectiveness of second-generation antipsychotics in patients with treatment-resistant schizophrenia: a review and meta-analysis of randomized trials. Am J Psychiatry 158:518–526, 2001

Chengappa KN, Vasile J, Levine J, et al: Clozapine: its impact on aggressive behavior among patients in a state psychiatric hospital. Schizophr Res 53:1–6, 2002

Chengappa KN, Parepally H, Brar JS, et al: A random-assignment, double-blind, clinical trial of once- vs twice-daily administration of quetiapine fumarate in patients with schizophrenia or schizoaffective disorder: a pilot study. Can J Psychiatry 48:187–194, 2003

Chong SA, Tan CH, Lee HS: Atrial ectopics with clozapine-risperidone combination. J Clin Psychopharmacol 17:130–131, 1997

Chong SA, Remington GJ, Bezchlibnyk-Butler KZ: Effect of clozapine on polypharmacy. Psychiatr Serv 51:250–252, 2000

Christison GW, Kirch DG, Wyatt RJ: When symptoms persist: choosing among alternative somatic treatments for schizophrenia. Schizophr Bull 17:217–245, 1991

Citrome L: Schizophrenia and valproate. Psychopharmacol Bull 37 (suppl 2):74–88, 2003

Citrome L, Volavka J, Czobor P, et al: Effects of clozapine, olanzapine, risperidone, and haloperidol on hostility among patients with schizophrenia. Psychiatr Serv 52:1510–1514, 2001

Cohen WJ, Cohen NH: Lithium carbonate, haloperidol, and irreversible brain damage. JAMA 230:1283–1287, 1974

Conley RR, Mahmoud R: A randomized double-blind study of risperidone and olanzapine in the treatment of schizophrenia or schizoaffective disorder. Am J Psychiatry 158:765–774, 2001

Conley RR, Kelly DL, Richardson CM, et al: The efficacy of high-dose olanzapine versus clozapine in treatment-resistant schizophrenia: a double-blind crossover study. J Clin Psychopharmacol 23:668–671, 2003

Correll CU, Leucht S, Kane JM: Lower risk for tardive dyskinesia associated with second-generation antipsychotics: a systematic review of 1-year studies. Am J Psychiatry 161: 414–425, 2004

Covell NH, Jackson CT, Evans AC, et al: Antipsychotic prescribing practices in Connecticut's public mental health system: rates of changing medications and prescribing styles. Schizophr Bull 28:17–29, 2002

Csernansky JG, Mahmoud R, Brenner R: A comparison of risperidone and haloperidol for the prevention of relapse in patients with schizophrenia. N Engl J Med 346:16–22, 2002

Davis JM: Overview: maintenance therapy in psychiatry, I: schizophrenia. Am J Psychiatry 132:1237–1245, 1975

Davis JM, Barter JT, Kane JM (eds): Antipsychotic Drugs. Baltimore, MD, Williams & Wilkins, 1989

Davis JM, Chen N, Glick ID: A meta-analysis of the efficacy of second-generation antipsychotics. Arch Gen Psychiatry 60:553–564, 2003

Dixon L, Weiden PJ, Delahanty J, et al: Prevalence and correlates of diabetes in national schizophrenia samples. Schizophr Bull 26:903–912, 2000

Donaldson SR, Gelenberg AJ, Baldessarini RJ: The pharmacologic treatment of schizophrenia: a progress report. Schizophr Bull 9:504–527, 1983

Ereshefsky L, Saklad SR, Tran-Johnson T, et al: Kinetics and clinical evaluation of haloperidol decanoate loading dose regimen. Psychopharmacol Bull 26:108–114, 1990

Ericksen SE, Hurt SW, Chang S: Haloperidol dose, plasma levels, and clinical response: a double-blind study [proceedings]. Psychopharmacol Bull 14:15–16, 1978

Farmer AE, Blewett A: Drug treatment of resistant schizophrenia: limitations and recommendations. Drugs 45:374–383, 1993

Freudenreich O, Goff DC: Antipsychotic combination therapy in schizophrenia: a review of efficacy and risks of current combinations. Acta Psychiatr Scand 106:323–330, 2002

Friedman J, Ault K, Powchik P: Pimozide augmentation for the treatment of schizophrenic patients who are partial responders to clozapine. Biol Psychiatry 42:522–523, 1997

Gaebel W, Frick U, Kopcke W, et al: Early neuroleptic intervention in schizophrenia: are prodromal symptoms valid predictors of relapse? Br J Psychiatry Suppl September(21):8–12, 1993

Gardos G: Are antipsychotic drugs interchangeable? J Nerv Ment Dis 159:343–348, 1974

Gattaz WF, Rost W, Hubner CK, et al: Acute and subchronic effects of low-dose bromocriptine in haloperidol-treated schizophrenics. Biol Psychiatry 25:247–255, 1989

Geddes J, Freemantle N, Harrison P, et al: Atypical antipsychotics in the treatment of schizophrenia: systematic overview and meta-regression analysis. BMJ 321:1371–1376, 2000

Gerlach J, Luhdorf K: The effect of L-dopa on young patients with simple schizophrenia, treated with neuroleptic drugs: a double-blind cross-over trial with Madopar and placebo. Psychopharmacologia 44:105–110, 1975

Glazer WM, Morgenstern H, Doucette JT: Predicting the long-term risk of tardive dyskinesia in outpatients maintained on neuroleptic medications. J Clin Psychiatry 54:133–139, 1993

Goff DC, Tsai G, Manoach DS, et al: Dose-finding trial of D-cycloserine added to neuroleptics for negative symptoms in schizophrenia. Am J Psychiatry 152:1213–1215, 1995

Goff DC, Henderson DC, Evins AE, et al: A placebo-controlled crossover trial of D-cycloserine added to clozapine in patients with schizophrenia. Biol Psychiatry 45:512–514, 1999a

Goff DC, Tsai G, Levitt J, et al: A placebo-controlled trial of D-cycloserine added to conventional neuroleptics in patients with schizophrenia. Arch Gen Psychiatry 56:21–27, 1999b

Green MF: What are the functional consequences of neurocognitive deficits in schizophrenia? Am J Psychiatry 153:321–330, 1996

Grundy SM, Cleeman JI, Merz CN, et al: Implications of recent clinical trials for the National Cholesterol Education Program Adult Treatment Panel III guidelines. Circulation 110(2):227–239, 2004

Gupta S, Sonnenberg SJ, Frank B: Olanzapine augmentation of clozapine. Ann Clin Psychiatry 10:113–115, 1998

Guttmacher MS: Phenothiazine treatment in acute schizophrenia; effectiveness: the National Institute of Mental Health Psychopharmacology Service Center Collaborative Study Group. Arch Gen Psychiatry 10:246–261, 1964

Harrigan EP, Miceli JJ, Anziano R, et al: A randomized evaluation of the effects of six antipsychotic agents on QTc, in the absence and presence of metabolic inhibition. J Clin Psychopharmacol 24:62–69, 2004

Harvey PD, Howanitz E, Parrella M, et al: Symptoms, cognitive functioning, and adaptive skills in geriatric patients with lifelong schizophrenia: a comparison across treatment sites. Am J Psychiatry 155:1080–1086, 1998

Healy D: The Creation of Psychopharmacology. Cambridge, MA, Harvard University Press, 2002

Henderson DC, Goff DC: Risperidone as an adjunct to clozapine therapy in chronic schizophrenics. J Clin Psychiatry 57:395–397, 1996

Henderson DC, Goff DC, Connolly CE, et al: Risperidone added to clozapine: impact on serum prolactin levels. J Clin Psychiatry 62:605–608, 2001

Heresco-Levy U, Javitt DC, Ermilov M, et al: Double-blind, placebo-controlled, crossover trial of glycine adjuvant therapy for treatment-resistant schizophrenia. Br J Psychiatry 169:610–617, 1996

Herz MI, Glazer WM, Mostert MA, et al: Intermittent vs maintenance medication in schizophrenia: two-year results. Arch Gen Psychiatry 48:333–339, 1991

Hogarty GE, Ulrich RF, Mussare F, et al: Drug discontinuation among long term, successfully maintained schizophrenic outpatients. Dis Nerv Syst 37:494–500, 1976

Hogarty GE, Schooler NR, Ulrich R, et al: Fluphenazine and social therapy in the aftercare of schizophrenic patients: relapse analyses of a two-year controlled study of fluphenazine decanoate and fluphenazine hydrochloride. Arch Gen Psychiatry 36:1283–1294, 1979

Hogarty GE, McEvoy JP, Munetz M, et al: Dose of fluphenazine, familial expressed emotion, and outcome in schizophrenia: results of a two-year controlled study. Arch Gen Psychiatry 45:797–805, 1988

Hogarty GE, McEvoy JP, Ulrich RF, et al: Pharmacotherapy of impaired affect in recovering schizophrenic patients. Arch Gen Psychiatry 52(1):29, 1995

IMS Health: IMS World Review 2004. Available at: http://www.imshealth.com/web/content/0,3148,64576068_63872702_70260998_70960214,00.html. Accessed October 3, 2005.

Inanaga K, Nakazawa Y, Inoue K, et al: Double-blind controlled study of L-dopa therapy in schizophrenia. Folia Psychiatr Neurol Jpn 29:123–143, 1975

Javitt DC, Zukin SR: Recent advances in the phencyclidine model of schizophrenia. Am J Psychiatry 148:1301–1308, 1991

Javitt DC, Zylberman I, Zukin SR, et al: Amelioration of negative symptoms in schizophrenia by glycine. Am J Psychiatry 151:1234–1236, 1994

Jeste DV, Rockwell E, Harris MJ, et al: Conventional vs. newer antipsychotics in elderly patients. Am J Geriatr Psychiatry 7:70–76, 1999

Johns CA, Thompson JW: Adjunctive treatments in schizophrenia: pharmacotherapies and electroconvulsive therapy. Schizophr Bull 21:607–619, 1995

Johnson DA, Ludlow JM, Street K, et al: Double-blind comparison of half-dose and standard-dose flupenthixol decanoate in the maintenance treatment of stabilised out-patients with schizophrenia. Br J Psychiatry 151:634–638, 1987

Jolley AG, Hirsch SR, Morrison E, et al: Trial of brief intermittent neuroleptic prophylaxis for selected schizophrenic outpatients: clinical and social outcome at two years. BMJ 301:837–842, 1990

Josiassen RC, Joseph A, Kohegyi E, et al: Clozapine augmented with risperidone in the treatment of schizophrenia: a randomized, double-blind, placebo-controlled trial. Am J Psychiatry 162(1):130–136, 2005

Kane J, Lieberman J (eds): Maintenance Pharmacotherapy in Schizophrenia. New York, Raven, 1987

Kane JM, Rifkin A, Quitkin F, et al: Fluphenazine vs placebo in patients with remitted, acute first-episode schizophrenia. Arch Gen Psychiatry 39:70–73, 1982

Kane JM, Rifkin A, Woerner M, et al: Low-dose neuroleptic treatment of outpatient schizophrenics, I: preliminary results for relapse rates. Arch Gen Psychiatry 40:893–896, 1983

Kane JM, Woerner M, Lieberman J: Tardive dyskinesia: prevalence, incidence, and risk factors. Psychopharmacology Suppl 2:72–78, 1985

Kane JM, Woerner M, Sarantakos S: Depot neuroleptics: a comparative review of standard, intermediate, and low-dose regimens. J Clin Psychiatry 47 (suppl):30–33, 1986

Kane J, Honigfeld G, Singer J, et al: Clozapine for the treatment-resistant schizophrenic: a double-blind comparison with chlorpromazine. Arch Gen Psychiatry 45:789–796, 1988a

Kane JM, Honigfeld G, Singer J, et al: Clozapine in treatment-resistant schizophrenics. Psychopharmacol Bull 24:62–67, 1988b

Kane JM, Davis JM, Schooler N, et al: A multidose study of haloperidol decanoate in the maintenance treatment of schizophrenia. Am J Psychiatry 159:554–560, 2002

Kane JM, Eerdekens M, Lindenmayer JP, et al: Long-acting injectable risperidone: efficacy and safety of the first long-acting atypical antipsychotic. Am J Psychiatry 160:1125–1132, 2003

Kapur S, Seeman P: Antipsychotic agents differ in how fast they come off the dopamine D2 receptors: implications for atypical antipsychotic action. J Psychiatry Neurosci 25:161–166, 2000

Kapur S, Seeman P: Does fast dissociation from the dopamine d(2) receptor explain the action of atypical antipsychotics? A new hypothesis. Am J Psychiatry 158:360–369, 2001

Karson CN, Weinberger DR, Bigelow L, et al: Clonazepam treatment of chronic schizophrenia: negative results in a double-blind, placebo-controlled trial. Am J Psychiatry 139:1627–1628, 1982

Kaye NS: Ziprasidone augmentation of clozapine in 11 patients. J Clin Psychiatry 64:215–216, 2003

Kellner R, Wilson RM, Muldawer MD, et al: Anxiety in schizophrenia: the responses to chlordiazepoxide in an intensive design study. Arch Gen Psychiatry 32:1246–1254, 1975

Kennedy E, Song F, Hunter R, et al: Risperidone versus typical antipsychotic medication for schizophrenia. Cochrane Database Syst Rev (2):CD000440, 2000

Kinon BJ, Lieberman JA: Mechanisms of action of atypical antipsychotic drugs: a critical analysis. Psychopharmacology (Berl) 124:2–34, 1996

Kinon BJ, Kane JM, Johns C, et al: Treatment of neuroleptic-resistant schizophrenic relapse. Psychopharmacol Bull 29:309–314, 1993

Kirkpatrick B, Kopelowicz A, Buchanan RW, et al: Assessing the efficacy of treatments for the deficit syndrome of schizophrenia. Neuropsychopharmacology 22:303–310, 2000

Kontaxakis VP, Havaki-Kontaxaki BJ, Stamouli SS, et al: Toxic interaction between risperidone and clozapine: a case report. Prog Neuropsychopharmacol Biol Psychiatry 26:407–409, 2002

Lee MS, Kim YK, Lee SK, et al: A double-blind study of adjunctive sertraline in haloperidol-stabilized patients with chronic schizophrenia. J Clin Psychopharmacol 18:399–403, 1998

Lehman AF, Kreynbuhl J, Buchanan RW, et al: The Schizophrenia Patient Outcomes Research Team (PORT): updated treatment recommendations 2003. Schizophr Bull 30:193–217, 2004a

Lehman AF. Lieberman JA, Dixon LB, et al: Practice guideline for the treatment of patients with schizophrenia (second edition). Am J Psychiatry 161:1–56, 2004b

Lerner V, Chudakova B, Kravets S, et al: Combined use of risperidone and olanzapine in the treatment of patients with resistant schizophrenia: a preliminary case series report. Clin Neuropharmacol 23:284–286, 2000

Leucht S, Pitschel-Walz G, Abraham D, et al: Efficacy and extrapyramidal side-effects of the new antipsychotics olanzapine, quetiapine, risperidone, and sertindole compared to conventional antipsychotics and placebo: a meta-analysis of randomized controlled trials. Schizophr Res 35:51–68, 1999

Leucht S, McGrath J, White P, et al: Carbamazepine for schizophrenia and schizoaffective psychoses. Cochrane Database Syst Rev (3):CD001258, 2002

Leucht S, Wahlbeck K, Hamann J, et al: New generation antipsychotics versus low-potency conventional antipsychotics: a systematic review and meta-analysis. Lancet 361:1581–1589, 2003

Levinson DF, Simpson GM, Singh H, et al: Fluphenazine dose, clinical response, and extrapyramidal symptoms during acute treatment. Arch Gen Psychiatry 47:761–768, 1990

Lieberman JA: Prediction of outcome in first-episode schizophrenia. J Clin Psychiatry 54 (suppl):13–17, 1993

Lieberman JA: Dopamine partial agonists: a new class of antipsychotic. CNS Drugs 18:251–267, 2004

Lieberman JA, Stroup TS, McEvoy JP, et al: Effectiveness of antipsychotic drugs in patients with chronic schizophrenia. N Engl J Med 353:1209–1223, 2005

Lindenmayer JP: New pharmacotherapeutic modalities for negative symptoms in psychosis. Acta Psychiatr Scand Suppl 388:15–19, 1995

Linnoila M, Viukari M, Kietala O: Effect of sodium valproate on tardive dyskinesia. Br J Psychiatry 129:114–119, 1976

Loebel AD, Lieberman JA, Alvir JM, et al: Duration of psychosis and outcome in first-episode schizophrenia. Am J Psychiatry 149:1183–1188, 1992

Luby ED, Cohen BD, Rosenbaum G, et al: Study of a new schizophrenomimetic drug: sernyl. AMA Arch Neurol Psychiatry 81:363–369, 1959

Lynch MR: Schizophrenia and the D1 receptor: focus on negative symptoms. Prog Neuropsychopharmacol Biol Psychiatry 16:797–832, 1992

Marder SR, Van Putten T, Mintz J, et al: Low- and conventional-dose maintenance therapy with fluphenazine decanoate: two-year outcome. Arch Gen Psychiatry 44:518–521, 1987

Marder SR, Essock SM, Miller AL, et al: Physical health monitoring of patients with schizophrenia. Am J Psychiatry 161:1334–1349, 2004

May PR, Tuma AH, Yale C, et al: Schizophrenia—a follow-up study of results of treatment. Arch Gen Psychiatry 33:481–486, 1976

McCreadie RG, MacDonald IM: High dosage haloperidol in chronic schizophrenia. Br J Psychiatry 131:310–316, 1977

Meaney AM, Smith S, Howes OD, et al: Effects of long-term prolactin-raising antipsychotic medication on bone mineral density in patients with schizophrenia. Br J Psychiatry 184:503–508, 2004

Meltzer HY: Treatment of the neuroleptic-nonresponsive schizophrenic patient. Schizophr Bull 18:515–542, 1992

Meltzer HY, Alphs L, Green AI, et al: Clozapine treatment for suicidality in schizophrenia: International Suicide Prevention Trial (InterSePT). Arch Gen Psychiatry 60:82–91, 2003

Miller AL, Craig CS: Combination antipsychotics: pros, cons, and questions. Schizophr Bull 28:105–109, 2002

Miller KK: Management of hyperprolactinemia in patients receiving antipsychotics. CNS Spectr 9 (8 suppl 7):28–32, 2004

Morgenstern H, Glazer WM: Identifying risk factors for tardive dyskinesia among long-term outpatients maintained with neuroleptic medications: results of the Yale Tardive Dyskinesia Study. Arch Gen Psychiatry 50:723–733, 1993

Mowerman S, Siris SG: Adjunctive loxapine in a clozapine-resistant cohort of schizophrenic patients. Ann Clin Psychiatry 8:193–197, 1996

Mullen J, Jibson MD, Sweitzer D: A comparison of the relative safety, efficacy, and tolerability of quetiapine and risperidone in outpatients with schizophrenia and other psychotic disorders: the Quetiapine Experience With Safety and Tolerability (QUEST) study. Clin Ther 23:1839–1854, 2001

Neborsky R, Janowsky D, Munson E, et al: Rapid treatment of acute psychotic symptoms with high- and low-dose haloperidol: behavioral considerations. Arch Gen Psychiatry 38:195–199, 1981

Perkins DO: Predictors of noncompliance in patients with schizophrenia. J Clin Psychiatry 63:1121–1128, 2002

Perovich RM, Lieberman JA, Fleischhacker WW, et al: The behavioral toxicity of bromocriptine in patients with psychiatric illness. J Clin Psychopharmacol 9:417–422, 1989

Plasky P: Antidepressant usage in schizophrenia. Schizophr Bull 17:649–657, 1991

Quitkin F, Rifkin A, Klein DF: Very high dosage vs standard dosage fluphenazine in schizophrenia: a double-blind study of nonchronic treatment-refractory patients. Arch Gen Psychiatry 32:1276–1281, 1975

Raskin S, Durst R, Katz G, et al: Olanzapine and sulpiride: a preliminary study of combination/augmentation in patients with treatment-resistant schizophrenia. J Clin Psychopharmacol 20:500–503, 2000

Reinstein M, Sirotovskaya L, Jones L: Effect of clozapine-quetiapine combination therapy on weight and glycaemic control. Clin Drug Invest 18:99–104, 1999

Rifkin A: Pharmacologic strategies in the treatment of schizophrenia. Psychiatr Clin North Am 16:351–363, 1993

Rifkin A, Quitkin F, Rabiner CJ, et al: Fluphenazine decanoate, fluphenazine hydrochloride given orally, and placebo in remitted schizophrenics, I: relapse rates after one year. Arch Gen Psychiatry 34:43–47, 1977

Rifkin A, Doddi S, Karajgi B, et al: Dosage of haloperidol for schizophrenia. Arch Gen Psychiatry 48:166–170, 1991

Robinson D, Woerner MG, Alvir JM, et al: Predictors of relapse following response from a first episode of schizophrenia or schizoaffective disorder. Arch Gen Psychiatry 56:241–247, 1999a

Robinson DG, Woerner MG, Alvir JM, et al: Predictors of treatment response from a first episode of schizophrenia or schizoaffective disorder. Am J Psychiatry 156:544–549, 1999b

Robinson DG, Woerner MG, Alvir JM, et al: Predictors of medication discontinuation by patients with first-episode schizophrenia and schizoaffective disorder. Schizophr Res 57:209–219, 2002

Rosse RB, Fay-McCarthy M, Kendrick K, et al: D-cycloserine adjuvant therapy to molindone in the treatment of schizophrenia. Clin Neuropharmacol 19:444–450, 1996

Schooler NR: Reducing dosage in maintenance treatment of schizophrenia: review and prognosis. Br J Psychiatry Suppl December (22):58–65, 1993

Schooler NR, Levine J, Severe JB, et al: Prevention of relapse in schizophrenia: an evaluation of fluphenazine decanoate. Arch Gen Psychiatry 37:16–24, 1980

Sheitman BB, Lindgren JC, Early J, et al: High-dose olanzapine for treatment-refractory schizophrenia. Am J Psychiatry 154:1626, 1997

Shiloh R, Zemishlany Z, Aizenberg D, et al: Sulpiride augmentation in people with schizophrenia partially responsive to clozapine: a double-blind, placebo-controlled study. Br J Psychiatry 171:569–573, 1997

Silver H, Nassar A: Fluvoxamine improves negative symptoms in treated chronic schizophrenia: an add-on double-blind, placebo-controlled study. Biol Psychiatry 31:698–704, 1992

Silver H, Barash I, Aharon N, et al: Fluvoxamine augmentation of antipsychotics improves negative symptoms in psychotic chronic schizophrenic patients: a placebo-controlled study. Int Clin Psychopharmacol 15:257–261, 2000

Siris SG: Adjunctive medication in the maintenance treatment of schizophrenia and its conceptual implications. Br J Psychiatry Suppl (22):66–78, 1993

Siris SG, van Kammen DP, Docherty JP: Use of antidepressant drugs in schizophrenia. Arch Gen Psychiatry 35:1368–1377, 1978

Siris SG, Bermanzohn PC, Mason SE, et al: Maintenance imipramine therapy for secondary depression in schizophrenia: a controlled trial. Arch Gen Psychiatry 51:109–115, 1994

Stroup TS, McEvoy JP, Swartz MS, et al: The National Institute of Mental Health Clinical Antipsychotic Trials of Intervention Effectiveness (CATIE) project: schizophrenia trial design and protocol development. Schizophr Bull 29:15–31, 2003

Stubbs JH, Haw CM, Staley CJ, et al: Augmentation with sulpiride for a schizophrenic patient partially responsive to clozapine. Acta Psychiatr Scand 102:390–393; discussion 393–394, 2000

Tollefson GD, Beasley CM Jr, Tran PV, et al: Olanzapine versus haloperidol in the treatment of schizophrenia and schizoaffective and schizophreniform disorders: results of an international collaborative trial. Am J Psychiatry 154:457–465, 1997

Tollefson GD, Birkett MA, Kiesler GM, et al: Double-blind comparison of olanzapine versus clozapine in schizophrenic patients clinically eligible for treatment with clozapine. Biol Psychiatry 49:52–63, 2001

Tran PV, Dellva MA, Tollefson GD, et al: Extrapyramidal symptoms and tolerability of olanzapine versus haloperidol in the acute treatment of schizophrenia. J Clin Psychiatry 58:205–211, 1997a

Tran PV, Hamilton SH, Kuntz AJ, et al: Double-blind comparison of olanzapine versus risperidone in the treatment of schizophrenia and other psychotic disorders. J Clin Psychopharmacol 17:407–418, 1997b

Tsai G, Yang P, Chung LC, et al: D-serine added to antipsychotics for the treatment of schizophrenia. Biol Psychiatry 44:1081–1089, 1998

Tsai GE, Yang P, Chung LC, et al: D-serine added to clozapine for the treatment of schizophrenia. Am J Psychiatry 156:1822–1825, 1999

U.S. Food and Drug Administration: Warning about hyperglycemia and atypical antipsychotic drugs. FDA Patient Safety News, Show #28, June 2004. Available at: http://www.accessdata.fda.gov/scripts/cdrh/cfdocs/psn/printer.cfm?id=229. Accessed December 6, 2005.

U.S. Preventive Services Task Force: Screening adults for lipid disorders: recommendations and rationale. Am J Prev Med 20:73–76, 2001

Van Putten T, May PR, Marder SR: Response to antipsychotic medication: the doctor's and the consumer's view. Am J Psychiatry 141:16–19, 1984

Van Putten T, Marder SR, Mintz J: A controlled dose comparison of haloperidol in newly admitted schizophrenic patients. Arch Gen Psychiatry 47:754–758, 1990

Volavka J, Cooper T, Czobor P, et al: Haloperidol blood levels and clinical effects. Arch Gen Psychiatry 49:354–361, 1992

Wang PS, Walker AM, Tsuang MT, et al: Dopamine antagonists and the development of breast cancer. Arch Gen Psychiatry 59:1147–1154, 2002

Wassef AA, Dott SG, Harris A, et al: Randomized, placebo-controlled pilot study of divalproex sodium in the treatment of acute exacerbations of chronic schizophrenia. J Clin Psychopharmacol 20:357–361, 2000

Weiden PJ, Mann JJ, Dixon L, et al: Is neuroleptic dysphoria a healthy response? Compr Psychiatry 30:546–552, 1989

Weissman EM: Antipsychotic prescribing practices in the Veterans Healthcare Administration—New York metropolitan region. Schizophr Bull 28:31–42, 2002

Wirshing DA, Wirshing WC, Kysar L, et al: Novel antipsychotics: comparison of weight gain liabilities. J Clin Psychiatry 60:358–363, 1999

Wolkowitz OM, Pickar D: Benzodiazepines in the treatment of schizophrenia: a review and reappraisal. Am J Psychiatry 148:714–726, 1991

Wyatt RJ: Early intervention for schizophrenia: can the course of the illness be altered? Biol Psychiatry 38:1–3, 1995

PSYCHOSOCIAL THERAPIES

MARVIN S. SWARTZ, M.D.

JOHN LAURIELLO, M.D.

ROBERT E. DRAKE, M.D., PH.D.

Major advances in the treatment of schizophrenia were heralded by the development of antipsychotic drugs in the 1950s and 1960s, which are clearly effective for the treatment of acute symptomatology and the prevention of relapse (Lauriello et al. 2003). However, long-term follow-up studies have consistently shown that the great majority of persons with schizophrenia continue to be plagued by residual psychotic symptoms, cognitive deficits, and other psychosocial problems, and only a small percentage of patients with schizophrenia recover completely.

Antipsychotic medications, including the new generation of antipsychotics, reduce positive symptoms and, to some extent, negative symptoms, but medications to date have had a limited effect on cognitive impairment and social and vocational functioning. For the great majority of patients, medications help with symptom control but do not clearly preserve or restore premorbid levels of social and vocational functioning and do not lead to normal functioning. Moreover, 20% or more of schizophrenic patients have psychotic symptoms that do not respond to antipsychotic medications, and many other patients have residual symptoms.

As a result of the limited effectiveness of antipsychotics, it is clear that most patients will need psychosocial therapies to address disabling residual symptoms, impaired social and vocational functioning, or risk of future relapse (Lauriello et al. 2003). Thus, a pressing need exists to develop empirically validated psychosocial interventions. This need has been addressed by the resurgence in research on treatment methods and systems of care for severely mentally ill patients.

In this chapter, we review the current state of key psychosocial interventions designed to augment and complement treatment with medications. Effective psychosocial treatments should not merely reduce overt psychotic symptoms or rates of hospitalization but also lead to gains in cognitive abilities and social skills, quality of life, and sustained competitive employment; reduction of comorbid substance abuse; and improvements in other domains. We review the major psychosocial treatment approaches that have a substantial evidence base. In addition, we highlight the trend toward optimizing patient preferences in the choice of treatment modality, including the increasing interest in peer-run or peer-assisted treatment approaches. We also highlight the dissemination of evidence-based practices in usual care settings spearheaded by the "Implementing Evidence-Based Practices for Severe Mental Illness Project" sponsored by the Robert Wood Johnson Foundation, the Center for Mental Health Services and Substance Abuse and Mental Health Services Administration, the National Alliance for the Mentally Ill, and state and local mental health organizations in several states (Torrey et al. 2001).

INDIVIDUAL PSYCHOTHERAPIES FOR SCHIZOPHRENIA

Although individual psychodynamic psychotherapy for schizophrenia has largely been abandoned, a summary of its role will provide a historical context for the discussion of other psychosocial treatments. For nearly 60 years, psychodynamically oriented psychotherapists assumed that the same basic treatment approaches applied to neurotic spectrum patients could be adapted to patients with severe psychosis. Case reports appeared to document that some patients diagnosed with schizophrenia improved with intensive insight-oriented treatment. In retrospect, some reports may have involved treatment of psychosis in the context of either a mood disorder or non-schizophrenia-spectrum disorders.

The effectiveness of individual psychodynamic psychotherapy for schizophrenia was tested in two landmark studies. May (1968) and colleagues sought to show the effectiveness of psychotherapy alone or in combination with medications. Moderately ill patients with schizophrenia were divided into five treatment groups: milieu therapy, individual therapy, antipsychotic treatment, electroconvulsive treatment, or antipsychotic treatment combined with individual psychotherapy. Antipsychotic treatment alone or in combination with individual psychotherapy showed superior response compared with the other groups. Next in order of effectiveness was electroconvulsive therapy, followed by individual psychotherapy or milieu treatment. Unexpectedly, the combination of antipsychotic medication and individual therapy conferred no advantage over antipsychotic medication alone. This study, however, was criticized for using relatively inexperienced therapists and a possibly inadequate dose of weekly psychotherapy.

Stanton and colleagues (1984) sought to address the criticisms of the May study by deploying experienced psychotherapists in more intensive treatment. Psychodynamically oriented psychotherapy was administered three times a week by experienced therapists and contrasted with weekly supportive psychotherapy. Both treatment

groups received antipsychotic medications administered by a psychopharmacologist blind to experimental condition. The intensive psychotherapy conditions showed no superiority compared with supportive psychotherapy and were associated with greater attrition, particularly with more severely symptomatic patients. Even among less symptomatic patients, the outcome favored the nonpsychodynamic treatment. The results of these studies and the growing influence of alternative models of psychotherapy have diminished the interest in the psychodynamic treatment of schizophrenia.

More recent approaches to individual therapy, informed by the "stress-vulnerability" hypothesis of schizophrenia, have received recent study and include individual personal therapy and cognitive-behavioral therapy (CBT). These psychotherapies attempt to ameliorate residual psychotic symptoms and prevent relapse by modifying individual patterns of stress and response to the illness.

PERSONAL THERAPY

Hogarty and colleagues (1995), at the University of Pittsburgh, developed *personal therapy*. They believed that patients with psychotic disorders could benefit by learning to anticipate and manage their episode-related affective arousal and sources of stress. Personal therapy was designed to be flexibly administered to follow the pace of the individual patient's progress, while maintaining standardization suitable for empirical study. The therapeutic approach used in personal therapy includes stress reduction and cognitive reframing techniques as well as vocational rehabilitation principles. Each weekly session of 30–45 minutes involves an approach that is individualized for the patient's stage of illness. In the initial phase of therapy, the focus is on educating the patient about the relation between stress and symptoms. The intermediate phase is designed to help patients develop relaxation and reframing techniques to reduce stress. The third phase offers patients an opportunity to use these skills in social and vocational settings, usually at about 18 months into treatment.

A 3-year trial of personal therapy (Hogarty et al. 1997a, 1997b) contrasted four treatment conditions: personal therapy, family therapy, supportive therapy, and family therapy combined with personal therapy. The trial found that personal therapy was no more effective than the other therapies in the primary outcome of relapse prevention. However, personal therapy was superior in social adjustment outcomes, with the greatest benefit occurring during the last 2 years of treatment. The study reported that only 60% of the patients in the personal therapy condition were able to progress to the third phase of therapy, in which skills were tested in real-world settings.

COGNITIVE-BEHAVIORAL THERAPY

CBT approaches to schizophrenia draw on previous work in depression and anxiety disorders. Largely led by investigators in Great Britain, studies have focused on the use of CBT to address residual psychotic symptoms, whereas more recent studies have sought to apply CBT to acute episodes. One approach, *coping strategy enhancement*, is used to decrease distress by teaching coping mechanisms by which the patient can distract himself or herself and ignore the content of some residual psychotic symptoms. CBT has been shown to reduce delusions that had persisted approximately 6 months but has had limited ability to reduce other symptoms or to improve social and vocational functioning (Tarrier et al. 1993).

Other CBT approaches attempt to decrease the severity of delusions by cognitively challenging the veracity of the delusions (Chadwick et al. 1994). Cognitive challenges are followed by a "behavioral experiment," which effectively tests the reality of delusional beliefs. Modifications of this approach have attempted to reduce persistent hallucinations that had appeared to be more resistant to CBT. Patients are directed to attend to individual characteristics of the hallucinations and their meaning and thus begin to see the internal origins of hallucinations (Bentall et al. 1994).

A study by Kuipers and colleagues (1998) randomized 60 individuals with schizophrenia to either a 9-month course of CBT plus usual care or usual care alone. Outcomes were assessed at the end of treatment and 9 months posttreatment. Patients receiving CBT had a significant reduction in overall symptom scores (29% for CBT group vs. 2% for control group), delusional distress, and frequency of hallucinations at the end of treatment; these differences continued to be significant 9 months after treatment ended.

Another study by Tarrier and colleagues (1998) compared CBT with supportive counseling and routine care alone and found significant reductions in delusions and hallucinations in the CBT group. At 12-month follow-up (Tarrier et al. 1999), CBT was still superior to the other treatment conditions. However, at 24 months, both CBT and supportive counseling groups were still superior to the control condition, but the CBT group had lost its advantage over the supportive therapy condition (Tarrier et al. 2000). Sensky and colleagues (2000) compared patients who received routine care in addition to CBT with a befriending intervention of equal intensity. In this study, both groups showed reduced psychotic symptoms after 9 months of treatment. However, at 9-month follow-up, symptom reduction was sustained in the CBT group but not in the comparison condition.

Psychoeducational medication management training, cognitive psychotherapy, cognitive therapy addressed to family members, and standard care were contrasted in various combinations in a study by Buchkremer and colleagues (1997). The intervention lasted 8 months, with follow-up assessments at 1 and 2 years. The treatment group combinations did not show a significant difference in psychopathological symptoms, compliance, or rehospitalization rates compared with the control group. However, the group that received all three interventions (psychoeducational medication management training, cognitive psychotherapy, and cognitive therapy addressed to family members) showed a trend toward fewer hospitalizations.

Tarrier and colleagues (1993) compared two forms of CBT: coping strategy enhancement and a problem-solving intervention for patients with medication-resistant symptoms. Both groups showed reductions in psychotic symptoms, with no significant differences between groups. Unfortunately, the study did not include a control condition, limiting the interpretability of these findings. Drury and colleagues (1996) attempted to test the efficacy of CBT in acute episodes and found that acutely psychotic inpatients receiving CBT in addition to antipsychotic medication experienced a significantly faster and more complete remission compared with a control group that spent equal hours with a therapist doing structured or supportive activities. At 9-month follow-up, the CBT group continued to report significantly fewer symptoms. One limitation of this study was that psychopathology measures were rated by unblinded treatment staff.

A brief CBT-based intervention known as compliance therapy, targeted at improved adherence to antipsychotic medication regimens in acutely psychotic inpatients, resulted in significant improvements in compliance, attitudes toward drug treatment, and insight into illness compared with control subjects receiving standard treatment (Kemp et al. 1996). These gains were still present at 6-month follow-up; however, the predicted improvements in social functioning or symptomatologies were not seen.

To date, CBT has not been shown to improve social or vocational functioning (Kuipers et al. 1997, 1998) or relapse rates (Tarrier et al. 1998), and studies reporting effects for negative symptoms generally have not found significant improvements associated with CBT (Buchkremer et al. 1997; Drury et al. 1996; Tarrier et al. 1998). In fact, patients with only negative symptoms have been excluded from CBT trials because of poor response (Garety et al. 2000). However, Sensky and colleagues (2000), in the study described previously, did find an improvement in negative symptoms in the CBT group at 9-month follow-up, suggesting that CBT may affect negative symptoms over time.

ILLNESS MANAGEMENT AND RECOVERY RESOURCE TOOL KIT

Other individually based approaches to treatment have focused on improving knowledge about mental illnesses—so-called psychoeducational programs. These programs provide information about mental illness, symptoms, the roles of stress and vulnerability, and approaches to treatment. Mueser and colleagues (2002) reviewed the controlled trials of psychoeducational models and found that three out of four controlled studies improved knowledge about mental illness, but only one of these had an appreciable effect on treatment adherence. The authors concluded that psychoeducation should play a role in other interventions but should not be expected to improve treatment outcomes without additional interventions.

Mueser and colleagues (2002) also reviewed other promising approaches to individual treatment and noted that four complementary approaches have a strong evidence base: 1) psychoeducational progams increase knowledge and awareness of illness, 2) behavioral tailoring approaches reduce behavioral barriers to adherence behaviors, 3) warning sign recognition treatment helps avert relapse, and 4) CBT reduces residual psychotic symptomatology. Mueser and colleagues combined these four approaches in a manualized combined intervention termed *Illness Management and Recovery*. The approach also has been developed into an evidence-based resource tool kit and is being disseminated as part of the national "Implementing Evidence-Based Practices Project" (see http://www.mentalhealthpractices.org). Although the approach is a logical and promising one, definitive study of this combined treatment modality awaits further testing.

FAMILY TREATMENT

Early approaches to family interventions in schizophrenia tended to view dysfunctional family behavior as causally related to schizophrenia. It is now widely accepted that familial dysfunction is largely secondary to the stress of living with a seriously ill relative. Nevertheless, family stress and distressed interactions do appear to have a significant effect on the course of illness. These distressed family interactions have been defined and referred to as *expressed emotion*.

Brown and Rutter (1966) developed the concept of expressed emotion to explain why some hospitalized patients with schizophrenia who had had a good response to pharmacological treatment relapsed soon after returning home. The construct of expressed emotion was empirically derived and refers to three related family behaviors:

high frequency of critical comments, hostility, and emotional overinvolvement. Patients with extensive contact with families with high expressed emotion have been found to have significantly higher rates of relapse despite adequate medication compliance (Kavanagh 1992; Leff et al. 1982). Research on expressed emotion has shown that it is a significant risk factor for relapse in many psychiatric and nonpsychiatric illnesses (Kavanagh 1992) and can be a factor in patient outcome in multiple care settings, social groups, or stressful treatment approaches (Moore et al. 1992; Snyder et al. 1994).

A more general view of the role of family relationships and schizophrenia is that persons with a chronic, relapsing illness tend to manifest exacerbations of illness with continued stress and that illness exacerbation creates stressful family relationships. Most controlled clinical interventions have documented the effectiveness of various family interventions for reducing relapse in the index patient (Leff 1996). Relapse rates for patients with schizophrenia whose families undergo psychoeducational and stress-modifying family treatment are approximately 24% compared with 64% for routine treatment (Mueser and Glynn 1998), similar to the magnitude of treatment effect seen with maintenance antipsychotic medication. Interventions that are longer in duration (typically longer than 9 months) appear to provide long-term relapse prevention and have been found to persist for 2 years (Mueser and Glynn 1998) or longer (Tarrier et al. 1994).

Reduction of high expressed emotion has been hypothesized to be the key ingredient in the efficacy of family interventions. In interventions with families with high expressed emotion, nonrelapsing patients were more likely to reside in families that had changed from high to low expressed emotion during treatment (Falloon et al. 1982; Hogarty et al. 1986; Leff et al. 1982; Tarrier et al. 1988). Critics of these studies pointed out that relatively few families in these studies were reassessed and that no clear correlation was found between reductions in expressed emotion and relapse. Critics further argued that a high expressed emotion status could be a consequence of relapse itself or patient illness severity and that proving a causal relation between expressed emotion and relapse required a controlled study, including interim expressed emotion assessments. Tarrier and colleagues' (1988) family study assessed expressed emotion at baseline, 4.5 months, and 9 months, but the reductions in expressed emotion found in the relatives in the experimental treatment also were found in the control condition.

The Treatment Strategies for Schizophrenia Study (Schooler et al. 1997) was one of the few large-scale studies investigating the efficacy of maintenance medication treatment combined with family intervention. The study found that standard dosing of depot antipsychotics is superior to both placebo and very-low-dose strategies for relapse prevention and that discontinuing medication and then restarting it when symptoms first appear is not effective at preventing relapse. The study also showed that relatively nonintensive multifamily psychoeducational monthly groups provided equal long-term relapse prevention compared with more intensive family treatment. These findings suggest the value of engaging families early in psychoeducational interventions that emphasize realistic expectations, support, detection of early warning signs of relapse, and medication compliance (American Psychiatric Association 1997).

McFarlane and colleagues (1996) studied schizophrenia patients at high risk for relapse because of histories of poor compliance, violence, and homelessness. Half of the patients and families received biweekly multifamily group treatment, and half received family intervention only during crises. No differences in relapse were seen for the two treatment groups (27% at 2 years), again suggesting that more intensive family treatment is not necessarily better.

Family intervention studies also have yielded negative findings. In a study of adolescent patients early in the illness, Linszen and colleagues (Linszen et al. 1996; Nugter et al. 1997) found that both the group receiving family treatment and the control group had equally low (16%–20%) overall relapse rates at 1 year, although the active comparison intervention involved a fairly intensive individual treatment approach. Similarly, in Hogarty and colleagues' (1997b) study of personal therapy, their family therapy arm offered no advantage over supportive therapy in preventing relapse, which was relatively low at 29% over 3 years. Similar to the Linszen study, the supportive therapy group in this study received enriched services, including biweekly sessions, minimum effective medication dosage, and case management. These studies illustrate that these interventions may lack adequate statistical power if the base relapse rate is low in the population selected or if the comparison treatment condition is too intensive. In studies with newer antipsychotic regimens with potentially lower relapse rates (Csernansky et al. 2002), the effects of family intervention may be more difficult to detect.

Family intervention studies also have improved outcomes in family stress, coping, and knowledge of schizophrenia (Barrowclough and Tarrier 1990; Dixon et al. 2001; Falloon et al. 1987; McFarlane et al. 1996; Zhang and Yan 1993). However, these improved outcomes may be highly correlated with reduced relapse, suggesting no independent effect of family intervention on these outcomes. The relation between relapse and social function-

ing has been assessed in two studies (Hogarty et al. 1997a; Schooler et al. 1997), in which relapsed subjects reentered their original treatment group once stabilized, and social functioning was assessed between relapses. Neither study found an advantage in social functioning for the experimental family treatment group. Interest in family treatment approaches should be stimulated by dissemination of a "Family Psychoeducation" resource tool kit through the national "Implementing Evidence-Based Practices Project" (Dixon et al. 2001).

SOCIAL SKILLS TRAINING

Even with the anticipated development of more efficacious medication regimens, most patients with schizophrenia will likely continue to have residual symptoms, cognitive impairments, and impaired social skills. Systematic research over the past several decades has sought to use psychosocial interventions to reduce functional impairments in schizophrenia. These psychiatric rehabilitation interventions draw on concepts from the rehabilitation of physical disabilities and use the principles of learning theory to improve the person's social competence and functioning in the domains of self-care, work, leisure, and family relationships. Social skills training (SST) is a carefully defined set of interventions specifically targeted toward acquisition of social functioning skills. There are currently three models of SST:

1. *Basic*—entails identifying and "overlearning" components of social interactions through repetition, with the expectation that these repertoires will be incorporated into natural interactions.
2. *Social problem solving*—attempts to correct deficits in receptive learning, processing, and sending skills according to the theory that faulty information processing is a key cause of social skills deficits.
3. *Cognitive remediation*—targets more fundamental cognitive impairments, including attention and planning. The model was based on the assumption that improving cognitive impairments will support more complex cognitive processes, leading to improved social skills.

BASIC MODEL

The basic SST model entails breaking down complex social repertoires into their basic elements, such as eye contact, speech volume, length of response, questioning, and other behaviors. Through repetitive practice and modeling by the therapist, new skills are acquired and then developed into a functional repertoire. The patient uses role-playing to practice integrating the social repertoires with the therapist and peers and is directed to practice in a real-world setting.

This model can be successfully implemented, with acquisition of social skills that persist anywhere between 6 and 12 months (Bellack and Mueser 1993). It is unclear whether the improvement in these social skills generalizes to improved symptomatology and reduced relapse rates. Investigators in Pittsburgh, Pennsylvania (Hogarty et al. 1986, 1991), found that patients receiving an intensive trial of SST combined with antipsychotic medications had a significantly lower relapse rate than did a group receiving only medications (30% vs. 46%). These gains persisted at 21 months but not at 24 months. This finding suggests that SST and other psychosocial interventions may require booster sessions or ongoing treatment to maintain a favorable effect.

Although the targeted skills in the basic model of SST can be acquired, generalization to the patient's natural environment has not been clearly shown (Bellack and Mueser 1993). Development of the social problem-solving model was intended to address these limitations.

Social Problem-Solving Model

The social problem-solving model assumes that impairments in information processing underlie the limited social competence present in many patients with schizophrenia. Specific domains of skill acquisition are broken down into modules on medication management, symptom management, recreation, basic conversation, and self-care. Patients can be assigned the modules that are the most salient. It is hoped that greater durability and generalization of social skills will be acquired through emphasis on learning, receiving, processing, and retaining skills. Marder and colleagues (1996) examined social adjustment among patients assigned to the problem-solving model compared with patients assigned to equally intensive supportive therapy and found a small but statistically significant advantage for the problem-solving intervention in two of six measures of social adjustment after 2 years. In a study comparing 6 months of treatment with either the problem-solving group model or equally intensive occupational therapy, Liberman and colleagues (1998) found that the problem-solving group had superior outcomes in 3 of 10 independent living skills that were maintained up to 18 months after completing the intervention. In this study, case managers assigned to each patient actively encouraged the patient to apply skills learned in the community, suggesting that generalization of skills may be fostered by community-based reinforcement.

Cognitive Remediation

Although patients with schizophrenia clearly have a wide range of cognitive impairments (Braff 1993), some deficits have been attributed to psychotic symptoms or medication side effects. Findings of cognitive impairments in persons at risk for schizophrenia, but not yet symptomatic or treated, make it unlikely that cognitive deficits are purely secondary to medication effects. Cognitive impairments associated with schizophrenia have not been definitively characterized, but some particular functions such as attention, memory, and planning appear to be more affected than others. Psychopharmacological interventions to ameliorate or prevent cognitive deficits are active areas of investigation. In addition, the practice of cognitive remediation of schizophrenia is an area of intensive investigation.

Given the limitations on the durability and generalizability of SST, researchers have sought to improve the impairments in elementary cognitive functions before teaching social skills as a way to "boost" the effectiveness of SST. Cognitive remediation shows some promise in improving performance and measures of vigilance and planning. However, insufficient evidence shows that these improvements generalize to other cognitive tests or particular social skills.

Integrated psychological treatment (Brenner et al. 1992), developed by researchers in Switzerland, is based on the theory that dysfunctions in lower and higher levels of cognitive deficits interact to diminish social competence, leading to increased stress resulting from difficult social interactions and to further impairment in cognitive functioning. Integrated psychological treatment includes sequential subprograms targeted to cognitive social functioning: the cognitive differentiation subprogram emphasizes treatment of basic cognitive skills through computer-based training in card sorting and concept formation; social perception and verbal communication subprograms refine these skills into verbal and social responses through social problem-solving exercises; and social skills and interpersonal problem-solving subprograms address more complex interpersonal problems through similar techniques to the motor skills models.

Outcome studies of cognitive remediation have been mixed. Controlled studies of integrated psychological treatment in schizophrenia have reported modest gains in elementary cognitive functions but no clear benefit for complex cognitive tasks or social and vocational functioning (Brenner et al. 1992). A study by Wykes and colleagues (1999) comparing intensive cognitive remediation and comparably intensive occupational therapy targeting deficits in executive functioning showed improvements in

3 of 12 cognitive measures but no direct improvements in social or vocational functioning or symptomatology. In a study of cognitive remediation before skills training, compared with a mirror image regimen, Hodel and Brenner (1994) found no advantage to initial treatment with cognitive remediation. No clear evidence to date indicates that integrated psychological treatment generalizes to improved symptomatology and social competence in real-world settings.

Ninety severely impaired long-term hospital patients were offered equally intensive 6-month duration cognitive remediation plus social problem-solving modules compared with supportive therapy also paired with social problem-solving modules (Spaulding et al. 1999). The cognitive remediation group had better outcomes in two of four measures of social competence and showed better acquisition of skills in two of four of the social problem-solving modules, suggesting that the cognitive remediation approach can enhance response to more standard skills training in very ill institutionalized patients.

An additional approach to SST is embodied by the clubhouse model of psychosocial rehabilitation. Originated in 1948 at Fountain House in New York City, the clubhouse model was developed as a collaborative community of professional staff and persons with mental illness (Anderson 1998; Macias et al. 2001). Community activities within the clubhouse focus on the work-ordered day, in which staff and patients work together to maintain clubhouse functions, with the expectation that patients will gain social and vocational skills and ultimately transition to competitive employment with the support of clubhouse-related transitional vocational programs. The clubhouse model has been widely disseminated, and efforts since the late 1970s have focused on enhancing program fidelity. Clubhouses are highly regarded among patients but have been subject to little empirical study. Nonetheless, they represent an important and likely predominant method of social skills enhancement in the United States.

Newly developing programs run by consumers based on self-help principles are also spreading rapidly in many states (Yanos et al. 2001). Many patients with serious mental illness have highlighted the importance of their participation in peer-run or self-help programs. Patients point to the role of self-help and peer-led services in promoting psychological well-being, empowerment, and sense of self-efficacy. There has been little empirical research on the effectiveness of self-help organizations and related interventions. Emerging empirical work on consumer-run and self-help services will elucidate the role of these services in community programs.

SUPPORTED EMPLOYMENT

The proportion of persons with chronic schizophrenia with competitive employment is 20% or lower (Bond et al. 2001a). Lack of sustainable living wages increases dependence on families and public assistance, contributes to low self-esteem and stigma, and often leads to a lack of daily structure and sense of purpose. With ever-shortening hospital stays, hospital-based vocational rehabilitation programs are no longer feasible, and vocational rehabilitation is largely community-based. Unfortunately, many approaches to vocational rehabilitation are not well suited to address the long-term impairment often associated with schizophrenia. In contrast to vocational rehabilitation programs in which patients are trained and then placed in the job, newer vocational models reverse that process.

In the late 1980s, new models of vocational rehabilitation, termed *supported employment*, were borrowed from the field of developmental disabilities. Supported employment focuses on individual placement after a rapid job search without extensive pre-employment assessment or training. After placement, patients are helped to learn skills and provided needed supports. Jobs often begin at just a few hours per week and increase over time. The focus is on mainstream jobs in the competitive labor market. Supported employment is provided in a wide variety of service contexts, including community mental health centers, community rehabilitation programs, clubhouses, and psychiatric rehabilitation centers.

A standardized approach to supported employment has been termed *individual placement and support*. The principles of individual placement and support have evolved as research shows how to improve employment outcomes (Becker and Drake 2003; Bond et al. 2001a, 2001b; Dixon et al. 2002; Drake et al. 1999; Lehman et al. 2002).

Key principles of the individual placement and support model include

1. *Competitive employment*—The goal of supported employment is competitive employment in work settings integrated into the community.
2. *Rapid job search*—Searching for jobs occurs early in the process of supported employment rather than following lengthy pre-employment assessment, training, or work trials.
3. *Integration of rehabilitation and mental health*—Vocational rehabilitation is considered an integral component of mental health treatment rather than a separate service. Optimally, employment specialists are integrated into multidisciplinary teams.

4. *Patient preferences*—Services are based on patients' preferences and choices rather than on providers' judgments.
5. *Continuous and comprehensive assessment*—Assessment occurs primarily in the course of community work experiences.
6. *Ongoing support*—Follow-along supports are tailored to the individual patient's needs and continued indefinitely.

Traditional vocational rehabilitation programs had limited success because workshop-based or sheltered employment skills were not generalizable to competitive employment settings (Bond et al. 2001a). In contrast, studies of the supported employment model have been consistently positive. Research has contrasted a traditional partial program to an integrated program of supported employment combined with case management. Subjects in the supported employment group significantly increased rates of competitive employment by 14%, whereas no improvement occurred in the control group (Drake et al. 1994). Two approaches to supportive employment—one with gradual entry and the other with accelerated job entry—were compared in another trial. Of the accelerated-entry patients, 56% were engaged in competitive employment compared with 29% of the gradual-entry group after 1 year (Bond et al. 1995).

Individual placement and support has shown effectiveness in diverse patient samples in New Hampshire and Washington, D.C. (Drake et al. 1999). An additional study compared individual placement and support with a standard psychosocial rehabilitation program in a population with severe mental illness and high rates of substance abuse and reported that the individual placement and support group was significantly more likely to obtain employment—42% versus 1%—although job retention was low, leveling off at 15%–20% (Lehman et al. 2002). The availability of a treatment manual for individual placement and support (Becker and Drake 1993) and a supported employment resource tool kit (Bond et al. 2001a) should stimulate further research into this treatment modality.

The benefits of supported employment have not fully extended to other nonvocational outcomes, such as improved self-esteem, improved quality of life, and reduction of symptoms and relapse. One noncontrolled study (Bell et al. 1996) indicated that patients who were paid in a Department of Veterans Affairs work placement program worked more hours, showed improvement in symptoms at follow-up, and had a reduced rate of hospitalization compared with unpaid patients. Fears that job stress would increase rates of relapse or other negative outcomes have not been borne out.

ASSERTIVE COMMUNITY TREATMENT

The dramatic shift in the locus of treatment from the hospital to the community had the unintended consequences of badly fragmenting the services and supports needed for persons with schizophrenia. In the posthospitalization era, services may be provided by a bewildering array of providers and agencies, including psychiatrists, nurses, pharmacists, social workers, vocational therapists, and housing providers. The traditionally constrained role of the case manager as a broker of community services often provides insufficient "glue" for the patients who lack the cognitive and social skills needed to integrate their own care.

As a response to service fragmentation, the assertive community treatment (ACT) program was originally developed by researchers in Madison, Wisconsin (Stein and Test 1980). ACT is currently the most carefully studied, defined, documented, and successful program being used in the delivery of services for persons with severe mental illness. In most ACT programs, patients are served by a multidisciplinary team that has a fixed caseload of patients and a high staff-to-patient ratio (1:10–12). ACT programs provide treatment, rehabilitation, and supports in the community 24 hours a day, 7 days a week. Services often provided include home delivery of medications, monitoring of physical and mental health, SST in the patient's natural environment, and support for family reintegration.

The landmark ACT study in Wisconsin (Stein and Test 1980) examined outcomes in a group of severely mentally ill patients assigned to ACT compared with a group discharged from the hospital to standard community care. The ACT group showed significant advantages in rates of hospitalization, employment, independent living, and family burden, with essentially no difference in costs; however, the advantages conferred by ACT did not persist after the patients were discharged from the experimental program. More than 25 control trials have shown the effectiveness of ACT in reducing hospitalization and other adverse outcomes and increasing patients' and their families' satisfaction (Burns and Santos 1995). Lehman et al. (1997) documented ACT's advantage over standard community care in a sample of homeless, chronically mentally ill persons. The superiority of ACT to comparison programs has been less consistent in studies of competitive employment, social functioning, quality of life, or other outcomes, prompting modification of ACT or leading to integration with other programs such as supported employment, family treatment, or dual-diagnosis treatment.

Bond and co-workers (2001b) reviewed the evidence on outcomes for ACT services (Table 18–1). Twenty-three control studies examined hospital outcomes for

TABLE 18–1. Studies comparing assertive community treatment with other interventions

	Selected outcome	Significantly better outcomes	Approximately equal outcomes	Significantly poorer outcomes
Hospital use	23	17	6	0
Housing stability	12	8	4	1
Symptoms	16	7	9	0
Quality of life	12	7	5	0
Social adjustment	13	3	10	0
Jail or arrest	10	2	7	1
Substance use	6	2	4	0
Taking medication as prescribed	4	2	2	0
Vocational outcomes	8	3	5	0
Consumer satisfaction	8	7	1	0

Source. Data from Bond et al. 2001b.

ACT patients and for those served by comparison programs. Seventeen trials found ACT to be superior in reducing hospital use. Similarly, of 12 studies examining residential stability, 8 studies found superior housing stability in the ACT condition, although one study found poorer outcomes for ACT patients. Of 16 studies that examined symptomatic outcomes in ACT programs, 7 trials found ACT to be superior. Quality of life was demonstrably superior in 7 of 12 control trials, and social adjustment improved in 3 of 13 trials. Jail or arrests were reduced in only 2 of 10 trials, and in one trial, poorer outcomes were found in the ACT condition. Substance abuse was improved in 2 of 6 trials. Medication adherence was improved in 2 of 4 studies. Vocational outcomes were improved in 3 of 8 studies. Consumer satisfaction was improved in 7 of 8 studies. Despite these impressive outcomes, these studies show that several outcome domains remain in which the performance of ACT could be improved, specifically in the areas of substance abuse, medication adherence, and vocational outcomes. New models of ACT, which integrate substance abuse treatment and supported employment, hold promise for improving these outcomes.

Because of the complexity of the services provided by ACT, it is difficult to answer several questions about its effectiveness, including

- What are the key ingredients that prevent relapse and hospitalization?

- Is ACT more cost-effective than other high-intensity services or modified ACT models?
- What minimum program intensity is needed to maintain gains?
- Which special populations of patients may require indefinite treatment?

It is clear, however, that programs that maintain good fidelity to the original ACT model have better outcomes (Scott and Dixon 1995). Dissemination of an ACT resource tool kit (Phillips et al. 2001) should strengthen interest in the fidelity of ACT in community programs.

INVOLUNTARY OUTPATIENT COMMITMENT AND RELATED PROCEDURES

In addition to the formal psychosocial interventions described earlier in this chapter, interest is growing in the use of legal tools designed to improve adherence with outpatient treatment such as involuntary civil commitment (Monahan et al. 2003). *Involuntary outpatient commitment,* one of these tools, is a controversial civil court procedure designed to benefit persons with serious mental illness who need ongoing psychiatric care and support to prevent relapse, hospital readmissions, homelessness, or incarceration but have difficulty following through with community-based treatment. Virtually all states in the United States permit some form of outpatient commitment. Forty states and the District of Columbia have explicit involuntary outpatient commitment statutes, and several states are currently considering enacting or modifying existing outpatient commitment legislation (Hiday 1992; McCafferty and Dooley 1990; Swartz et al. 1995; Torrey and Kaplan 1995).

Involuntary outpatient commitment may be distinguished from other related mechanisms of court-mandated treatment, including conditional release or guardianship. Under conditional release from a hospital, an involuntarily committed patient is released to community care under the ongoing supervision of the hospital, and this treatment is usually restricted to previously hospitalized and involuntarily committed patients. A limited number of naturalistic studies of conditional release indicate that it does appear to be effective in reducing rehospitalization and violent behavior (O'Keefe et al. 1997). Under guardianship, the court appoints a guardian for a patient adjudicated to be incompetent. The guardian consents to treatment for the patient, who then may be compelled to adhere to treatment, including forced medication and hospitalization. Geller et al. (1998) found that mandated treatment under guardianship appeared to reduce rehospitalizations and total hospital days.

Involuntary outpatient commitment orders typically require compliance with recommended outpatient treatment (i.e., keeping scheduled appointments with a mental health provider). Some outpatient commitment statutes stop short of permitting forced medication of legally competent individuals. In every jurisdiction, outpatient commitment orders are of limited duration. In North Carolina, a psychiatrist may recommend to the court that an outpatient be involuntarily committed initially not longer than 90 days, after which a hearing must be held to renew the order for up to 180 days. When a person under involuntary outpatient commitment fails to comply with treatment, the responsible clinician may request that law officers transport the individual to an outpatient facility for persuasion to accept treatment or evaluation for inpatient commitment (Swartz et al. 1995).

Naturalistic studies of involuntary outpatient commitment taken as a whole support the effectiveness of the procedure in reducing hospitalization and improving other outcomes, although all existing naturalistic studies had major design limitations (Fernandez and Nygard 1990; Hiday and Scheid-Cook 1987, 1989, 1991; Keilitz 1990; Moloy 1992; Ridgely et al. 2002). Two randomized controlled studies of involuntary outpatient commitment in North Carolina (Swartz et al. 1995) and New York City (Stead-man et al. 2001) provided conflicting views of the effectiveness of involuntary outpatient commitment. In North Carolina, where an involuntary outpatient commitment statute was well established, subjects under involuntary outpatient commitment who were ordered by the court to 180 days or more of involuntary outpatient commitment and were provided frequent outpatient services had decreased hospital readmissions, violence, victimization, family strain, and arrests and improved quality of life and treatment adherence, but subjects with short periods of involuntary outpatient commitment generally did not benefit (Borum et al. 1999; Compton et al. 2003; Hiday et al. 2002; Swanson et al. 1997, 2000, 2001, 2003; Swartz et al. 1999, 2001a, 2001b, 2002a, 2002b, 2003; Wagner et al. 2003). Critics of this study point out that neither the length of the outpatient commitment order nor the treatment intensity was controlled in the design, limiting the strength of the findings. In New York, the outpatient commitment study was part of a 3-year pilot program to test and evaluate outpatient commitment as a first step toward considering permanent outpatient commitment legislation for the state (Steadman et al. 2001). The study found no significant statistical differences between the control and experimental groups in follow-up hospitalizations, arrests, quality of life, symptoms, homelessness, or other outcomes. Critics of this study point out that during the start-up phase of the pilot program, implementation and enforcement of outpatient commitment were inadequate, and the study had a small sample size, making it difficult to detect meaningful differences between experimental groups.

Additional studies of involuntary outpatient commitment are needed to evaluate its effectiveness definitively, although some critics argue that involuntary outpatient commitment should not be used at all because it is coercive, may discourage patients from voluntarily seeking treatment, and would be unnecessary if optimal community-based treatment were universally available. Although these studies appear to provide contrary findings, both show wide variability in the implementation and practice of involuntary outpatient commitment. These differences render findings across studies difficult to compare and interpret. Even within North Carolina, where the findings of effectiveness of involuntary outpatient commitment have been most consistent, the "dose" of involuntary outpatient commitment varied widely as did the services provided to patients. Given that most states in the United States and several other countries explicitly permit involuntary outpatient commitment, attempts to study further the effectiveness of outpatient commitment are warranted if involuntary outpatient commitment is to be used appropriately.

CONCLUSION

Although antipsychotic medications were major advancements in schizophrenia therapeutics and helped make possible the era of deinstitutionalization, merely preventing rehospitalization can no longer be viewed as the final goal of treatment. Many patients can be maintained as outpatients despite persistent psychotic symptoms, pervasive negative symptoms, and poor social competence, but these residual impairments can no longer be regarded as acceptable outcomes. Newer antipsychotic drugs may significantly improve compliance, treatment of symptoms, and possibly relapse rates and overall outcome compared with the first generation of antipsychotics. Pharmacological interventions aimed at deficit symptoms may become available in the future as well.

Psychosocial interventions clearly will retain a pivotal place in the modern therapeutic armamentarium. Relatively simple interventions such as sustained family interventions and more comprehensive ACT programs are demonstrably effective in preventing relapse and hospital recidivism, and patients with treatment-resistant psychotic symptoms may benefit from new modalities of CBT. For patients with persistent negative symptoms and impaired social competence, SST shows great promise and should be more broadly available to such patients. As empirically validated therapies continue to emerge, implementation of these new treatment strategies in usual care settings will require careful attention.

It is also important to acknowledge emerging trends in psychosocial services and research—even though many newer approaches have not been definitively studied. Newer interventions are based on commonsense approaches to helping patients adapt and adjust to serious psychiatric disorders. These approaches generally involve use of education, skills training, and natural supports to help people learn to manage their own illnesses, to improve their functioning in normal adult roles, to reintegrate into their communities, and to pursue improved quality of life. These model approaches also place a primary focus on developing trusting, collaborative relationships between practitioners and patients to help patients pursue their own goals. Even though these approaches are termed *recovery-oriented* treatments, they share a hopeful outlook regarding long-term outcomes, a focus on patient preferences for outcomes and choice of interventions, and a focus on helping people to achieve community integration and to function in the real-life settings of their choice.

REFERENCES

American Psychiatric Association: Practice guidelines for the treatment of patients with schizophrenia. Am J Psychiatry 154:1–63, 1997

Anderson SB: We Are Not Alone: Fountain House and the Development of Clubhouse Culture. New York, Fountain House, 1998

Barrowclough C, Tarrier N: Social functioning in schizophrenic patients, I: the effects of expressed emotion and family intervention. Soc Psychiatry Psychiatr Epidemiol 25:125–129, 1990

Becker DR, Drake RE: A Working Life: The Individual Placement and Support (IPS) Program. Concord, New Hampshire–Dartmouth Psychiatric Research Center, 1993

Becker DR, Drake RE: A Working Life for People With Severe Mental Illness. New York, Oxford University Press, 2003

Bell MD, Lysaker PH, Milstein RM: Clinical benefits of paid work activity in schizophrenia. Schizophr Bull 22:51–67, 1996

Bellack AS, Mueser KT: Psychosocial treatment for schizophrenia. Schizophr Bull 19:317–336, 1993

Bentall RP, Haddock G, Slade PD: Cognitive therapy for persistent auditory hallucinations: from theory to therapy. Behav Ther 25:51–66, 1994

Bond GR, Dietzen LL, McGrew JH, et al: Accelerating entry into supported employment for persons with severe psychiatric disabilities. Rehabil Psychol 40:91–111, 1995

Bond GR, Becker DR, Drake RE, et al: Implementing supported employment as an evidence-based practice. Psychiatr Serv 52:313–322, 2001a

Bond GR, Drake RE, Mueser KT, et al: Assertive community treatment for people with severe mental illness. Disease Management and Health Outcomes 9:141–159, 2001b

Borum R, Swartz MS, Riley S, et al: Consumer perceptions of involuntary outpatient commitment. Psychiatr Serv 50:1489–1491, 1999

Braff DL: Information processing and attention dysfunctions in schizophrenia. Schizophr Bull 19:233–259, 1993

Brenner HD, Hodel B, Roder V, et al: Treatment of cognitive dysfunctions and behavioral deficits in schizophrenia. Schizophr Bull 18:21–26, 1992

Brown GW, Rutter M: The measurement of family activities and relationships: a methodological study. Hum Relat 2 (suppl):10–15, 1966

Buchkremer G, Klingberg S, Holle R, et al: Psychoeducational psychotherapy for schizophrenic patients and their key relatives or care-givers: results of a 2-year follow-up. Acta Psychiatr Scand 96:483–491, 1997

Burns BJ, Santos AB: Assertive community treatment: an update of randomized trials. Psychiatr Serv 46:669–675, 1995

Chadwick PD, Lowe CF, Horne P, et al: Modifying delusions: the role of empirical testing. Behav Ther 25:35–49, 1994

Compton SN, Swanson JW, Wagner HR, et al: Involuntary outpatient commitment and homelessness in persons with severe mental illness. Ment Health Serv Res 5:27–38, 2003

Csernansky JG, Mahmoud R, Brenner R: A comparison of risperidone and haloperidol for the prevention of relapse in patients with schizophrenia. N Engl J Med 346:16–22, 2002

Dixon L, McFarlane WR, Lefley H, et al: Evidence-based practices for services to families of people with psychiatric disabilities. Psychiatr Serv 52:903–910, 2001

Dixon L, Hoch JS, Clark R, et al: Cost-effectiveness of two vocational rehabilitation programs for persons with severe mental illness. Psychiatr Serv 53:1118–1124, 2002

Drake RE, Becker DR, Biesanz JC, et al: Rehabilitative day treatment vs supported employment, I: vocational outcomes. Community Ment Health J 30:519–532, 1994

Drake RE, McHugo GJ, Bebout RR, et al: A randomized clinical trial of supported employment for inner-city patients with severe mental disorders. Arch Gen Psychiatry 56:627–633, 1999

Drury V, Birchwood M, Cochrane R, et al: Cognitive therapy and recovery from acute psychosis: a controlled trial, I: impact on psychotic symptoms. Br J Psychiatry 169:593–601, 1996

Falloon IR, Boyd JL, McGill CW, et al: Family management in the prevention of exacerbations of schizophrenia: a controlled study. N Engl J Med 306:1437–1440, 1982

Falloon IR, McGill CW, Boyd JL, et al: Family management in the prevention of morbidity of schizophrenia: social outcome of a two-year longitudinal study. Psychol Med 17:59–66, 1987

Fernandez GA, Nygard S: Impact of involuntary outpatient commitment on the revolving-door syndrome in North Carolina. Hosp Community Psychiatry 41:1001–1004, 1990

Garety PA, Fowler D, Kuipers E: Cognitive-behavioral therapy for medication-resistant symptoms. Schizophr Bull 26:73–86, 2000

Geller J, Grudzinskas AJ Jr, McDermeit M, et al: The efficacy of involuntary outpatient treatment in Massachusetts. Adm Policy Ment Health 25:271–285, 1998

Hiday VA: Coercion in civil commitment: process, preferences, and outcome. Int J Law Psychiatry 15:359–377, 1992

Hiday VA, Scheid-Cook TL: The North Carolina experience with outpatient commitment: a critical appraisal. Int J Law Psychiatry 10:215–232, 1987

Hiday VA, Scheid-Cook TL: A follow-up of chronic patients committed to outpatient treatment. Hosp Community Psychiatry 40:52–59, 1989

Hiday VA, Scheid-Cook TL: Outpatient commitment for revolving door patients: compliance and treatment. J Nerv Ment Dis 179:83–88, 1991

Hiday VA, Swartz MS, Swanson JW, et al: Impact of outpatient commitment on victimization of people with severe mental illness. Am J Psychiatry 159:1403–1411, 2002

Hodel B, Brenner HD: Cognitive therapy with schizophrenic patients: conceptual basis, present state, future directions. Acta Psychiatr Scand Suppl 384:108–115, 1994

Hogarty GE, Anderson CM, Reiss DJ, et al: Family psychoeducation, social skills training, and maintenance chemotherapy in the aftercare treatment of schizophrenia, I: one-year effects of a controlled study on relapse and expressed emotion. Arch Gen Psychiatry 43:633–642, 1986

Hogarty GE, Anderson CM, Reiss DJ, et al: Family psychoeducation, social skills training, and maintenance chemotherapy in the aftercare treatment of schizophrenia, II: two-year effects of a controlled study on relapse and adjustment. Environmental-Personal Indicators in the Course of Schizophrenia (EPICS) Research Group. Arch Gen Psychiatry 48: 340–347, 1991

Hogarty GE, Kornblith SJ, Greenwald D, et al: Personal therapy: a disorder-relevant psychotherapy for schizophrenia. Schizophr Bull 21:379–393, 1995

Hogarty GE, Greenwald D, Ulrich RF, et al: Three-year trials of personal therapy among schizophrenic patients living with or independent of family, II: effects on adjustment of patients. Am J Psychiatry 154:1514–1524, 1997a

Hogarty GE, Kornblith SJ, Greenwald D, et al: Three-year trials of personal therapy among schizophrenic patients living with or independent of family, I: description of study and effects on relapse rates. Am J Psychiatry 154:1504–1513, 1997b

Kavanagh DJ: Recent developments in expressed emotion and schizophrenia. Br J Psychiatry 160:601–620, 1992

Keilitz I: Empirical studies of involuntary outpatient civil commitment: is it working? Ment Phys Disabil Law Rep 14: 368–379, 1990

Kemp R, Hayward P, Applewhaite G, et al: Compliance therapy in psychotic patients: randomized controlled trial. BMJ 312:345–349, 1996

Kuipers E, Garety P, Fowler D, et al: London-East Anglia randomized controlled trial of cognitive-behavioural therapy for psychosis, I: effects of the treatment phase. Br J Psychiatry 171:319–327, 1997

Kuipers E, Fowler D, Garety P, et al: London-East Anglia randomized controlled trial of cognitive-behavioural therapy for psychosis, III: follow-up and economic evaluation at 18 months. Br J Psychiatry 173:61–68, 1998

Lauriello J, Lenroot R, Bustillo JR: Maximizing the synergy between pharmacotherapy and psychosocial therapies for schizophrenia. Psychiatr Clin North Am 26:191–211, 2003

Leff J: First perceptions of treatment: the physician-family patient network. Journal of Practical Psychiatry and Behavioral Health 2:10–15, 1996

Leff J, Kuipers L, Berkowitz R, et al: A controlled trial of social intervention in the families of schizophrenia patients. Br J Psychiatry 141:121–134, 1982

Lehman AF, Dixon LB, Kernan E, et al: A randomized trial of assertive community treatment for homeless persons with severe mental illness. Arch Gen Psychiatry 54:1038–1043, 1997

Lehman AF, Goldberg R, Dixon LB, et al: Improving employment outcomes for persons with severe mental illnesses. Arch Gen Psychiatry 59:165–172, 2002

Liberman RP, Wallace CJ, Blackwell G, et al: Skills training versus psychosocial occupational therapy for persons with persistent schizophrenia. Am J Psychiatry 155:1087–1091, 1998

Linszen D, Dingemans P, Van der Does JW, et al: Treatment, expressed emotion and relapse in recent onset schizophrenic disorders. Psychol Med 26:333–342, 1996

Macias C, Barreira P, Alden M, et al: The ICCD benchmarks for clubhouses: a practical approach to quality improvement in psychiatric rehabilitation. Psychiatr Serv 52:207–213, 2001

Marder SR, Wirshing WC, Mintz J, et al: Two-year outcome of social skills training and group psychotherapy for outpatients with schizophrenia. Am J Psychiatry 153:1585–1592, 1996

May PRA: Treatment of Schizophrenia: A Comparative Study of Five Treatment Models. New York, Science House, 1968

McCafferty G, Dooley J: Involuntary outpatient commitment: an update. Ment Phys Disabil Law Rep 14:277–287, 1990

McFarlane WR, Dushay RA, Stastny P, et al: A comparison of two levels of family aided assertive community treatment. Psychiatr Serv 47:744–750, 1996

Moloy KA: Analysis: Critiquing the Empirical Evidence: Does Involuntary Outpatient Commitment Work? Washington, DC, Mental Health Policy Resource Center, 1992

Monahan J, Swartz M, Bonnie RJ: Mandated treatment in the community for people with mental disorders. Health Aff (Millwood) 22:28–38, 2003

Moore E, Ball RA, Kuipers L: Expressed emotion in staff working with the long-term adult mentally ill. Br J Psychiatry 161:802–808, 1992

Mueser KT, Glynn SM: Family intervention for schizophrenia, in Best Practice: Developing and Promoting Empirically Supported Interventions. Edited by Dobson KS, Craig KE. Newbury Park, CA, Sage, 1998, pp 157–186

Mueser KT, Corrigan PW, Hilton DW, et al: Illness management and recovery: a review of the research. Psychiatr Serv 53:1272–1284, 2002

Nugter A, Dingemans P, Van der Does JW, et al: Family treatment, expressed emotion and relapse in recent onset schizophrenia. Psychiatry Res 72:23–31, 1997

O'Keefe C, Potensa DP, Mueser KT: Treatment outcomes for severely mentally ill patient on conditional discharge to community-based treatment. J Nerv Ment Dis 185:409–411, 1997

Phillips SD, Burns BJ, Edgar ER, et al: Moving assertive community treatment into standard practice. Psychiatr Serv 52:771–779, 2001

Ridgely S, Borum R, Petrilla J: The Effectiveness of Outpatient Commitment. Santa Monica, CA, RAND, 2002

Schooler NR, Keith SJ, Severe JB, et al: Relapse and rehospitalization during maintenance treatment of schizophrenia: the effects of dose reduction and family treatment. Arch Gen Psychiatry 54:453–463, 1997

Scott JE, Dixon LB: Assertive community treatment and case management for schizophrenia. Schizophr Bull 21:657–668, 1995

Sensky T, Turkington D, Kingdon D, et al: A randomized controlled trial of cognitive-behavioral therapy for persistent symptoms in schizophrenia resistant to medication. Arch Gen Psychiatry 57:165–172, 2000

Snyder KS, Wallace CJ, Mor K, et al: Expressed emotion by residential care operators and the residents' symptoms and quality of life. Hosp Community Psychiatry 45:1141–1143, 1994

Spaulding WD, Reed D, Sullivan M, et al: Effects of cognitive treatment in psychiatric rehabilitation. Schizophr Bull 25:657–676, 1999

Stanton AH, Gunderson JG, Knapp PH, et al: Effects of psychotherapy in schizophrenia, I: designed implementation of a controlled study. Schizophr Bull 10:520–563, 1984

Steadman HJ, Gounis K, Dennis D, et al: Assessing the New York City involuntary outpatient commitment pilot program. Psychiatr Serv 52:330–336, 2001

Stein LI, Test MA: Alternative to mental hospital treatment, I: conceptual model, treatment program, and clinical evaluation. Arch Gen Psychiatry 37:392–397, 1980

Swanson JW, Swartz MS, George LK, et al: Interpreting the effectiveness of involuntary outpatient commitment: a conceptual model. J Am Acad Psychiatry Law 25:5–16, 1997

Swanson JW, Swartz MS, Borum R, et al: Involuntary outpatient commitment and reduction of violent behaviour in persons with severe mental illness. Br J Psychiatry 176:324–331, 2000

Swanson JW, Borum R, Swartz MS, et al: Can involuntary outpatient commitment reduce arrests among persons with severe mental illness? Criminal Justice and Human Behavior 28:156–189, 2001

Swanson JW, Swartz MS, Elbogen EB, et al: Effects of involuntary outpatient commitment on subjective quality of life in persons with severe mental illness. Behav Sci Law 21:473–491, 2003

Swartz MS, Burns BJ, Hiday VA, et al: New directions in research on involuntary outpatient commitment. Psychiatr Serv 46:381–385, 1995

Swartz MS, Swanson JW, Wagner HR, et al: Can involuntary outpatient commitment reduce hospital recidivism? Findings from a randomized trial in severely mentally ill individuals. Am J Psychiatry 156:1968–1975, 1999

Swartz MS, Swanson JW, Hiday VA, et al: A randomized controlled trial of outpatient commitment in North Carolina. Psychiatr Serv 52:330–336, 2001a

Swartz MS, Swanson JW, Wagner HR, et al: Effects of involuntary outpatient commitment and depot antipsychotics on treatment adherence in persons with severe mental illness. J Nerv Ment Dis 189:583–592, 2001b

Swartz MS, Swanson JW, Monahan J: Endorsement of personal benefit of outpatient commitment among persons with severe mental illness. Psychol Public Policy Law 9:70–93, 2002a

Swartz MS, Wagner HR, Swanson JW, et al: The perceived coerciveness of involuntary outpatient commitment: findings from an experimental study. J Am Acad Psychiatry Law 30:207–217, 2002b

Swartz MS, Swanson JW, Wagner HR, et al: Assessment of four stakeholder groups' preferences concerning outpatient commitment for persons with schizophrenia. Am J Psychiatry 160:1139–1146, 2003

Tarrier N, Barrowclough C, Vaughn C, et al: The community management of schizophrenia: a controlled trial of a behavioural intervention with families to reduce relapse. Br J Psychiatry 153:532–542, 1988

Tarrier N, Beckett R, Harwood S, et al: A trial of two cognitive-behavioural methods of treating drug-resistant residual psychotic symptoms in schizophrenic patients, I: outcome. Br J Psychiatry 162:524–532, 1993

Tarrier N, Barrowclough C, Porceddu K, et al: The Salford Family Intervention Project: relapse rates of schizophrenia at five and eight years. Br J Psychiatry 165:829–832, 1994

Tarrier N, Yusupoff L, Kinney C, et al: Randomised controlled trial of intensive cognitive behaviour therapy for patients with chronic schizophrenia. BMJ 317:303–307, 1998

Tarrier N, Wittkowski A, Kinney C, et al: Durability of the effects of cognitive-behavioural therapy in the treatment of chronic schizophrenia: 12-month follow-up. Br J Psychiatry 174:500–504, 1999

Tarrier N, Kinney C, McCarthy E, et al: Two-year follow-up of cognitive-behavioral therapy and supportive counseling in the treatment of persistent symptoms in chronic schizophrenia. J Consult Clin Psychol 68:917–922, 2000

Torrey EF, Kaplan R: A national survey of the use of outpatient commitment. Psychiatr Serv 46:778–784, 1995

Torrey WC, Drake RE, Dixon L, et al: Implementing evidence-based practices for persons with severe mental illnesses. Psychiatr Serv 52:45–50, 2001

Wagner HR, Swartz MS, Swanson JW, et al: Does involuntary outpatient commitment lead to more intensive treatment? Psychol Public Policy Law 9:70–93, 2003

Wykes T, Reeder C, Corner J, et al: The effects of neurocognitive remediation on executive processing in patients with schizophrenia. Schizophr Bull 25:291–307, 1999

Yanos PT, Primavera LH, Knight EL: Consumer-run service participation, recovery of social functioning, and the mediating role of psychological factors. Psychiatr Serv 52:493–500, 2001

Zhang M, Yan H: Effectiveness of psychoeducation of relatives of schizophrenia patients: a prospective cohort study of five cities of China. Int J Ment Health 22:47–59, 1993

THE PRODROME

ELIZABETH M. TULLY, M.D.

THOMAS H. MCGLASHAN, M.D.

Schizophrenia is a severe, lifelong neuropsychiatric disorder that can affect children, adolescents, and adults. The typical onset occurs in young adults in their late adolescence or early 20s, and the diagnosis usually follows a dramatic psychotic episode or "first break." However, signs and symptoms heralding the disorder are often present months to years before the diagnosis is made.

This period of onset—or *prodrome*—is of great interest to researchers because it may hold the key to improved prediction and identification of cases. This could lead to application of earlier treatment and thereby possibly prevent, delay, or attenuate the first episode of psychosis. The schizophrenia prodrome is currently the subject of intensive investigation in several centers in the United States and around the world.

In this chapter, we review essential literature describing the prodrome of schizophrenia, including the development of instruments that can identify individuals who are vulnerable to psychoses, the potential for intervention, and the promise of treating schizophrenia earlier in life.

DEFINITIONS

Prodrome derives from the Greek word *prodromos* or *precursor*. In clinical medicine, *prodrome* refers to those early signs and symptoms that precede the characteristic manifestations of the acute, full-blown illness. For example, hepatitis A is described as having a variable, systemic prodrome of 1–2 weeks marked by fever, headache, nausea and vomiting, arthralgias, myalgias, and anorexia. In addition, the individual may complain of nonspecific fatigue. Later, the constellation of clinical jaundice, right-upper-quadrant pain, and the confirmatory finding of anti–hepatitis A virus immunoglobulin M in serum makes the diagnosis of hepatitis A definitive.

The schizophrenia prodrome is currently defined as an early or prepsychotic state that represents a deviation from the usual behavior and experience of an individual (Yung and McGorry 1996). Therefore, the prodrome can be regarded as both a state and a process leading up to the full-blown illness. The prodrome is a retrospective concept by definition.

Schizophrenia can be divided into three phases that delineate the development of psychosis over time (see Figure 19–1). The first phase—the *premorbid phase*—is a period of normality for most persons who ultimately develop schizophrenia. When deficits exist, they usually begin at birth and usually are subtle, stable, and asymptomatic. In the second—or *prodromal*—phase, symptoms occur with increasing severity beginning after puberty. This phase lasts between 2 and 5 years on average (Beiser et al. 1993; Loebel et al. 1992). Global functioning declines in an obvious downward, usually accelerating tra-

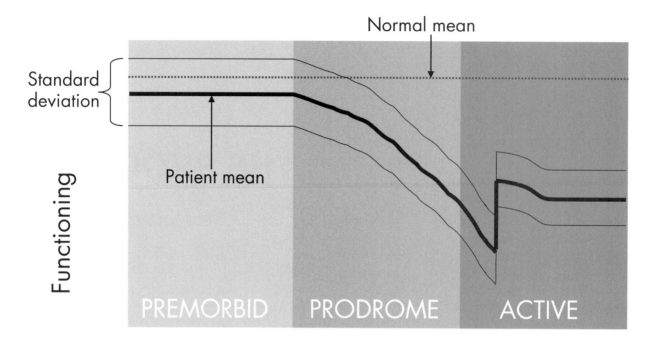

FIGURE 19–1.　Schematic representation of the early course of illness in schizophrenic patients.

Time is shown on the ordinate and global functioning on the abscissa. The dotted lines represent 100% of age-adjusted, average normal functioning. The bolder curve illustrates the average course of a group of patients with schizophrenia over premorbid, prodromal, and psychotic (active) phases. Functioning generally declines rapidly during the prodromal phase, as well as early in the psychotic phase. The duration of time between onset of psychosis and the first antipsychotic treatment is known as the duration of untreated psychosis. Variability in course is expressed by the upper and lower hairline time course curves that are meant to illustrate the wide range that is observed across patients throughout the course of illness.

jectory. According to retrospective reports, about 80%–90% of patients with schizophrenia remember their prodromal phase (Hafner et al. 1994). The third phase—the *psychotic phase*—is ushered in with frankly psychotic symptoms. At this point, patients feel convinced that their hallucinations and delusions are real. Their earlier insight in the prodromal phase, consisting of recognition of attenuated psychotic experiences as false, is now lost.

The psychotic phase marks the first episode of schizophrenia. The DSM-IV-TR (American Psychiatric Association 2000) criteria for schizophrenia require at least two characteristic psychotic symptoms as well as social/occupational dysfunction and duration of at least 6 months. For most patients, the severity of the illness continues to increase for several years before reaching a stable plateau (Davidson and McGlashan 1997).

Prevention of schizophrenia can be discussed in relation to primary, secondary, and tertiary prevention efforts.

Primary prevention tries to reduce the incidence of new cases in the population. In schizophrenia research, *primary prevention* refers to intervention in the premorbid phase. Examples of intervention in this phase are improving prenatal care, reducing environmental insults (Mednick and Schulsinger 1968), and reducing mean paternal age (Malaspina et al. 2002). *Secondary prevention* aims to reduce the prevalence of the disorder. In the case of schizophrenia, prevalence could be reduced by efforts to delay onset of early signs and symptoms of the disorder. Finally, *tertiary prevention* aims to reduce morbidity, course progression, and mortality. Tertiary prevention begins by treating schizophrenia as soon as possible after onset to reduce the duration of untreated psychosis and minimize the damage that active psychosis can wreak on the patient's job, social life, and family functioning. International research has found the average duration of untreated psychosis to be between 1 and 2 years (McGlashan 1999).

Early detection of schizophrenia with active intervention can advance prevention of the disorder, especially its secondary and tertiary forms.

HISTORY OF CLINICAL RESEARCH EFFORTS

The prodromal phase of schizophrenia has been recognized since the early twentieth century by Bleuler (1911/1950). Emil Kraepelin (1919/1971) described the onset of mostly negative and nonspecific symptoms followed by positive symptoms and then the first psychotic episode. According to the Kraepelinian view, the sequence of deterioration is immutable. From 1984 to 1988, the Falloon project in Buckingham County, England, taught primary care practitioners to recognize early warning signs of schizophrenia derived from the prodromal signs outlined in DSM-III (American Psychiatric Association 1980). Such persons were treated with a psychoeducational, family-based, problem-solving psychosocial intervention, which may have delayed onset and contributed to a lower incidence and prevalence of florid episodes of schizophrenia (Falloon et al. 1996). Falloon applied a behavioral family therapy, education, and home-based monitoring model of treatment to patients in the prodromal phase.

Since these early years, other investigators in Australia, the United States, Canada, and Europe have described the prodrome or the period from the first sign of illness to the first mental health contact, even though they used different diagnostic definitions and methodology (McGlashan et al. 2001). McGorry and colleagues (2002) founded the Personal Assessment and Crisis Evaluation (PACE) Clinic in Melbourne, Australia, to study and treat prodromal patients. An international colloquium of investigators interested in the early course convened in Stavanger, Norway, in 1995. This event led to publication of the first contemporary collected works from this perspective (McGlashan 1996) and formation of the International Early Psychosis Association.

Research efforts can be divided into study of the preonset and early post-onset phases of schizophrenia. Preonset studies include early premorbid, late premorbid, and prodromal phases. Post-onset studies include investigations of the duration of untreated psychosis and neuropsychology in first-episode schizophrenia. Introduction of antipsychotic treatment in the pre-onset or prodromal phase aims both to treat active symptoms and to prevent progression of the illness, as does reduction of untreated psychosis in the post-onset phase. Treatment in the prodromal, pre-onset phase aims to decrease prodromal symptoms and to reduce prevalence (secondary prevention) by delaying onset or averting it entirely.

CLINICAL FEATURES AND DIAGNOSTIC CRITERIA

Prodromal symptoms are nonspecific and nonpsychotic. They are usually preceded by a period of normal, or at least nonsymptomatic, functioning in the premorbid phase. However, in some cases of early-onset schizophrenia, the onset occurs abruptly without any apparent prodrome, whereas in other cases, especially those in which there is an early childhood onset, no premorbid phase characterized by normal functioning occurs. In other variations of very early onset, the premorbid phase is abnormal but asymptomatic, although a gradual decline in functioning occurs. Variability in the course of functioning is also characteristic of schizophrenia in its later phases.

Unfortunately, detection of cases in the early premorbid phase remains an elusive objective. It has been recognized for years that some individuals who develop schizophrenia have subtle social, behavioral, and intellectual deficits such as impaired motor development and coordination, neurological soft signs, lower intelligence, and a broad range of social problems. Among the possible vulnerability markers predicting adult schizophrenia spectrum disorders in the premorbid phase is an attention deficit measured by the Continuous Performance Test (Cornblatt 2000). Although attentional, behavioral, and neuromotor abnormalities are noted in children who later develop schizophrenia, these factors are probably insufficient to cause the illness or even to serve as reliable and specific markers for it.

The natural history of the prodrome is characterized by nonspecific early symptoms of depression and anxiety followed by or concurrent with negative symptoms, including apathy, social withdrawal, and cognitive changes affecting concentration and attention. These symptoms are then succeeded by the positive symptoms of suspiciousness, ideas of reference, and perceptual abnormalities, which often serve as harbingers of the first episode (Hafner and Maurer 2001).

Prodromal patients as a group have several clinical characteristics in common. They and their families especially recognize and are distressed by their symptoms. The patients are both cognitively and functionally impaired. Their Global Assessment of Functioning (GAF) scale scores can be less than 50 on a scale of 1–100, indicating serious symptoms (Miller et al. 2003). These patients have often sought psychiatric treatment in the past and may have received psychotropic medications, including antipsychotics (Addington et al. 2002).

Several prodromal assessment instruments now provide opportunities to study the prodrome prospectively. Chapman et al. (1994) used prospectively established criteria to screen numerous American university students. The instrument rates psychotic and quasi-psychotic symptoms on a continuum of deviancy from normal to floridly psychotic on "psychosis proneness" scales. Students who scored high on Perceptual Aberration or Magical Ideation scales (5.5%) developed psychosis compared with control subjects who scored lower (1.3%). The difference was statistically significant but had low positive predictive value.

The PACE Clinic in Melbourne has applied a "close-in" strategy to identify individuals at risk for psychosis and avoid false-positive results (McGorry et al. 2002). In this approach, researchers focus on those individuals who are at high risk for developing psychosis in the near future because of developmental stage, genetic predisposition, and early mental status changes that indicate impending psychosis. Three categories of selection criteria are used in PACE. Category one requires at least one attenuated, or subthreshold, positive psychotic symptom: ideas of reference, odd beliefs or magical thinking, perceptual disturbance, odd thinking and speech, paranoid ideation, and odd behavior or appearance. Category two criteria consist of brief, limited intermittent psychotic symptoms that spontaneously resolve within a week. Category three combines functional decline in the previous year and genetic risk (a first-degree relative with schizotypal personality disorder or psychotic disorder). A structured interview, the Comprehensive Assessment of At Risk Mental States (CAARMS), is used to determine whether criteria are met. An initial sample of 21 individuals yielded an annual conversion rate to psychosis of 21% (Yung et al. 1996), and a second sample of 49 individuals reported a 41% annual conversion rate (Yung et al. 2003). This group most recently reported follow-up data on a cohort of 104 individuals meeting "ultra-high-risk" criteria (Yung et al. 2004). By 6 months, 29 subjects had developed psychosis (Kaplan-Meier risk estimate=27%), and by 12 months, 36 subjects had progressed to psychosis (Kaplan-Meier risk estimate=35%).

McGlashan and his team at Yale University formed the Prevention Through Risk Identification, Management and Education (PRIME) Clinic. They created assessment instruments modeled after the Australian description of prodromal types to rate prodromal symptoms: the Scale of Prodromal Symptoms (SOPS) and the Structured Interview for Prodromal Syndromes (SIPS) (McGlashan et al. 2001). The SOPS is contained within

the SIPS, and the two are designed to diagnose prodromal syndromes and to rate the severity of prodromal symptoms. The SIPS is designed for use by experienced clinicians who have had specific training in the use of the instrument. These criteria identify a symptomatic patient group that is at high risk for progression to first-episode psychosis within the next year.

The SOPS and SIPS are used both to diagnose the prodrome and to assess change systematically in prodromal psychopathology over time. They were originally developed to accomplish three goals: 1) to define the presence or absence of psychosis, 2) to define the presence or absence of one or more of the three prodromal states defined by Yung et al. (1996), and 3) to measure severity of prodromal symptoms cross-sectionally and longitudinally. In accordance with DSM-IV-TR, the SOPS and SIPS define psychosis and two of three prodromal states by positive symptoms. Five positive psychotic symptoms are delusions, paranoia, grandiosity, hallucinations, and disorganized speech. The corresponding five prodromal positive symptoms are unusual thought content, suspiciousness, expansiveness, perceptual abnormalities, and circumstantial speech that is difficult to follow but not incoherent.

The psychosis threshold requires at least one of the five positive symptoms at a psychotic level of intensity, and it must be present for more than half the days over 1 month. The severity of the prodrome is further quantified by negative, disorganized, and general psychiatric symptoms. The negative domain includes social isolation or withdrawal, avolition, decreased emotional expression, decreased expression of self, decreased ideational richness, and deterioration of role functioning. The disorganized domain includes odd behavior or appearance, bizarre thinking, difficulties with focus and attention, and impairment in personal hygiene and social awareness. The general domain includes sleep disturbance, dysphoric mood, motor disturbances, and impaired stress tolerance.

During the interview, a family psychiatric history, a rating of schizotypal personality disorder, and the GAF Scale score are also obtained. The diagnostic criteria for prodromal syndromes (Table 19–1) describe three prodromal subgroups based on attenuated positive symptoms, brief psychotic symptoms, and genetic risk plus functional deterioration. In our experience, most prodromal patients meet the attenuated positive symptoms criteria. A few meet the genetic risk plus functional deterioration criteria without meeting the criteria for attenuated positive symptoms. The brief psychotic symptoms subtype appears to be rare.

Both the CAARMS and the SIPS have shown good interrater reliability and predictive validity for conversion to

TABLE 19-1.   Diagnostic criteria for prodromal syndromes and for psychosis

Prodromal syndromes	Diagnostic criteria
Attenuated positive symptoms syndrome	1. Abnormal unusual thought content, suspiciousness, grandiosity, perceptual abnormalities, and/or organization of communication that is below the threshold of frank psychosis. AND 2. These symptoms have begun or worsened in the past year. AND 3. These symptoms occur at least once per week for the last month. AND 4. Psychosis ruled out.
Brief intermittent psychosis syndrome	1. Frankly psychotic unusual thought content, suspiciousness, grandiosity, perceptual abnormalities, and/or organization of communication. BUT 2. These symptoms have begun in the past 3 months. AND 3. The symptoms occur currently at least several minutes per day at least once per month. AND 4. Psychosis ruled out.
Genetic risk plus recent deterioration	1. First-degree relative with history of any psychotic disorder. OR 2. Schizotypal personality disorder in patient. AND 3. Substantial functional decline in the past year. AND 4. Psychosis ruled out.
Rule out psychosis	1. Frankly psychotic unusual thought content, suspiciousness, grandiosity, perceptual abnormalities, and/or organization of communication. AND 2. Symptoms are disorganizing or dangerous. OR 3. Symptoms occur more than 1 hour per day more than four times per week in the past month.

psychosis (Miller et al. 2002; Yung et al. 1996). For example, rater agreement in differentiating prodromal from nonprodromal patients was 93% with the SIPS, and the validity study reported that 46% of the prodromal patients had converted to schizophrenic psychosis at 6 months and 54% at 12 months. A preliminary validation study of the Prodromal States Questionnaire as an initial screening instrument reported good concurrent validity with a diagnosis of the prodrome by the SIPS (Loewy and Cannon 2002).

EPIDEMIOLOGY

The incidence of schizophrenia is approximately 1 new patient per year per 10,000 population, and the prevalence is 1% of the population worldwide. The gender distribution of schizophrenia is approximately equal in men and women. Although meticulous epidemiological studies of the prodrome have not yet been done, it is believed that the incidence of prodromal patients will mirror that of patients with schizophrenia (approximately 1 per 10,000) but that prodromal patients will be on average 1–2 years younger. Recruitment efforts to date have been more successful with younger prodromal patients, possibly explaining the tendency for a predominance of males in prodromal samples because of their earlier age at onset. Finally, to the extent that current prodromal criteria cannot identify and eliminate false-positive cases, not all prodromal samples will develop schizophrenia. Until criteria become more specific, the prodrome will continue to include patients with disorders other than schizophrenia as well as people with no disorders at all.

GENETICS, NEUROPATHOLOGY, NEUROIMAGING, AND NEUROPSYCHOLOGICAL TESTING

The pathogenesis of the prodrome and of schizophrenia remains an enigma. The neurodevelopmental hypothesis of schizophrenia etiology currently prevails, although alternative models have been proposed to account for schizophrenia's long latency, fluctuating course, and heterogeneity of disease expression. Environmental stress and other unknown neurobiological mechanisms may play intertwining roles in this process. Genetic studies of schizophrenia have failed to find a major gene. In fact, only 15% of the children of parents with schizophrenia develop schizophrenia themselves. Offspring of discordant monozygotic twins have equivalent risks of schizophrenia, yet mean schizophrenia concordance rates are only 48% in identical twins (Onstad et al. 1991).

Although the cause of the schizophrenia prodrome remains a mystery, several factors associated with risk of schizophrenia spectrum disorders have been identified. Possible contributory factors include maternal influenza during gestation, obstetrical complications, various neurointegrative deficits in infancy, motor coordination dysfunction in childhood, attention deficit, social isolation, and problematic teacher-rated behaviors in adolescence. Stress from early separations and dysfunctional family environments also may play a role in enhanced risk (Olin and Mednick 1996).

No pathognomonic laboratory or neuropathological examinations are available to detect the prodrome. Although cerebral gray matter volume deficits have been found in several cortical regions on magnetic resonance imaging studies (Pantelis et al. 2003), substantial overlap is seen between pathological cases and control groups. Of 20 subjects scanned longitudinally, the 10 individuals who had developed psychosis showed progressive reductions in gray matter in the left parahippocampal, fusiform, orbitofrontal, and cerebellar cortices and the cingulate gyri. Those who did not develop psychosis only had changes in cerebellum. Neuroimaging of a high-risk prodromal sample in Melbourne, Australia (Phillips et al. 2002), found left hippocampal volumes that were intermediate between those of normal and schizophrenia contrast groups. Normal hippocampal volume in this high-risk group predicted conversion to psychosis. Over the next year following conversion, significant reductions were reported in left medial temporal, left frontal, and left cerebellar volumes. Serial neuroimaging may help to elucidate prediction of conversion to psychosis in the future.

The prodrome has no typical neuropsychological profile, but a range of neuropsychological deficits are characteristic of established schizophrenia (Heinrichs 2001), and cognitive deficits are present in the post-onset phase. Addington and Addington (2002) reported that the cognitive functioning of 150 first-episode subjects admitted to the Calgary Early Psychosis Program remained in the impaired range despite significant improvement on some memory tasks with treatment. Hawkins et al. (2004) reported that the neuropsychological performance of prodromal patients falls between the deficit levels reported in first-episode and chronic schizophrenia samples and the normal level of healthy control subjects.

DIFFERENTIAL DIAGNOSIS OF THE PRODROME

The prodrome signals the impending onset of disorders other than schizophrenia, making the differential diagnosis of the prodrome a critical and challenging exercise. It is important to rule out general medical conditions that can mimic a prodromal state and/or progress to frankly psychotic symptoms, such as Cushing's disease, delirium, certain seizure disorders, lupus, and various types of drug intoxication. Drug dependence, such as chronic marijuana use in particular, may lead to amotivation, dysphoria, perceptual abnormalities, and paranoia. Several major psychiatric disorders also must be considered in the differential diagnosis:

- *Major depression with psychotic features.* Depressive symptoms are common in the prodrome and throughout the natural history of schizophrenia. Most prodromal patients, however, do not meet full diagnostic criteria for major depression and complain of emotional numbness rather than true sadness or sustained irritability. In addition, depression with psychotic features is often associated with melancholia and older age.
- *Schizotypal personality disorder.* Schizotypal personality traits are present from an early age and are enduring but stable aspects of functioning. This disorder can coexist with the prodrome, but the two conditions are distinguished mostly by course. Symptoms in the prodrome are progressive, not static.
- *Borderline personality disorder.* Brief psychotic episodes under stress accompanied by a pattern of intense, unstable relationships; impulsivity; and self-mutilation indicate a diagnosis of borderline personality disorder. These traits are present usually from an early age and are unlikely to show sudden emergence in young adulthood.

- *Pervasive developmental disorder.* Patients with this disorder have a pattern of odd behaviors, impaired communication, and poor reciprocal social interaction skills, which are usually evident in early childhood. Although this condition may resemble the prodrome in some ways, it is usually associated with mental retardation and other general medical conditions, such as congenital and chromosomal abnormalities.
- *Posttraumatic stress disorder.* The characteristic symptoms involve reexperiencing a traumatic event and a variety of autonomic, dysphoric, and cognitive complaints. However, unlike prodromal symptoms, posttraumatic stress disorder develops after a psychologically traumatic event that is generally outside the range of usual human experience.
- *Obsessive-compulsive disorder (OCD).* Severe cases of OCD can be difficult to distinguish from the prodrome. Prodromal patients usually do not show compulsive behaviors or preoccupation with the classic OCD themes of contamination or inadvertent harm to others, and they do not experience OCD symptoms as ego-dystonic.
- *Attention-deficit/hyperactivity disorder (ADHD).* Although attention deficits are common in the prodrome, patients with true ADHD usually are identified before age 7 years. ADHD is highly comorbid with oppositional defiant disorder, learning disorder, and depression rather than psychotic-like symptoms.

Prodromal symptoms may be interpreted by parents and families as normal adolescent development. Indeed, hallucinatory experiences have been reported by healthy young people, and there may be a continuum of psychotic symptoms in the population (Johns and van Os 2001). Transient prodromelike symptoms can occur in young adult populations without the prodrome, but these symptoms are not usually accompanied by significant functional impairment.

CASE HISTORIES

The following disguised case vignettes from our PRIME Prodromal Research Clinic illustrate patients whose symptoms meet the criteria for one of the three prodromal syndromes described earlier. Prodromal patients can meet criteria for a prodromal syndrome alone or two or three syndromes simultaneously.

CASE ONE: ATTENUATED POSITIVE SYMPTOMS SYNDROME

Simon, a single, 22-year-old, Caucasian man, attended college full time. For the past 8 months, he had become increasingly concerned about an image he sensed near him whenever he was in the bathroom of his apartment washing his face or showering. The image was that of a shadowy, vaguely female figure whose presence was triggered by running water. He was frightened by the image and felt she was "spiteful" and wished for his death by falling in the bathroom. Simon knew that it was not real, but it bothered him. He wanted treatment to eliminate the image and other images he first reported sensing in his childhood. The image appeared almost every time he entered the bathroom, so he avoided showering and washed only half of his face at a time.

In his evaluation, Simon acknowledged that his friends regarded him as "weird" because of his preoccupation with themes such as the moral messages hidden in the music he played, the decline of civilization, and the special meaning he obtained from games of chess. He felt unmotivated, had subtle difficulty completing his schoolwork despite maintaining a high grade point average, and procrastinated on his personal activities of daily living. He needed frequent prompts from his roommate. He felt confusion once or twice a month, during which time he forgot what he was talking about mid sentence, and his friends had noticed. In fact, his girlfriend frequently complained to him that he was not the same.

Simon worried that other students wanted to exclude him from certain social groups and that he could overcome this by changing his hairstyle and style of clothing in ways he could not explain. These concerns occurred approximately once every 2 weeks, and he believed that he was probably imagining them. He complained of feeling unmotivated and different from how he felt when he was younger.

Simon was judged to meet the attenuated positive symptoms criteria. The attenuated positive symptoms included perceptual abnormalities (sensing images in the room) and suspiciousness (people excluding him and talking negatively about him).

CASE TWO: BRIEF INTERMITTENT PSYCHOTIC SYNDROME

Calvin, a 16-year-old, African American sophomore, lived with his parents and older sister. There was no family history of psychotic illness. In the seventh grade, Calvin became depressed and withdrawn and complained of difficulties concentrating and problems with sleep. The parents attributed these problems to adjustment to junior high school, but the depressive symptoms resurfaced in his sophomore year.

During his initial evaluation, Calvin was guarded and had constricted affect. He said that people at school disliked him and wanted to hurt him for reasons he could not specify. With detailed questioning, Calvin admitted that he avoided two classmates because he thought he heard them calling him "a homo." He felt at that time that he was in danger of being assaulted by them but admitted that they probably had not called him "a homo" or intended to attack him. However, he reported similar experiences, lasting only a few minutes and not leading to confrontation, four to five other times over the past 3 months. Calvin also had mild conceptual disorganization manifested as occasional circumstantial thinking but no other unusual thought content or grandiosity. His grades had slipped from mostly A's to mostly C's. His parents worried that if his performance continued to decline, he might have to repeat his sophomore year.

Calvin was judged to meet the brief intermittent psychotic syndrome criteria. He had moments of paranoia that were of delusional intensity but not acutely disorganizing or dangerous and too brief to meet duration criteria for presence of psychosis.

CASE THREE: GENETIC RISK AND FUNCTIONAL DETERIORATION PRODROMAL SYNDROME

Tanya, a single, 19-year-old, Caucasian woman, worked at a fast-food restaurant and attended cosmetology classes part time. She was the middle of three sisters, one of whom had been hospitalized for schizophrenia. Tanya had felt depressed for at least a year prior to her referral and had been taking both a psychostimulant for ADHD and an antidepressant at various times with only moderate success. She reported trouble concentrating, had mismanaged her finances to the point that many checks had been returned for insufficient funds, and was involved in chronic fights with her mother, which she regretted. One month prior to referral, Tanya thought she heard her name being called repetitively, and once in the month before her referral, she thought she heard the compact disc player playing when it was turned off.

Tanya was unmotivated to do anything except spend time with her boyfriend and mostly stayed alone in her room listening to music. She let leftover food accumulate on every surface in her bedroom. Tanya was on the verge of being fired at work because of absenteeism, and she frequently did not attend beauty school. She complained of not having feelings when it was normal to have them. Tanya was brought for evaluation by her parents, who expressed concern that she was showing symptoms similar to those they had seen before her older sister's psychotic break.

Tanya was a passive participant in the evaluation but endorsed depression and avolition. Although she acknowledged the concerns of her parents and promised to start engaging in more productive activities "tomorrow," the family noted that tomorrow never came. Tanya said that she did not believe that hearing her name called and hearing the compact disc player playing when it was turned off were real events and said that it was "all in my head."

The number and strength of Tanya's negative symptoms and her dramatic decrease in occupational, educational, and social functioning were striking. Her GAF scale score was judged to have declined at least 40 points in the past year. This functional decline plus the family history of schizophrenia in a first-degree relative satisfied the genetic risk and functional deterioration prodromal syndrome. Her positive symptoms appeared either too mild or too infrequent to meet attenuated positive symptoms or brief psychotic symptoms criteria.

FAMILY INTERVIEWS

A recent qualitative research study of the evolution of symptoms in prodromal patients divided 20 individuals into a "never normal" group and a larger subgroup called the "declining" group according to themes emerging in family interviews (Corcoran et al. 2003). The "never normal" group was typically described as having multiple problems since birth, whereas the other group was described as declining from an essentially normal baseline. In addition to the families' concerns about the degree of temporal change in the "declining" group, they may have attributed behavior and personality changes to street drug use, the wrong friends, adolescent turmoil, or various environmental stressors.

The suffering of the families often intensifies during the prodrome as they grapple with the deteriorating behavior of the prodromal patient. Parents feel incompetent, bewildered, and grief-stricken. We present several examples of parents' descriptions of prodromal patients from the PRIME Clinic.

FATHER OF MICHAEL, AGE 17

He has changed. When I saw him come out of our house holding the .22, I knew. I asked him what he was doing with it, and he ignored me, walked away. The neighbor found another .22 in the guitar case he had with him the night he stole their car. The police came. He was driving around for no reason by himself at 2:30 A.M. The neighbor didn't press charges. I don't allow guns in my home. When Michael was younger, I let him and his brother plink at some cans in the woods behind our house, and we watched them. He was never interested in hunting. What is he doing? We don't know. He wants to join the military, but I told him he can forget that.

He stays in his room, but before he used to be part of the family gatherings; now we're the enemy somehow. He was friendly to everyone, like the mayor. Now he has just one friend, a troubled boy like one of those kids who shot up Columbine. He is disrespectful and really awful to his mother. Her heart is broken. His brothers and sisters weren't like this at his age; they are all fine. He won't do anything we ask; that's all gone. He's completely different. Always just that blank look, and then he walks off. We thought it was drugs, but the psychiatrist we took him to had him tested, and everything was negative. He has ADHD and used to take the medication, but now he refuses. He did better in school on it, but now he takes completed homework and projects I helped him with to school and never turns them in. He just doesn't care. We are really worried; we've got to do something.

MOTHER OF NIKEESHA, AGE 13

She needs help. She wants help, too. She says, "Mama, please take me to the doctor." She's up half the night, talking to herself and laughing for hours. It can go on all night. I can't get her up for school in the morning, and it's all the time now; I can't get her to do anything. I give her the shoes because she's just walking around, and I yell, "Put them on!" I come back, and she's over here, fooling around, looking at stuff, shoes not on, still half-dressed. Won't take a shower unless I nag. Won't eat, just picks. She's in her own world. She doesn't talk to herself in the school because she knows the other kids are going to notice, so she can control it when she wants to. The teachers say she's quiet and does her work. At home, she did chores, but here lately, nothing—she doesn't hear me. It's getting worse and worse. She never goes out of the house. She says she doesn't hear voices, but what is she laughing at? What?

MOTHER OF BRUCE, AGE 16

The other kids make fun of him at school. He's like a loner. He has no friends, and he fights with his sister because he takes an hour in the bathroom with the OCD stuff, and she's gotta go to work. He takes everything so seriously. His grade point average has always been high. He wants to be perfect. He does great in track, but that's all he does. He worries all the time that he's fat and not fit enough. He's losing weight, too. Then he told me about the voices, so I was really concerned, and I cried. He says he's not sure they're real, but they worry me. He gets depressed. He says sometimes he thinks about wishing he were dead and can see a type of vision about hurting himself. He's got this whole confusing God thing going on. He feels like God talks to him, and he isn't going to listen to us, except the commandments say honor thy father and mother. He gets real mad at me if there's some skin showing, like maybe my top shows my shoulders a little, because he can't stand any sex stuff at all. He's never had a girlfriend. You just can't reach him; his father tries, but he ends up yelling at Bruce. We don't know what to do. It's getting worse bit by bit I think.

COURSE AND PROGNOSIS

Diagnostic criteria for the prodrome can be used to predict psychosis within the next 12 months according to a patient's presenting symptoms (Table 19–1). Two groups have each published similar criteria. The PACE Clinic in Melbourne has shown a prospective risk of conversion or positive predictive value of 40.8% within the first 12 months in 49 prodromal patients (Yung et al. 2003). Most recently, a follow-up study of 104 "ultra-high-risk" patients reported that 34.6% of the patients developed frank psychotic symptoms within 12 months (Yung et al. 2004). The PRIME Clinic in New Haven, Connecticut, has

shown a prospective risk of conversion of 50% within the first 12 months in 14 prodromal patients. Of the 20 patients who received nonprodromal diagnoses at the PRIME Clinic, none has converted (Miller et al. 2002).

Despite the high positive predictive value of current prodromal diagnostic criteria, false-positive diagnoses occur. False-positive diagnoses are likely to occur with disorders such as major depression, bipolar disorder, OCD, and schizotypal personality disorder. In the PRIME Clinic sample, most of the patients who did not progress to schizophrenia remained prodromal, and only a few experienced remission of prodromal symptoms within 12 months. Although false-negative diagnoses are also likely to occur, we have thus far found that patients who had not initially met prodromal criteria did not progress to psychosis within the next year. Examination of larger groups of patients over several years will undoubtedly help clarify the extent of false-positive and false-negative diagnoses.

Current prodromal diagnostic criteria identify mostly late prodromal patients who are at imminent risk for progression to psychosis and do not capture all patients who are truly prodromal. Patients who do not initially meet full criteria should be asked to return for a new assessment if their symptoms worsen because a few such patients have subsequently progressed to the point of meeting prodromal criteria (Miller et al. 2002).

TREATMENT

TREATMENT STUDIES

Two controlled studies involving treatment of prodromal symptoms with atypical antipsychotic medications have been done. In the first trial, prodromal patients were randomly assigned to receive open-label risperidone and cognitive-behavioral therapy (CBT) plus usual care ($n=32$) or usual care alone ($n=28$) (McGorry et al. 2002) for 6 months. The major dependent variable was onset of psychosis. Risperidone 1–2 mg/day plus antidepressants and anxiolytics as needed were given to the medication group. The patients receiving risperidone also received CBT in 12–24 sessions, but the usual-care patients did not. Six-month conversion to psychosis rates were 9.7% for risperidone plus CBT and 35.7% for usual care ($P< 0.05$). Risperidone was stopped after 6 months, and patients were followed up for 6 more months. Some patients converted to psychosis during the medication-free follow-up interval.

The results of the study provide strong support for the ability of an atypical antipsychotic medication in conjunction with CBT to postpone, rather than eliminate, progression to psychosis among prodromal patients. More-over, no significant differences were observed in severity of illness ratings at fixed 6-month intervals for each of the treatment groups after treatment had been discontinued.

The finding that those patients randomly assigned to receive risperidone converted to psychosis after risperidone was discontinued suggests that treatment delays but does not prevent onset. It also suggests the need for more studies of longer-term medication administration. Because the medication and CBT were bundled together, it is unknown whether the beneficial effects could be attributed to risperidone separately, to CBT separately, or to the combined effects of both treatments. Also, because of the open-label design of the study, the placebo effect of the medication could not be assessed.

McGlashan et al. (2003) conducted a double-blind, placebo-controlled trial of olanzapine in 60 prodromal patients. This trial consisted of a four-site North American study comparing the safety and efficacy of olanzapine ($n=31$) with placebo ($n=29$) in the treatment of prodromal symptoms. In this study, individual and family psychosocial interventions were given to each patient in both arms of the trial. Olanzapine was given at dosages ranging from 5 to 15 mg/day, with a mean maximum dosage of 10.2 mg/day. Analyses of the first 8 weeks of treatment with the SOPS indicated that the patients randomly assigned to receive olanzapine improved from baseline significantly over 8 weeks. The 1-year results showed that 16 patients became psychotic, including 11 from the placebo group (McGlashan 2004) and 5 from the olanzapine group. Eight of the 16 patients converted within the first month from baseline. Weight gain was significantly greater in the olanzapine group, but the adverse events, including extrapyramidal side effects, were generally the same for both groups. The results of more extended analyses are pending at this time.

These trials underscore important ethical dilemmas—the risk of not intervening medically in the prodromal phase for true prodromal patients at imminent risk for psychosis versus the risk of unnecessary treatment for false-positive prodromal patients. The primary risks for prodromal patients concern medication side effects, stigma, and placebo (McGlashan 2001). Medication side effects of the new-generation antipsychotics are mild to moderate, although long-term adverse effects are unknown. Moreover, the benefits can be significant. Clinicians may delay diagnosis of schizophrenia for fear of socially stigmatizing the patient. At the PRIME Clinic, prodromal patients are told that they are "at risk" for psychosis but that psychosis is not inevitable. Although some patients have denied that anything is wrong, none have experienced seriously negative consequences from the

"at-risk" designation. Patients who are truly prodromal and given placebo in a medication trial may be considered at even greater risk, if in fact antipsychotic medication could delay or even prevent onset of psychosis. However, evidence for such a clear benefit is only beginning to accumulate. The current state of our clinical knowledge regarding treatment of the prodrome reflects the concept of "equipoise," or a state of genuine clinical uncertainty regarding the relative merits of early detection and treatment of the prodrome.

TREATMENT RECOMMENDATIONS

Early identification and treatment of the prodrome at the PRIME Clinic have had several benefits, including reduced psychosocial morbidity. Patients and their families express relief that the condition is recognized, monitored, and treated with minimal disruption of daily life and usually on an outpatient basis. Social withdrawal and isolation are reduced, and families receive emotional support and education about the prodrome.

We recommend active follow-up care for prodromal patients at frequent intervals. Although the length of follow-up will vary with the needs of the individual, establishment of a treatment alliance with the patient and the family is critical for extended diagnostic evaluation, overall stress reduction, and timely crisis intervention. We also recommend a detailed assessment of global functioning at baseline and at periodic intervals not only to guide treatment but also to reduce strain in the family by setting reasonable goals.

We recommend supportive therapy for the patient, family therapy, psychoeducation, and liaison with other treating physicians and therapists. Safety issues, including substance abuse, poor self-care, and suicidal and homicidal behavior, must be vigorously addressed. Comorbid disorders should be treated.

Treatment of the prodrome with conventional antipsychotics currently being used in the treatment of schizophrenia is still in its research phase and is not recommended for standard treatment. From a research perspective, drugs that target mechanisms of action such as excessive oxidative stress and hypofunction of the N-methyl-D-aspartate subtype of glutamate receptors may be beneficial, including glycine, omega-3 fatty acid supplementation, and lamotrigine.

Even though we favor a measured and hopeful approach to the family's concerns about the future of the prodromal patient, a frank discussion about the options of more intensive treatment, community resources, and case management services should be introduced sooner rather than later if conversion occurs.

Certainly, establishment of early-detection programs within larger mental health units will identify prodromal patients and provide many rich opportunities for treatment research in this extremely interesting clinical population. The shadowy path that arcs from birth to the first psychotic episode is likely to be further illuminated by accumulating knowledge of the phases of the prodrome.

REFERENCES

Addington J, Addington D: Cognitive functioning in first episode psychosis: predictors of outcome. Presentation at the Third International Conference on Early Psychosis, Copenhagen, Denmark, September 2002

Addington J, van Mastrigt S, Hutchinson J, et al: Pathways to care: help seeking behaviour in first episode psychosis. Acta Psychiatr Scand 106:358–364, 2002

American Psychiatric Association: Diagnostic and Statistical Manual of Mental Disorders, 3rd Edition. Washington, DC, American Psychiatric Association, 1980

American Psychiatric Association: Diagnostic and Statistical Manual of Mental Disorders, 4th Edition, Text Revision. Washington, DC, American Psychiatric Association, 2000

Beiser M, Erikson D, Flemming JAE, et al: Establishing the onset of psychotic illness. Am J Psychiatry 150:1349–1354, 1993

Bleuler E: Dementia Praecox or the Group of Schizophrenias (1911). Translated by Zinkin J. New York, International Universities Press, 1950

Chapman LJ, Chapman JP, Kwapil TR, et al: Putatively psychosis-prone subjects 10 years later. J Abnorm Psychol 103: 171–183, 1994

Corcoran C, Davidson L, Sills-Shahar R, et al: A qualitative research study of the evolution of symptoms in individuals identified as prodromal to psychosis. Psychiatr Q 74:313–332, 2003

Cornblatt B: Vulnerability markers in the premorbid phase. Presentation at the Second International Conference on Early Psychosis, New York, April 2, 2000

Davidson L, McGlashan TH: The varied outcomes of schizophrenia. Can J Psychiatry 42:34–43, 1997

Falloon IRH, Kydd RR, Coverdale JH, et al: Early detection and intervention for initial episodes of schizophrenia. Schizophr Bull 22:271–282, 1996

Hafner H, Maurer K: The prodromal phase of psychosis, in Early Intervention in Psychotic Disorders. Edited by Miller T, Mednick SA, McGlashan TH, et al. Amsterdam, Kluwer Academic, 2001, pp 71–100

Hafner H, Maurer K, Loffler W, et al: The epidemiology of early schizophrenia: influence of age and gender on onset and early course. Br J Psychiatry Suppl 23:29–38, 1994

Hawkins KA, Addington J, Keefe RSE, et al: Neuropsychological status of subjects at high risk for a first episode of psychosis. Schizophr Res 67:115–122, 2004a

Heinrichs RW: In Search of Madness. New York, Oxford University Press, 2001, pp 54–85

Johns LC, van Os J: The continuity of psychotic experiences in the general population. Clin Psychol Rev 21(8): 1125–1141, 2001

Kraepelin E: Dementia Praecox and Paraphrenia (1919). Translated by Barclay RM. New York, Robert E Krieger Publishing, 1971

Loebel AD, Lieberman JA, Alvir JMJ, et al: Duration of psychosis and outcome in first-episode schizophrenia. Am J Psychiatry 149:1183–1188, 1992

Loewy R, Cannon TD: The Prodromal States Questionnaire (PSQ): self-report of prodromal psychotic symptoms. Poster presented at the Third International Conference on Early Psychosis, Copenhagen, Denmark, September 2002

Malaspina D, Brown A, Goetz D, et al: Schizophrenia risk and paternal age: a potential role for de novo mutations in schizophrenia vulnerability genes. CNS Spectr 7:26–29, 2002

McGlashan TH: Early detection and intervention in schizophrenia: editor's introduction. Schizophr Bull 22:197–199, 1996

McGlashan TH: Duration of untreated psychosis in first-episode schizophrenia: marker or determinant of course? Biol Psychiatry 46:899–907, 1999

McGlashan TH: Psychosis treatment prior to psychosis onset: ethical issues. Schizophr Res 51:47–54, 2001

McGlashan TH: Olanzapine for treatment of the schizophrenia prodrome: 2-year results of a randomized placebo-controlled study (abstract). Biol Psychiatry 55(suppl):226, 2004

McGlashan TH, Miller TJ, Woods SW, et al: Instrument for the assessment of prodromal symptoms and states, in Early Intervention in Psychotic Disorders. Edited by Miller T, Mednick SA, McGlashan TH, et al. Amsterdam, Kluwer Academic 2001, pp 135–149

McGlashan TH, Zipursky RB, Perkins D, et al: The PRIME North America randomized double-blind clinical trial of olanzapine versus placebo in patients at risk of being prodromally symptomatic for psychosis, I: study rationale and design. Schizophr Res 61:7–18, 2003

McGorry PD, Yung AR, Phillips LJ: "Closing in": what features predict the onset of first-episode psychosis within an ultra-high-risk group?, in The Early Stages of Schizophrenia. Edited by Zipursky RB, Schulz SC. Washington, DC, American Psychiatric Publishing, 2002, pp 3–31

Mednick SA, Schulsinger F: Some premorbid characteristics related to breakdown in children with schizophrenic mothers, in Transmission of Schizophrenia. Edited by Rosenthal D, Kety SS. New York, Pergamon, 1968, pp 267–291

Miller TJ, McGlashan TH, Rosen JL, et al: Prospective diagnosis of the initial prodrome for schizophrenia based on the Structured Interview for Prodromal Syndromes: preliminary evidence of interrater reliability and predictive validity. Am J Psychiatry 159:863–865, 2002

Miller TJ, Zipursky RB, Perkins, D, et al: The PRIME North America randomized double-blind clinical trial of olanzapine versus placebo in patients at risk of being prodromally symptomatic for psychosis, II: baseline characteristics of the "prodromal" sample. Schizophr Res 61:19–30, 2003

Olin SC, Mednick SA: Risk factors of psychosis: identifying vulnerable populations premorbidly. Schizophr Bull 22:223–240, 1996

Onstad S, Skre I, Torgersen S, et al: Twin concordance for DSM-III-R schizophrenia. Acta Psychiatr Scand 83:395–401, 1991

Pantelis C, Velakoulis D, McGorry PD, et al: Neuroanatomical abnormalities before and after onset of psychosis: a cross-sectional and longitudinal MRI comparison. Lancet 361:281–288, 2003

Phillips LJ, Velakoulis D, Pantelis C, et al: Nonreduction in hippocampal volume is associated with higher risk of psychosis. Schizophr Res 58(2–3):145–158, 2002

Yung AR, McGorry PD: The prodromal phase of first-episode psychosis: past and current conceptualizations. Schizophr Bull 22:353–370, 1996

Yung AR, McGorry PD, McFarlane CA, et al: Monitoring and care of young people at incipient risk of psychosis. Schizophr Bull 22:283–303, 1996

Yung AR, Phillips LJ, Yuen HP, et al: Psychosis prediction: 12 month follow up of a high-risk ("prodromal") group. Schizophr Res 60:21–32, 2003

Yung AR, Phillips LJ, Yuen HP, et al: Risk factors for psychosis in an ultra high-risk group: psychopathology and clinical features. Schizophr Res 67:131–142, 2004

FIRST EPISODE

Diana O. Perkins, M.D., M.P.H.

Jeffrey A. Lieberman, M.D.

Shon Lewis, M.D.

In this chapter, we review the clinical features that characterize the premorbid, prodromal, and first-episode phases of schizophrenia. We also discuss the current understanding of optimal treatment of the first episode. In particular, recognition and treatment of psychosis soon after illness onset may improve outcomes; however, treatment delay continues to be a public health concern. Pharmacological treatment continues to be the cornerstone of treatment, but other modalities, including individual, group, and family therapies, may increase the likelihood of full recovery.

STAGES OF ILLNESS

PREMORBID

The psychoses that define schizophrenia (also the related schizoaffective and schizophreniform disorders) emerge in adolescence or early adulthood for about 70% of affected individuals (Alda et al. 1996; Hafner and Nowotny 1995). Vulnerability to schizophrenia may be a result of a combination of genetic and environmental factors that cause altered brain development during fetal life or shortly after birth (see Chapter 4, "Prenatal and Perinatal Factors," this volume). The clinical manifestations of this altered brain development are subtle but detectable. Longitudinal studies of the offspring of individuals with schizophrenia consistently find that impairments in attention, verbal memory, executive function, motor skills, social function, and school function in childhood predict subsequent risk of schizophrenia (Niemi et al. 2003).

Many (Cannon et al. 1999; Fuller et al. 2002; Isohanni et al. 2000; Zammit et al. 2004) but not all (Cannon et al. 2002; Jones et al. 1994) population-based cohort studies found that academic performance in childhood was similar for individuals who later developed schizophrenia and those who did not. One study found that for individuals who later developed schizophrenia, performance on standardized academic tests in eleventh grade significantly declined from performance in fourth and eighth grade (Fuller et al. 2002). Prospective studies of individuals at high risk for schizophrenia because they have a first-degree relative with psychosis generally find that these high-risk individuals have lower IQ in childhood, but to some extent, the lower IQ is related to environmental rather than genetic factors (Niemi et al. 2003). The Edinburgh High-Risk Study found that for the 5 subjects who developed psychosis, IQ had declined at follow-up from baseline (asymptomatic) evaluation, whereas no change in IQ occurred in the 54 high-risk subjects who did not develop psychosis (Cosway et al. 2000). Several high-risk studies have found attentional deficits present in childhood (Niemi et al. 2003). For example, in the New York High-Risk Project, 58% (7 of 12) of the subjects who developed a psychotic disorder had attentional deficits compared with only 22% (15 of 67) of the high-risk subjects who did not develop a psychotic disorder (Ott et al. 1998). The authors noted that the severity of deficits was stable at each assessment period.

Several studies have found that IQ or performance on standardized tests of academic performance declines during adolescence prior to the emergence of frank psychosis (Ang and Tan 2004; Fuller et al. 2002; Zammit et al. 2004). In the retrospective study of performance on standardized scholastic tests described earlier, these same students who had been performing close to average in grade and middle school were performing significantly below average by eleventh grade on tests of reading (40th percentile), language (37th percentile), and sources of information (41st percentile) (Fuller et al. 2002). A decline in cognitive function likely underlies this decline in academic performance and may be the earliest symptomatic manifestation of illness onset.

Studies have found that deficits in self-reported social and organizational ability and in measured intellectual function are predictive of later development of schizophrenia (Davidson et al. 1999). However, the rate of development of schizophrenia is relatively low: about 1 in 10,000 individuals in the general population per year. Risk prediction leads to concern about both false-positive and false-negative results. The predictive accuracy may be quantified by the specificity (to identify correctly who *will not* become ill out of all of those who *do not* eventually become ill) and sensitivity (to identify correctly who *will* become ill from all those who *do* eventually become ill) of the criteria. A set of criteria with low sensitivity will miss many people who are indeed at risk. Of perhaps more concern with criteria used to identify a person as at risk for developing a psychotic disorder is the specificity, because falsely identifying someone as "at risk" may lead to undue worry and concern, potentially be stigmatizing, and result in inappropriate treatment. The success of risk prediction is always limited by the underlying rate of illness. Because schizophrenia is relatively rare, with an estimated lifetime risk of 1 per 100, even criteria with high specificity (e.g., >0.90) will have many more false-positive than true-positive results (Perkins 2000, 2004).

PRODROMAL

Subjectively experienced prodromal symptoms may herald the development of psychosis by a few weeks to a few years. Symptoms include frequent misperceptions, such as seeing things out the corner of one's eye or hearing knocking or whistling noises. Prodromal symptoms also include subdelusional changes in thought process and content (e.g., becoming very suspicious of others) or ideas of reference. Individuals also may complain of worsening problems with easy distractibility and poor attentional abilities. These symptoms may impair ability to function at school, work, or in social situations, and the functional difficulties are often what bring the person to clinical attention (J. Addington et al. 2002). Much of the decline in social and occupational function associated with schizophrenia occurs during the prodrome, prior to the onset of frank psychosis (Hafner et al. 1999; Yung and McGorry 1996). Recent efforts have had some success at identifying individuals in the prodromal stage, prior to the onset of a full psychotic syndrome (Miller et al. 2003; Yung et al. 2004).

EMERGENCE OF PSYCHOSIS (FIRST EPISODE)

Typically, schizophrenic psychotic disorders, including schizophrenia, schizoaffective disorder, and schizophreniform disorder, begin in adolescence or early adulthood. Epidemiological studies estimate the average age at onset in women to be about 29 years, somewhat older than the average age at onset in men (25 years) (Hafner et al. 1998; Jablensky and Cole 1997). Onset occurs for most individuals (about 75%) between ages 15 and 30 (Heiden and Hafner 2000). Age at onset may vary in specific populations. For example, both men and women who have a first-degree relative with a psychotic disorder have a younger age at onset (Gorwood et al. 1995). In addition, some evidence over the past century suggests that age at onset may be later (Di Maggio et al. 2001; Stompe et al. 2000).

The symptoms of schizophrenia emerge gradually, over many months to years, for about half of affected individuals and abruptly, over days or weeks, for the other half of affected individuals (Harrison et al. 2001). As the symptoms of schizophrenia emerge and the illness progresses, profound decrements in social and vocational function may occur. The diagnosis of schizophrenia requires hallucinations, delusions, or disorganization, but it is often the other associated impairments in cognitive function and the severity of negative symptoms that most contribute to social and vocational impairments (M.F. Green et al. 2000). The clinical progression of schizophrenia occurs during the initial decade of illness, followed by relative clinical stability (Hafner and an der Heiden 1997).

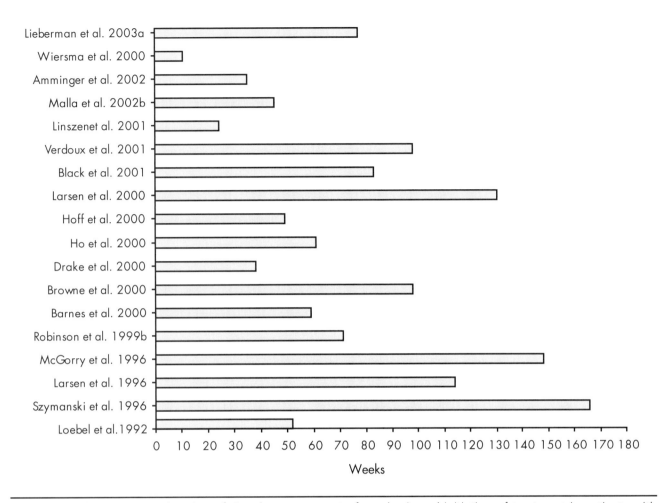

FIGURE 20–1. Mean duration of time between onset of psychosis and initiation of treatment in patients with schizophrenia.

THE PROBLEM OF TREATMENT DELAY

Considerable delay often occurs between the onset of psychotic symptoms and treatment initiation (duration of untreated psychosis). In most communities, an average of a year or more elapses from the time psychosis first occurs to first treatment, whereas the median time to treatment is shorter (about 3–4 months) (Larsen et al. 2001) (see Figure 20–1). The reasons for treatment delays are not well understood. In part, delay is a result of lack of recognition of the symptoms of psychosis as a mental illness by the patient and significant others (Lincoln and McGorry 1995; Lincoln et al. 1998; Perkins et al. 1999). However, it appears that despite the presence of frank psychotic symptoms, the patient, family, and health care provider may not recognize the illness as psychosis (J. Addington et al. 2002).

For several reasons, treatment delay is currently one of the most serious deficiencies in the clinical management of schizophrenia. First, the emerging psychotic and other symptoms of schizophrenia impair social and occupational or school function, with significant functional decline occurring in the first few years of illness. The onset of illness in the late teens to 20s for most affected individuals is a crucial time for psychosocial development. Emerging psychosis often derails normal development, and early intervention may minimize functional losses. Second, psychosis is associated with behavioral disturbances that later may be viewed as embarrassing or that are criminal and have legal consequences. Third, the onset of psychosis is a period when individuals are at increased risk for aggressive behaviors toward others, property, or themselves (Milton et al. 2001). Although little systematic study of this issue has been done, it stands to reason that the sooner psychosis is appropriately treated, the lower the risk for psychosis-related aggressive behaviors.

Duration of untreated psychosis has emerged as an independent predictor of likelihood and extent of recovery from an initial first episode and thus may be a potentially modifiable prognostic factor. A meta-analysis of 42 research reports from 28 studies found that shorter duration of untreated psychosis was associated with greater response to antipsychotic treatment, including improvement in severity of global psychopathology, positive symptoms, negative symptoms, and functional outcomes (Perkins et al. 2005). These associations were independent of the effect of other variables also associated with prognosis, including premorbid function. The effect persists into the chronic stage of illness, affecting outcomes after 15 years of illness.

Clinical programs that provide early intervention have been less systematically investigated but may reduce the likelihood of hospitalization and improve outcome. Recent specialized programs directed at the education of community and health care providers have proven successful in dramatically reducing treatment delays. For example, the Norwegian Early Treatment and Intervention in Psychosis project involved a comprehensive multimedia educational program targeting general population, health professionals, and schools and establishment of a rapid early intervention treatment team (Johannessen et al. 2001). Before the program, duration of untreated psychosis was, on average, 114 weeks (median=26 weeks). Following the program, duration of untreated psychosis was reduced, on average, to 26 weeks (median=5 weeks) ($P < 0.0005$) (Larsen et al. 2000).

In a follow-up study, duration of untreated psychosis and symptom severity were compared between two areas, one that received intense community and professional education (Rogaland County, Norway) and the other that did not (Oslo County, Norway, and Roskilde County, Denmark). Both areas had specialized first-episode treatment programs. Median duration of untreated psychosis in the intervention city was 5 weeks compared with 16 weeks in the nonintervention city (P=0.003). In addition, symptom severity was significantly lower and 3-month clinical outcome was significantly better in the intervention program (Melle et al. 2004). Similar programs exist elsewhere, including the first such program in Australia (Early Psychosis Prevention and Intervention Centre [EPPIC]) (McGorry et al. 1996). In the EPPIC, duration of untreated psychosis was reduced and outcomes were better for individuals with shorter duration of untreated psychosis (Harrigan et al. 2003). Cost of care was reduced 30% in the first year of treatment, mainly as a result of reduced hospital days (Mihalopoulos et al. 1999). Several other first-episode programs in the United Kingdom, Canada, Europe, and Asia have successfully reduced duration of untreated psychosis (Scholten et al. 2003).

TREATMENT OF THE FIRST EPISODE

GENERAL PRINCIPLES

The first episode of schizophrenia is usually frightening and even traumatic for the patient and his or her family because of the symptoms of the illness and, at times, the coercive, confusing, or unpleasant treatment interventions. Initial treatment should not only address the psychotic symptoms but also minimize subjective distress and focus on establishing a therapeutic alliance. For most patients, antipsychotic treatment results in remission of positive symptoms. Following the initial clinical response to antipsychotics and other treatments, functional recovery is emphasized. Residual symptoms, including cognitive impairments and negative symptoms, may impede functional recovery. Comorbid disorders, especially substance use disorders, should be identified and addressed. Relapse risk is very high, even in patients with good symptomatic and functional recovery, but long-term maintenance treatment with antipsychotic drugs substantially reduces the risk of relapse. Specialized first-episode treatment programs emphasize rapid entry into the health care system and intense services, including optimal pharmacotherapy, community-based services, individual and family therapeutic interventions, and assertive outreach to engage and maintain the patient in treatment.

ANTIPSYCHOTIC CHOICE AND DOSING

All antipsychotics are effective at reducing or eliminating positive symptoms; however, there may be individual differences in both symptomatic response and the experience of side effects. Compared with the first-generation antipsychotics, the second-generation antipsychotics have a decreased risk of neurological side effects, especially tardive dyskinesia, and better subjective tolerability (Lehman et al. 2004b). With the exception of clozapine, which is reserved for patients with treatment-resistant disorder because of its side-effect profile, there is no evidence of clinically meaningful differences in efficacy among the second-generation antipsychotics (Lehman et al. 2004b). However, several controlled studies now suggest greater efficacy of at least some second-generation compared with first-generation antipsychotics (Davis et al. 2003; Lieberman et al. 2005).

In addition, new data are consistent with the theory that second-generation antipsychotics may offer neuroprotection, at least to some patients. A multisite, randomized, double-blind comparison of haloperidol and olanzapine in 262 first-episode patients diagnosed with schizophrenia compared brain structural volumes during

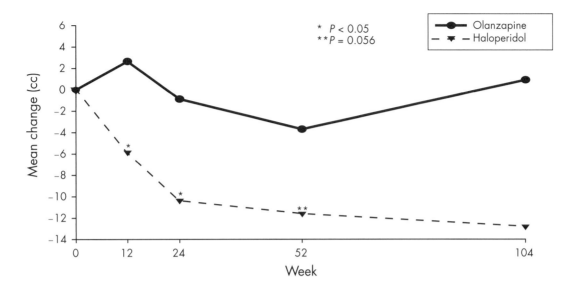

FIGURE 20–2. Whole-brain gray matter magnetic resonance imaging volumes for patients with schizophrenia, by treatment group, for observed cases.

For whole-brain gray matter volume, haloperidol-treated patients had a significant—both within-group ($P<0.002$) and between-group ($P<0.006$)—volume loss compared with olanzapine-treated patients at all time points.

the first 2 years of treatment (Lieberman et al. 2005). Olanzapine-treated subjects did not show significant decreases in whole-brain gray matter volumes over the follow-up period, unlike haloperidol-treated subjects (see Figure 20–2). For comparison purposes, healthy subjects from four sites underwent the same brain imaging. Haloperidol-treated subjects showed significant reductions in whole-brain gray matter volume, whereas olanzapine-treated subjects and healthy comparison subjects did not show volume reductions (see Figure 20–3). Better clinical outcomes, including improved neurocognitive function and less negative symptom severity, were associated with less reduction in gray matter volumes. This study offers preliminary evidence that second-generation antipsychotics may have long-term benefits, although it is not clear from the results whether the differences between olanzapine and haloperidol in gray matter volumes reflect haloperidol-associated toxicity or a neuroprotective effect of olanzapine.

In first-episode patients, the second-generation antipsychotics that have been systematically studied show reduced risk of neurological side effects but increased risk of other side effects, including weight gain, lipid abnormalities, and prolactin elevation (Emsley 1999; Lieberman et al. 2003b). Quetiapine, aripiprazole, and ziprasidone may be associated with reduced risk of weight gain and endocrine and metabolic disturbances, but these agents have not yet been systematically studied in first-episode

patients (Walter et al. 2001).

The dose of antipsychotic needed to achieve positive symptom remission in first-episode patients is typically lower than the dose needed in chronically ill patients, and use of lower doses often minimizes side-effect risk (Chakos et al. 1996; Cullberg 1999). For example, in a case series of 35 patients who received very-low-dose haloperidol (1 mg/day for first 6 weeks, mean dose at 12 weeks= 1.8 mg/day), 66% had remission of positive symptoms by 12 weeks of treatment. This response rate is similar to response rates in other first-episode studies, with very low risk of extrapyramidal side effects (Oosthuizen et al. 2004). Similarly, in a dose-finding study with first-generation antipsychotics, first-episode patients developed parkinsonian symptoms at much lower doses than did chronically ill patients (McEvoy et al. 1991). A recent study of 49 acutely psychotic, neuroleptic-naive patients with schizophrenia, schizophreniform disorder, or schizoaffective disorder found that 2 or 4 mg/day of risperidone was equally efficacious, with an advantage for the lower dosage in fine motor functioning (Merlo et al. 2002). Consistent with these studies, the American Psychiatric Association "Practice Guideline for the Treatment of Patients With Schizophrenia" and the Schizophrenia Patient Outcomes Research Team recommend that patients in a first psychotic episode should be given doses that are about half of the dose used in chronically ill populations (Lehman et al. 2004a, 2004b).

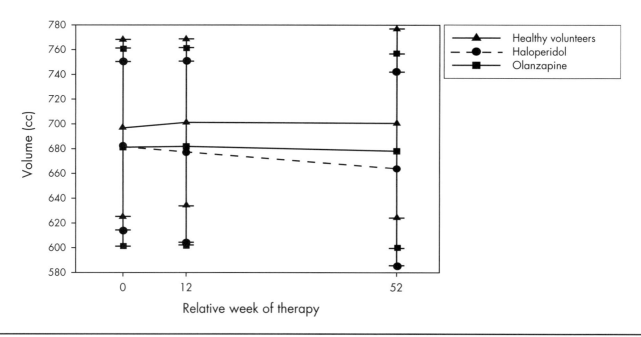

FIGURE 20–3. Whole-brain gray matter magnetic resonance imaging (MRI) volumes for patients, by treatment group, and for healthy volunteers.

Baseline, week 12, and week 52 (means±SDs) magnetic resonance images of healthy volunteers (*n*=58) and patients (*n*=75) from four sites were analyzed. Pairwise analyses: Least-squares mean changes in volume of the whole-brain gray matter in the haloperidol group differed significantly from those of olanzapine-treated patients (week 12, *P*<0.001; week 52, *P*<0.008) and healthy volunteers (week 12, *P*<0.001; week 52, *P*<0.003) at each time point.

The median time to positive symptom remission is about 3 months, but many patients will require 6–12 months to realize the maximal benefit of the antipsychotic (Loebel et al. 1992). Clinicians need to avoid pressures to escalate the dose past reasonable target doses, especially in the first few weeks of treatment. Early dose escalation increases the risk of poorly tolerated side effects without the likelihood of more rapid or better symptom response. Furthermore, because the first episode is a time when patients form their attitudes about treatment, efforts that minimize unpleasant side effects may influence patients' willingness to take medications long term. In a study of first-episode patients, the only variable that predicted whether patients would attend a follow-up assessment was antipsychotic dose, with those taking higher doses less likely to comply (Jackson et al. 2001).

POSITIVE SYMPTOMS

Studies consistently find positive symptom remission or near remission with both first- and second-generation antipsychotics. For example, in 70 first-episode patients who received first-generation antipsychotics, positive symptoms remitted by 1 year for 83%, with mean and median time to remission of 36 and 11 weeks, respectively

(Robinson et al. 1999b). A more recent randomized, double-blind clinical trial in 160 first-episode patients found that most patients had achieved positive symptom remission by 1 year with clozapine (81%) or chlorpromazine (79%) (Lieberman et al. 2003a). Subjects randomized to clozapine responded more quickly and remained in remission longer than did those receiving chlorpromazine, however, suggesting some advantage for the second-generation antipsychotic. The positive symptom responsivity of first-episode patients is also found in community treatment programs; in one clinical program, 37 of 53 (70%) patients taking primarily second-generation antipsychotics achieved complete positive symptom remission by 1 year (Malla et al. 2002a).

NEGATIVE AND COGNITIVE SYMPTOMS

Negative and cognitive symptoms of schizophrenia generally take longer to respond compared with positive symptoms and may not substantially benefit from antipsychotic treatment. In addition, the relative refractoriness of negative and cognitive symptoms may contribute to the less than optimal functional recovery that is often observed in first-episode patients (J. Addington et al. 2003; Kopala et al. 1996; Lieberman et al. 2003b; Verdoux et al. 2002).

First-generation antipsychotics may, to some extent, benefit cognitive function and negative symptoms (Davis et al. 2003; Mishara and Goldberg 2004); second-generation antipsychotics offer somewhat greater benefits. For example, a double-blind, randomized trial compared olanzapine and haloperidol in 167 first-episode patients with schizophrenia, schizoaffective disorder, or schizophreniform disorder (Keefe et al. 2004). After 12 weeks of treatment, significantly greater improvement in cognitive function, as measured by a weighted composite score of measures of verbal fluency, motor function, working memory, verbal memory, and vigilance, was seen in olanzapine-treated patients compared with haloperidol-treated patients, but cognitive function improved with both treatments. Similarly, in this same study, olanzapine-treated patients, compared with haloperidol-treated patients, had greater improvement in negative symptom severity (Lieberman et al. 2003b). Naturalistic studies generally find cognitive and negative impairments to be stable, at least in the early stage of illness, although a subgroup of patients with poor prognosis may experience decline in cognitive function (Addington et al. 2003; Stirling et al. 2003; Townsend et al. 2002).

RESIDUAL SYMPTOMS

Level of functional recovery is correlated with severity of residual negative and cognitive symptoms and to a lesser extent with residual positive symptoms (Malla et al. 2002b). Residual positive symptoms are often addressed by sequential trials of different antipsychotics because patients may have profound individual differences in response to any given antipsychotic. Clozapine or the addition of adjunctive treatments (e.g., valproate) also may benefit residual positive symptoms in some patients (Casey et al. 2003; Lehman et al. 2004b). Nonpharmacological strategies, specifically cognitive-behavioral therapy, have shown efficacy for residual positive symptoms in clinical trials (Haddock et al. 1998).

Little systematic study is available to guide clinicians when confronted with residual mood lability, dysphoria, or anxiety in first-episode patients. Benzodiazepines are effective in treating anxiety, but their use is limited if comorbid substance abuse or substance use disorder is present (Wolkowitz and Pickar 1991). Mood stabilizers, including anticonvulsants and lithium, are widely used in patients with schizophrenia, and some evidence indicates that they also may reduce impulsivity and aggression (Lehman et al. 2004b).

On presentation with an acute psychotic episode, first-episode patients often have mood symptoms (D. Addington et al. 1998). Depressive symptoms often will resolve as psychotic symptoms remit (Koreen et al. 1993); however, a postpsychotic depression may develop. The sparse available clinical trial data give mixed results for the value of antidepressants in patients with schizophrenia, even those whose symptoms meet full major depression syndrome criteria (D. Addington et al. 2002; Levinson et al. 1999). Most clinicians will recommend an antidepressant trial if significant depressive symptoms are present, given the relative safety of most antidepressants in common use (Lehman et al. 2004b).

For most first-episode patients, negative symptoms are secondary to either antipsychotic side effects (e.g., parkinsonian-related akinesia or apathy), depression (e.g., social withdrawal, anhedonia), or the effects of illness on self-esteem (e.g., poor motivation due to concerns about failure). Treatment thus should address the underlying cause. Residual primary negative symptoms (e.g., deficit syndrome) are difficult to treat, with no proven options. Medications under study include those that affect the *N*-methyl-D-aspartate receptor, such as glycine (Heresco-Levy et al. 1999), D-cycloserine (Goff et al. 1999), and neurosteroids (Strous et al. 2003).

Few proven treatments are available to address residual cognitive symptoms as well. The second-generation antipsychotics improve neurocognitive function in first-episode patients compared with first-generation antipsychotics, with the effect likely to be clinically meaningful (Emsley 1999; Keefe et al. 2004).

SUICIDE

The suicide risk is high in patients with schizophrenia, with about 1 of 10 patients eventually dying by suicide. More than half of these suicides occur within the first 5 years of illness (Verdoux et al. 2001). In addition, a significant minority (approximately 15%–25%) of first-episode patients make a suicide attempt prior to treatment (J. Addington et al. 2004; Cohen et al. 1994; Steinert et al. 1999). Although the presence of depression in the presenting psychotic episode or in the postpsychotic period is an important risk factor for suicide, patients with schizophrenia may attempt suicide in the absence of prominent depressive symptoms as a result of hallucinations, paranoia, disorganization, or other symptoms considered more primary to psychosis or other factors.

Evidence indicates that first-episode treatment programs reduce suicide risk in recovering first-episode patients (J. Addington et al. 2004), although in a randomized controlled trial, suicidality was not reduced in patients treated in a specialized first-episode treatment program (Nordentoft et al. 2002). Clozapine is indicated for the treatment of suicidality in patients with schizophrenia

(Meltzer et al. 2003). Although its use in first-episode schizophrenia has been studied recently (Lieberman et al. 2003a), clozapine is not considered at this time a first-line drug for first-episode schizophrenia given the risk of life-threatening complications. It should be considered early in the course of treatment only in patients whose symptoms are unresponsive to other second-generation antipsychotic drugs or whose suicidality remains a prominent residual symptom.

SUBSTANCE USE DISORDERS

Substance use and substance use disorders are common in first-episode patients (A.I. Green et al. 2004). Use of certain substances, particularly marijuana and psychostimulants, may be environmental factors that affect vulnerability to psychosis and impair recovery (Andreasson et al. 1987; Hambrecht and Hafner 2000; Linszen et al. 1994). Illicit substance use is also associated with poor adherence to treatment and thus is associated with increased relapse risk (Coldham et al. 2002; A.I. Green et al. 2004; Hudson et al. 2004). Thorough evaluation and targeted treatment of substance use is thus a critical component of first-episode treatment. The use of pharmacological strategies is not well researched, and clinicians often turn to strategies proven to be useful in substance-dependent patient populations (Noordsy and Green 2003).

MAINTENANCE PHASE TREATMENT

RELAPSE PREVENTION

Even with recovery from a first psychotic episode, the risk of eventual relapse is very high. Longitudinal studies generally find that by 1 year after recovery, about one-third of patients have experienced relapse, and by 2 years, two-thirds have relapsed. With sufficient follow-up periods, more than 90% of patients will experience recurrence of symptoms.

Relapse risk is greatly diminished by maintenance antipsychotic treatment (Robinson et al. 1999a). With multiple episodes of psychosis, some proportion of patients fail to recover, at least to the same degree as with their first episode (Lieberman et al. 1996). This process of psychotic relapse, treatment failure, and incomplete recovery leads many patients to a chronic course of illness (Lieberman 1999). The deterioration process occurs predominantly in the early phases of the illness, especially during the first 5–10 years after the initial episode.

However, even with strong evidence of the risk of relapse without antipsychotic medication, no clear consensus has been reached on the recommended duration of treatment for patients who have recovered from a first episode of schizophrenia. The American Psychiatric Association "Practice Guideline for the Treatment of Patients With Schizophrenia" (Lehman et al. 2004b) recommends the following:

> In arriving at a plan of treatment with remitted first-episode patients, clinicians should engage patients in discussion of the long-term potential risks of maintenance treatment with the prescribed antipsychotic versus risk of relapse (e.g., effect of relapse on social and vocational function, risk of dangerous behaviors with relapse, and risk of developing chronic treatment-resistant symptoms). Prudent treatment options that clinicians may discuss with remitted patients include either 1) indefinite antipsychotic maintenance medication or 2) medication discontinuation with close follow-up and a plan of antipsychotic reinstitution with symptom recurrence. (p. 26)

Specialized first-episode treatment programs find relatively low relapse rates. In a Dutch program in which 76 patients recovering from a first episode of psychosis had received treatment, only 15% had experienced symptom exacerbation after 15 months of treatment (Linszen et al. 1998). After 15 months of initial treatment, follow-up care was provided in the community. Within 5 years of initial recovery, 52% had at least one relapse, and 25% experienced chronic residual symptoms.

During both the acute phase and, more importantly, the maintenance phase of treatment, close monitoring for medication side effects is necessary. Regular monitoring should be done for abnormal involuntary movements and parkinsonian symptoms, sexual side effects, weight gain, metabolic status (e.g., glucose, cholesterol, triglycerides), and sedation (Lehman et al. 2004b).

FUNCTIONAL RECOVERY

First-episode patients treated in routine clinical settings typically have a deteriorating illness course despite good initial symptomatic response. For example, in a study of 349 patients followed up to 15 years after their first onset of schizophrenia, 17% had no disability at follow-up, whereas 24% still had severe disability, and the remaining 59% had varying degrees of disability (Wiersma et al. 1998). Although little systematic investigation has been done, specialized first-episode treatment programs may improve functional outcomes (J. Addington et al. 2003; Carbone et al. 1999; Linszen et al. 1998; Malla et al. 2003). Optimal maintenance pharmacological treatment may be required for functional recovery, but in some patients, medications will not be sufficient, and other treatment modalities will be needed.

MODEL FIRST-EPISODE PROGRAMS

The best psychosocial interventions for first-episode patients remain unknown, although specialized first-episode treatment programs may use a combination of strategies with some indication of success. The goals of treatment are symptomatic and functional recovery. In addition to optimal pharmacological therapy, as discussed earlier, model programs include family therapy, individual therapies, and group therapies. Many programs include an intense treatment model that is a modification of Assertive Community Treatment (ACT). Ongoing studies are investigating the effect of various therapies on outcome. The results of preliminary studies are mixed, with some but not all studies indicating benefit from one or more elements of first-episode treatment programs (Jackson et al. 2001; Jorgensen et al. 2000; Kuipers et al. 2004; Leavey et al. 2004; Nordentoft et al. 2002). The potential of these programs to improve overall prognosis for a substantial number of patients warrants further investigation.

CONCLUSION

Early treatment of schizophrenia and related psychotic disorders is likely to minimize risk of the complications of untreated psychosis, including dangerous behaviors and functional impairments. Intervention soon after the onset of illness may increase the likelihood of recovery. Pharmacotherapy should be optimized, and family and individual psychotherapy should be considered, to increase the likelihood of functional recovery. Once remission from the first episode is reached, the clinician and patient face the difficult issue of maintenance treatment duration. Despite remission, relapse risk is very high. Clinically useful predictors of the small minority who maintain remission without pharmacotherapy have not yet been identified, and the optimal length of maintenance treatment for recovered patients is not known. Prevention of recurrent relapse may reduce risk of clinical deterioration.

Second-generation or atypical antipsychotics represent an advance in the treatment of first-episode schizophrenia, with evidence for greater tolerability with equal or better therapeutic efficacy compared with first-generation antipsychotics in this population. Future research will help to characterize the efficacy of atypical antipsychotics relative to one another and define the effect of their use on the long-term outcomes of schizophrenia; however, available evidence and consensus expert opinion support their use as first-line treatment in first-episode schizophrenia (Lehman et al. 2004a).

There is movement toward developing specialized programs to treat individuals in the early course of illness.

The term *critical period* refers to the initial few years of illness, when attitudes and beliefs toward illness are developed and initial treatment occurs. Intense treatment, including family, group, and individual therapies, and assertive community outreach during this critical period may reduce the risk of suicide and relapse and may increase symptomatic and functional recovery.

REFERENCES

Addington D, Addington J, Patten S: Depression in people with first-episode schizophrenia. Br J Psychiatry Suppl 172:90–92, 1998

Addington D, Addington J, Patten S, et al: Double-blind, placebo-controlled comparison of the efficacy of sertraline as treatment for a major depressive episode in patients with remitted schizophrenia. J Clin Psychopharmacol 22:20–25, 2002

Addington J, van Mastrigt S, Hutchinson J, et al: Pathways to care: help seeking behaviour in first episode psychosis. Acta Psychiatr Scand 106:358–364, 2002

Addington J, Leriger E, Addington D: Symptom outcome 1 year after admission to an early psychosis program. Can J Psychiatry 48:204–207, 2003

Addington J, Williams J, Young J, et al: Suicidal behaviour in early psychosis. Acta Psychiatr Scand 109:116–120, 2004

Alda M, Ahrens B, Lit W, et al: Age of onset in familial and sporadic schizophrenia. Acta Psychiatr Scand 93:447–450, 1996

Amminger GP, Edwards J, Brewer WJ, et al: Duration of untreated psychosis and cognitive deterioration in first-episode schizophrenia. Schizophr Res 54(3):223–230, 2002

Andreasson S, Allebeck P, Engstrom A, et al: Cannabis and schizophrenia: a longitudinal study of Swedish conscripts. Lancet 2:1483–1486, 1987

Ang YG, Tan HY: Academic deterioration prior to first episode schizophrenia in young Singaporean males. Psychiatry Res 121:303–307, 2004

Barnes TR, Hutton SB, Chapman MJ, et al: West London first-episode study of schizophrenia: clinical correlates of duration of untreated psychosis. Br J Psychiatry 177:207–211, 2000

Black K, Peters L, Rui Q, et al: Duration of untreated psychosis predicts treatment outcome in an early psychosis program. Schizophr Res 47(2–3):215–222, 2001

Browne S, Clarke M, Gervin M, et al: Determinants of quality of life at first presentation with schizophrenia. Br J Psychiatry 176:173–176, 2000

Cannon M, Jones P, Huttunen MO, et al: School performance in Finnish children and later development of schizophrenia: a population-based longitudinal study. Arch Gen Psychiatry 56:457–463, 1999

Cannon M, Caspi A, Moffitt TE, et al: Evidence for early childhood, pan-developmental impairment specific to schizophreniform disorder: results from a longitudinal birth cohort. Arch Gen Psychiatry 59:449–456, 2002

Carbone S, Harrigan S, McGorry PD, et al: Duration of untreated psychosis and 12-month outcome in first-episode psychosis: the impact of treatment approach [see comments]. Acta Psychiatr Scand 100:96–104, 1999

Casey DE, Daniel DG, Wassef AA, et al: Effect of divalproex combined with olanzapine or risperidone in patients with an acute exacerbation of schizophrenia. Neuropsychopharmacology 28:182–192, 2003

Chakos MH, Alvir JM, Woerner MG, et al: Incidence and correlates of tardive dyskinesia in first episode of schizophrenia. Arch Gen Psychiatry 53:313–319, 1996

Cohen S, Lavelle J, Rich CL, et al: Rates and correlates of suicide attempts in first-admission psychotic patients. Acta Psychiatr Scand 90:167–171, 1994

Coldham EL, Addington J, Addington D: Medication adherence of individuals with a first episode of psychosis. Acta Psychiatr Scand 106:286–290, 2002

Cosway R, Byrne M, Clafferty R, et al: Neuropsychological change in young people at high risk for schizophrenia: results from the first two neuropsychological assessments of the Edinburgh High Risk Study. Psychol Med 30:1111–1121, 2000

Cullberg J: Integrating intensive psychosocial therapy and low dose medical treatment in a total material of first episode psychotic patients compared to "treatment as usual": a 3 year follow-up. Med Arh 53:167–170, 1999

Davidson M, Reichenberg A, Rabinowitz J, et al: Behavioral and intellectual markers for schizophrenia in apparently healthy male adolescents. Am J Psychiatry 156:1328–1335, 1999

Davis JM, Chen N, Glick ID: A meta-analysis of the efficacy of second-generation antipsychotics. Arch Gen Psychiatry 60:553–564, 2003

Di Maggio C, Martinez M, Menard JF, et al: Evidence of a cohort effect for age at onset of schizophrenia. Am J Psychiatry 158:489–492, 2001

Drake RJ, Haley CJ, Akhtar S, et al: Causes and conseqences of duration of untreated psychosis in schizophrenia. Br J Psychiatry 177:511–515, 2000

Emsley RA: Risperidone in the treatment of first-episode psychotic patients: a double-blind multicenter study. Risperidone Working Group. Schizophr Bull 25:721–729, 1999

Fuller R, Nopoulos P, Arndt S, et al: Longitudinal assessment of premorbid cognitive functioning in patients with schizophrenia through examination of standardized scholastic test performance. Am J Psychiatry 159:1183–1189, 2002

Goff DC, Tsai G, Levitt J, et al: A placebo-controlled trial of D-cycloserine added to conventional neuroleptics in patients with schizophrenia. Arch Gen Psychiatry 56:21–27, 1999

Gorwood P, Leboyer M, Jay M, et al: Gender and age at onset in schizophrenia: impact of family history. Am J Psychiatry 152:208–212, 1995

Green AI, Tohen MF, Hamer RM, et al: First episode schizophrenia-related psychosis and substance use disorders: acute response to olanzapine and haloperidol. Schizophr Res 66:125–135, 2004

Green MF, Kern RS, Braff DL, et al: Neurocognitive deficits and functional outcome in schizophrenia: are we measuring the "right stuff"? Schizophr Bull 26:119–136, 2000

Haddock G, Tarrier N, Spaulding W, et al: Individual cognitive-behavior therapy in the treatment of hallucinations and delusions: a review. Clin Psychol Rev 18:821–838, 1998

Hafner H, an der Heiden W: Epidemiology of schizophrenia. Can J Psychiatry 42:139–151, 1997

Hafner H, Nowotny B: Epidemiology of early onset schizophrenia. Eur Arch Psychiatry Clin Neurosci 245:80–92, 1995

Hafner H, an der Heiden W, Behrens S, et al: Causes and consequences of the gender difference in age at onset of schizophrenia. Schizophr Bull 24:99–113, 1998

Hafner H, Loffler W, Maurer K, et al: Depression, negative symptoms, social stagnation and social decline in the early course of schizophrenia. Acta Psychiatr Scand 100:105–118, 1999

Hambrecht M, Hafner H: Cannabis, vulnerability, and the onset of schizophrenia: an epidemiological perspective. Aust N Z J Psychiatry 34:468–475, 2000

Harrigan SM, McGorry PD, Krstev H: Does treatment delay in first-episode psychosis really matter? Psychol Med 33:97–110, 2003

Harrison G, Hopper K, Craig T, et al: Recovery from psychotic illness: a 15- and 25-year international follow-up study. Br J Psychiatry 178:506–517, 2001

Heiden W, Hafner H: The epidemiology of onset and course of schizophrenia. Eur Arch Psychiatry Clin Neurosci 250:292–303, 2000

Heresco-Levy U, Javitt DC, Ermilov M, et al: Efficacy of high-dose glycine in the treatment of enduring negative symptoms of schizophrenia. Arch Gen Psychiatry 56:29–36, 1999

Ho BC, Andreasen NC, Flaum M, et al: Untreated initial psychosis: its relation to quality of life and symptom remission in first-episode schizophrenia. Am J Psychiatry 157(5):808–815, 2000

Hoff AL, Sakuma M, Razi K, et al: Lack of association between duration of untreated illness and severity of cognitive and structural brain deficits at the first episode of schizophrenia. Am J Psychiatry 157(11):1824–1828, 2000

Hudson TJ, Owen RR, Thrush CR, et al: A pilot study of barriers to medication adherence in schizophrenia. J Clin Psychiatry 65:211–216, 2004

Isohanni M, Jones P, Kemppainen L, et al: Childhood and adolescent predictors of schizophrenia in the Northern Finland 1966 birth cohort—a descriptive life-span model. Eur Arch Psychiatry Clin Neurosci 250:311–319, 2000

Jablensky A, Cole SW: Is the earlier age at onset of schizophrenia in males a confounded finding? Results from a cross-cultural investigation. Br J Psychiatry 170:234–240, 1997

Jackson H, McGorry P, Henry L, et al: Cognitively oriented psychotherapy for early psychosis (COPE): a 1-year follow-up. Br J Clin Psychol 40 (pt 1):57–70, 2001

Johannessen JO, McGlashan TH, Larsen TK, et al: Early detection strategies for untreated first-episode psychosis. Schizophr Res 51:39–46, 2001

Jones P, Rodgers B, Murray R, et al: Child development risk factors for adult schizophrenia in the British 1946 birth cohort. Lancet 344:1398–1402, 1994

Jorgensen P, Nordentoft M, Abel MB, et al: Early detection and assertive community treatment of young psychotics: the Opus Study Rationale and design of the trial. Soc Psychiatry Psychiatr Epidemiol 35:283–287, 2000

Judge AM, Perkins DO, Nieri J, et al: Pathways to care in first episode psychosis: a pilot study on help-seeking precipitants and barriers to care. Journal of Mental Health 14(5): 465–469, 2005

Keefe RS, Seidman LJ, Christensen BK, et al: Comparative effect of atypical and conventional antipsychotic drugs on neurocognition in first-episode psychosis: a randomized, double-blind trial of olanzapine versus low doses of haloperidol. Am J Psychiatry 161:985–995, 2004

Kopala LC, Fredrikson D, Good KP, et al: Symptoms in neuroleptic-naive, first-episode schizophrenia: response to risperidone. Biol Psychiatry 39:296–298, 1996

Koreen AR, Siris SG, Chakos M, et al: Depression in first-episode schizophrenia [see comments]. Am J Psychiatry 150:1643–1648, 1993

Kuipers E, Holloway F, Rabe-Hesketh S, et al: An RCT of early intervention in psychosis: Croydon Outreach and Assertive Support Team (COAST). Soc Psychiatry Psychiatr Epidemiol 39:358–363, 2004

Larsen JK, Johannessen JO, Guldberg CA, et al: Early intervention programs in first-episode psychosis and reduction of duration of untreated psychosis. Schizophr Res 36:344–345, 2000

Larsen TK, McGlashan TH, Moe L: First-episode schizophrenia, I: early course parameters. Schizophr Bull 22(2):241–256, 1996

Larsen TK, Friis S, Haahr U, et al: Early detection and intervention in first-episode schizophrenia: a critical review. Acta Psychiatr Scand 103:323–334, 2001

Leavey G, Gulamhussein S, Papadopoulos C, et al: A randomized controlled trial of a brief intervention for families of patients with a first episode of psychosis. Psychol Med 34: 423–431, 2004

Lehman AF, Kreyenbuhl J, Buchanan RW, et al: The Schizophrenia Patient Outcomes Research Team (PORT): updated treatment recommendations 2003. Schizophr Bull 30:193–217, 2004a

Lehman AF, Lieberman JA, Dixon LB, et al: Practice guideline for the treatment of patients with schizophrenia (second edition). Am J Psychiatry 161 (2 suppl):1–56, 2004b

Levinson DF, Umapathy C, Musthaq M: Treatment of schizoaffective disorder and schizophrenia with mood symptoms. Am J Psychiatry 156:1138–1148, 1999

Lieberman JA: Is schizophrenia a neurodegenerative disorder? A clinical and neurobiological perspective. Biol Psychiatry 46:729–739, 1999

Lieberman JA, Alvir JM, Koreen A, et al: Psychobiologic correlates of treatment response in schizophrenia. Neuropsychopharmacology 14:13S–21S, 1996

Lieberman JA, Phillips M, Gu H, et al: Atypical and conventional antipsychotic drugs in treatment-naive first-episode schizophrenia: a 52-week randomized trial of clozapine vs chlorpromazine. Neuropsychopharmacology 28:995–1003, 2003a

Lieberman JA, Tollefson G, Tohen M, et al: Comparative efficacy and safety of atypical and conventional antipsychotic drugs in first-episode psychosis: a randomized, double-blind trial of olanzapine versus haloperidol. Am J Psychiatry 160:1396–1404, 2003b

Lieberman JA, Tollefson GD, Charles C, et al: Antipsychotic drug effects on brain morphology in first-episode psychosis. Arch Gen Psychiatry 62:361–370, 2005

Lincoln CV, McGorry P: Who cares? Pathways to psychiatric care for young people experiencing a first episode of psychosis. Psychiatr Serv 46:1166–1171, 1995

Lincoln C, Harrigan S, McGorry PD: Understanding the topography of the early psychosis pathways: an opportunity to reduce delays in treatment. Br J Psychiatry Suppl 172: 21–25, 1998

Linszen DH, Dingemans PM, Lenior ME: Cannabis abuse and the course of recent-onset schizophrenic disorders. Arch Gen Psychiatry 51:273–279, 1994

Linszen D, Lenior M, de Haan L, et al: Early intervention, untreated psychosis and the course of early schizophrenia. Br J Psychiatry Suppl 172:84–89, 1998

Linszen DH, Dingemans P, Lenior M: Early intervention and a five-year follow-up in young adults with a short duration of untreated psychosis: ethical implications. Schizophr Res 51 (1):55–61, 2001

Loebel AD, Lieberman JA, Alvir JM, et al: Duration of psychosis and outcome in first-episode schizophrenia. Am J Psychiatry 149:1183–1188, 1992

Malla AK, Norman RM, Manchanda R, et al: Status of patients with first-episode psychosis after one year of phase-specific community-oriented treatment. Psychiatr Serv 53:458–463, 2002a

Malla AK, Norman RM, Manchanda R, et al: Symptoms, cognition, treatment adherence and functional outcome in first-episode psychosis. Psychol Med 32:1109–1119, 2002b

Malla A, Norman R, McLean T, et al: A Canadian programme for early intervention in non-affective psychotic disorders. Aust N Z J Psychiatry 37:407–413, 2003

McEvoy JP, Hogarty GE, Steingard S: Optimal dose of neuroleptic in acute schizophrenia: a controlled study of the neuroleptic threshold and higher haloperidol dose. Arch Gen Psychiatry 48:739–745, 1991

McGorry PD, Edwards J, Mihalopoulos C, et al: EPPIC: an evolving system of early detection and optimal management. Schizophr Bull 22:305–326, 1996

Melle I, Larsen TK, Haahr U, et al: Reducing the duration of untreated first-episode psychosis: effects on clinical presentation. Arch Gen Psychiatry 61:143–150, 2004

Meltzer HY, Alphs L, Green AI, et al: Clozapine treatment for suicidality in schizophrenia: International Suicide Prevention Trial (InterSePT). Arch Gen Psychiatry 60:82–91, 2003

Merlo MC, Hofer H, Gekle W, et al: Risperidone, 2 mg/day vs. 4 mg/day, in first-episode, acutely psychotic patients: treatment efficacy and effects on fine motor functioning. J Clin Psychiatry 63:885–891, 2002

Mihalopoulos C, McGorry PD, Carter RC: Is phase-specific, community-oriented treatment of early psychosis an economically viable method of improving outcome? Acta Psychiatr Scand 100:47–55, 1999

Miller TJ, McGlashan TH, Rosen JL, et al: Prodromal assessment with the structured interview for prodromal syndromes and the scale of prodromal symptoms: predictive validity, interrater reliability, and training to reliability. Schizophr Bull 29:703–715, 2003

Milton J, Amin S, Singh SP, et al: Aggressive incidents in first-episode psychosis. Br J Psychiatry 178:433–440, 2001

Mishara AL, Goldberg TE: A meta-analysis and critical review of the effects of conventional neuroleptic treatment on cognition in schizophrenia: opening a closed book. Biol Psychiatry 55:1013–1022, 2004

Niemi LT, Suvisaari JM, Tuulio-Henriksson A, et al: Childhood developmental abnormalities in schizophrenia: evidence from high-risk studies. Schizophr Res 60:239–258, 2003

Noordsy DL, Green AI: Pharmacotherapy for schizophrenia and co-occurring substance use disorders. Curr Psychiatry Rep 5:340–346, 2003

Nordentoft M, Jeppesen P, Abel M, et al: OPUS study: suicidal behaviour, suicidal ideation and hopelessness among patients with first-episode psychosis: one-year follow-up of a randomised controlled trial. Br J Psychiatry Suppl 43:S98–S106, 2002

Oosthuizen P, Emsley R, Jadri TH, et al: A randomized, controlled comparison of the efficacy and tolerability of low and high doses of haloperidol in the treatment of first-episode psychosis. Int J Neuropsychopharmacol 7:125–131, 2004

Ott SL, Spinelli S, Rock D, et al: The New York High-Risk Project: social and general intelligence in children at risk for schizophrenia. Schizophr Res 31:1–11, 1998

Perkins DO: Markers for schizophrenia. Am J Psychiatry 157:1527, 2000

Perkins DO: Evaluating and treating the prodromal stage of schizophrenia. Curr Psychiatry Rep 6:289–295, 2004

Perkins DO, Gu H, Boteva K, et al: Relationship between duration of untreated psychosis and outcome in first-episode schizophrenia: a critical review and meta-analysis. Am J Psychiatry 162(10):1785–1804, 2005

Robinson D, Woerner MG, Alvir JM, et al: Predictors of relapse following response from a first episode of schizophrenia or schizoaffective disorder. Arch Gen Psychiatry 56:241–247, 1999a

Robinson DG, Woerner MG, Alvir JM, et al: Predictors of treatment response from a first episode of schizophrenia or schizoaffective disorder [see comments]. Am J Psychiatry 156:544–549, 1999b

Scholten DJ, Malla AK, Norman RM, et al: Removing barriers to treatment of first-episode psychotic disorders. Can J Psychiatry 48:561–565, 2003

Steinert T, Wiebe C, Gebhardt RP: Aggressive behavior against self and others among first-admission patients with schizophrenia. Psychiatr Serv 50:85–90, 1999

Stirling J, White C, Lewis S, et al: Neurocognitive function and outcome in first-episode schizophrenia: a 10-year follow-up of an epidemiological cohort. Schizophr Res 65:75–86, 2003

Stompe T, Ortwein-Swoboda G, Strobl R, et al: The age of onset of schizophrenia and the theory of anticipation. Psychiatry Res 93:125–134, 2000

Strous RD, Maayan R, Lapidus R, et al: Dehydroepiandrosterone augmentation in the management of negative, depressive, and anxiety symptoms in schizophrenia. Arch Gen Psychiatry 60:133–141, 2003

Szymanski SR, Cannon TD, Gallacher F, et al: Course of treatment response in first-episode and chronic schizophrenia. Am J Psychiatry 153(4):519–525, 1996

Townsend LA, Norman RM, Malla AK, et al: Changes in cognitive functioning following comprehensive treatment for first episode patients with schizophrenia spectrum disorders. Psychiatry Res 113:69–81, 2002

Verdoux H, Liraud F, Gonzales B, et al: Predictors and outcome characteristics associated with suicidal behaviour in early psychosis: a two-year follow-up of first-admitted subjects. Acta Psychiatr Scand 103:347–354, 2001

Verdoux H, Liraud F, Assens F, et al: Social and clinical consequences of cognitive deficits in early psychosis: a two-year follow-up study of first-admitted patients. Schizophr Res 56:149–159, 2002

Walter G, Wiltshire C, Anderson J, et al: The pharmacologic treatment of the early phase of first-episode psychosis in youths. Can J Psychiatry 46:803–809, 2001

Wiersma D, Nienhuis FJ, Slooff CJ, et al: Natural course of schizophrenic disorders: a 15-year followup of a Dutch incidence cohort. Schizophr Bull 24:75–85, 1998

Wiersma D, Wanderling J, Dragomirecka E, et al: Social disability in schizophrenia: its development and prediction over 15 years in incidence cohorts in six European centres. Psychol Med 30(5):1155–1167, 2000

Wolkowitz OM, Pickar D: Benzodiazepines in the treatment of schizophrenia: a review and reappraisal. Am J Psychiatry 148:714–726, 1991

Yung AR, McGorry PD: The prodromal phase of first-episode psychosis: past and current conceptualizations. Schizophr Bull 22:353–370, 1996

Yung AR, Phillips LJ, Yuen HP, et al: Risk factors for psychosis in an ultra high-risk group: psychopathology and clinical features. Schizophr Res 67:131–142, 2004

Zammit S, Allebeck P, David AS, et al: A longitudinal study of premorbid IQ score and risk of developing schizophrenia, bipolar disorder, severe depression, and other nonaffective psychoses. Arch Gen Psychiatry 61:354–360, 2004

TREATMENT OF CHRONIC SCHIZOPHRENIA

ALEXANDER L. MILLER, M.D.

JOSEPH P. MCEVOY, M.D.

DILIP V. JESTE, M.D.

STEPHEN R. MARDER, M.D.

The advent of new-generation antipsychotics, led by clozapine, and of psychosocial interventions that demonstrably improve patient functioning and quality of life has made optimal treatment of chronic schizophrenia very different now than it was a couple of decades ago. Clinicians have several therapeutic options for which solid evidence of efficacy exists. The goals of treatment can and should be loftier than keeping patients out of the hospital and adequately managing medication side effects. However, a relatively small minority of patients become symptom-free and without need for medication or other interventions. Thus, long-term treatment of schizophrenia typically means long-term engagement of patients and clinicians in efforts to optimize outcomes and minimize morbidity and suffering. This is an ongoing problem-solving exercise, in which both patients and treatments change over time. There are seldom single answers that are best for everyone. Rather, for any individual, a range of treatment choices must be tailored to his or her needs and circumstances.

The goal of this chapter is to highlight some of the issues that arise repeatedly in treating chronic schizophrenia and to discuss the evidence and observations that can help guide treatment selection. We first describe a set of principles for treating the multiple facets of schizophrenia over the course of illness after the first episode. Then we address a series of frequently asked questions faced by psychiatrists in their daily work with patients with schizophrenia. The literature on evidence-based practices in schizophrenia is dominated by studies of acute treatments and interventions. Long-term studies are extraordinarily difficult to conduct because of the expense and high dropout rates. Moreover, during long-term studies, new treatments arise, and health care delivery systems change, confounding efforts to attribute patient outcomes to any single intervention or set of interventions. Therefore, we are often in the position of extrapolating from relatively short-term studies and relying on expert opinion regarding long-term approaches to treatment of chronic schizophrenia.

PRINCIPLES OF LONG-TERM TREATMENT

DIAGNOSIS

The diagnosis of schizophrenia has major implications for treatment and prognosis, as well as for eligibility for public assistance programs. DSM-IV-TR (American Psychiatric Association 2000) diagnostic criteria for schizophrenia are reasonably clear-cut and are unlikely to change substantially until we have reliable and valid biological tests (e.g., genetic analyses) to replace or supplement history and clinical observation. Especially in the early years of illness, however, diagnosis may be confounded by substance abuse, prominent affective symptoms, denial of symptoms, and the hope that the illness is something other than schizophrenia. Moreover, clinicians are understandably reluctant to label patients with the diagnosis of a devastating illness until they feel assured of its accuracy. However, correctly making the diagnosis is a critical step in developing a treatment plan to optimize quality of life and reduce the negative effects of the illness. Thus, diagnosis should be an ongoing process. As the course of illness and response to treatment unfold, diagnosis must be updated.

INTEGRATION OF TREATMENTS

The major conclusion of the New Freedom Commission on Mental Health (2003) was that the mental health care system in the United States is fragmented and in chaos. Thus, the patient with chronic schizophrenia often must deal with multiple different providers of care and resources. Given that some degree of cognitive impairment and disorganization is characteristic of the illness (Palmer et al. 1997), an individual with schizophrenia negotiating the way through the multiple systems faces a daunting, even impossible, task. Thus, the treatment plan must be integrative, not one that compartmentalizes treatment according to provider profession, without regard to how the pieces fit together. Because physician time is relatively expensive, the task of integrating elements of care often falls to nonphysicians, with physicians cast in the role of prescribing medications and supervising other members of the treatment team. In the context of an illness that affects all aspects of the patient's life, however, prescribing cannot occur in a vacuum of knowledge about living environment, resources, and social circumstances, all of which can hugely affect prescribing decisions. Conversely, psychotropic medications, and their side effects, can profoundly affect progress toward other goals, such as work and independent living.

TREATMENT PLANS

The treatment plan is a vital communication tool among those responsible for the patient's treatment. It should reflect all treatment goals, specify the mechanisms to achieve them, and assign primary responsibility for each to members of the treatment team. Progress toward goals should be documented. Changing circumstances for the patient or regarding treatment options require updating the treatment plan. The treatment plan is a synthesis of treatment team and patient goals for treatment that should be determined collaboratively. For example, a patient may not view absence of symptoms as an important treatment goal but may readily agree that talking to himself interferes with his socialization goals. The process of mutually identifying and agreeing on treatment goals is discussed more in a later section on adherence.

DOCUMENTATION

A recent study of medical record documentation of psychotic symptoms and medication side effects in patients with schizophrenia found that symptom documentation was incomplete 55% of the time and that side-effect documentation was incomplete 85% of the time, when chart documentation was compared with direct patient observations made by trained investigators (Cradock et al. 2001). The study was done in typical mental health clinics, in which physician turnover is often high and patients with unscheduled visits are seen by someone other than their regular physician. Under these conditions, if the chart does not convey the information needed to make rational prescribing decisions, the potential for erratic and inconsistent decision making is enormous, and physician time is inefficiently spent trying to extract historical treatment details from patients and their families.

Although documentation is an individual responsibility, much of the care of patients with chronic schizophrenia occurs in organizations such as hospitals and clinics. There is an organizational responsibility to work with practitioners to identify which critical elements of information are needed (and how often) and then to structure paper or electronic record keeping to facilitate documentation of these elements. Documentation requirements must deal with the realities of clinical care. For example, a half-hour assessment protocol is inconsistent with seeing patients every 20 minutes.

USE OF "EFFECTIVE" TREATMENTS

The evidence-based treatments described in preceding chapters of this book have been the focus of efficacy and effectiveness (real-world) trials. When an individual patient does not respond to one of these treatments, there are two possible reasons: 1) the treatment was ineffective for the patient, or 2) the treatment was ineffectively delivered. Distinguishing between these possibilities can be difficult or impossible but is well worth the effort. An ineffective treatment is not a future option, whereas an ineffectively delivered treatment could be of great value if used correctly.

Ineffective use of medications can be by patient (not taken as prescribed) or by prescriber (incorrect dose or inadequate duration of dose). Similarly, ineffective use of nonmedication interventions can be by patient (inadequate participation) or by provider (incorrect application of intervention). Again, good documentation of treatment is essential for evaluating provider variables. Partial or total nonadherence by patients to psychosocial treatment is usually easy to recognize because adherence means being physically present and participating in the activity. Taking oral medications as an outpatient, in contrast, typically occurs in the absence of clinicians and often with no supervision. Recent studies indicate that clinicians tend to overestimate schizophrenic patient adherence to taking antipsychotic medications (Byerly et al. 2003) and that partial adherence is very common (Lacro et al. 2002). Long-acting (depot) injectable antipsychotics are an option for one component of inadequate medication adherence.

Context

Patients with schizophrenia are affected by physical environment and by family and social environments. Many of these contextual factors can be improved (or made less stressful) by proven therapeutic interventions that change the patient's family, work, or physical environment (e.g., Drake et al. 1996; Pitschel-Walz et al. 2001; Velligan et al. 2000). In addition, the patient's own view and understanding of his or her illness is important. Denial of illness is a strong predictor of medication nonadherence and of relapse (Perkins 2002; Zygmunt et al. 2002). Thus, the treatment team should evaluate and, as indicated, work to change the context within which the patient operates, including patient understanding and perceptions.

COMMON CLINICAL QUESTIONS

What Are the Options for Antipsychotic Treatment Failures?

Much of the debate about antipsychotic use centers around selection of "first-line" choices and whether first-genera-

tion antipsychotics still belong in this category. In an illness that, for most patients, needs treatment for decades, however, decisions about how to handle treatment failures are far more frequent than decisions about what to start at the outset of the illness. Moreover, even though a large majority of patients with chronic schizophrenia in the United States are now taking second-generation antipsychotics, many have had one or more trials of first-generation antipsychotics in the past. Thus, the most common clinical decision about what to do next is for the patient who has failed or been intolerant of at least one first-generation antipsychotic and at least one second-generation antipsychotic.

Most of the voluminous literature on randomized controlled trials of the efficacy of antipsychotics in chronic schizophrenia consists of parallel-group studies comparing antipsychotics with one another or with placebo. This study design yields no information about how to treat those who do poorly on their assigned treatment. By far, the highest-quality evidence for how to treat antipsychotic medication failures comes from multiple studies of clozapine that showed its unique value for treatment-refractory schizophrenia (Kane et al. 1988, 2001).

Findings from several studies of switching between antipsychotics have been published and typically show that patients do better on a new antipsychotic (Casey et al. 2003a; C.T. Lee et al. 2002; Weiden et al. 1997, 2003). Unfortunately, most of these studies are designed to address the question of how best to switch from current medications to a new one rather than quantifying the benefits of switching. To answer the latter question, the study needs to include a group that is not switched so that the effects of time and natural variation in illness severity can be controlled for. Published switch studies that lack this comparison group do not inform us if improved outcomes after switching are a result of the new medication or other factors.

Various expert consensus guidelines and algorithms have attempted to guide clinicians in selecting a rational sequence of medication treatments for chronic schizophrenia (Altamura et al. 1997; "Canadian Clinical Practice Guidelines for the Treatment of Schizophrenia" 1998; Frances et al. 1996; Kane et al. 2003b; McEvoy et al. 1999; Miller et al. 1999, 2004; Pearsall et al. 1998; Lehman et al. 2004; Smith and Docherty 1998; Stahl 1999). The recommendations in these guidelines and algorithms are based on a mixture of established evidence and expert opinion. An antipsychotic algorithm based solely on data from two or more methodologically sound randomized controlled efficacy trials for schizophrenia would have two recommendations: 1) begin with an approved antipsychotic that does not carry a "black box" warning from

TABLE 21–1.   Evidence of antipsychotic efficacy at different stages of schizophrenia

Stage of illness	Strong evidence	Moderate evidence	Weak evidence
First episode	Treat with antipsychotic	Use newer antipsychotic	Choice of specific antipsychotic
Failure of first antipsychotic		Use another antipsychotic (other than clozapine)	Choice of specific antipsychotic
Failure of second antipsychotic	Use clozapine		Use another antipsychotic (other than clozapine)
Failure of third antipsychotic	Use clozapine		
Failure of clozapine		Augment clozapine	
Failure of clozapine augmentation			Use another antipsychotic or combination of antipsychotics

the U.S. Food and Drug Administration (FDA), and 2) use clozapine for treatment-refractory schizophrenia. Clinicians, however, want to know whether to start with a newer or an older antipsychotic, whether a newer antipsychotic may work when an older one has not and vice versa, how many different trials are warranted before clozapine should be used, and what to do for those whose symptoms respond poorly to clozapine. Expert opinion is fairly uniform in several of these areas, yet convincing new data could change these opinions dramatically. Thus, for example, recent guidelines and algorithms generally recommend newer-generation antipsychotics ahead of first-generation antipsychotics for first-episode treatment, mainly for reasons of safety and tolerability. Much-needed data on effects of these agents on long-term course of illness and general health could, however, strongly reinforce or contradict this recommendation. A synthesis of recommendations from antipsychotic guidelines and algorithms that rates quality of evidence for the recommendations is presented in Table 21–1.

WHAT ARE THE OPTIONS FOR THE PATIENT WITH TREATMENT-REFRACTORY SCHIZOPHRENIA?

The terms *treatment refractory* and *treatment resistant* usually refer to persistent positive symptoms in a person who has had two or more adequate antipsychotic trials (Buckley et al. 2001). Functional impairment is not specified but implied. That is, residual psychotic symptoms that have little or no effect on day-to-day functioning are not viewed as warranting aggressive changes in therapy to totally eliminate them.

As noted in an earlier chapter (see Chapter 17, "Pharmacotherapies," this volume), studies of the efficacy of clozapine for treatment-refractory schizophrenia indicate that this medication should be tried in *every* patient in this category. However, these same studies indicate that about

half the group will have an inadequate response. It is important to use blood levels to verify that an adequate trial of clozapine has been given. Evidence suggests that a plasma clozapine concentration of 350 ng/mL or more is needed for optimal effectiveness (Perry 2001).

If 20% of patients with schizophrenia have a treatment-refractory disorder and half do not respond to clozapine, then 10% of all patients with schizophrenia have an illness for which no randomized controlled trials show efficacy of treatments available in the United States. Those who refuse clozapine or cannot tolerate it must be added to this 10%. Thus, most clinicians who see more than a few patients with schizophrenia probably have multiple patients who fall into this category.

Because the literature is so sparse, most treatment guidelines have no recommendations for treating this population. There is some evidence (including one randomized controlled trial), however, for the value of clozapine augmentation with another antipsychotic (Friedman et al. 1997; Henderson and Goff 1996; Mowerman and Siris 1996; Shiloh et al. 1997). Some evidence also supports clozapine augmentation with electroconvulsive therapy (Benatov et al. 1996; Fink 1998; Kales et al. 1999; Kupchik et al. 2000; Landy 1991; Safferman and Munne 1992) or with lamotrigine (see subsection "What About Other Agents Combined With Antipsychotics?" later in this chapter). Thus, when expert groups have addressed the issue, clozapine augmentation is the first-choice recommendation for those patients with an inadequate response to clozapine (McEvoy et al. 1999; Miller et al. 1999, 2004). The greatest number of reports is on augmentation with another antipsychotic. Use of a clozapine-augmenting agent with potent dopamine receptor–blocking activity has pharmacological appeal, but no actual evidence shows that this property is important to successful augmentation, and evidence from animal studies indicates that addition of dopamine receptor antagonists will increase the risk of extrapyramidal side effects (EPS) and tardive dyskinesia (Kapur et al. 2002).

For patients who refuse clozapine, medication options are to administer an antipsychotic that has not already been used (including a first-generation antipsychotic if the patient has no history of failure to respond to one from this group) or a combination of agents. At a recent consensus conference, expert opinion was that a trial of a different single antipsychotic should precede use of combinations, mainly because of safety considerations and the greater likelihood that monotherapy will be better adhered to (Miller et al. 2004). A patient history of having had a partial response to an earlier antipsychotic trial would suggest that this agent should be one of the components of a trial of combined antipsychotics.

Nonmedication interventions may be very useful for patients with refractory symptoms. There is growing evidence that cognitive treatment can modify problematic behavioral responses to persistent psychosis (Cormac et al. 2002). Family and other caregivers can benefit from support, support groups, and multiple family therapy (Dixon et al. 2001).

What Is the Evidence Regarding Combination Antipsychotic Treatments?

In the United States, 10%–20% of patients with schizophrenia are simultaneously taking more than one antipsychotic drug, which is referred to as *combination antipsychotics* or *antipsychotic polypharmacy* (Miller and Craig 2002). The evidence for efficacy of antipsychotic combinations was recently summarized by Stahl and Grady (2004). On the basis of all published reports as of the end of 2003, the total number of patients receiving combinations with clozapine was 276, whereas the number receiving all other combinations was 77. By contrast, when newer antipsychotics are presented to the FDA for approval, several thousand patients have been treated with them.

Absence of evidence for efficacy of combination antipsychotics does not mean that they are ineffective for individual patients, but it does mean that clinicians should carefully evaluate the effects of the combination relative to monotherapies, including clozapine, and document their superiority. Reasons for not using combination antipsychotics unnecessarily include added side-effect burden, increased risk of harmful drug–drug interactions, decreased adherence, difficulties in making rational dose adjustments, and increased costs (Miller and Craig 2002). Combinations often start as short-term measures (added as needed or for cross-titration) that become indefinitely extended. The added value of the combination, if any, can be established only by showing that outcomes are better

for the combination than for either medication alone. Another consideration in assessing a combination is that its effectiveness may be a result of a higher total dose of antipsychotic, which could have been achieved more simply by increasing the dose of the first antipsychotic. Unless it has been documented, before adding the second agent, that dose increases of the first agent were ineffective, there is no way to distinguish between these possibilities.

What About Other Agents Combined With Antipsychotics?

Psychotropics other than another antipsychotic can be combined with an antipsychotic for treatment of a host of coexisting symptoms and syndromes, as noted in the chapters on coexisting conditions (see Chapter 12, "Co-occurring Substance Use and Other Psychiatric Disorders," and Chapter 22, "Nonpsychiatric Comorbid Disorders," this volume). Here, we focus on use of agents to enhance antipsychotic efficacy for core symptoms of schizophrenia.

Data on augmentation of antipsychotics with other agents are scarce. Initial positive reports on reductions in psychopathology by open-label combination of clozapine with lamotrigine (Dursun and Deakin 2001; Dursun et al. 1999) were recently confirmed in a randomized controlled trial, although the magnitude of the improvement was quite small (Tiihonen et al. 2003). Augmentation of risperidone or olanzapine with divalproex was found to reduce positive symptoms more than adding placebo to these antipsychotics in the initial weeks of treating acute episodes, but the difference was no longer detectable after 4 weeks (Casey et al. 2003b). Efforts to treat negative symptoms of schizophrenia with antidepressants have produced mixed results, with little evidence of much effect on "core" negative symptoms (R.W. Buchanan et al. 1996, 1998).

Which Acute Patient Characteristics Influence Choice of Treatment?

The second edition of the American Psychiatric Association "Practice Guideline for the Treatment of Patients With Schizophrenia" (Lehman et al. 2004) states that the goals of treatment of an acute psychotic exacerbation include

> To prevent harm, control disturbed behavior, reduce the severity of psychosis and associated symptoms (e.g., agitation, aggression, negative symptoms, affective symptoms), determine and address the factors that led to the occurrence of the acute episode, effect a rapid return to the best level of functioning, develop an alliance with the

patient and family, formulate short- and long-term treatment plans, and connect the patient with appropriate aftercare in the community. (p. 3)

Once diagnosis is established, treatment with an antipsychotic should begin promptly. The patient's past experiences with antipsychotic medications, in terms of both therapeutic benefit and tolerability, may help in selecting a particular agent. The usual dosage ranges for the available antipsychotics are listed in Table 17–1 in Chapter 17 ("Pharmacotherapies"). During the first few days of treatment, adjunctive benzodiazepines can be very helpful in decreasing agitation and subjective distress and can improve sleep. Affective features that accompany acute exacerbations frequently clear with antipsychotic treatment alone. However, if depression persists, an antidepressant can be added. Persistent agitation and hostility can be addressed with a mood stabilizer or β-blocker.

Clinicians must immediately assess risk for dangerousness to self or others in patients experiencing an acute exacerbation of psychosis. Prior suicide attempts, depressed mood, hopelessness, and suicidal ideation all elevate the risk for suicide attempts and should lead to heightened monitoring by staff. Prior violence to others, current violent impulses, comorbid substance use disorder, current intoxication, and unmedicated psychosis all predict increased short-term risk for violence (Borum et al. 1996). The goal of risk assessment is to establish any information that should lead to clinical concern; clinical concern should lead directly to clinical intervention (e.g., treatment of psychosis, detoxification, or hospitalization).

Acute psychotic exacerbations occur for a variety of reasons during the long-term course of schizophrenia. Initially, it is useful to determine whether the exacerbation resulted from a period of nonadherence with prescribed antipsychotic medication. Patients whose exacerbations are related to medication nonadherence tend to have low levels of insight and often require involuntary commitment to receive treatment (McEvoy et al. 1984). Recovery may take weeks to months after antipsychotic treatment is reinstituted. As the patient recovers, the clinician should explore with the patient what led him or her to discontinue the prescribed medication (e.g., side effects, cost, felt he or she did not need it), attempt to resolve the issues involved, and develop a collaborative plan.

Patients with acute psychotic exacerbations despite adherence to antipsychotic treatment tend to have higher levels of insight, to be subjectively distressed, and to seek treatment on a voluntary basis. Independent, external stresses often can be identified (e.g., death of a supportive relative), or an episode of substance abuse may have occurred. These patients usually will recover within days in a protected setting if their current antipsychotic is simply continued at its original dose, although a brief temporary increase in dose or the addition of a benzodiazepine for a few days may be helpful. Psychosocial interventions to relieve the external stressors, or referral for substance use treatment, may be indicated (McEvoy et al. 1984).

In the current environment of short-term inpatient, or even outpatient, treatment of acute psychotic exacerbations, the clinician must maintain contact with the patient's family and those involved in the patient's living, vocational, and social situations to attempt to coordinate an adequate support system. Some patients have a history of medication adherence, no history of substance use or violence, and a stable living situation. However, some challenging patients commonly have more than one of the following features: homelessness, comorbid substance use, violence, and frequent rehospitalization or incarcerations. The fundamental treatment goals for these patients are ensured antipsychotic treatment and stable housing. Unless an exceptionally dedicated assertive community treatment team is available to find these patients every day and deliver oral antipsychotic treatment to them, the use of a long-acting injectable antipsychotic is indicated. Homeless patients do not have a safe place to store medication or a stable daily routine into which taking medication can be woven.

WHICH LONG-TERM PATIENT CHARACTERISTICS INFLUENCE CHOICE OF TREATMENT?

In the context of treating chronic schizophrenia, long-term patient characteristics refer to demographic or relatively enduring features of the patient that clinicians should attend to in selecting treatments. A key task of psychiatric practice is selection and adaptation of evidence-based treatments to optimize their use for individual patients. Because age is such an important factor, we discuss it as a separate issue later in this chapter.

Selection of long-term medication treatment should take into account the patient's current and past physical and medical conditions, as well as family medical history. Antipsychotic drugs present a spectrum of side effects (see Table 17–2 in Chapter 17, this volume) that can help guide medication choice.

In promoting informed decision making and medication adherence, discussion of potential side effects of medication options with patients is a critical step in the medication selection process. Characteristics such as obesity, high blood pressure, family history of sudden death, high sensitivity to side effects, family history of diabetes, and cardiac conditions can help guide choice of antipsychotic

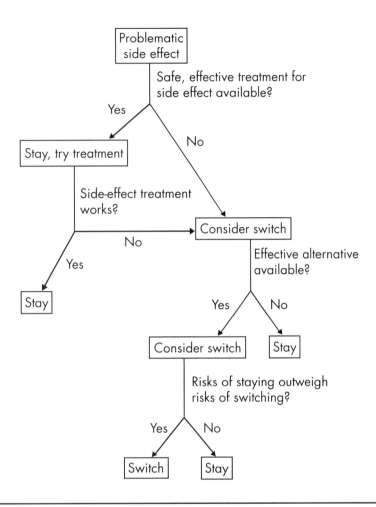

FIGURE 21–1. Flowchart for deciding whether a patient whose condition has been stabilized with an antipsychotic that has a problematic side effect should be maintained on that medication or switched to another antipsychotic.

medication. Ultimately, however, the primary goal of medication is optimal treatment of schizophrenia. Avoidance of unwanted side effects is extremely important, but relief of suffering and disability caused by the illness is paramount. Thus, clinicians frequently end up facing the dilemma of treating patients who are doing the best they have ever done while taking a medication but have a side effect (e.g., weight gain) that is physically and medically problematic.

No rules exist for these situations, but logic can be used to find an individualized solution to the dilemma. Clinicians and patients should collaboratively examine several questions: Are there effective, tolerable, safe treatments for the side effect? Are there medication alternatives with a reasonable chance of success? On the basis of history and current circumstances, what are the risks of unsuccessful treatment with a different antipsychotic? These questions should be periodically revisited as new information about treatments and side effects emerges and patient circumstances change. Although the evidence

is scanty, pessimism about the ability of patients with chronic schizophrenia to benefit from behavior change programs does not seem warranted. A recent report, for example, showed quite good effects of a weight-control program for managing weight gain associated with second-generation antipsychotics (Vreeland et al. 2003). Figure 21–1 presents a decision tree to help guide medication decision making for the person with chronic schizophrenia who is well stabilized but has problematic side effects.

HOW SHOULD MEDICATION ADHERENCE PROBLEMS BE EVALUATED AND TREATED?

Potential causes of relapse in chronic schizophrenia are manifold, but inadequate adherence to prescribed medication regimens always should be considered as a contributing factor. Most patients fall somewhere on the spectrum between complete medication adherence and total nonadherence. This raises the question of how much adherence is enough. A cutoff of taking less than 75%–80%

of the prescribed doses is often used to define inadequate adherence, but the empirical basis for this is not strong. Some data suggest that as adherence declines below 100%, a direct relation is seen between degree of nonadherence and level of symptoms (Docherty et al. 2003). Dose of medication, relative to minimally effective dose, obviously makes a difference if missed doses are sporadic rather than grouped. That is, if a patient taking double his or her minimally effective dose misses half of each daily dose, the net result approximates the minimally effective dose, whereas the same degree of nonadherence in a patient prescribed his or her minimally effective dose would result in clearly subtherapeutic dosing.

No "gold standard" exists for assessing outpatient oral medication adherence (Velligan et al. 2003). Objective measures, such as pill counts, blood levels, or use of devices that record opening of the pill container, have practical limitations in terms of time and effort or expense. Moreover, these methods require patients to remember to bring their containers or when to take their last dose before having blood drawn. Physician and patient estimates of adherence are far easier to obtain, but recent studies have found that both groups significantly overestimate pill taking, relative to objective measures (Byerly et al. 2003; Lam et al. 2003). Thus, a clinician examining a previously stable patient whose symptoms have worsened is often without any reliable way of determining whether decreased medication adherence is a contributing factor or whether medication effectiveness has decreased. Increasing the dose of medication may be effective in either circumstance; thus, improvement after a dose increase should not be construed as clear evidence that the patient's dose–response curve has changed. A blood level measurement after the patient has restabilized while taking the same medication may be useful as a baseline measure against which to compare blood levels at the time of any future relapses. If a patient's illness worsens with no change in the treatment regimen, then careful questioning about the details of medication taking and side effects is warranted. If a patient cannot describe when, where, and what medicines are taken, nonadherence may be the problem. Similarly, if there are no side effects, or if previously reported side effects are suddenly denied or have become more tolerable, the patient may not be taking the medication.

Repeated relapses, with improvements during periods of controlled supervision of medications and worsening when medication administration is not supervised, are strongly suggestive of adherence problems. Many factors can contribute to inadequate medication adherence, but a few deserve special mention here because of their frequency:

- Substance abuse involving drugs and/or alcohol is common in schizophrenia and can result in poor medication adherence. Direct inquiries about substance abuse to patients and those in frequent contact with them can be supplemented with blood and urine testing.
- Problems with side effects can contribute to erratic taking of medications, and patients may incorrectly attribute dysphoric experiences to medication side effects. Exploration of the contribution of side effects, real or perceived, to medication nonadherence is worthwhile.
- Availability of medications can interfere with medication adherence. Sometimes the issue is cost, but often the long waits and relatively remote pharmacies stand in the way of better adherence. For patients with an illness that affects motivation and planning abilities, the role of systemic barriers to obtaining and refilling medication prescriptions is always a consideration.

Several psychosocial interventions to improve medication adherence in schizophrenia have been evaluated. One controlled study of compliance therapy found that identifying patient goals and aspirations and relating them to treatment outcomes affected by medications improved medication adherence (Kemp et al. 1998). However, this finding was not confirmed in a recent replication study (O'Donnell et al. 2003). Both studies began with inpatients, but the earlier study included outpatient follow-up sessions, which may have contributed to the differing results.

Boczkowski et al. (1985) found that behavioral tailoring resulted in significantly greater increases in adherence than did psychoeducation:

> The investigator helped each participant tailor his prescribed regimen so that it was better adapted to his personal habits and routines. This involved identifying a highly visible location for the placement of medications and pairing the daily medication intake with specific routine behavior of the participant. Each participant was given a self-monitoring spiral calendar, which featured a dated slip of paper for each dose of the neuroleptic. The participant was instructed to keep the calendar near his medications and to tear off a slip each time he took a pill. (p. 668)

Supervision of outpatients by family members or friends can enhance compliance (A. Buchanan 1992; McEvoy et al. 1989b). Case workers and assertive community treatment teams can deliver and oversee taking of medications, as can operators of residential facilities.

Sometimes hospital-based, legally sanctioned coercion is needed to ensure that medications are delivered.

Unfortunately, available evidence suggests that the patients who most resist treatment and require coercion show little or no improvement in acknowledgment of illness and need for treatment when they are forcibly treated, even though their psychiatric symptoms diminish significantly (Marder et al. 1984; McEvoy et al. 1989a). Therefore, after discharge, these patients are unlikely to continue with treatment when the choice is again theirs in the outpatient setting. However, outpatient commitment has been shown to improve medication adherence in this group, as discussed in Chapter 18 ("Psychosocial Therapies") (Swartz et al. 2001).

For patients who have adherence problems with oral medications but are willing to continue taking medications, the clinician can consider changing to a different, better-tolerated oral medication or to a depot preparation. On average, patients find the newer antipsychotics more tolerable (Hellewell 2002), yet the evidence thus far is that better tolerability results in only modest gains in adherence (Dolder et al. 2002). Depot preparations have the virtues of certainty of administration and immediate knowledge of missed doses. The magnitude of the relapse-prevention advantage of using depot antipsychotics has varied considerably across studies, depending on study design and type of patients enrolled (Adams et al. 2001; Schooler 2003), but outcomes generally have been superior to oral treatment with the same medication. The introduction of the first depot preparation of a second-generation antipsychotic—risperidone—gives clinicians a useful new depot option (Kane et al. 2003a).

UNCOMMON SYNDROMES

POLYDIPSIA–HYPONATREMIA

Polydipsia–hyponatremia is a common syndrome among chronically hospitalized psychotic patients, especially those with schizophrenia. The literature review of De Leon et al. (1994) suggested that more than 20% of chronically hospitalized patients have polydipsia, and one-quarter of these (5% of the total) also have hyponatremia. In a subsequent prospective epidemiological study of a state hospital, De Leon et al. (1996) found that 26% of the total chronically hospitalized population had polydipsia and that 5% also had hyponatremia. Nursing and other clinical staff can often identify patients who are drinking excessive amounts of water. A urine-specific gravity less than 1.009 is suggestive of polydipsia. If a patient appears to have polydipsia, it may be useful to carefully check weights between 7:00 and 8:00 A.M., after the patient

voids and before breakfast, and again between 3:00 and 4:00 P.M., with the patient wearing similar clothing. The normalized diurnal weight gain is the percentage of weight gained between morning and afternoon, calculated by dividing the day's weight gain by the morning weight. A normalized diurnal weight gain less than 1.2% is normal. A normalized diurnal weight gain greater than 4% carries a serious risk of water intoxication.

Polydipsia–hyponatremia may lead to urological (bladder dilatation), cardiovascular (congestive heart failure), or central nervous system (seizures) complications (Delva et al. 2002). Abnormalities in the release of antidiuretic hormone or atrial natriuretic peptide do not fully explain the polydipsia–hyponatremia syndrome (Kawai et al. 2001; Verghese et al. 1998). However, in the presence of polydipsia, events that can lead to increased release of antidiuretic hormone (heavy cigarette smoking, vomiting, head injury, psychotic exacerbation, or drugs such as carbamazepine) may lead to hyponatremia (Kawai et al. 2001). Patients with polydipsia who have developed hyponatremia should have their weights checked several times daily. A gain of 10% or more of their baseline weight (first morning weight after voiding) should lead to fluid restriction.

Clozapine is the one pharmacological treatment that has shown consistent therapeutic benefit for patients with polydipsia–hyponatremia (H.S. Lee et al. 1991; Spears et al. 1996; Verghese et al. 1998); clozapine produces decreased fluid intake and urine volume and increased serum sodium and osmolality. Other pharmacological agents, including other second-generation antipsychotics, angiotensin-converting enzyme inhibitors, clonidine, β-blockers, naloxone, and democlocycline, have been tried but have not shown replicable benefit (Delva et al. 2002). Patients who develop severe hyponatremia need medical treatment in an intensive care unit. The serum sodium levels should be raised gradually over several days to avoid risk of osmotic demyelination syndrome (Edoute et al. 2003).

CATATONIA

Catatonia is a syndrome of motor and behavioral abnormalities that may accompany a wide range of psychotic, mood, or medical disorders (Rosebush and Mazurek 1999). Examination for catatonia is not a part of the routine mental status or physical examinations, and catatonia can be missed. The Catatonia Rating Scale has been developed and tested for this purpose (Braunig et al. 2000). In patients with schizophrenia, catatonia is predominantly characterized by grimacing, jerky movements, mannerisms, rituals, exaggerated responsiveness, and posturing.

It is important to correctly recognize catatonic hypomotility because hypomotility is associated with considerable morbidity, including dehydration, infection, malnutrition, and thromboembolism (Rosebush and Mazurek 1999). Intramuscular or intravenous benzodiazepines usually will relieve catatonic hypomotility within minutes and preclude or limit the need for maintenance intravenous or nasogastric tube feeding and catheterization. Electroconvulsive therapy can benefit those patients with hypomotility not relieved by benzodiazepines.

INTEGRATING PHARMACOTHERAPY AND PSYCHOSOCIAL TREATMENT

Long-term treatment in chronic schizophrenia should be based on a recovery model that seeks to optimize an individual's overall well-being. The recovery orientation focuses on improving functional outcomes, including vocational, social, and educational outcomes, and quality of life. Because improvements in these outcomes almost always require both psychosocial treatments or rehabilitation and pharmacotherapy, these two modalities of treatment should be integrated in long-term strategies.

The treatment literature provides some guidance regarding approaches to combining treatments. Psychosocial treatments are most likely to be effective when symptoms have been adequately treated with drugs. A large multicenter study found that psychosocial treatments could actually lead to a worse outcome when outpatients with schizophrenia were given a placebo (Hogarty et al. 1974). In addition, psychosocial treatments are more effective when medication adherence is ensured by a long-acting injectable antipsychotic (Hogarty et al. 1979). Another study with social skills training found that patients who received a type of pharmacotherapy that minimized the proportion of time that they were in a psychotic state also showed the greatest improvements in social adjustment (Marder et al. 1996).

The introduction of the second-generation antipsychotics also has provided information suggesting that pharmacological strategies can promote psychosocial treatments and rehabilitation. The strongest evidence has emerged from a Department of Veterans Affairs Cooperative Study that compared clozapine and haloperidol (Rosenheck et al. 1998). The use of psychosocial treatments was monitored during the study. Patients who received clozapine were more likely to participate in psychosocial treatments. This interaction of second-generation antipsychotics and psychosocial treatments is supported by a study that found that patients who received

risperidone and a more intensive form of social skills training tended to have better outcomes relative to treatment with haloperidol and the same social skills training (Marder et al. 2003). Taken together, these studies suggest that second-generation antipsychotics, perhaps because of reduced EPS, improved adherence, or improved effects on cognition or negative symptoms, may facilitate productive use of psychosocial treatments.

TREATMENT OF CHRONIC SCHIZOPHRENIA IN OLDER PATIENTS

The number of elderly people with schizophrenia is expected to more than double over the next three decades (Palmer et al. 1999). Several unique clinical features associated with aging make treatment in older patients a challenge as well as an opportunity to help improve their functioning and quality of life. In this section, we focus on characteristics that distinguish the treatment of chronic schizophrenia in older adults.

DIAGNOSIS

Most older patients with schizophrenia had their onset of illness in adolescence or early adulthood and thus have had many years of experience with the illness. A little more than 20% of the patients with schizophrenia manifest symptoms of the illness for the first time in middle or old age (Harris and Jeste 1988). Inconsistencies in nosology and a tendency to attribute late-onset psychoses to "organic" factors or to mood disorders have led to diagnostic confusion in these cases.

The International Late-Onset Schizophrenia Group (Howard et al. 2000) concluded that two separate categories had face validity and clinical utility: 1) late-onset schizophrenia (mostly middle-age onset—i.e., during the fifth, sixth, or seventh decade of life) and 2) very-late-onset schizophrenia-like psychosis (onset during or after the seventh decade). Patients meeting strict clinical criteria for late-onset schizophrenia are similar to those with early-onset schizophrenia in clinical symptomatology, family history, cognitive deficits, nonspecific brain imaging abnormalities, course of illness, and treatment response and do not manifest mood disorders or dementia when followed up over several years (Jeste et al. 1997). Also, several important and consistent differences between early- and late-onset schizophrenia suggest that the latter should be identified as a distinct subtype of schizophrenia. Such differences include a much higher prevalence of late-onset schizophrenia in women, its association with paranoid subtype, less severe negative symptoms and cognitive impairment, and a need for lower doses of antipsychotics.

Very-late-onset schizophrenia-like psychosis, a heterogeneous group of disorders, differs from both early- and late-onset schizophrenia in that it is associated with sensory impairment, social isolation, visual hallucinations, and, usually, progressive cognitive decline but is not characterized by formal thought disorder, affective blunting, or family history of schizophrenia.

COURSE

The course of schizophrenia in late life varies considerably. Whereas a small minority of patients experience complete or nearly complete remission of symptoms, and a small minority worsen to the level of dementia, most patients have a relatively stable course, with significant improvement in psychotic symptoms (Bleuler 1972/1978; Cohen et al. 2000; Jeste et al. 2003b). The rate of aging-associated cognitive decline in older community-dwelling schizophrenic patients is similar to that in age-comparable nonschizophrenic individuals (Eyler Zorrilla et al. 2000; Heaton et al. 2001). However, because patients with schizophrenia generally have a greater degree of premorbid cognitive deficits, they continue to be more impaired than nonschizophrenic subjects in later life as well. In contrast to younger adults, physical comorbidity is a greater problem than illicit substance abuse in older patients with schizophrenia.

PHARMACOKINETICS AND PHARMACODYNAMICS: AGE-RELATED CHANGES

Older patients show greater variability of response and greater sensitivity to medications than do younger adults (Jeste et al. 2005). Elderly patients tend to have higher blood levels and to be more sensitive to the therapeutic and adverse effects of antipsychotic medications compared with their younger counterparts, implying that lower dosages than those used in younger patients may be optimal. The "start low and go slow" approach to starting new medications is often appropriate for older patients.

CONTEXT

Most older people with schizophrenia are not institutionalized and do not live with families. Common residences for them include assisted living facilities (e.g., a board-and-care home) or quasi-independent settings such as single-room-occupancy hotels. The level and quality of health care provided in these settings vary widely and gen-

erally range from inadequate to poor. A treating psychiatrist needs to review the entire biopsychosocial situation to ensure that all general medical conditions are evaluated and treated appropriately, no unnecessary polypharmacy is found, and the patient has access to various available forms of social assistance.

BASELINE EVALUATION

Before an antipsychotic is started in an elderly person, a comprehensive medical and psychosocial evaluation is recommended. Physical comorbidity and polypharmacy (including the use of prescribed and over-the-counter medications, nutritional supplements, and herbal supplements) frequently complicate treatment in older patients. Cognitive and sensory deficits may interfere with adherence to prescribed medication regimens. Elderly patients may unintentionally take incorrect doses of medications or follow erroneous dosing schedules.

SELECTION OF AN ANTIPSYCHOTIC

Special considerations in an elderly person include the potential adverse consequences of adding an antipsychotic to a preexisting medication regimen or effects on a comorbid physical illness. Second-generation antipsychotics are preferred to conventional ones given the high risk of EPS and tardive dyskinesia in older persons. One exception to this rule is a patient who has been taking a first-generation antipsychotic for many years, is stable, does not have distressing side effects, and does not want to risk switching to another antipsychotic. In terms of choosing among different second-generation antipsychotics, no studies show greater efficacy of one over the others in elderly patients. Therefore, the selection is determined primarily by the side-effect profiles of individual antipsychotics in the context of a given patient's medical status, other pharmacological regimen, and relevant psychosocial considerations (including medication costs).

Recently, the FDA issued a "black box" warning regarding increased mortality with atypical antipsychotics in elderly patients with dementia-related psychosis. Whether this increased risk extends to elderly patients with schizophrenia is unknown.

Table 21–2 lists the clinically significant side effects of antipsychotics and those antipsychotics more commonly associated with these effects in elderly patients. This table may help the clinician to decide which agents to avoid in a given patient. For example, the patients in whom urinary retention needs to be avoided, such as those with prostatic hypertrophy, should not be given the antipsychotics that are more likely to produce anticholinergic ef-

TABLE 21–2.   Side effects associated with different antipsychotics in elderly patients

Side effect	Antipsychotics more commonly associated with these effects
Sedation	Typical antipsychotics, clozapine, olanzapine, quetiapine, aripiprazole

Anticholinergic effects
  Central (confusion, disorientation, agitation, delirium)
  Peripheral (constipation, urinary retention, glaucoma, dry mouth)
	Thioridazine, chlorpromazine, clozapine

Orthostatic hypotension	Low-potency first-generation antipsychotics, clozapine, quetiapine (others in high doses)
Extrapyramidal symptoms	High-potency first-generation antipsychotics, risperidone (olanzapine in high doses)
Weight gain	First-generation antipsychotics, clozapine, olanzapine (high doses of risperidone and quetiapine)
Hyperprolactinemia (sexual dysfunction, osteoporosis)	First-generation antipsychotics (especially haloperidol), risperidone
Cerebrovascular accidents in elderly patients with dementia	Risperidone, olanzapine,[a] aripiprazole
Increased mortality in elderly patients with dementia	All atypical antipsychotics

[a]This is based on recent analyses of combined databases with these agents; a cause-and-effect relation between these agents and cerebrovascular events has not yet been established.

fects. An increased incidence of diabetes has been noted with at least some of the newer antipsychotics. This potential complication of antipsychotic treatment is discussed in Chapter 17 ("Pharmacotherapies").

First-Generation Antipsychotics

Although there is a relative dearth of literature on the effects of first-generation or typical antipsychotics in elderly patients, these drugs have been shown to be at least moderately effective in the treatment of schizophrenia (Jeste et al. 2003a) or psychosis of Alzheimer's disease (Katz et al. 2003; Street et al. 2000) in elderly patients. Discontinuation of antipsychotics has been found to be associated with a high incidence of psychotic relapse. In six double-blind, controlled studies that included middle-aged and elderly patients, the mean rate of relapse for patients whose first-generation antipsychotic was withdrawn was 40% over an average 6-month follow-up period, whereas that for patients maintained on those antipsychotics was 11% (Jeste et al. 1993).

The risk of EPS and tardive dyskinesia with first-generation antipsychotics is much greater in older than in younger patients. The cumulative annual incidence of

tardive dyskinesia with first-generation antipsychotics has been found to be sixfold higher (i.e., about 30%; Jeste et al. 1999b) in later life than in younger adults. Other side effects of particular concern in elderly patients include sedation, anticholinergic effects, and postural hypotension.

Second-Generation Antipsychotics

Second-generation, or atypical, antipsychotic medications have rapidly become the first-line treatment for older patients with psychotic disorders in the United States. Controlled data on the efficacy and safety of the second-generation antipsychotics in older patients with schizophrenia are lacking. Nonetheless, available data suggest that the second-generation antipsychotics may be at least as efficacious as and better tolerated than the conventional antipsychotics, mainly because of a lower risk of both EPS and tardive dyskinesia (Jeste et al. 1999b; Madhusoodanan et al. 2000; Sajatovic et al. 2000; Street et al. 2000). Use of clozapine is mainly restricted to patients with treatment-resistant symptoms.

In the only large-scale, double-blind comparative study of second-generation antipsychotics in elderly patients with schizophrenia published to date, risperidone at a median dosage of 2 mg/day was found to be as effective as olanzapine at a median dosage of 10 mg/day (Jeste et al. 2003a). Subjects came from both inpatient and outpatient settings. Both drugs produced significant improvement in psychiatric symptoms from baseline, with a low incidence of EPS, in this 8-week trial. The two drugs did not differ in therapeutic or adverse effects, except that clinically significant weight gain (≥7% of baseline body weight) occurred in 14% of the olanzapine-treated patients compared with 5% of the risperidone-treated patients.

Side Effects

The risk of developing tardive dyskinesia has been shown to be significantly lower for patients taking second-generation antipsychotics than for those taking first-generation antipsychotic medications (Dolder and Jeste 2003; Jeste et al. 1999a). Side effects of second-generation antipsychotics that are of concern in elderly persons include sedation, orthostatic hypotension, EPS (at higher dose ranges), weight gain, and type 2 diabetes mellitus.

Sedation is one of the most common side effects of antipsychotic drugs in older patients, especially with clozapine, olanzapine, quetiapine, and aripiprazole. Sedation can be helpful for the elderly patient with insomnia or severe agitation. It may, however, increase the risk of falls and fractures. Excessive sedation may occur when antipsychotics are administered in combination with other central nervous system depressants.

Anticholinergic side effects of antipsychotics (especially with clozapine) in the presence of the age-related decrease in cholinergic function can lead to serious problems by worsening disorientation, confusion, constipation, urinary retention, glaucoma, visual hallucinations, and agitation. Concomitant use of other medications with anticholinergic side effects (e.g., antiparkinsonian medications) increases the risk of severe toxicity.

Other side effects are particularly relevant for older patients. Important cardiovascular side effects include orthostatic hypotension, particularly with clozapine and quetiapine, and QTc prolongation with ziprasidone. In terms of weight gain, elderly patients who are frail or poorly nourished may benefit from this effect; however, weight gain also may aggravate preexisting cardiovascular disease or osteoarthritis in this population. Hyperprolactinemia with first-generation antipsychotics and risperidone may lead to sexual dysfunction and may compromise bone-mineral density and increase the incidence of osteoporosis.

Reports of a higher incidence of serious cerebrovascular events (strokes and transient ischemic attacks) with risperidone and olanzapine and of increased mortality with olanzapine in elderly patients with dementia (Katz et al. 2003; "Dear Doctor" letter from Eli Lilly to physicians, dated February 27, 2004) have led to labeling changes and have appropriately increased clinical concern about these issues. However, at this time, no cause-and-effect relation between the antipsychotics and those adverse effects has been established. It is expected that further research will clarify the clinical significance of these findings.

Monitoring medication side effects. Given the elevated risk of most side effects, older patients should be assessed more frequently than younger adults are. Elderly patients would be considered to be in the high-risk category for the recommended monitoring of most side effects listed in the chapter on pharmacological treatments of schizophrenia and should be monitored carefully (see Chapter 17, "Pharmacotherapies").

Dosing

The starting dose in older patients generally should be one-quarter to one-half of the usual starting dose for younger adults. The required dose of an antipsychotic for an older patient tends to correlate inversely with current age and with age at onset of illness. Thus, a good guideline is the older a patient is, the lower the recommended dose should be. Patients with late-onset schizophrenia typically require a lower dose than comparably aged early-onset patients; for patients with very-late-onset schizophrenia-like psychosis, even lower doses may be warranted (Howard et al. 2000). Occasionally, however, a treatment-resistant older patient may need amounts comparable to those given to younger adults. As chronically ill patients who have been taking antipsychotics for many years continue to age, their dose requirements often decrease. Doses should, therefore, be monitored according to the clinical needs of a given patient at a given time. The length of treatment trial in an elderly patient should generally be longer (6–10 weeks) than that in a younger adult, with slower dose increases.

The recommended average dosage ranges (mg/day) for elderly patients with schizophrenia are shown in Table 21–3.

Switching Medications

As discussed earlier, a frequent dilemma facing clinicians involves whether and how best to switch patients who have been taking a first-generation antipsychotic for several years to a second-generation agent. Sometimes, a similar issue arises when a patient does not respond adequately to or develops unacceptable adverse effects with

TABLE 21–3. Recommended average dosage ranges (mg/day) for elderly patients with schizophrenia

Drug	Initial dosage	Maintenance dosage
Risperidone	0.5–1	1.5–3
Olanzapine	5–7.5	7.5–12.5
Quetiapine	25–50	100–300
Clozapine	25–50	75–200
Aripiprazole	5–15	15–25

a second-generation antipsychotic and may need to be switched to a different second-generation drug. Such a decision should be made after an informed discussion with the patient and his or her caregiver, as appropriate. When switching antipsychotics is indicated, it should be done gradually and over a much longer period than in younger adults (except in the instance of life-threatening adverse events). The dose of the antipsychotic to be discontinued should be slowly decreased while the new agent is slowly titrated up (Jeste et al. 1999b). Generally, the dose should be reduced by no more than 25% at a time, with further dose reductions staggered over a period of several weeks. During the time of dose reduction of an older drug, the new agent should be started at a low dose and increased slowly. The lowest effective maintenance dose should be used once the patient is clinically stable.

Concomitant Medications

Depressive symptoms are common and also functionally disruptive in older persons with schizophrenia (Jin et al. 2001). In such cases, an antidepressant may be added. No comparative trials of antidepressants in this population have yet been published, but citalopram has been found to be useful and relatively safe in a small open-label study of older patients with schizophrenia (Kasckow et al. 2001). Several other nonantipsychotic drugs have been used with varying success in older patients, although no controlled studies have been published.

INTEGRATING PHARMACOLOGICAL AND PSYCHOSOCIAL TREATMENTS

Recent work has shown the benefits of integrated cognitive-behavioral social skills training (Granholm et al. 2005) and of functional adaptation skills training (Patterson et al. 2003) in improving daily functioning in older patients with schizophrenia. A special emphasis is required in terms of educating patients (and their caregivers) about medication adherence, in view of the fact that most older patients are receiving complex regimens of multiple medications.

REFERENCES

Adams CE, Fenton MKP, Quraishi S, et al: Systematic meta-review of depot antipsychotic drugs for people with schizophrenia. Br J Psychiatry 179:290–299, 2001

Altamura AC, Barnas C, Bitter I, et al: Treatment of schizophrenic disorders: algorithms for acute pharmacotherapy. International Journal of Psychiatry in Clinical Practice 1 (suppl 1):S25–S30, 1997

American Psychiatric Association: Diagnostic and Statistical Manual of Mental Disorders, 4th Edition, Text Revision. Washington, DC, American Psychiatric Association, 2000

Benatov R, Sirota P, Megged S: Neuroleptic-resistant schizophrenia treated with clozapine and ECT. Convuls Ther 12:117–121, 1996

Bleuler M: The Schizophrenic Disorders: Long-Term Patient and Family Studies (1972). Translated by Clemens SM. New Haven, CT, Yale University Press, 1978

Boczkowski JA, Zeichner A, DeSanto N: Neuroleptic compliance among chronic schizophrenic outpatients: an intervention outcome report. J Consult Clin Psychol 53:666–671, 1985

Borum R, Swartz M, Swanson J: Assessing and managing violence risk in clinical practice. Journal of Practical Psychiatry and Behavioral Health 4:205–215, 1996

Braunig P, Kruger S, Shugar G, et al: The Catatonia Rating Scale, I: development, reliability, and use. Compr Psychiatry 41:147–158, 2000

Buchanan A: A two-year prospective study of treatment compliance in patients with schizophrenia. Psychol Med 22:787–797, 1992

Buchanan RW, Kirkpatrick B, Bryant N, et al: Fluoxetine augmentation of clozapine treatment in patients with schizophrenia. Am J Psychiatry 153:1625–1627, 1996

Buchanan RW, Breier A, Kirkpatrick B, et al: Positive and negative symptom response to clozapine in schizophrenic patients with and without the deficit syndrome. Am J Psychiatry 155:751–760, 1998

Buckley P, Miller AL, Olsen J, et al: When symptoms persist: clozapine augmentation strategies. Schizophr Bull 27:615–628, 2001

Byerly M, Fisher R, Rush AJ, et al: Comparison of clinician vs. electronic monitoring of antipsychotics adherence in schizophrenia. Paper presented at the 156th annual meeting of the American Psychiatric Association, San Francisco, CA, May 17–22, 2003

Canadian clinical practice guidelines for the treatment of schizophrenia. The Canadian Psychiatric Association. Can J Psychiatry 43 (suppl 2):25S–40S, 1998

Casey DE, Carson WH, Saha AR: Switching patients to aripiprazole from other antipsychotic agents: a multicenter randomized study. Psychopharmacology 166:391–399, 2003a

Casey DE, Daniel DG, Wassef AA, et al: Effect of divalproex combined with olanzapine or risperidone in patients with an acute exacerbation of schizophrenia. Neuropsychopharmacology 28:182–192, 2003b

Cohen CI, Cohen GD, Blank K, et al: Schizophrenia and older adults: an overview: directions for research and policy. Am J Geriatr Psychiatry 8:19–28, 2000

Cormac I, Jones C, Campbell C: Cognitive behaviour therapy for schizophrenia. Cochrane Database Syst Rev (1): CD000524, 2002

Cradock J, Young AS, Sullivan G: The accuracy of medical record documentation in schizophrenia. J Behav Health Serv Res 28:456–465, 2001

De Leon J, Verghese C, Tracy JI, et al: Polydipsia and water intoxication in psychiatric patients: a review of the epidemiological literature. Biol Psychiatry 35:408–419, 1994

De Leon J, Dadvand M, Canuso C, et al: Polydipsia and water intoxication in a long-term psychiatric hospital. Biol Psychiatry 40:28–34, 1996

Delva NH, Chang A, Hawken ER, et al: Effects of clonidine in schizophrenic patients with primary polydipsia: three single case studies. Prog Neuropsychopharmacol Biol Psychiatry 26:387–392, 2002

Dixon LB, McFarlane WR, Lefley H, et al: Evidence-based practices for services to families of people with psychiatric disabilities. Psychiatr Serv 52:903–910, 2001

Docherty NM, Grogg A, Kozma C, et al: Antipsychotic maintenance in schizophrenia: partial compliance and clinical outcome (abstract). Schizophr Bull 60 (suppl):281, 2003

Dolder CR, Jeste DV: Incidence of tardive dyskinesia with typical versus atypical antipsychotics in very high risk patients. Biol Psychiatry 53:1142–1145, 2003

Dolder CR, Lacro JP, Jeste DV: Antipsychotic medication adherence: is there a difference between typical and atypical agents? Am J Psychiatry 159:103–108, 2002

Drake RE, McHugo GJ, Becker DR, et al: The New Hampshire study of supported employment for people with severe mental illness. J Consult Clin Psychol 64:391–399, 1996

Dursun SM, Deakin JFW: Augmenting antipsychotic treatment with lamotrigine or topiramate in patients with treatment-resistant schizophrenia: a naturalistic case-series outcome study. J Psychopharmacol 15:297–301, 2001

Dursun SM, McIntosh D, Milliken H: Clozapine plus lamotrigine in treatment-resistant schizophrenia. Arch Gen Psychiatry 56:950, 1999

Edoute Y, Davids MR, Johnston C, et al: An integrative physiological approach to polyuria and hyponatremia: a "double-take" on the diagnosis and therapy in a patient with schizophrenia. Q J Med 96:531–540, 2003

Eyler Zorrilla LT, Heaton RK, McAdams LA, et al: Cross-sectional study of older outpatients with schizophrenia and healthy comparison subjects: no differences in age-related cognitive decline. Am J Psychiatry 157:1324–1326, 2000

Fink M: ECT and clozapine in schizophrenia. J ECT 14:223–226, 1998

Frances A, Docherty JP, Kahn DA, et al: Expert Consensus Guidelines Series: Treatment of schizophrenia. J Clin Psychiatry 57 (suppl 12B):5–58, 1996

Friedman JH, Ault K, Powchik P: Pimozide augmentation for the treatment of schizophrenic patients who are partial responders to clozapine. Biol Psychiatry 42:522–523, 1997

Granholm E, Periveliotis D, McQuaid JR, et al: A randomized controlled trial of cognitive behavioral social skills training for middle-aged and older outpatients with chronic schizophrenia. Am J Psychiatry 162:520–529, 2005

Harris MJ, Jeste DV: Late onset schizophrenia: an overview. Schizophr Bull 14:39–55, 1988

Heaton RK, Gladsjo JA, Palmer BW, et al: Stability and course of neuropsychological deficits in schizophrenia. Arch Gen Psychiatry 58:24–32, 2001

Hellewell JS: Patients' subjective experiences of antipsychotics: clinical relevance. CNS Drugs 16:457–471, 2002

Henderson DC, Goff DC: Risperidone as an adjunct to clozapine therapy in chronic schizophrenics. J Clin Psychiatry 57:395–397, 1996

Hogarty GE, Goldberg SC, Schooler NR: Drug and sociotherapy in the aftercare of schizophrenia patients. Arch Gen Psychiatry 31:609–618, 1974

Hogarty GE, Schooler NR, Ulrich R, et al: Fluphenazine and social therapy in the aftercare of schizophrenic patients: relapse analyses of a two-year controlled study of fluphenazine decanoate and fluphenazine hydrochloride. Arch Gen Psychiatry 36:1283–1294, 1979

Howard R, Rabins PV, Seeman MV, et al: Late-onset schizophrenia and very-late-onset schizophrenia-like psychosis: an international consensus. Am J Psychiatry 157:172–178, 2000

Jeste DV, Lacro JP, Gilbert PL, et al: Treatment of late-life schizophrenia with neuroleptics. Schizophr Bull 19:817–830, 1993

Jeste DV, Symonds LL, Harris MJ, et al: Non-dementia non-praecox dementia praecox? Late-onset schizophrenia. Am J Geriatr Psychiatry 5:302–317, 1997

Jeste DV, Lacro JP, Baile A, et al: Lower incidence of tardive dyskinesia with risperidone compared with haloperidol in older patients. J Am Geriatr Soc 47:716–719, 1999a

Jeste DV, Rockwell E, Harris MJ, et al: Conventional vs. newer antipsychotics in elderly patients. Am J Geriatr Psychiatry 7:70–76, 1999b

Jeste DV, Barak Y, Madhusoodanan S, et al: An international multisite double-blind trial of the atypical antipsychotic risperidone and olanzapine in 175 elderly patients with chronic schizophrenia. Am J Geriatr Psychiatry 11:638–647, 2003a

Jeste DV, Twamley EW, Eyler Zorrilla LT, et al: Aging and outcome in schizophrenia. Acta Psychiatr Scand 107:336–343, 2003b

Jeste DV, Dolder CR, Nayak GV, et al: Atypical antipsychotics in elderly patients with dementia or schizophrenia: review of recent literature. Harv Rev Psychiatry 13(6):340–351, 2005

Jin H, Zisook S, Palmer BW, et al: Association of depressive symptoms with worse functioning in schizophrenia: a study of older outpatients. J Clin Psychiatry 62:797–803, 2001

Kales HD, Dequardo JR, Tandon R: Combined electroconvulsive therapy and clozapine in treatment-resistant schizophrenia. Prog Neuropsychopharmacol Biol Psychiatry 23:547–556, 1999

Kane J, Honigfeld G, Singer J, et al: Clozapine for the treatment-resistant schizophrenic: a double-blind comparison versus chlorpromazine/benztropine. Arch Gen Psychiatry 45:789–796, 1988

Kane JM, Marder SR, Schooler NR, et al: Clozapine and haloperidol in moderately refractory schizophrenia: a 6-month randomized and double-blind comparison. Arch Gen Psychiatry 58:965–972, 2001

Kane JM, Eerdekens M, Lindenmayer JP, et al: Long-acting injectable risperidone: efficacy and safety of the first long-acting atypical antipsychotic. Am J Psychiatry 160:1125–1132, 2003a

Kane JM, Leucht S, Carpenter D, et al: Expert Consensus Guidelines Series: Optimizing pharmacologic treatment of psychotic disorders, introduction: methods, commentary, and summary. J Clin Psychiatry 64 (suppl 12):1–100, 2003b

Kapur S, McClelland RA, VanderSpek SC, et al: Increasing D2 affinity results in the loss of clozapine's atypical antipsychotic action. Neuroreport 13:831–835, 2002

Kasckow JW, Mohamed S, Thallasinos A, et al: Citalopram augmentation of antipsychotic treatment in older schizophrenia patients. Int J Geriatr Psychiatry 16:1163–1167, 2001

Katz IR, Jeste DV, Pollock BG, et al: Commentary: treating aggressive behavior in the elderly. J Clin Psychiatry 64(suppl):S12–S16, 2003

Kawai N, Baba A, Suzuki T, et al: Roles of arginine vasopressin and atrial natriuretic peptide in polydipsia-hyponatremia of schizophrenic patients. Psychiatr Res 101:39–45, 2001

Kemp R, Kirov G, Everitt B, et al: Randomized controlled trial of compliance therapy: 18 month follow-up. Br J Psychiatry 172:413–419, 1998

Kupchik M, Spivak B, Mester R, et al: Combined electroconvulsive-clozapine therapy. Clin Neuropharmacol 23:14–16, 2000

Lacro JP, Dunn LB, Dolder CR, et al: Prevalence of and risk factors for medication nonadherence in patients with schizophrenia: a comprehensive review of recent literature. J Clin Psychiatry 63:892–909, 2002

Lam FYW, Velligan DI, DiCocco M, et al: Comparative assessment of antipsychotic adherence by concentration monitoring, pill count and self-report (abstract). Schizophr Bull 60 (suppl):313, 2003

Landy DA: Combined use of clozapine and electroconvulsive therapy. Convuls Ther 9:176–180, 1991

Lee CT, Conde BJ, Mazlan M, et al: Switching to olanzapine from previous antipsychotics: a regional collaborative multicenter trial assessing 2 switching techniques in Asia Pacific. J Clin Psychiatry 63:569–576, 2002

Lee HS, Kwon KY, Alphs LD, et al: Effect of clozapine on psychogenic polydipsia in chronic schizophrenia. J Clin Psychopharmacol 11:222–223, 1991

Lehman AF, Lieberman JA, Dixon LB, et al: Practice guideline for the treatment of patients with schizophrenia, second edition. Am J Psychiatry 161 (2 suppl):1–56, 2004

Madhusoodanan S, Brenner R, Cohen CI: Risperidone for elderly patients with schizophrenia or schizoaffective disorder. Psychiatr Ann 30:175–180, 2000

Marder SR, Swann E, Winsdale WJ, et al: A study of medication refusal by involuntary patients. Hosp Community Psychiatry 35:724–726, 1984

Marder SR, Wirshing WC, Mintz J, et al: Two-year outcome of social skills training and group psychotherapy for outpatients with schizophrenia. Am J Psychiatry 153:1585–1592, 1996

Marder SR, Glynn SM, Wirshing WC, et al: Maintenance treatment of schizophrenia with risperidone or haloperidol: 2-year outcomes. Am J Psychiatry 160:1405–1412, 2003

McEvoy JP, Howe AC, Hogarty GE: Differences in the nature of relapse and subsequent inpatient course between medication compliant and noncompliant schizophrenic patients. J Nerv Ment Dis 172:412–416, 1984

McEvoy JP, Appelbaum PS, Apperson LJ, et al: Why must some schizophrenic patients be involuntarily committed? The role of insight. Compr Psychiatry 30:13–17, 1989a

McEvoy JP, Freter S, Everett G, et al: Insight and the clinical outcome of schizophrenic patients. J Nerv Ment Dis 177:48–51, 1989b

McEvoy JP, Scheifler PI, Frances A: Expert Consensus Guideline Series: Treatment of schizophrenia 1999. J Clin Psychiatry 60 (suppl 11):1–80, 1999

Miller AL, Craig CS: Combination antipsychotics: pros, cons, and questions. Schizophr Bull 28:105–109, 2002

Miller AL, Chiles JA, Chiles JK, et al: The Texas Medication Algorithm Project (TMAP) Schizophrenia Algorithms. J Clin Psychiatry 60:649–657, 1999

Miller AL, Hall CS, Buchanan RW, et al: The Texas Medication Algorithm Project antipsychotic algorithm for schizophrenia: 2003 update. J Clin Psychiatry 65:500–508, 2004

Mowerman S, Siris SG: Adjunctive loxapine in a clozapine-resistant cohort of schizophrenic patients. Ann Clin Psychiatry 8:193–197, 1996

New Freedom Commission on Mental Health: Achieving the promise: transforming mental health care in America. 2003. Available at http://www.mentalhealthcommission.gov.

O'Donnell C, Donohoe G, Sharkey L, et al: Compliance therapy: a randomised controlled trial in schizophrenia. BMJ 327 (7419):834, 2003

Palmer BW, Heaton RK, Paulsen JS, et al: Is it possible to be schizophrenic yet neuropsychologically normal? Neuropsychology 11:437–446, 1997

Palmer BW, Heaton SC, Jeste DV: Older patients with schizophrenia: challenges in the coming decades. Psychiatr Serv 50:1178–1183, 1999

Patterson TL, McKibbin C, Taylor M, et al: Functional Adaptation Skills Training (FAST): a pilot psychosocial intervention study in middle-aged and elderly patients with chronic psychotic disorders. Am J Geriatr Psychiatry 11: 17–23, 2003

Pearsall R, Glick ID, Pickar D, et al: A new algorithm for treating schizophrenia. Psychopharmacol Bull 34:349–353, 1998

Perkins DO: Predictors of noncompliance in patients with schizophrenia. J Clin Psychiatry 63:1121–1128, 2002

Perry PJ: Therapeutic drug monitoring of antipsychotics. Psychopharmacol Bull 35:19–29, 2001

Pitschel-Walz G, Leucht S, Bauml J, et al: The effect of family interventions on relapse and rehospitalization in schizophrenia—a meta-analysis. Schizophr Bull 27:73–92, 2001

Rosebush PI, Mazurek MF: Catatonia: re-awakening to a forgotten disorder. Mov Disord 14:395–397, 1999

Rosenheck R, Tekell J, Peters J, et al: Does participation in psychosocial treatment augment the benefit of clozapine? Department of Veterans Affairs Cooperative Study Group on Clozapine in Refractory Schizophrenia. Arch Gen Psychiatry 55:618–625, 1998

Safferman AZ, Munne R: Combining clozapine with ECT. Convuls Ther 8:141–143, 1992

Sajatovic M, Madhusoodanan S, Buckley P: Schizophrenia in the elderly: guidelines for its recognition and treatment. CNS Drugs 13:103–115, 2000

Schooler NR: Relapse and rehospitalization: comparing oral and depot antipsychotics. J Clin Psychiatry 64 (suppl 16):14–17, 2003

Shiloh R, Zemishlany Z, Aizenberg D, et al: Sulpiride augmentation in people with schizophrenia partially responsive to clozapine: a double-blind, placebo-controlled study. Br J Psychiatry 171:569–573, 1997

Smith TE, Docherty JP: Standards of care and clinical algorithms for treating schizophrenia. Psychiatr Clin North Am 21:203–220, 1998

Spears NM, Leadbetter RA, Shutty MS: Clozapine treatment in polydipsia and intermittent hyponatremia. J Clin Psychiatry 57:123–128, 1996

Stahl SM: Selecting an atypical antipsychotic by combining clinical experience with guidelines from clinical trials. J Clin Psychiatry 60 (suppl 10):31–41, 1999

Stahl SM, Grady MM: A critical review of atypical antipsychotic utilization: comparing monotherapy with polypharmacy and augmentation. Curr Med Chem 11:313–327, 2004

Street JS, Tollefson GD, Tohen M, et al: Olanzapine for psychotic conditions in the elderly. Psychiatr Ann 30:191–196, 2000

Swartz MS, Swanson JW, Hiday VA, et al: A randomized controlled trial of outpatient commitment in North Carolina. Psychiatr Serv 52:325–329, 2001

Tiihonen J, Hallikainen T, Ryynanen OP, et al: Lamotrigine in treatment-resistant schizophrenia: a randomized placebo-controlled crossover trial. Biol Psychiatry 54:1241–1248, 2003

Velligan DI, Bow-Thomas CC, Huntzinger D, et al: Randomized controlled trial of the use of compensatory strategies to enhance adaptive functioning in outpatients with schizophrenia. Am J Psychiatry 157:1317–1323, 2000

Velligan DI, DiCocco M, Castillo DA, et al: Obstacles in assessing adherence to oral antipsychotic medications (abstract). Schizophr Res 60:330, 2003

Verghese C, Abraham G, Nair C, et al: Absence of changes in antidiuretic hormone, angiotensin II, and atrial natriuretic peptide with clozapine treatment of polydipsia-hyponatremia: 2 case reports. J Clin Psychiatry 59:415–419, 1998

Vreeland B, Minsky S, Menza M, et al: A program for managing weight gain associated with atypical antipsychotics. Psychiatr Serv 54:1155–1157, 2003

Weiden PJ, Aquila R, Dalheim L, et al: Switching antipsychotic medications. J Clin Psychiatry 58 (suppl 10):63–72, 1997

Weiden PJ, Simpson GM, Potkin SG, et al: Effectiveness of switching to ziprasidone for stable but symptomatic outpatients with schizophrenia. J Clin Psychiatry 64:580–588, 2003

Zygmunt A, Olfson M, Boyer CA, et al: Interventions to improve medication adherence in schizophrenia. Am J Psychiatry 159:1653–1664, 2002

NONPSYCHIATRIC COMORBID DISORDERS

LISA DIXON, M.D., M.P.H.

ERICK MESSIAS, M.D., M.P.H., PH.D.

KAREN WOHLHEITER, M.S.

Several studies documented markedly increased mortality rates among persons with schizophrenia. The life expectancy of persons with schizophrenia is on average reduced by 9–10 years (Tsuang et al. 1980). Although suicide is responsible for a significant share of this increased mortality, increased medical morbidity and substance use also contribute. Such comorbidity also influences the care of schizophrenic patients by complicating treatment and affecting prognosis. For example, comorbid substance use disorders are associated with negative outcomes such as increased psychotic symptoms, poorer treatment compliance, violence, homelessness, medical problems, poor money management, and greater use of crisis-oriented services (Dixon 1999). In improving the health status and quality of life of persons with schizophrenia, it is imperative to enhance our understanding and management of comorbidity.

In this chapter, we review the findings regarding the presence of substance use disorders and medical conditions among patients with schizophrenia. First, we review general models to understanding comorbid conditions.

Second, we address nicotine dependence and substance-related disorders. Third, we review the most common medical comorbidities associated with schizophrenia. Finally, we discuss how these issues affect the treatment of schizophrenia.

MODELS OF COMORBIDITY

Comorbidity is defined as the occurrence of two or more diagnostic categories in the same individual at the same time. Four models have been used to explain the higher rate of substance use comorbidity in schizophrenia (Mueser et al. 1995). These same models can be applied to further our understanding of somatic comorbidities in schizophrenia.

In the *secondary disorder model*, the presence of schizophrenia leads to an increased vulnerability to substance abuse for either self-medication, social facilitation, or pleasure enhancement and to an increased risk for somatic comorbidities, either through medication side effects or

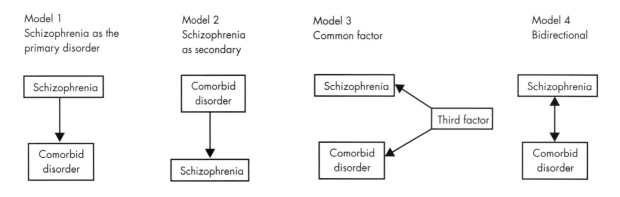

FIGURE 22–1.   Models of comorbidity.

through behavioral inclinations. Risk of diabetes, for example, could be increased by antipsychotic drugs or by poor dietary habits or decreased physical activities.

In the *secondary psychiatric disorder model*, the psychiatric presentation is a result of the comorbid condition. Most studies point to the possibility of substance abuse acting as a precipitator of psychotic symptoms in those with a psychobiological vulnerability, not as a causal factor. No evidence shows that this path could occur in medical conditions (i.e., having such conditions causes schizophrenia). However, in some cases, medical conditions such as partial seizures or systemic lupus erythematosus could lead to psychotic symptoms, mimicking schizophrenia.

In the *common factor model*, the increased rate of schizophrenia and other conditions is the result of a shared etiological factor. This third variable could be either a genetic common vulnerability or a shared environmental risk factor. For example, some have hypothesized a shared genetic risk between diabetes and schizophrenia given the increased family history of diabetes found in some early studies (Mukherjee et al. 1989b).

In the *bidirectional model*, schizophrenia and the comorbid conditions interact in such a way that either disorder influences the occurrence of the other. An example of this model is when patients with schizophrenia use psychoactive substances to counter symptoms and experience worsening of psychotic symptoms as a result of the substance use.

The four models of comorbidity in schizophrenia are depicted in Figure 22–1.

NICOTINE DEPENDENCE

Patients with schizophrenia are much more likely to be smokers compared with the general population (Dalack et

al. 1998; Ziedonis et al. 1994). An estimated 70%–90% of persons with schizophrenia smoke, whereas the estimated prevalence in the United States general population is 25% (Bergen and Caporaso 1999). Also, those with schizophrenia who smoke tend to smoke more heavily, use cigarettes with a higher level of nicotine, and quit less frequently (Lohr and Flynn 1992). Cigarette smoking in persons with schizophrenia may be an attempt to self-medicate negative symptoms (Dalack et al. 1998). Nicotine dependence is also associated with a reduction in the serum level of some antipsychotic medications (Lyon 1999), mostly by induction of cytochrome P450 1AC promoted by the "tar" (polynuclear aromatic hydrocarbons) present in cigarettes (Ziedonis and Nickou 2001). As such, serum levels of haloperidol, fluphenazine, thiothixene, clozapine, and olanzapine are decreased in patients who smoke cigarettes (Ziedonis and Nickou 2001). International studies have proposed the role of social and economic determinants in smoking behavior in schizophrenia as well (Srinivasan and Thara 2002).

Patients with schizophrenia are more likely to initiate smoking after age 20 and are more likely to be daily smokers than are other individuals (de Leon et al. 2002). A differential pattern of response to nicotine in subjects with schizophrenia, in tests of sensory gating and eye tracking measures, points to the presence of abnormalities in the nicotinic system in schizophrenia (Sherr et al. 2002).

Cigarette smoking has been associated with a variety of medical conditions in the general population, with similar effects expected in persons with schizophrenia. The adverse effects of cigarette smoking on pregnancy outcomes are well known, and as expected, smoking seems to be associated with adverse pregnancy outcomes in women with schizophrenia (Nilsson et al. 2002). Higher prevalence of chronic obstructive pulmonary disease also has been found among those with schizophrenia (Himmelhoch et al. 2004).

A controlled clinical trial has shown a role for bupropion and atypical antipsychotics in smoking cessation for individuals with schizophrenia (George et al. 2002). There is some indication that clozapine reduces smoking in schizophrenia, although the mechanisms for this action remain unknown (Procyshyn et al. 2001, 2002). Given the hypothesis of an abnormality in the nicotinic system in persons with schizophrenia (Sherr et al. 2002), nicotine replacement strategies likely will play an important role in treating cigarette smoking in this population. It is important to note that in patients who stop or reduce smoking, the dosage of antipsychotic medication may need to be adjusted to compensate for the induction previously caused by cigarettes. Further research is needed to assess the effectiveness of smoking cessation programs for persons with schizophrenia.

SUBSTANCE USE DISORDERS

Substance use disorders are the most common comorbid conditions in schizophrenia (Ziedonis and Nickou 2001). As many as half of patients with schizophrenia are affected by alcohol or drug use disorders (Bellack and DiClemente 1999; Dixon 1999; Fowler et al. 1998; Regier et al. 1990). Substance use disorders may be an important disease modifier because they tend to affect patients with less severe clinical characteristics (Dixon et al. 1991). Patients with deficit schizophrenia (i.e., patients with primary and enduring negative symptoms) are less likely to use drugs, except marijuana and alcohol (Kirkpatrick et al. 1996). Patients with schizophrenia report abusing drugs for the same reasons as the general population does (e.g., "getting high," relieving depression, and relaxing) (Dixon et al. 1991).

A study based on a sample from the Epidemiologic Catchment Area survey found that patients with schizophrenia follow three patterns related to substance use: no use, cannabis and alcohol use, and polysubstance abuse (Cuffel et al. 1993). That same study found that patients with either pattern of substance use were more likely to be younger, to be male, and to have depressive symptoms.

Persons with schizophrenia who have a comorbid substance use disorder often have many negative outcomes, such as more frequent and longer periods of hospitalization, more pronounced psychotic symptoms, more severe cerebral gray matter volume deficits (Mathalon et al. 2003), poorer treatment adherence, more depressive symptoms, higher risk of suicide, violence, legal problems, incarceration, severe financial problems, family burden, housing instability, and increased risk for HIV infection (Drake and Wallach 1989; Drake et al. 1989) and hepatitis infection,

particularly hepatitis C (Rosenberg et al. 2001). Those outcomes are particularly striking in light of the association of drug use with less severe clinical characteristics. This contrast shows the role of drug use as a major disease modifier in schizophrenia.

MARIJUANA USE

Persons with schizophrenia are at high risk for marijuana abuse (DeQuardo et al. 1994). A review of the evidence on the role of cannabinoids in the development of schizophrenia concluded that use of marijuana leads to a twofold increase in the relative risk of later onset of schizophrenia; however, the authors also concluded that "cannabis use appears to be neither a sufficient nor a necessary cause for psychosis" (Arseneault et al. 2004, p. 110). Furthermore, cannabis abuse has been proposed as a precipitant of psychotic episodes in persons with schizophrenia (Linszen et al. 1994). Its use also may increase the risk for tardive dyskinesia (Zaretsky et al. 1993). Pharmacologically, marijuana has anticholinergic effects that may lead some patients with schizophrenia to use it to relieve the extrapyramidal side effects of some antipsychotic medications (Ziedonis and Nickou 2001).

ALCOHOL USE

Alcohol has been shown to exert some of its effect by inhibiting the response of the N-methyl-D-aspartate (NMDA) receptor, a receptor system implicated in schizophrenia, which leads to disruption in glutamatergic neurotransmission (Tsai et al. 1995), and by modulating γ-aminobutyric acid (GABA)$_A$ receptors in the central nervous system (CNS) (Morrow et al. 2001). Persons with schizophrenia are more likely to abuse alcohol compared with the general population (Regier et al. 1990). Alcohol seems to have a destabilizing social effect, and those with an alcohol-related disorder are more likely to have unstable housing, conceptual disorganization, denial of mental illness, and rehospitalization (Osher et al. 1994). Among persons with schizophrenia, suspiciousness is associated with a higher risk of alcohol dependence, particularly in males (Messias and Bienvenu 2003).

COCAINE USE

Cocaine use is associated with release of dopamine in the human brain, particularly in the orbitofrontal area, an area associated with motivated behavior and drive (Volkow and Fowler 2000). Chronic exposure to cocaine thus is associated with changes in the orbitofrontal, striatal, and thalamic areas (Volkow and Fowler 2000).

Persons with schizophrenia are more likely to use cocaine than are people in the general population. Patients with schizophrenia who abuse cocaine have been found to have less severe negative symptoms, younger age at first hospitalization, and higher rates of paranoid subtype (Lysaker et al. 1994).

SUBSTANCE USE DISORDERS IN SCHIZOPHRENIA: AN INTEGRATIVE APPROACH

Patients with symptoms being considered for a schizophrenia diagnosis always should be evaluated for substance use disorders as part of their clinical workup. Furthermore, the presence of a substance use disorder in a patient with schizophrenia should shape the treatment recommendations. A comprehensive and integrative approach to substance use disorder in schizophrenia has been shown to reduce abuse and to help attain remission (Drake and Mueser 2000, 2001; Drake et al. 1998). This treatment modality involves assertive outreach, case management, a stagewise motivational approach for patients who do not recognize the need for substance abuse treatment, behavioral interventions for those who are trying to attain or maintain abstinence, family interventions, housing, rehabilitation, and pharmacology (Lehman et al. 2004). Because of the problem of lack of insight about substance dependence, the first step in the treatment implementation should be devoted to motivation building rather than abstinence achievement, which is the long-term goal. One way to motivate a patient with schizophrenia to stop using drugs and alcohol is to help him or her recognize the role of this behavior in interfering with personal goals and interpersonal relationships (Drake and Mueser 2001). Two other elements to inform substance use disorder treatment in persons with schizophrenia are 1) conceptualizing treatment as an ongoing process and 2) a harm reduction model.

These elements have been integrated in the Behavioral Therapy for Substance Abuse in Schizophrenia (BTSAS) model, which was developed to address specific problems pertinent to this population (Bennett et al. 2001). The treatment protocol contains six main components:

1. A urinalysis contingency designed to enhance motivation to change and increase the salience of goals
2. Structured goal setting to identify realistic, short-term goals for decreased substance use
3. Motivational interviewing to enhance motivation to reduce use
4. Social skills and drug refusal skills to enable patients to develop relationships with people who do not use drugs, to enable patients to refuse social pressure to use sub-

stances, and to provide success experiences that can increase self-efficacy for change
5. Education about the reasons for substance use and the particular dangers of substance use for people with severe and persistent mental illness to shift the decisional balance toward decreased use
6. Relapse prevention training that focuses on behavioral skills for coping with urges and dealing with high-risk situations and lapses

BTSAS was specifically structured to reduce the load on memory and attention and to minimize demands on higher-level cognitive processes. It is administered in small groups twice per week for 6 months (Bellack and DiClemente 1999; Bellack and Gearon 1998; Bennett et al. 2001).

MEDICAL ILLNESSES

Persons with schizophrenia also are at higher risk for some medical illnesses that deserve attention, particularly diabetes, infectious diseases (especially sexually transmitted diseases), and respiratory conditions, such as emphysema and chronic bronchitis. Data from the Schizophrenia Patient Outcomes Research Team (PORT) showed higher than expected rates of diabetes, heart disease, respiratory illness, and sexually transmitted diseases in this population (Dixon et al. 1999). Comparison of data from a sample of persons with schizophrenia treated in community settings with data from a matched national sample found that those with schizophrenia had a higher prevalence of respiratory conditions, such as chronic obstructive pulmonary disease and asthma, diabetes, and liver disease (Sokal et al. 2004). Contributors to this increased risk include higher rates of obesity (Allison et al. 1999), cigarette smoking (Dalack et al. 1998), and medication side effects (Jeste et al. 1996). The presence of an increased risk for diabetes and cardiovascular disorders in this population has raised the possibility of a "metabolic syndrome" affecting patients with schizophrenia (Ryan and Thakore 2002).

The social withdrawal associated with schizophrenia is a factor that could prevent self-care and treatment-seeking behavior for physical complaints (Goldman 1999). Patients with schizophrenia also perceive more barriers to treatment of medical conditions (Dickerson et al. 2003), which may lead to lack of preventive services that could have affected the prevalence of certain conditions. Furthermore, research indicates that schizophrenia is a factor in decreasing the likelihood of receiving preventive medical care and in making fewer visits for chronic medical conditions (Folsom et al. 2002).

DIABETES MELLITUS

Antipsychotic medication seems to play a role in the origin of diabetes in persons with schizophrenia; however, there has been some report of increased diabetes prevalence in persons with diabetes before the introduction of antipsychotic compounds (Dixon et al. 2000). Furthermore, drug-naive patients also have been shown to have more highly impaired fasting glucose tolerance, to be more insulin resistant, and to have higher levels of plasma glucose, insulin, and cortisol than do healthy comparison subjects (Ryan et al. 2003).

Although type 2 diabetes is a highly prevalent chronic medical condition diagnosed in approximately 4.5% of the United States population (Centers for Disease Control and Prevention 2005), those with schizophrenia have an estimated prevalence of 16%–25% (Dixon et al. 2000; Mukherjee et al. 1996; Newcomer et al. 2002; Subramaniam et al. 2003).

Atypical antipsychotics, particularly clozapine, quetiapine, and olanzapine, seem to be associated with an increased risk for developing diabetes (Koro et al. 2002; Sernyak et al. 2002). Other risk factors for diabetes in persons with schizophrenia include sedentary lifestyle, obesity, poor diet, and high smoking rates.

Much like schizophrenia, diabetes mellitus is a chronic condition that requires following a complex set of treatment recommendations, including behavior change and medication use. Schizophrenia symptoms, as well as cognitive limitations, limited family and social supports, and poor treatment adherence, affect the outcome of diabetes in persons with schizophrenia, and those factors might be amenable to modification by careful, and comprehensive, treatment planning.

Diabetes also may have specific effects among persons with schizophrenia, as shown in its role as a risk factor for tardive dyskinesia (Mukherjee et al. 1989a; Woerner et al. 1993).

Acute Complications

Severe hyperglycemia is associated with symptoms such as polyuria, polydipsia, weight loss, and blurred vision. The most important acute complication of diabetes mellitus is diabetic ketoacidosis, defined as low serum pH (≤7.35), low serum bicarbonate (≤15), and an anion gap, concomitant with ketonemia (Henderson and Ettinger 2003). Diabetic ketoacidosis is a life-threatening situation and requires immediate action on the part of the clinician.

Chronic Complications

Long-term complications of diabetes include retinopathy (with potential loss of vision), nephropathy (leading to renal failure), peripheral neuropathy (increased risk of foot ulcers, amputation, and Charcot's joints), autonomic neuropathy (cardiovascular, gastrointestinal, and genitourinary dysfunction), and greatly increased risk of atheroma affecting large vessels (increased risk of macrovascular complications of stroke, myocardial infarction, or peripheral vascular disease).

Metabolic Syndrome

Problems with glucose metabolism are one component of the metabolic syndrome, which encompasses three or more of the following (National Institutes of Health 2001):

1. Abdominal obesity: waist circumference >102 cm in men and >88 cm in women
2. Elevated serum triglycerides: ≥150 mg/dL
3. Low high-density lipoprotein cholesterol: <40 mg/dL in men and <50 mg/dL in women
4. High blood pressure: ≥130/85 mm Hg
5. Impaired fasting glucose: ≥110 mg/dL

Clinicians treating schizophrenia should be aware of the metabolic syndrome because it appears to be more prevalent in persons with schizophrenia (Heiskanen et al. 2003; Ryan and Thakore 2002), and it has been associated with increased all-cause mortality rate, and coronary heart disease, in middle-aged men (Lakka et al. 2002).

Treatment Implications: Importance of Intensive Glucose Control

Intensive glucose control has been shown to reduce the rate of complications from diabetes (UK Prospective Diabetes Study Group 1998). Much like schizophrenia treatment, diabetes care should be thought of in an integrative and multicomponent fashion. Diabetes treatment should have a multidimensional approach that may include education, counseling, monitoring, self-management, and pharmacological treatment with insulin or oral antidiabetic agents.

HIV AND AIDS

Concern has been growing about the rates at which HIV and other sexually transmitted diseases have spread among those with chronic and severe mental illness (McKinnon et al. 1997). Individuals with schizophrenia are at an increased risk for HIV infection compared with the general population. The current best estimate of HIV prevalence among individuals those with a severe mental illness is between 2% and 5%, and this rate varies according to location, being highest in large urban centers (5%) versus nonmetropolitan areas (2%) (Rosenberg et al. 2001). This prevalence estimate is about eight times the overall estimated United States population prevalence (Rosenberg et al. 2001).

Women with schizophrenia are at particularly high risk for HIV infection—the male-to-female ratio is 4:3, in contrast with the 5:1 ratio reported in the general population (Rosenberg et al. 2001).

Contributing factors to this increased prevalence include injection drug use and unsafe sexual practices (Rosenberg et al. 2001). Data suggest that persons with severe mental illness are more likely to engage in high-risk sexual behavior and less likely to change their health behaviors (Davidson et al. 2001; McDermott et al. 1994).

VIRAL HEPATITIS

The seroprevalence of hepatitis B virus (HBV) and hepatitis C virus (HCV) among those with severe mental illness is much higher than in the general population. Current estimates are 23.4% for HBV and 19.6% for HCV; these rates are 5 and 11 times the prevalence rates in the general population for these infections, respectively (Rosenberg et al. 2001). Contributing factors to the increased prevalence of these infections include unsafe sexual practices and drug use (Davidson et al. 2001).

Chronic Complications

Hepatocellular carcinoma is a long-term complication of hepatitis B and C (Kaplan and Reddy 2003). Hepatitis C infection also increases the risk of cirrhosis (Yoho et al. 2003). The simultaneous infection with hepatitis B and C, for which injection drug users are at increased risk, is associated with further increases in cirrhosis risk. Other complications of viral hepatitis include fulminant hepatitis (massive hepatic necrosis), spontaneous reactivations, and chronic hepatitis.

Clinicians must think of long-term monitoring of hepatitis viruses in persons with schizophrenia, particularly because this population is exposed to other hepatotoxic agents, such as alcohol and some antipsychotic medications. As an example, 1% of the patients taking chlorpromazine will develop intrahepatic cholestasis with jaundice 1–4 weeks into the treatment (Dienstag and Isselbacher 2005).

OTHER CONDITIONS ASSOCIATED WITH SCHIZOPHRENIA

Osteoporosis

Patients with schizophrenia have been noted to have more osteoporosis than do people in the general population (Halbreich and Palter 1996). Reasons for this decrease in bone mineral densities include increased level of smoking, antipsychotic-induced decreases in testosterone and estrogen, hyperprolactinemia and hypercortisolemia (Halbreich and Palter 1996), and dietary and behavioral features associated with schizophrenia.

Respiratory Diseases

Persons with schizophrenia have a higher prevalence of respiratory diseases, such as asthma, emphysema, and chronic bronchitis, when compared with the general population (Sokal et al. 2004). Some studies have reported that individuals with schizophrenia have higher mortality rates from all respiratory diseases compared with the general population (Buda et al. 1988; Joukamaa et al. 2001). Part of this association is likely to come from the higher rates of cigarette smoking, which points to opportunities of preventive strategies in this population.

Polydipsia and Hyponatremia

Polydipsia is the intake of more than 3 L/day of fluid, and it may be primary or secondary to medical conditions or medication side effects (Brookes and Ahmed 2002). The estimated prevalence for psychiatric populations is between 5% and 20% (Brookes and Ahmed 2002; de Leon et al. 1994). Polydipsia may lead to serious metabolic imbalances, such as water intoxication (i.e., severe hyponatremia—serum sodium<120 mmol/L), which is potentially fatal because the cerebral edema can result in delirium, seizures, coma, and death. Characteristics associated with the risk of polydipsia among psychiatric populations include chronicity, schizophrenia diagnosis, smoking, some medications, male gender, and white race (de Leon et al. 1994).

Before a diagnosis of psychosis-induced polydipsia is reached, other causes, such as diabetes mellitus, diabetes insipidus, chronic renal failure, malignancy, pulmonary disease, hypocalcemia, and hypokalemia, should be excluded.

Pharmacological interventions to treat polydipsia are few and with questionable efficacy (Brookes and Ahmed 2002), although there is some indication that clozapine may help (Verghese et al. 1996). Fluid restriction, along with sodium replacement, is the most recommended treatment (Verghese et al. 1996).

TABLE 22–1. Summary of recommended monitoring and psychoeducational measures for patients with schizophrenia

Issue	Recommendation
Weight gain	• Mental health providers should monitor body mass index (BMI) for patients with schizophrenia. • The relative risk of weight gain for the different antipsychotic medications should be a consideration in drug selection for patients who have a BMI>25. • Unless a patient is underweight (BMI<18.5), a weight gain of 1 BMI unit indicates a need for an intervention.
Diabetes	• A baseline measure of glucose should be obtained for all patients before starting a new antipsychotic. • Patients who have significant risk factors for diabetes should have fasting glucose or hemoglobin A_{1C} monitored 4 months after starting an antipsychotic and then yearly. • Psychiatrists should be aware of the symptoms of new-onset diabetes (including weight change, polyuria, polydipsia) and should monitor their presence at regular intervals.
HIV and viral hepatitis	• Clinicians should ask about sexual practices and injection drug use. • Clinicians should educate about safe sexual practices and needle use. • Health care providers should address drug use.
Hyperlipidemia	• Mental health providers should be aware of the lipid profiles for all patients with schizophrenia. • As a group, individuals with schizophrenia should be considered to be at high risk for coronary heart disease. • Psychiatrists should follow National Cholesterol Education Program guidelines (http://www.nhlbi.nih.gov/about/ncep/) or U.S. Preventive Services Task Force guidelines (http://www.ahcpr.gov/clinic/ajpmsuppl/lipidrr.htm) for screening and treating patients who are at high risk for cardiovascular disease.
Chronic lung disease	• Mental health providers should assess level of cigarette smoking and consider intervention. • Clinicians should inquire about respiratory symptoms.
QT prolongation	• Clinicians should *not* prescribe thioridazine, mesoridazine, or pimozide for patients with known heart disease, a personal history of syncope, a family history of sudden death at an early age (younger than 40, especially if both parents had sudden death), or prolonged QTc syndrome. • If ziprasidone is prescribed for patients with the risk factors described in the previous recommendation, an electrocardiogram should be evaluated at baseline, and a subsequent electrocardiogram is indicated if a patient presents with symptoms (e.g., syncope).

Source. Adapted from Marder et al. 2004.

CONDITIONS NEGATIVELY ASSOCIATED WITH SCHIZOPHRENIA

Rheumatoid Arthritis

There have been several reports of a lower than expected prevalence rate of rheumatoid arthritis in patients with schizophrenia. A review of the epidemiological evidence supported this finding (Eaton et al. 1992). This association points to the hypothesis of there being an autoimmune component to schizophrenia. The proper identification of rheumatoid arthritis, a condition linked with autoimmune pneumonia, as opposed to the much more prevalent arthritic syndrome, more associated with degenerative joint disease, is one of the main limitations to

studies on this relation. A recent community-based study failed to show an association between arthritis and schizophrenia (Sokal et al. 2004).

Cancer

There has been some indication that patients with schizophrenia might have a lower than expected cancer incidence (Allebeck 1989; Mortensen 1994). Some investigators have suggested that this could be related to an antineoplastic effect of antipsychotic medication, but larger epidemiological samples are needed to test this hypothesis. Conversely, studies indicate that patients with schizophrenia have higher mortality from lung cancer (Brown et al. 2000).

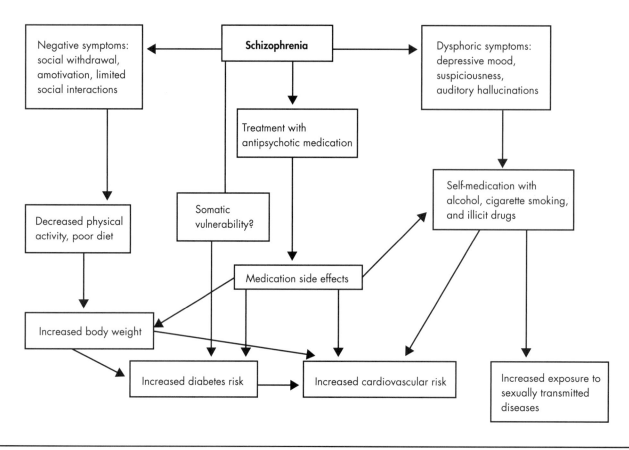

FIGURE 22–2. Possible pathways to comorbid conditions in schizophrenia.

TREATMENT CONSIDERATIONS

MEDICAL COMORBIDITIES: REDUCING BARRIERS TO HEALTH CARE

As reviewed in this chapter, persons with schizophrenia are at higher risk for specific somatic diseases compared with the general population. Among these diseases are diabetes, chronic respiratory disorders, and sexually transmitted diseases. These conditions share two features: they are potentially preventable, and they demand lifelong monitoring and treatment after they develop. Reducing barriers to health care to persons with schizophrenia is necessary to address both of these features. In this context, psychiatrists and the mental health team should strive to work in conjunction and coordination with their counterparts in medical care.

Besides reducing barriers to primary care, clinicians treating schizophrenia should remain alert because of the high presence of multiple risk factors in this population. As such, clinicians should consider regular (e.g., semiannual) monitoring of fasting glucose or hemoglobin A1c to detect emerging diabetes, especially in those with obesity.

Prevention of weight gain should be a high priority because losing weight is difficult for many patients. A summary of recommended monitoring and psychoeducational measures is presented in Table 22–1.

HIV AND HEPATITIS: RISK REDUCTION STRATEGIES

Elements shown to be effective in risk reduction programs for HIV and hepatitis include (Wainberg et al. 2003):

- Information and skills training in sexual assertiveness, negotiation, problem solving, use of condoms, and risk self-management
- Intensive sessions (6–15 hours) to achieve reduction in risk behavior
- Training of participants to become AIDS educators or advocates
- Booster or maintenance sessions
- Gender sensitivity training
- Inclusion of sexually abstinent patients in training programs as a way to validate this choice for other patients choosing to remain abstinent

CONCLUSION

Medical and substance use comorbidity plays a substantial role in the lives of persons with schizophrenia, and a comprehensive approach to comorbidity in schizophrenia is needed. In Figure 22–2, we summarize some of the systemic factors associated with comorbid conditions in schizophrenia. This model could be used as a means to identify the different points at which one might intervene to avoid comorbidities and help patients with schizophrenia live longer and healthier. These comorbidities pose substantial challenges for the treatment system in the care of persons with a core disease that is itself socially and cognitively disabling. However, the care system and physicians must be mindful of the higher comorbidity rate among persons with schizophrenia. Although more research is necessary, such attention is likely to positively influence long-term outcomes for the schizophrenia population.

REFERENCES

Allebeck P: Schizophrenia: a life-shortening disease. Schizophr Bull 15:81–89, 1989

Allison DB, Fontaine KR, Heo M, et al: The distribution of body mass index among individuals with and without schizophrenia. J Clin Psychiatry 60:215–220, 1999

Arseneault L, Cannon M, Witton J, et al: Causal association between cannabis and psychosis: examination of the evidence. Br J Psychiatry 184:110–117, 2004

Bellack AS, DiClemente CC: Treating substance abuse among patients with schizophrenia. Psychiatr Serv 50:75–80, 1999

Bellack AS, Gearon JS: Substance abuse treatment for people with schizophrenia. Addict Behav 6:749–766, 1998

Bennett ME, Bellack AS, Gearon JS: Treating substance abuse in schizophrenia: an initial report. J Subst Abuse Treat 20:163–175, 2001

Bergen AW, Caporaso N: Cigarette smoking. J Natl Cancer Inst 91:1365–1375, 1999

Brookes G, Ahmed AG: Pharmacological treatments for psychosis-related polydipsia. Cochrane Database Syst Rev (3): CD003544, 2002

Brown S, Inskip H, Barraclough B: Causes of the excess mortality of schizophrenia. Br J Psychiatry 177:212–217, 2000

Buda M, Tsuang MT, Fleming JA: Causes of death in DSM-III schizophrenics and other psychotics (atypical group): a comparison with the general population. Arch Gen Psychiatry 45:283–285, 1988

Centers for Disease Control and Prevention: National Diabetes Fact Sheet. Atlanta, GA, National Center for Chronic Disease Prevention and Health Promotion, 2005. Available at: http://www.cdc.gov/diabetes/pubs/estimates.htm Accessed September 21, 2005.

Cuffel BJ, Heithoff KA, Lawson W: Correlates of patterns of substance abuse among patients with schizophrenia. Hosp Community Psychiatry 44:247–251, 1993

Dalack GW, Healy DJ, Meador-Woodruff JH: Nicotine dependence in schizophrenia: clinical phenomena and laboratory findings. Am J Psychiatry 155:1490–1501, 1998

Davidson S, Judd F, Jolley D, et al: Risk factors for HIV/AIDS and hepatitis C among the chronic mentally ill. Aust N Z J Psychiatry 35:203–209, 2001

de Leon J, Verghese C, Tracy JI, et al: Polydipsia and water intoxication in psychiatric patients: a review of the epidemiological literature. Biol Psychiatry 35:408–419, 1994

de Leon J, Diaz FJ, Rogers T, et al: Initiation of daily smoking and nicotine dependence in schizophrenia and mood disorders. Schizophr Res 56:47–54, 2002

DeQuardo JR, Carpenter CF, Tandon R: Patterns of substance abuse in schizophrenia: nature and significance. J Psychiatr Res 28:267–275, 1994

Dickerson FB, McNary SW, Brown CH, et al: Somatic healthcare utilization among adults with serious mental illness who are receiving community psychiatric services. Med Care 41:560–570, 2003

Dienstag J, Isselbacher K: Toxic and drug-induced hepatitis, in Harrison's Principles of Internal Medicine, 16th Edition. Edited by Kasper DL, Fauci AS, Longo DL, et al. New York, McGraw-Hill, 2005, pp 1838–1844

Dixon L: Dual diagnosis of substance abuse in schizophrenia: prevalence and impact on outcomes. Schizophr Res 35(suppl): S93–S100, 1999

Dixon L, Haas G, Weiden PJ, et al: Drug abuse in schizophrenic patients: clinical correlates and reasons for use. Am J Psychiatry 148:224–230, 1991

Dixon L, Postrado L, Delahanty J, et al: The association of medical comorbidity in schizophrenia with poor physical and mental health. J Nerv Ment Dis 187:496–502, 1999

Dixon L, Weiden P, Delahanty J, et al: Prevalence and correlates of diabetes in national schizophrenia samples. Schizophr Bull 26:903–912, 2000

Drake RE, Mueser KT: Psychosocial approaches to dual diagnosis. Schizophr Bull 26:105–118, 2000

Drake RE, Mueser KT: Managing comorbid schizophrenia and substance abuse. Curr Psychiatry Rep 3:418–422, 2001

Drake RE, Wallach MA: Substance abuse among the chronic mentally ill. Hosp Community Psychiatry 40:1041–1046, 1989

Drake RE, Osher FC, Wallach MA: Alcohol use and abuse in schizophrenia: a prospective community study. J Nerv Ment Dis 177:408–414, 1989

Drake RE, Mercer-McFadden C, Mueser KT, et al: Review of integrated mental health and substance abuse treatment for patients with dual disorders. Schizophr Bull 24:589–608, 1998

Eaton WW, Hayward C, Ram R: Schizophrenia and rheumatoid arthritis: a review. Schizophr Res 6:181–192, 1992

Folsom DP, McCahill M, Bartels SJ, et al: Medical comorbidity and receipt of medical care by older homeless people with schizophrenia or depression. Psychiatr Serv 53:1456–1460, 2002

Fowler IL, Carr VJ, Carter NT, et al: Patterns of current and lifetime substance use in schizophrenia. Schizophr Bull 24:443–455, 1998

George TP, Vessicchio JC, Termine A, et al: A placebo controlled trial of bupropion for smoking cessation in schizophrenia. Biol Psychiatry 52:53–61, 2002

Goldman LS: Medical illness in patients with schizophrenia. J Clin Psychiatry 60 (suppl 21):10–15, 1999

Halbreich U, Palter S: Accelerated osteoporosis in psychiatric patients: possible pathophysiological processes. Schizophr Bull 22:447–454, 1996

Heiskanen T, Niskanen L, Lyytikainen R, et al: Metabolic syndrome in patients with schizophrenia. J Clin Psychiatry 64:575–579, 2003

Henderson D, Ettinger E: Glucose intolerance and diabetes in schizophrenia, in Medical Illness and Schizophrenia. Edited by Meyer J, Nasrallah H. Washington, DC, American Psychiatric Publishing, 2003, pp 99–114

Himmelhoch S, Kreyenbuhl J, Lehman A, et al: Prevalence of chronic obstructive pulmonary disease among individuals with serious mental illness. Am J Psychiatry 161:2317–2319, 2004

Jeste DV, Gladsjo JA, Lindamer LA, et al: Medical comorbidity in schizophrenia. Schizophr Bull 22:413–430, 1996

Joukamaa M, Heliovaara M, Knekt P, et al: Mental disorders and cause-specific mortality. Br J Psychiatry 179:498–502, 2001

Kaplan DE, Reddy KR: Rising incidence of hepatocellular carcinoma: the role of hepatitis B and C: the impact on transplantation and outcomes. Clin Liver Dis 7:683–714, 2003

Kirkpatrick B, Amador XF, Flaum M, et al: The deficit syndrome in the DSM-IV Field Trial, I: alcohol and other drug abuse. Schizophr Res 20:69–77, 1996

Koro CE, Fedder DO, L'Italien GJ, et al: Assessment of independent effect of olanzapine and risperidone on risk of diabetes among patients with schizophrenia: population based nested case-control study. BMJ 325(7358):243, 2002

Lakka H, Laaksonen D, Lakka T, et al: The metabolic syndrome and total and cardiovascular disease mortality in middle-aged men. JAMA 288:2709–2716, 2002

Lehman AF, Lieberman JA, Dixon LB, et al: Practice guideline for the treatment of patients with schizophrenia (second edition). Am J Psychiatry 161 (2 suppl):1–56, 2004

Linszen DH, Dingemans PM, Lenior ME: Cannabis abuse and the course of recent-onset schizophrenic disorders. Arch Gen Psychiatry 51:273–279, 1994

Lohr J, Flynn K: Smoking and schizophrenia. Schizophr Res 8:93–102, 1992

Lyon ER: A review of the effects of nicotine on schizophrenia and antipsychotic medications. Psychiatr Serv 50:1346–1350, 1999

Lysaker P, Bell M, Beam-Goulet J, et al: Relationship of positive and negative symptoms to cocaine abuse in schizophrenia. J Nerv Ment Dis 182:109–112, 1994

Marder SR, Essock SM, Miller AL, et al: Physical health monitoring of patients with schizophrenia. Am J Psychiatry 161:1334–1349, 2004

Mathalon DH, Pfefferbaum A, Lim KO, et al: Compounded brain volume deficits in schizophrenia-alcoholism comorbidity. Arch Gen Psychiatry 60:245–252, 2003

McDermott BE, Sautter FJ Jr, Winstead DK, et al: Diagnosis, health beliefs, and risk of HIV infection in psychiatric patients. Hosp Community Psychiatry 45:580–585, 1994

McKinnon K, Carey MP, Cournos F: Research on HIV, AIDS, and severe mental illness: recommendations from the NIMH National Conference. Clin Psychol Rev 17:327–331, 1997

Messias E, Bienvenu OJ: Suspiciousness and alcohol use disorders in schizophrenia. J Nerv Ment Dis 191:387–390, 2003

Morrow AL, VanDoren MJ, Penland SN, et al: The role of GABAergic neuroactive steroids in ethanol action, tolerance and dependence. Brain Res Brain Res Rev 37:98–109, 2001

Mortensen PB: The occurrence of cancer in first admitted schizophrenic patients. Schizophr Res 12:185–194, 1994

Mueser KT, Bennett M, Kushner M: Epidemiology of substance use disorders among persons with chronic mental illness, in Double Jeopardy. Edited by Lehman A, Dixon L. Chur, Switzerland, Harwood Academic Publishers, 1995, pp 9–26

Mukherjee S, Roth SD, Sandyk R, et al: Persistent tardive dyskinesia and neuroleptic effects on glucose tolerance. Psychiatry Res 29:17–27, 1989a

Mukherjee S, Schnur DB, Reddy R: Family history of type 2 diabetes in schizophrenic patients. Lancet 1(8636):495, 1989b

Mukherjee S, Decina P, Bocola V, et al: Diabetes mellitus in schizophrenic patients. Compr Psychiatry 37:68–73, 1996

National Institutes of Health: Third Report of the National Cholesterol Education Program Expert Panel on Detection, Evaluation and Treatment of High Blood Cholesterol in Adults (Adult Treatment Panel III). Bethesda, MD, National Institutes of Health, 2001

Newcomer JW, Haupt DW, Fucetola R, et al: Abnormalities in glucose regulation during antipsychotic treatment of schizophrenia. Arch Gen Psychiatry 59:337–345, 2002

Nilsson E, Lichtenstein P, Cnattingius S, et al: Women with schizophrenia: pregnancy outcome and infant death among their offspring. Schizophr Res 58:221–229, 2002

Osher FC, Drake RE, Noordsy DL, et al: Correlates and outcomes of alcohol use disorder among rural outpatients with schizophrenia. J Clin Psychiatry 55:109–113, 1994

Procyshyn RM, Ihsan N, Thompson D: A comparison of smoking behaviours between patients treated with clozapine and depot neuroleptics. Int Clin Psychopharmacol 16:291–294, 2001

Procyshyn RM, Tse G, Sin O, et al: Concomitant clozapine reduces smoking in patients treated with risperidone. Eur Neuropsychopharmacol 12:77–80, 2002

Regier DA, Farmer ME, Rae DS, et al: Comorbidity of mental disorders with alcohol and other drug abuse: results from the Epidemiologic Catchment Area (ECA) Study. JAMA 264:2511–2518, 1990

Rosenberg SD, Goodman LA, Osher FC, et al: Prevalence of HIV, hepatitis B, and hepatitis C in people with severe mental illness. Am J Public Health 91:31–37, 2001

Ryan MC, Thakore JH: Physical consequences of schizophrenia and its treatment: the metabolic syndrome. Life Sci 71:239–257, 2002

Ryan MC, Collins P, Thakore JH: Impaired fasting glucose tolerance in first-episode, drug-naive patients with schizophrenia. Am J Psychiatry 160:284–289, 2003

Sernyak MJ, Leslie DL, Alarcon RD, et al: Association of diabetes mellitus with use of atypical neuroleptics in the treatment of schizophrenia. Am J Psychiatry 159:561–566, 2002

Sherr JD, Myers C, Avila MT, et al: The effects of nicotine on specific eye tracking measures in schizophrenia. Biol Psychiatry 52:721–728, 2002

Sokal J, Messias E, Dickerson FB, et al: Comorbidity of medical illnesses among adults with serious mental illness who are receiving community psychiatric services. J Nerv Ment Dis 192:421–427, 2004

Srinivasan TN, Thara R: Smoking in schizophrenia—all is not biological. Schizophr Res 56:67–74, 2002

Subramaniam M, Chong SA, Pek E: Diabetes mellitus and impaired glucose tolerance in patients with schizophrenia. Can J Psychiatry 48:345–347, 2003

Tsai G, Gastfriend DR, Coyle JT: The glutamatergic basis of human alcoholism. Am J Psychiatry 152:332–340, 1995

Tsuang MT, Woolson RF, Fleming JA: Premature deaths in schizophrenia and affective disorders: an analysis of survival curves and variables affecting the shortened survival. Arch Gen Psychiatry 37:979–983, 1980

UK Prospective Diabetes Study Group: Intensive blood-glucose control with sulphonylureas or insulin compared with conventional treatment and risk of complications in patients with type 2 diabetes. Lancet 352:837–853, 1998

Verghese C, de Leon J, Josiassen RC: Problems and progress in the diagnosis and treatment of polydipsia and hyponatremia. Schizophr Bull 22:455–464, 1996

Volkow ND, Fowler JS: Addiction, a disease of compulsion and drive: involvement of the orbitofrontal cortex. Cereb Cortex 10:318–325, 2000

Wainberg M, Cournos F, McKinnon K, et al: HIV and hepatitis C in patients with schizophrenia, in Medical Illness and Schizophrenia. Edited by Meyer J, Nasrallah H. Washington, DC, American Psychiatric Publishing, 2003, pp 115–140

Woerner MG, Saltz BL, Kane JM, et al: Diabetes and development of tardive dyskinesia. Am J Psychiatry 150:966–968, 1993

Yoho RA, Cruz LL, Mazaheri R, et al: Hepatitis C: a review. Plast Reconstr Surg 112:597–605, 2003

Zaretsky A, Rector NA, Seeman MV, et al: Current cannabis use and tardive dyskinesia. Schizophr Res 11:3–8, 1993

Ziedonis D, Nickou C: Substance abuse in patients with schizophrenia, in Schizophrenia and Comorbid Conditions: Diagnosis and Treatment. Edited by Hwang MY, Bermanzohn PC. Washington, DC, American Psychiatric Publishing, 2001, pp 187–221

Ziedonis DM, Kosten TR, Glazer WM, et al: Nicotine dependence and schizophrenia. Hosp Community Psychiatry 45:204–206, 1994

TREATMENT OF SCHIZOPHRENIA IN THE PUBLIC SECTOR

JOHN E. KRAUS, M.D., PH.D.

T. SCOTT STROUP, M.D., M.P.H.

Theoretically, treatment of schizophrenia in the public sector should be no different from the "best practice" evidence-based treatments (both pharmacological and psychosocial rehabilitative) described elsewhere in this book. However, reality more often than not impinges on theory in the form of budgetary constraints, shortage of trained professionals, patient noncompliance with treatments, transportation deficiencies, low or no availability of insurance or other funding sources, and lack of community resources, among other barriers. Thus, treatment of schizophrenia in the public sector represents the individual development, within each treatment site, of a "good enough" treatment model that ultimately may be based on the cobbling together of disparate resources.

An attempt to discuss the treatment of schizophrenia in the public sector in a generic manner is further complicated by the multiple various settings and systems that at some level provide public treatment: state hospitals, the federal Department of Veterans Affairs (VA) system, forensic treatment settings (both state and federal), community mental health centers (CMHCs), and jails and prisons. Even within specific types of treatment settings, clinical practice may vary by county, state, or country. Further-

more, the types of schizophrenia patients served vary significantly in each treatment setting, such as forensic versus nonforensic or inpatient versus community-based treatment. Therefore, in this chapter, we broadly address challenges in treating schizophrenia in the public sector, focusing primarily on systems of care in the United States.

SCHIZOPHRENIA AND THE PUBLIC SECTOR

Chronic schizophrenia is commonly associated with low socioeconomic status. The concept of *downward drift* has long been present in schizophrenia research and is relevant to the many individuals with schizophrenia who are indigent. Dunham (1965) posited that the large proportion of patients with schizophrenia in the lower socioeconomic groups results from an inability (because of the illness) to move into a higher socioeconomic bracket or from the downward drift to the lowest bracket. This disadvantaged position in socioeconomic status (complicated by unemployment or underemployment) can be a persistent outcome related to the illness (Agerbo et al. 2004).

Additionally, evidence suggests that disadvantaged socioeconomic status may increase the risk of illness or, at the least, be present before the first treatment contact (Harrison et al. 2001; Tien and Eaton 1992).

Compounding the problem of low socioeconomic status (which eliminates the option of "self-pay" private treatment settings) is the problem of underinsurance among persons with severe mental illness. In the United States, up to 44% of those with mental illness lack health insurance (Landerman et al. 1994; Rupp 1991; Yanos et al. 2004). Even if patients have some form of health insurance, private insurance usually is more restrictive in coverage for mental illness than in coverage for medical illness, and benefits may be quickly exhausted. The result is that far more people end up with no psychiatric coverage than end up with no coverage for medical illnesses and thus have no access to the pool of mental health providers who accept private or public (Medicare, Medicaid) insurance. These "psychiatrically indigent" patients often come to the attention of treatment providers in emergency or crisis situations and are subsequently referred to state hospitals or to community hospitals that have provider contracts with counties or states for indigent care. Socioeconomically disadvantaged and underinsured persons are ultimately dependent on public sector mental health services.

PUBLIC SECTOR DEFINED

Mental health services can be defined as public if they are supported by public funds. Funds raised by taxes may be allocated for mental health services in yearly budgets of states, counties, and larger cities (typically as a subset of funding for a health and human services department). Additionally, services provided by taxpayer dollars in the form of entitlement programs qualify as public. These services include treatment rendered under the federal health insurance program of Medicare and the state Medicaid programs (also supported in large part by federal funds).

Medicare was enacted in 1966 to provide health insurance for persons older than 65 or with a disability. Medicare, like many private insurance policies, treats mental illness differently from medical illness. It requires higher copayments for mental health services, an arrangement that has been called "blatantly discriminatory" by the American Psychiatric Association. Medicare also limits the total number of lifetime days allotted to a patient in a psychiatric hospital rather than allowing for an annual "spell of illness" (as it does for medical illness).

Psychiatric hospitals are exempt from the diagnosis-related groups (DRGs) payment methodology that applies to medical illness. DRG payment is based on norms for inpatient treatment lengths of stay, and hospitals are paid for an episode of treatment rather than on a bed-day basis. The reason for the exemption of psychiatric services is that a mental illness diagnosis alone is not an adequate predictor of length of stay in a psychiatric unit. However, a modification of DRG payment method for mental illness has shown some success at the state level (Frank and McGuire 1994; McGuire et al. 1990).

Medicaid, also enacted in 1966, is a medical assistance program for certain individuals and families with low incomes and resources. Medicaid is targeted for children, pregnant women, and persons who are blind or disabled. Adults with schizophrenia must show disability to qualify for Medicaid. Being classified as disabled is a difficult bureaucratic process for persons with severe mental illness, and the assistance of social workers and case managers is often required. Medicaid does not pay for hospitalization in state psychiatric hospitals because of an Institutes of Mental Disease (IMD) exclusion, which was intended to ensure that the states continue to pay for state hospital care. However, Medicaid will pay for acute psychiatric treatment rendered in general hospitals (assuming that the low Medicaid payments are accepted by that hospital). Medicaid also will pay for medications, although limits are often placed on the number of prescriptions that may be filled in a defined period (e.g., six prescriptions per month). Of particular relevance to the treatment of schizophrenia is that in many states, costs for second-generation or atypical antipsychotics are very near the top of Medicaid expenditures for prescription medications. For example, in North Carolina, atypical antipsychotics rank second only to proton-pump inhibitors in terms of class of drug with the highest costs. Such costs have led some states to create preferred drug lists (or modified formularies) whereby medications with the lowest cost are used first, and higher-cost medications require preapproval.

Care for persons who are medically indigent (uninsured) or underinsured is often subsidized by county and state governments when these patients are not eligible for or have not yet qualified for entitlement programs (Medicaid, Medicare). The most obvious examples are funds for state psychiatric hospitals and CMHCs. Public funding of mental health programs is therefore highly dependent on the economic status of the state or county at any given time; in other words, the current strength of the taxpayer base. The economic downturn of the early 2000s led to, at best, freezes and, at worst, cuts in budget allocations for health and human services, cuts that quickly "trickled down" to mental health and substance abuse treatment programs. For example, in fiscal year 2003, 32 of 38 state mental health agencies reported budget cuts of up to 12.5% (National Association of State Mental Health Program Directors Research Institute 2003). Of particular concern, 68% of states reduced services and 61% reduced the number of persons served to deal with budget cuts (National Association of State Mental Health Program Directors Research Institute 2003). It is important to emphasize that the ability of a given public mental health system to provide a "best practices" or "evidence-based" service delivery model is inexorably tied to the availability of funds.

Finally, other taxpayer-supported institutions that provide medical and mental health care may be considered public. These include the VA hospitals and clinics and the criminal justice system (jails and prisons), now one of the largest mental health providers. State prisons and jails have similar service delivery sensitivity to state budgetary constraints.

SYSTEMS OF CARE AND PERSONS SERVED

Schizophrenic patients can enter the public system in many ways. The particular setting in which treatment occurs often depends on where a patient falls within a spectrum of treatment populations. Public sector treatment populations include persons without any insurance; persons who lack health insurance that provides for mental health treatment; persons with a history of military service; persons found guilty of a crime and requiring incarceration; persons found incapable of proceeding to trial because of a mental illness; persons found not guilty by reason of insanity; and persons in regions without any private providers (e.g., rural areas). Specific systems of care have evolved in response to each patient population's specific needs.

COMMUNITY MENTAL HEALTH CENTERS

The development of CMHCs was spurred by legislative activity at the federal level. The Mental Health Study Act of 1955 was passed partly in response to the substandard conditions identified in many state hospitals (highlighted in a 1948 motion picture called *The Snake Pit*). The Mental Health Study Act led to recognition of the need for community care of persons with severe mental illness, that care should be regional and in smaller hospitals, and that nonhospital care and rehabilitative services should be expanded. Related legislation included the Mental Retardation Facilities and Community Mental Health Centers Construction Act of 1963 and the Community Mental Health Center Amendments of 1975. The 1963 act sought

to ensure provision of the basic mental health services of inpatient treatment, emergency services, partial hospitalization, outpatient services, and consultation/education. The 1975 amendments added additional services to the basic core of the 1963 act: care for children and the elderly, continuing mental health care for persons discharged from hospitals, screening services prior to hospital admission, substance abuse services, and transitional housing.

In concert with this federal legislation was the development of CMHCs, whose program design was based on a core set of guiding principles (Lamb 1999). A CMHC serves a specific catchment area, a geographic region that defines a CMHC's or state hospital's population of responsibility. The goal is to allow treatment close to a patient's home, which also facilitates family visits and participation. Comprehensive services are offered that target a range of diagnoses, age groups, treatment modalities (e.g., pharmacological, psychological, rehabilitative), and general needs (e.g., housing, vocational services, disability application). To offer these services, teams must be multidisciplinary, usually consisting of a psychiatrist team leader and various combinations of psychologists, nurses, social workers, rehabilitative therapists, and case workers. Ideally, services provide continuity of care to ease transition from various service settings; for example, from hospital to supported living (e.g., group home) and from supported living to independent living. The efficacy of programs should be continually reevaluated and measured, and improvement is always the goal. To this end, input from patients is necessary. Research into treatment modalities and outcome of care is sometimes incorporated, but this is a feature in only a minority of programs. Data from such research are helpful in improving patient care, prioritizing services, eliminating ineffective or redundant practices, and supporting funding increases for effective programs. Finally, most community mental health systems have limited their scope of service to specific target populations, often defined by a certain threshold of severity of illness. Schizophrenic patients are always included in target populations. Persons with schizophrenia treated in CMHCs usually have no health insurance, lack insurance to pay for private mental health services, or live in areas where appropriate private services are not available.

Persons with schizophrenia, even if they have insurance with mental health benefits or the ability to pay out of pocket, still may receive treatment in CMHCs if they live in underserved (typically rural) areas. In rural areas, public services may be the only treatment option because of the lack of qualified professionals engaged in private practice. The situation is particularly severe for child, adolescent, and geriatric patients with schizophrenia. Even within the public sector, the number of qualified providers is insufficient (Pion et al. 1997), and the vast majority of rural counties have no practicing psychiatrists (National Advisory Committee on Rural Health 1993). Such shortages result in schizophrenic patients receiving treatment by general medical doctors and relying heavily on social services (U.S. Department of Health and Human Services 1999). The need for specialized care may result in hospitalization hundreds of miles from home, usually in a state psychiatric hospital. "Telemental health," or the use of telecommunications and videoconferencing technology to diagnose and treat mental illness, has been proposed as one potential solution to this problem (Monnier et al. 2003).

A few CMHC services have obtained the status of "best practice." One of these is the Assertive Community Treatment (ACT) team model. The goal of ACT is to provide services to patients who would otherwise receive treatment in the hospital without shifting the burden of care to families or other caregivers (Dixon 2000; Scott and Dixon 1995; Stein and Test 1980; Stein et al. 1975). Providers go to the patient, be it at home or at work, to deliver treatment, which may include anything from medication management to assistance with activities of daily living. Such active contact is of particular importance in treating a disease such as schizophrenia, in which lack of insight into illness and symptoms may affect up to 50% of patients, leading to treatment noncompliance, missed appointments, and relapse (Sevy et al. 2004; Smith et al. 2004). ACT teams have been found to be superior to usual care in terms of retaining patients in treatment (Herinckx et al. 1997), preventing hospitalization (Essock and Kontos 1995), and increasing the likelihood of stable housing (Morse et al. 1997). Related to the ACT model is the concept of case management, in which one person, usually a social worker or paraprofessional mental health provider, is responsible for coordinating the care of a patient. Case managers typically serve as "brokers" who help their patients navigate the maze of mental health and social services that may be available. Many case managers also provide a variety of supportive services directly.

Assisting patients in obtaining supportive housing also has been shown to decrease hospitalization and homelessness and to increase social and occupational functioning and quality of life (Hawthorne et al. 1994; Okin et al. 1995). Examples include long-term group residences, or "group homes," which have on-site staff, and cooperative apartments, where staff members are not on-site but visit regularly (Herz and Marder 2002).

Treatment adherence can be enhanced to some degree by the use of outpatient commitments, which require patients to attend their mental health treatment appoint-

ments or risk being brought in involuntarily for evaluation. Although outpatient commitment statutes typically have no provision to force outpatients to take medicines, this method has been shown to increase adherence to treatment (Swanson et al. 2003). However, it also can be viewed as overly coercive by patients (Elbogen et al. 2003; Swartz et al. 2003).

Given the extensive literature supporting the use of antipsychotics to treat schizophrenia and the growing database regarding specific community interventions to improve functional outcomes (ACT, supportive housing, supportive employment), the current consensus is that community treatment of schizophrenia can and should be evidence based (Drake et al. 2000, 2001; W.C. Torrey et al. 2001). Use of practice guidelines (Kane et al. 2003; Lehman et al. 2004) should result in improved patient outcomes and standardization of treatment practices regardless of geographic locale or training background. Use of these guidelines also should aid in prioritizing services in the setting of stagnant or reduced funding.

STATE PSYCHIATRIC HOSPITALS

State psychiatric hospitals provide both acute and long-term patient care to the same populations of patients that receive treatment in the CMHCs (i.e., indigent, underinsured, or residing in a rural or otherwise underserved area). The current trend is toward a reduction in the overall size of state hospitals, shifting the vast majority of care to the community (i.e., outpatient care). The current focus of most state hospitals is on acute crisis stabilization and rapid discharge to community care, with discharge planning starting shortly after admission. Although downsizing of state psychiatric hospitals has been occurring over the last few decades (coincident with the expansion of CMHCs), recent developments have hastened the rate. In July 1999, the U.S. Supreme Court issued the *Olmstead v. L. C.* decision. In its decision, the Court interpreted Title II of the Americans with Disabilities Act (ADA) as requiring states to administer services "in the most integrated setting appropriate to the needs of qualified individuals with disabilities" (28 C.F.R. 35.130[d] [1998]). Inherent in the decision was the concept of treating persons with mental illness in the least restrictive environment, with state hospitals being considered more restrictive than community treatment. In the opinion of the Court,

> states are required to place persons with mental disabilities in community settings rather than in institutions when the State's treatment professionals have determined that community placement is appropriate, the transfer from institutional care to a less restrictive set-

ting is not opposed by the affected individual, and the placement can be reasonably accommodated, taking into account the resources available to the State and the needs of others with mental disabilities. (Olmstead v. L.C. 1999)

The decision has forced states to critically evaluate how persons with severe mental illness are treated in state hospital settings and how resources should be allocated in the community.

Who remains in state psychiatric hospitals? Involuntary commitment criteria require proof of dangerousness to self or others; thus, persons who remain in state psychiatric hospitals for long-term treatment are those who cannot safely be discharged to community care. For these patients, no community service setting can reproduce the elements of the hospital treatment environment that help to maintain patient safety. The availability of specific resources can vary widely among communities; often, residential centers that have 24-hour supervision by trained mental health staff are in short supply, and very few, if any, locked residential facilities are available. How the latter represents a less restrictive setting than a state psychiatric hospital is unclear.

Various factors contribute to the likelihood that a patient with schizophrenia will be hospitalized (Fogel 1999). These include severe impairment in function, active general medical conditions, history of criminal behavior associated with psychosis, persistent noncompliance with treatment outside of the hospital setting, lack of financial and social supports, and—perhaps chief among these—recurrent aggressive or self-injurious behavior. Schizophrenic patients who remain in state psychiatric hospitals for a prolonged period often have an illness complicated by persistent violent behavior. Violent patients have longer hospital stays (Citrome et al. 1994), and assaultive behavior is more common than self-injurious behaviors on long-term psychiatric units (Kraus and Sheitman 2004). The use of clozapine to reduce violent behavior in this patient population has been supported by several retrospective studies (Chengappa et al. 1999, 2002; Kraus and Sheitman 2005). Environmental (e.g., ward crowding) (Ng et al. 2001; Nijman and Rector 1999) and psychosocial rehabilitative interventions (e.g., "treatment malls") (Kraus et al. 2004) also have been shown to affect rates and severity of violent behavior. By necessity, state hospitals have become specialists in the management of both acutely and chronically dangerous, violent patients.

Treatment in state psychiatric hospitals is similar to treatment delivered in the community, with the exception of the key differences of centralized treatment locale, locked wards, and the ability to use involuntary forced medication treatment protocols. Persons admitted to the hospital with an acute exacerbation of schizophrenia require reinstitution or adjustment of antipsychotic therapy, appropriate levels of observation to ensure patient (and others') safety, and an environment that is conducive to symptom reduction (e.g., low stimulation, trained staff to offer reassurance and support). Most state psychiatric hospitals allow for involuntary forced emergency treatment—that is, antipsychotic (and often anxiolytic) medication is given despite patient refusal when threat of harm to patient, staff, or others is imminent if treatment were to be delayed. Medication is usually administered intramuscularly, but rapidly dissolving formulations of atypical antipsychotics have facilitated the use of oral medications in some situations. Despite court findings supporting the right of committed patients to refuse treatment, involuntary forced treatment also may occur in nonemergency situations when it is determined that the patient requires antipsychotic medication to allow for active participation in treatment planning or to prevent further deterioration. The intensity of review for the use of nonemergency forced treatment varies by state and ranges from the agreement of the treatment team together with a second consulting physician to review boards that examine each individual case and render a decision for or against forced treatment to the requirement for a judgment of incompetence and the appointment of a legal guardian (Simon 2003).

Aside from pharmacotherapy, state hospitals provide psychosocial rehabilitative services. Specialists in occupational therapy, vocational therapy, recreational therapy, and psychology assist in developing individualized treatment (or "programming") for each patient. One recent trend, which has received a fairly high level of popularity despite the relative lack of research into its effectiveness, is the "treatment mall." Treatment malls are centralized, off-unit areas where multiple groups and activities are offered to patients in the context of an individualized treatment schedule. Groups are often interdisciplinary and are usually composed of both male and female patients. Although the mall model currently lacks substantial empirical data, it makes some intrinsic sense. The goal is to provide a more normalized, structured experience (e.g., "going to the mall" is similar to going to work or school) and to ease transition back to community living. The centralization of services also facilitates rational use of manpower and reduces duplication of effort.

Most state psychiatric hospitals include medical services for the identification and treatment of comorbid medical conditions. Incorporation of medical services is particularly important for persons with schizophrenia because these patients have increased mortality and behaviors that elevate risk for medical disease (such as smoking, obesity, and sedentary lifestyle) (Lambert et al. 2003). Additionally, a greater burden of medical problems contributes to more severe psychiatric symptoms in schizophrenic patients (Dixon et al. 1999). Given that half of schizophrenic patients have at least one comorbid medical condition (Green et al. 2003; see also Chapter , "Nonpsychiatric Comorbid Disorders," this volume), medical treatment planning, on both the inpatient and the outpatient level, is an essential aspect of schizophrenia management in the public sector.

DEPARTMENT OF VETERANS AFFAIRS SERVICES

Schizophrenic patients who served in a branch of the United States military may be eligible for mental health treatment through the VA medical centers. The level of benefits varies depending on the designated priority group (e.g., those with greater than 50% service-connected disability are defined as priority group 1). One must have "veteran status" prior to obtaining any benefits. To qualify for this status, the individual must have 24 months of active military service, although there are some exceptions (e.g., discharge due to disability). Services covered under the VA medical benefits package include inpatient and outpatient mental health and substance abuse treatment. Prescription drugs are available under the VA national formulary system.

The VA mental health care system offers many of the services described earlier for CMHCs and state hospitals. Somewhat unique to the VA as a public mental health system is its ability to collect and store large amounts of data (particularly pharmacy data) and the ability to initiate multicenter clinical trials within a single service provider network. The VA system usually has better data management capabilities than other public systems, and, as a consequence, information about many patients can be tracked and analyzed.

Analysis of VA pharmacy record databases have yielded information on prescribing practices of atypical antipsychotics, including potential racial disparities (Copeland et al. 2003), dosing and switching practices (Owen et al. 2003; Sernyak et al. 2003a, 2003b), polypharmacy (Leslie and Rosenheck 2001), and costs associated with atypical antipsychotic use (Byerly et al. 2003). The VA system also draws from a national population base, allowing for centralized research with a large number of patients within a single-payer public system. Large clinical trials have investigated the use of clozapine in schizophrenic patients, examining not just clinical response (Rosenheck et al. 1998a) but also quality of life (Cramer et al. 2001), effect on health care costs (Rosenheck et al. 1999), effect on

family (Rosenheck et al. 2000), and role in psychosocial rehabilitation (Rosenheck et al. 1998b). Comparative trials have added information about treatment with typical and atypical antipsychotics (Rosenheck et al. 1997, 2003), as well as data regarding the efficacy of a variety of psychosocial interventions including life skills training (Brown and Munford 1983), intensive community care (Rosenheck et al. 1995), and paid employment (Bell et al. 1996). Information management and centralized provider status have facilitated research into "real world" issues related to schizophrenia in the VA system; thus, a strong argument can be made for updating computer and data management systems and for developing research coalitions in other public settings.

JAIL, PRISON, AND FORENSIC TREATMENT SETTINGS

The criminal justice system, particularly jails and prisons, has become one of the largest providers of mental health care in the United States because of the numerous mentally ill individuals within these facilities. For example, a 2002 survey of Tennessee jails reported that 17.8% of the inmate population had a mental illness (Diehl and Hiland 2003). A 1999 report by the U.S. Department of Justice estimated that at least 16% of the inmates in jails and prisons had a serious mental illness, including schizophrenia, bipolar disorder, and major depressive disorder (Ditton 1999). Of the mentally ill inmates, 53% were in prison for a violent offense (Ditton 1999). Incredibly, 44% of 2,585 mentally ill persons surveyed by the National Alliance for the Mentally Ill reported having been detained or arrested by the criminal justice system in their lifetime (Hall et al. 2003). A recent Human Rights Watch Report (2003) estimated that on any given day, 70,000 inmates in United States prisons are psychotic.

Given the high prevalence of mental illness among inmates, Gilligan (2001) has referred to the prisons as the "last mental hospital." Thus, jails and prisons "by default" become one of the largest public providers of mental health treatment. Part of the explanation for the large number of mentally ill persons in legal custody is the "criminalization" of mental illness, whereby persons who show dangerous and possibly illegal behaviors, as a consequence of their mental illness, are directed toward the criminal justice system rather than referred for mental health treatment (Quanbeck et al. 2003; E.F. Torrey 1995; Treffert 1981).

In addition to the general jail and prison inmate population is the forensic psychiatry treatment population. These persons, who have had contact with the criminal justice system, fall into two major categories. The first group comprises those who cannot proceed to trial because their mental illness precludes their understanding of the legal and judiciary process. The focus of psychiatric treatment for these patients is competency restoration, or treatment of the offender's mental illness to such a degree that he or she can understand the legal situation and participate in court proceedings (Bertman et al. 2003; R.D. Miller 2003). The second group comprises those who have been deemed not guilty by reason of insanity; that is, determination has been made that the severity of symptoms of mental illness precluded individual responsibility for a criminal act. In practice, most people found not guilty by reason of insanity have a diagnosis of schizophrenia or schizoaffective disorder. For example, almost two-thirds of the patients in an outpatient program for offenders found not guilty by reason of insanity had a diagnosis of a primary psychotic disorder (Kravitz and Kelly 1999). Such patients receive treatment for their mental illness, but release back to community care, despite successful psychiatric treatment, can be complicated by the notoriety of the index offense and the difficulty in predicting future violent behavior (Patterson and Wise 1998). Finally, in those who are found guilty but mentally ill (Palmer and Hazelrigg 2000), the verdict requires that a convicted offender serve the full sentence designated for the crime, with the expectation that treatment for mental illness will be provided.

DUAL DIAGNOSIS PATIENTS

A patient population group shared among all the public treatment settings is the dually diagnosed group; that is, schizophrenic patients with a comorbid substance abuse problem (Mueser et al. 1990). The Epidemiologic Catchment Area Study reported that 47% of the persons with a lifetime diagnosis of schizophrenia or schizophreniform disorder also met lifetime criteria for substance dependence (Regier et al. 1990). Patients with both schizophrenia and a substance use problem have a worse prognosis, with complications of more frequent relapses and hospitalizations (RachBeisel et al. 1999) related to treatment noncompliance (Owen et al. 1996). Drake and colleagues (Drake and Mueser 2001; Drake et al. 2004) emphasized that treatment of schizophrenia complicated by a substance use disorder should be based on an integration of treatment modalities, as opposed to participation in separate programs. In integrated dual diagnosis programs, an individual's mental and substance use disorders are treated by the same clinician, who has been trained to assess and treat both problems. The substance abuse treatments in integrated programs are designed specifically for persons with severe and persistent mental illness, having a slower pace

and a longer-term perspective than programs that focus on only substance abuse. Integrated programs emphasize the need for pharmacotherapy to treat the mental illness (as opposed to the blanket prohibition of any psychoactive medications in some substance abuse programs).

PREVENTION PROGRAMS

Most public and community mental health programs have prevention programs at the secondary and tertiary levels. *Secondary prevention* is essentially treatment of the acute condition, with the goal of restoring function to premorbid levels. Components of secondary prevention include early identification of illness and then symptomatic and functional recovery (treatment). The finding that psychotic symptoms appear on average a year or more before first treatment contact (Larsen et al. 2001) suggests that identification strategies are not optimal. *Tertiary prevention* includes rehabilitative efforts geared toward avoiding adverse consequences of the illness (e.g., disability).

Very few public mental health systems have primary prevention programs related to schizophrenia, in which an effort is made to help persons at risk avoid the onset of psychosis. Recent research regarding identification and treatment of prodromal symptoms provides a rationale for developing primary prevention models in schizophrenia treatment (McGlashan 2003; McGlashan et al. 2003; T.J. Miller et al. 2003). Persons who are at high risk for schizophrenia have attenuated psychotic symptoms; brief, limited, and intermittent psychotic symptoms; or trait and state risk factors (e.g., having a first-degree relative with schizophrenia or having schizotypal personality disorder) (Brewer et al. 2003; Yung and McGorry 1996). Persons meeting strict high-risk criteria have a rate of progression to psychotic disorder of 40% over 12 months (Yung et al. 2003). Early pharmacotherapy and psychotherapy targeted toward this group have been found to reduce the risk of transition to psychosis (McGorry et al. 2002). Additionally, antipsychotic treatment results in symptomatic relief in prodromal patients, although this group is highly sensitive to the side effects of antipsychotic medication (with greater weight gain with olanzapine treatment than with placebo) (Woods et al. 2003). In an effort to improve and standardize diagnosis of a schizophrenia prodromal syndrome, the Structured Interview for Prodromal Syndromes has been developed (T.J. Miller et al. 2003).

The current evidence suggests that early identification and treatment of persons at risk for schizophrenia is possible and results in improved outcome. Less clear is the optimal public health approach to cost-effectively identify these persons in community populations and the risk-benefit ratio of antipsychotic drug treatment in this population.

CONCLUSION

Treatment of schizophrenia in the public sector varies depending on service location and target population. The quality and quantity of service provided are based on economic constraints and the availability of qualified professionals. Ideally, treatment of schizophrenia in the public sector prioritizes interventions that have shown efficacy in reducing relapse and need for hospitalization while increasing patient psychosocial functioning (i.e., evidence-based or best practices). These interventions include, at a minimum, antipsychotic medication, assertive outreach (ACT), supportive housing, case management, and integrated services for treating coexisting substance use or medical problems.

Individual service settings must further prioritize to maximize cost-benefit ratios based on the realities of their own financial and provider situations as well as their target population. Service settings must define outcome measures (e.g., hospitalization, homelessness, medication compliance) and assess the effect of their chosen interventions on these measures. Effective interventions can be further supported, and less effective interventions can be refined or abandoned. Research results derived from such analyses should contribute to the development of evidence-based practice. Thus, data management and analysis are crucial aspects of public treatment settings.

Service settings should have the capacity to treat patients in all phases of illness, from acute exacerbation of psychotic symptoms to remission. Ultimately, the goal for all patients is treatment in the least restrictive setting and the development of optimal functioning and recovery.

REFERENCES

Agerbo E, Byrne M, Eaton WW, et al: Marital and labor market status in the long run in schizophrenia. Arch Gen Psychiatry 61:28–33, 2004

Bell MD, Lysaker PH, Milstein RM: Clinical benefits of paid work activity in schizophrenia. Schizophr Bull 22:51–67, 1996

Bertman LJ, Thompson JW Jr, Waters WF, et al: Effect of an individualized treatment protocol on restoration of competency in pretrial forensic inpatients. J Am Acad Psychiatry Law 31:27–35, 2003

Brewer WJ, Wood SJ, McGorry PD, et al: Impairment of olfactory identification ability in individuals at ultra-high risk for psychosis who later develop schizophrenia. Am J Psychiatry 160:1790–1794, 2003

Brown MA, Munford AM: Life skills training for chronic schizophrenics. J Nerv Ment Dis 171:466–470, 1983

Byerly MJ, Weber M, Brooks D, et al: Cost evaluation of risperidone compared with olanzapine. Psychiatr Serv 54:742–744, 2003

Chengappa KN, Ebeling T, Kang JS, et al: Clozapine reduces severe self-mutilation and aggression in psychotic patients with borderline personality disorder. J Clin Psychiatry 60:477–484, 1999

Chengappa KN, Vasile J, Levine J, et al: Clozapine: its impact on aggressive behavior among patients in a state psychiatric hospital. Schizophr Res 53:1–6, 2002

Citrome L, Green L, Fost R: Length of stay and recidivism on a psychiatric intensive care unit. Hosp Community Psychiatry 45:74–76, 1994

Copeland LA, Zeber JE, Valenstein M, et al: Racial disparity in the use of atypical antipsychotic medications among veterans. Am J Psychiatry 160:1817–1822, 2003

Cramer J, Rosenheck R, Xu W, et al: Detecting improvement in quality of life and symptomatology in schizophrenia. Schizophr Bull 27(2):227–234, 2001

Diehl S, Hiland E: A Survey of County Jails in Tennessee: Four Years Later—A Descriptive Study of Services to People With Mental Illness and Substance Abuse Problems. Nashville, Tennessee Mental Health Planning and Policy Council, Tennessee Department of Mental Health and Developmental Disabilities, February 2003, pp 1–39

Ditton PM: Mental Health and Treatment of Inmates and Probationers (NCJ 174463). Washington, DC, U.S. Department of Justice, July 1999

Dixon L: Assertive community treatment: twenty-five years of gold. Psychiatr Serv 51:759–765, 2000

Dixon L, Postrado L, Delahanty J, et al: The association of medical comorbidity in schizophrenia with poor physical and mental health. J Nerv Ment Dis 187:496–502, 1999

Drake RE, Mueser KT: Managing comorbid schizophrenia and substance abuse. Curr Psychiatry Rep 3:418–422, 2001

Drake RE, Mueser KT, Torrey WC, et al: Evidence-based treatment of schizophrenia. Curr Psychiatry Rep 2:393–397, 2000

Drake RE, Goldman HH, Leff HS, et al: Implementing evidence-based practices in routine mental health service settings. Psychiatr Serv 52:179–182, 2001

Drake RE, Mueser KT, Brunette MF, et al: A review of treatments for people with severe mental illnesses and co-occurring substance use disorders. Psychiatr Rehabil J 27:360–374, 2004

Dunham HW: Community and Schizophrenia: An Epidemiological Analysis. Detroit, MI, Wayne State University Press, 1965

Elbogen EB, Swanson JW, Swartz MS: Effects of legal mechanisms on perceived coercion and treatment adherence among persons with severe mental illness. J Nerv Ment Dis 191:629–637, 2003

Essock SM, Kontos N: Implementing assertive community treatment teams. Psychiatr Serv 46:679–683, 1995

Fogel BS: Neuropsychiatry in public mental health settings, in Neuropsychiatry and Mental Health Services. Edited by Ovsiew F. Washington, DC, American Psychiatric Press, 1999, pp 47–68

Frank RG, McGuire TG: Establishing a capitation policy for mental health and substance abuse services in healthcare reform. Behav Healthc Tomorrow 3:36–39, 1994

Gilligan J: The last mental hospital. Psychiatr Q 72:45–61, 2001

Green AI, Canuso CM, Brenner MJ, et al: Detection and management of comorbidity in patients with schizophrenia. Psychiatr Clin North Am 26:115–139, 2003

Hall LL, Graf AC, Fitzpatrick MJ, et al: Shattered Lives: Results of a National Survey of NAMI Members Living With Mental Illnesses and Their Families. Arlington, VA, National Alliance for the Mentally Ill, July 2003

Harrison G, Gunnell D, Glazebrook C, et al: Association between schizophrenia and social inequality at birth: case-control study. Br J Psychiatry 179:346–350, 2001

Hawthorne WB, Fals-Stewart W, Lohr JB: A treatment outcome study of community-based residential care. Hosp Community Psychiatry 45:152–155, 1994

Herinckx HA, Kinney RF, Clarke GN, et al: Assertive community treatment versus usual care in engaging and retaining clients with severe mental illness. Psychiatr Serv 48:1297–1306, 1997

Herz MI, Marder SR: Schizophrenia: Comprehensive Treatment and Management. Philadelphia, PA, Lippincott Williams & Wilkins, 2002

Human Rights Watch Report: Ill-Equipped: U.S. Prisons and Offenders With Mental Illness, 2003. Available at: http://www.hrw.org/reports/2003/usa1003.

Kane JM, Leucht S, Carpenter D, et al: Expert consensus guideline series: Optimizing pharmacologic treatment of psychotic disorders: introduction: methods, commentary, and summary. J Clin Psychiatry 64 (suppl 12):5–19, 2003

Kraus JE, Sheitman BB: Characteristics of violent behavior in a large state psychiatric hospital. Psychiatr Serv 55:183–185, 2004

Kraus JE, Sheitman BB: Clozapine reduces violent behavior in heterogeneous diagnostic groups. J Neuropsychiatry Clin Neurosci 17:36–44, 2005

Kraus JE, Webster SL, Sheitman BB: The introduction of a psychosocial intervention, a "treatment mall," has a gender dependent effect on the need for restrictive interventions (abstract). J Neuropsychiatry Clin Neurosci 16:226, 2004

Kravitz HM, Kelly J: An outpatient psychiatry program for offenders with mental disorders found not guilty by reason of insanity. Psychiatr Serv 50:1597–1605, 1999

Lamb HR: Public psychiatry and prevention, in The American Psychiatric Press Textbook of Psychiatry, 3rd Edition. Edited by Hales RE, Yudofsky SC, Talbot JA. Washington, DC, American Psychiatric Press, 1999, pp 1535–1554

Lambert TJ, Velakoulis D, Pantelis C: Medical comorbidity in schizophrenia. Med J Aust 178 (suppl):S67–S70, 2003

Landerman LR, Burns BJ, Swartz MS, et al: The relationship between insurance coverage and psychiatric disorder in predicting use of mental health services. Am J Psychiatry 151:1785–1790, 1994

Larsen TK, Friis S, Haahr U, et al: Early detection and intervention in first-episode schizophrenia: a critical review. Acta Psychiatr Scand 103:323–334, 2001

Lehman AF, Lieberman JA, Dixon LB, et al: Practice guideline for the treatment of patients with schizophrenia, second edition. Am J Psychiatry 161 (2 suppl):1–56, 2004

Leslie DL, Rosenheck RA: Use of pharmacy data to assess quality of pharmacotherapy for schizophrenia in a national health care system: individual and facility predictors. Med Care 39:923–933, 2001

McGlashan TH: Commentary: Progress, issues, and implications of prodromal research: an inside view. Schizophr Bull 29:851–858, 2003

McGlashan TH, Zipursky RB, Perkins D, et al: The PRIME North America randomized double-blind clinical trial of olanzapine versus placebo in patients at risk of being prodromally symptomatic for psychosis, I: study rationale and design. Schizophr Res 61:7–18, 2003

McGorry PD, Yung AR, Phillips LJ, et al: Randomized controlled trial of interventions designed to reduce the risk of progression to first-episode psychosis in a clinical sample with subthreshold symptoms. Arch Gen Psychiatry 59:921–928, 2002

McGuire TG, Mosakowski WS, Radigan LS: Designing a state level prospective payment system for inpatient psychiatric services in Medicaid. Adm Policy Ment Health 18:43–54, 1990

Miller RD: Hospitalization of criminal defendants for evaluation of competence to stand trial or for restoration of competence: clinical and legal issues. Behav Sci Law 21:369–391, 2003

Miller TJ, McGlashan TH, Rosen JL, et al: Prodromal assessment with the structured interview for prodromal syndromes and the scale of prodromal symptoms: predictive validity, interrater reliability, and training to reliability. Schizophr Bull 29:703–715, 2003

Monnier J, Knapp RG, Frueh BC: Recent advances in telepsychiatry: an updated review. Psychiatr Serv 54:1604–1609, 2003

Morse GA, Calsyn RJ, Klinkenberg WD, et al: An experimental comparison of three types of case management for homeless mentally ill persons. Psychiatr Serv 48:497–503, 1997

Mueser KT, Yarnold PR, Levinson DF, et al: Prevalence of substance abuse in schizophrenia: demographic and clinical correlates. Schizophr Bull 16:31–56, 1990

National Advisory Committee on Rural Health: Sixth Annual Report on Rural Health. Rockville, MD, U.S. Department of Health and Human Services, 1993

National Association of State Mental Health Program Directors Research Institute. State Profile Highlights, No. 03–01. Alexandria, VA, National Association of State Mental Health Program Directors, May 2003, pp 1–6

Ng B, Kumar S, Ranclaud M, et al: Ward crowding and incidents of violence on an acute psychiatric inpatient unit. Psychiatr Serv 52:521–525, 2001

Nijman HL, Rector G: Crowding and aggression on inpatient psychiatric wards. Psychiatr Serv 50:830–831, 1999

Okin RL, Borus JF, Baer L, et al: Long-term outcome of state hospital patients discharged into structured community residential settings. Psychiatr Serv 46:73–78, 1995

Olmstead v L.C. (98–536) 527 U.S. 581 (1999); 138 F3d 893

Owen RR, Fischer EP, Booth BM, et al: Medication noncompliance and substance abuse among patients with schizophrenia. Psychiatr Serv 47:853–858, 1996

Owen RR, Fischer EP, Kirchner JE, et al: Clinical practice variations in prescribing antipsychotics for patients with schizophrenia. Am J Med Qual 18:140–146, 2003

Palmer CA, Hazelrigg M: The guilty but mentally ill verdict: a review and conceptual analysis of intent and impact. J Am Acad Psychiatry Law 28:47–54, 2000

Patterson RF, Wise BF: The development of internal forensic review boards in the management of hospitalized insanity acquittees. J Am Acad Psychiatry Law 26:661–664, 1998

Pion GM, Keller P, McCombs H: Final Report of the Ad Hoc Rural Mental Health Provider Work Group: Mental Health Providers in Rural and Isolated Areas. Rockville, MD, Center for Mental Health Services, Substance Abuse and Mental Health Services Administration, U.S. Department of Health and Human Services, October 1997

Quanbeck C, Frye M, Altshuler L: Mania and the law in California: understanding the criminalization of the mentally ill. Am J Psychiatry 160:1245–1250, 2003

RachBeisel J, Scott J, Dixon L: Co-occurring severe mental illness and substance use disorders: a review of recent research. Psychiatr Serv 50:1427–1434, 1999

Regier DA, Farmer ME, Rae DS, et al: Comorbidity of mental disorders with alcohol and other drug abuse: results from the Epidemiologic Catchment Area (ECA) Study. JAMA 264:2511–2518, 1990

Rosenheck R, Neale M, Leaf P, et al: Multisite experimental cost study of intensive psychiatric community care. Schizophr Bull 21:129–140, 1995

Rosenheck R, Cramer J, Xu W, et al: A comparison of clozapine and haloperidol in hospitalized patients with refractory schizophrenia. Department of Veterans Affairs Cooperative Study Group on Clozapine in Refractory Schizophrenia. N Engl J Med 337:809–815, 1997

Rosenheck R, Lawson W, Crayton J, et al: Predictors of differential response to clozapine and haloperidol. Veterans Affairs Cooperative Study Group on Clozapine in Refractory Schizophrenia. Biol Psychiatry 44:475–482, 1998a

Rosenheck R, Tekell J, Peters J, et al: Does participation in psychosocial treatment augment the benefit of clozapine? Department of Veterans Affairs Cooperative Study Group on Clozapine in Refractory Schizophrenia. Arch Gen Psychiatry 55:618–625, 1998b

Rosenheck R, Cramer J, Allan E, et al: Cost-effectiveness of clozapine in patients with high and low levels of hospital use. Department of Veterans Affairs Cooperative Study Group on Clozapine in Refractory Schizophrenia. Arch Gen Psychiatry 56:565–572, 1999

Rosenheck R, Cramer J, Jurgis G, et al: Clinical and psychopharmacologic factors influencing family burden in refractory schizophrenia. Department of Veterans Affairs Cooperative Study Group on Clozapine in Refractory Schizophrenia. J Clin Psychiatry 61:671–676, 2000

Rosenheck R, Perlick D, Bingham S, et al: Effectiveness and cost of olanzapine and haloperidol in the treatment of schizophrenia: a randomized controlled trial. JAMA 290:2693–2702, 2003

Rupp A: Underinsurance for severe mental illness. Schizophr Bull 17:401–405, 1991

Scott JE, Dixon LB: Assertive community treatment and case management for schizophrenia. Schizophr Bull 21:657–668, 1995

Sernyak MJ, Dausey D, Desai R, et al: Prescribers' nonadherence to treatment guidelines for schizophrenia when prescribing neuroleptics. Psychiatr Serv 54:246–248, 2003a

Sernyak MJ, Leslie D, Rosenheck R: Use of system-wide outcomes monitoring data to compare the effectiveness of atypical neuroleptic medications. Am J Psychiatry 160:310–315, 2003b

Sevy S, Nathanson K, Visweswaraiah H, et al: The relationship between insight and symptoms in schizophrenia. Compr Psychiatry 45:16–19, 2004

Simon RI: The law and psychiatry, in The American Psychiatric Publishing Textbook of Clinical Psychiatry, 4th Edition. Edited by Hales RE, Yudofsky SC. Washington, DC, American Psychiatric Publishing, 2003, pp 1585–1628

Smith TE, Hull JW, Huppert JD, et al: Insight and recovery from psychosis in chronic schizophrenia and schizoaffective disorder patients. J Psychiatr Res 38:169–176, 2004

Stein LI, Test MA: Alternative to mental hospital treatment, I: conceptual model, treatment program, and clinical evaluation. Arch Gen Psychiatry 37:392–397, 1980

Stein LI, Test MA, Marx AJ: Alternative to the hospital: a controlled study. Am J Psychiatry 132:517–522, 1975

Swanson JW, Swartz MS, Elbogen EB, et al: Effects of involuntary outpatient commitment on subjective quality of life in persons with severe mental illness. Behav Sci Law 21:473–491, 2003

Swartz MS, Swanson JW, Hannon MJ: Does fear of coercion keep people away from mental health treatment? Evidence from a survey of persons with schizophrenia and mental health professionals. Behav Sci Law 21:459–472, 2003

Tien AY, Eaton WW: Psychopathologic precursors and sociodemographic risk factors for the schizophrenia syndrome. Arch Gen Psychiatry 49:37–46, 1992

Torrey EF: Jails and prisons—America's new mental hospitals. Am J Public Health 85:1661–1662, 1995

Torrey WC, Drake RE, Dixon L, et al: Implementing evidence-based practices for persons with severe mental illnesses. Psychiatr Serv 52:45–50, 2001

Treffert DA: Legal "rites": criminalizing the mentally ill. Hillside J Clin Psychiatry 3:123–137, 1981

U.S. Department of Health and Human Services: Mental Health: A Report of the Surgeon General. Rockville, MD, U.S. Department of Health and Human Services, Public Health Service, 1999

Woods SW, Breier A, Zipursky RB, et al: Randomized trial of olanzapine versus placebo in the symptomatic acute treatment of the schizophrenic prodrome. Biol Psychiatry 54:453–464, 2003

Yanos PT, Lu W, Minsky S, et al: Correlates of health insurance among persons with schizophrenia in a statewide behavioral health care system. Psychiatr Serv 55:79–82, 2004

Yung AR, McGorry PD: The initial prodrome in psychosis: descriptive and qualitative aspects. Aust N Z J Psychiatry 30: 587–599, 1996

Yung AR, Phillips LJ, Yuen HP, et al: Psychosis prediction: 12-month follow up of a high-risk ("prodromal") group. Schizophr Res 60:21–32, 2003

INDEX

Page numbers printed in **boldface** type refer to tables or figures.

AA. *See* Arachidonic acid

Abnormal connectivity hypothesis, 180

Abnormal Involuntary Movement Scale (AIMS), 310

Abstract thinking difficulties, 207

ACC. *See* Anterior cingulate cortex

N-Acetylaspartate (NAA), 73, 142, 157

Acquired immunodeficiency syndrome (AIDS), 387–388, 389
    risk reduction strategies for, 390

ACT (assertive community treatment), 334–335, **335**, 337, 361, 398

Acute paranoid disorder, 196

ADA (Americans with Disabilities Act), 398

ADHD (attention-deficit/hyperactivity disorder), 127, 205, 347, 348

Adherence to treatment, 367, 370, 371–373
    assessment of, 372
    in community mental health centers, 398
    compliance therapy for, 329, 372
    cutoff for, 371–372
    depot antipsychotics and, 314, 367, 373
    strategies for improvement of, 372–373
    among substance-abusing patients, 372

Adolescents. *See* Children and adolescents at risk for schizophrenia

Adoption studies, 40, 41–42

Aesclepiades of Prusa, 4

Aetius of Amida, 5

Affective disorder(s)
    with psychotic features, 197, 346
    vs. schizophrenia, 213

Affective symptoms of schizophrenia
    depression, 209–211, 227–229
    flattened or blunted affect, 2, **2**, 12, 85, 167, 188, 189, 190, 194, **195**, 202
    inappropriate affect, 201

relation of cognitive deficits to, 253

Age at onset, 20, **20**, 85, 187, 290, 353, 354, 374
    gender differences in, 290
    social functioning and, 276

Aggressive behavior. *See* Hostility/aggression

Agranulocytosis, clozapine-induced, 304, 305, 307, 316

AIDS (acquired immunodeficiency syndrome), 387–388, **389**
    risk reduction strategies for, 390

AIMS (Abnormal Involuntary Movement Scale), 310

Akathisia, 304, 308–309
    vs. anxiety, 212
    management of, 309, **309**
    monitoring for, 309
    vs. psychotic agitation, 308
    suicidality and, 309
    tardive, 310
    time of onset of, 308

ALA (alpha-linolenic acid), 122–123

Alcohol use disorders, 224, 385
    anxiety and, 212
    disulfiram for, 226
    hallucinations in, 214
    naltrexone for, 226
    prognostic significance of, 296
    suicidal behavior and, 211

Alcohol Use Scale, 225

Alexander of Tralles, 5, 6

Alienation, 4

Alienists, 4–5, 10

Alogia, 167, 188, 202, 203

Alpha-linolenic acid (ALA), 122–123

Alzheimer, Alois, 13, 137, 151

Alzheimer's disease, 99, 139, 152, 173, 175, 376

Amantadine, **309**

Amenorrhea, 312

American Psychiatric Association's "Practice Guideline for the Treatment of Patients With Schizophrenia," 313, 357, 360, 369

Americans with Disabilities Act (ADA), 398

α-Amino-3-hydroxy-5-methyl-4-isoxazolepropionic acid (AMPA) receptors, 97, 98–99, 102, 144, 155, **156**

D-Amino acid oxidase (DAAO), 101

Amino acid transporters, 97

γ-Aminobutyric acid (GABA), 72, 73, 75, 76, 85, 87

    alcohol effects on, 385

    α5 receptors for, 179

    GABAergic system deficits, 155

        in anterior cingulate cortex, 158

    nonpyramidal neurons and neurotransmitter function of, 152

    regulation of dopamine production by, 179

    in working memory circuit, 159

Amisulpride, 88, 89, 312

Amotivation/avolition, 167, 188, 190, 194, **195**, 203, 252

AMPA (α-amino-3-hydroxy-5-methyl-4-isoxazolepropionic acid) receptors, 97, 98–99, 102, 144, 155, **156**

AMPAkines, 99

Amphetamine

    psychosis induced by, 87–88, 145, 214

        historical description of, 87

        long-term sensitization to, 88

        in nonschizophrenic subjects, 87–88

        in patients with schizophrenia, 88

        steps in development of, 87

    striatal dopamine release induced by, 90–91, **91–92**

        ketamine effects on, 104–106, **105**

Amygdala, 178–179

Anandamide, 126

Anergia, 203

Anhedonia, 85, 190, 194, **195**

Anorgasmia, 312

Anterior cingulate cortex (ACC)

    abnormalities in schizophrenia, 158

        frontotemporal deficits and, 159

        gray matter volume reductions, 171

    dopamine tracts in, 157

    GABA$_A$ receptor binding in, 155

    integrative functions of, 158

    neuronal density in, 153

    prefrontal–anterior cingulate circuitry, 158

Antiadrenergic effects of antipsychotics, 304

Anticholinergic effects of antipsychotics, 304, **306**

    in elderly patients, **376**

Anticonvulsants, 318

Antidepressants, 229, 303, 317

    for elderly patients, 378

    for negative symptoms of schizophrenia, 369

    for obsessive-compulsive disorder, 234–235

    for patients with comorbid substance abuse, 226

    for posttraumatic stress disorder, 233

    for social phobia, 232

    tricyclic, 317

Antidiuretic hormone, 373

Antioxidant defense systems (AODs), **120**, 123

Antioxidant supplementation, 127–129

Antipsychotics, 88–89, 303–316. *See also specific drugs*

    adherence to treatment with, 371–373

    administration routes for, 315

    adverse effects of, 117–118, 304, **306**, 357

        cardiovascular effects, 312–313

        deciding whether to switch to another antipsychotic due to, 371, **371**

        effect on treatment adherence, 372

        in elderly patients, 375–376, **376**, 377

        extrapyramidal side effects, 308–310, **309**

        maintenance treatment and, 313

        metabolic effects, 310–312, **311**

        monitoring for, 309, 310, 311, **311, 389**

        neuroleptic dysphoria, 313

        sedation, 312–313

    augmentation of, 369

    availability of, 372

    combinations of, 315, 319, 369

    criteria for response to, 316

    D$_2$ receptor occupancy of, 85, 88–89

        clinical response related to, 88, 89

        for first- vs. second-generation drugs, 89, 304

    dosage of, **305**, 315

        in elderly patients, 377, **378**

        in first-episode patients, 357

        for rapid neuroleptization, 315

    effect on cognitive deficits, 251, 253–254, 316

    effect on oxidative stress, 124

    effect on positive and negative symptoms, 303, 304, 316

    effect on prognosis, **294**, 296–297

    effect on social and vocational functioning, 277, 327

    efficacy of, 117, 313–314, 356

        at different stages of illness, **368**

    in elderly patients, 375–378

    factors influencing response to, 316

    failure of, 367–368, **368**

    for first-episode psychosis, 356–359

    first-generation (typical), 304–305, **305**

        history and development of, 303–304

        mechanism of action of, 88–89, 304

    guidelines and algorithms for sequence of, 367–368

    half-lives of, **305**

limitations of, 118

long-acting injectable (depot) formulations of, **314,** 314–315

maintenance treatment with, 313

membrane phospholipid effects of, 123, 124

NMDA agonists combined with, 100, **101**

polypharmacy with, 315, 319, 369

in prodromal period, 349–350

psychosocial therapies and, 327–337

reduction in baseline symptoms after initiation of, 117

for relapse prevention, 313

relative potency of, 304, **305**

second-generation (atypical), **305,** 305–308

   aripiprazole, 308

   clozapine, 305–307

   effectiveness of, 313–314

   history and development of, 304

   mechanisms of action of, 89, 304

   olanzapine, 307–308

   quetiapine, 308

   risperidone, 307

   ziprasidone, 308

switching between, 367

   in elderly patients, 377–378

targeted, intermittent therapy with, 313

time to therapeutic effect of, 315

use in patients with comorbid disorders

   depression, 228–229

   obsessive-compulsive disorder, 234–235

   panic disorder, 231

   social phobia, 232

   substance use disorders, 226

use in state psychiatric hospitals, 399

use in Veterans Affairs medical centers, 400

value of global market for, 303

Anxiety symptoms and disorders, 211–212, 230–235

comorbid anxiety disorders, 212

definition of, 211

differential diagnosis of, 230

effects on quality of life, 212

obsessive-compulsive disorder and symptoms, 9, 212, 213, 233–235

panic attacks and panic disorder, 231

prevalence of, 230

social phobia, 212, 231–232

trauma and posttraumatic stress disorder, 232–233

Anxiolytics, 303

AODs (antioxidant defense systems), **120,** 123

Apathy, 85, 203

Apoptosis, 125, 138, 144

Appearance of patient, 201

Arachidonic acid (AA), 118–121, **120,** 125

antipsychotic effects on levels of, 123

defective conversion of n-6 fatty acids to, 123

eicosanoids derived from, 126

neurodevelopmental effects of deficits of, 125

niacin-induced flushing and, 127

in peripheral tissues, 120–121

symptom severity and, 126

tardive dyskinesia and, 126

2-Arachidonoylglycerol, 126

Aretaeus of Cappadocia, 5, 11, 31

Aripiprazole, 304, 308

adverse effects of, **306,** 308

dosage and half-life of, **305**

in elderly patients, **378**

history and development of, 308

mechanism of action of, 89, 308

in patients with substance use disorders, 226

Aristotle, 4, 6

Arnold, Thomas, 9

Aspartate, 97

Asperger's syndrome, 127, 262

ASQ (Attributional Style Questionnaire), 265, 266

Assaultive behavior. *See* Hostility/aggression

Assertive community treatment (ACT), 334–335, **335,** 337, 361, 398

Assessment instruments, 17, 189

Abnormal Involuntary Movement Scale, 310

Alcohol Use Scale, 225

Attributional Style Questionnaire, 265, 266

Bell Sysaker Emotion Recognition Task, 270

Brief Psychiatric Rating Scale, 99, 191, 228, 307, 319

Buss-Durkee Hostility Inventory, 209

Calgary Depression Rating Scale for Schizophrenia, 210–211

California Verbal Learning Test, 247

Catatonia Rating Scale, 373

Clinical Global Impression, 307

Composite International Diagnostic Interview, 17

Comprehensive Assessment of At Risk Mental States, 344

Comprehensive Assessment of Symptoms and History, 189

Continuous Performance Test, 205, 246, 343

   "AX" version of, 70, 100, 246

Dartmouth Assessment of Lifestyle Instrument, 225

Diagnostic Interview Schedule, 17, 189

Digit Symbol Test, 247

Disability Assessment Scale, 290, 292

Drug Use Scale, 225

Facial Emotion Identification Task, 270

Global Assessment of Functioning Scale, 290, **293,** 343, 344

Global Assessment Scale, 290

Internal, Personal, and Situational Attributions Questionnaire, 265, 266

Assessment instruments (continued)
   Iowa Tests, 249
   Mini-Mental State Examination, 100
   Overt Aggression Scale, 209
   Positive and Negative Syndrome Scale, 99, 100, 194, **196,**
      205, 206, 209, 231
   Present State Examination, 17, 18, 189
   Prodromal States Questionnaire, 345
   Scale for the Assessment of Negative Symptoms, 191, 194,
      195, 206
   Scale for the Assessment of Positive Symptoms, 191, 194,
      194, 205, 206
   Scale of Prodromal Symptoms, 344
   Schedule for Affective Disorders and Schizophrenia, 189
   Schedule for Deficit Syndromes, 204, **204**
   Schedules for Clinical Assessment in Neuropsychiatry, 17,
      18
   Structured Clinical Interview for DSM-III-R, 17
   Structured Clinical Interview for DSM-IV, 189
   Structured Interview for Prodromal Syndromes, 344–345,
      401
   Trail Making Parts A and B tests, 255
   Wechsler Adult Intelligence Scale, 247, 264
   Wisconsin Card Sorting Test, 70, 100, 202, 247, 252, 254
   Yale-Brown Obsessive Compulsive Scale, 234
Association studies, 46
Asthma, 388
Atrial natriuretic peptide, 373
Attention-deficit/hyperactivity disorder (ADHD), 127, 205,
      347, 348
Attentional problems, 70, 205, 208, 246
Attenuated positive symptoms syndrome, 347
Attributional style, **262,** 265–267
   deciding which attributions to code, 266
   definition of, 265
   in depressed persons, 265
   measurement of, 265, 266
   mechanisms by which persecutory beliefs lead to, 266–267
   self-discrepancy theory and, 267
   self-serving and personalizing biases, 265–266
   unanswered questions about, 266–267
Attributional Style Questionnaire (ASQ), 265, 266
Auditorization of thoughts, 200
Auditory hallucinations, 199–200
Autism, 127, 262, 263
Autoimmune diseases, **28,** 28–29
Autonomic dysfunction, in neuroleptic malignant syndrome,
      309
Avenzoar of Seville, 6
Averrhoës of Cordoba, 6
Avicenna, 6

Avolition/amotivation, 167, 188, 190, 194, **195,** 203, 252
AX version of Continuous Performance Test (AX-CPT), 70,
      100, 246

Baillarger, Jules, 12
Bartholomaeus Anglicus, 6
Basal ganglia, 173–174
Basic fibroblast growth factor, 119
Báthory, Erzsébet, 7
Battie, William, 9
Bax/Bcl-2 ratio, 144
BDD (body dysmorphic disorder), 214
BDNF (brain-derived neurotrophic factor), 76, 119
Behavioral symptoms, 2, **2,** 190, **194,** 200–201
Behavioral Therapy for Substance Abuse in Schizophrenia
      (BTSAS), 386
Bell Sysaker Emotion Recognition Task, 270
Bentall, Richard, 265–267
Benzodiazepines, 317, 370
   for catatonic hypomobility, 374
   for panic disorder, 231
   for patients with comorbid substance use disorders, 226
Benztropine mesylate, **309**
Bernard de Gordon, 6
Bethlem, 9
Biblical conceptions of "madness," 2, 3
Bipolar disorder, 213
Birth complications. *See* Obstetrical complications
Bleuler, Eugen, 1, 10, 13, 69, 167, 187, 201, 211, 343
Blood pressure monitoring, **311,** 313
BMI (body mass index), 311, **311**
Body dysmorphic disorder (BDD), 214
Body mass index (BMI), 311, **311**
Borderline personality disorder, 346
Bosch, Hieronymus, 32
BPRS (Brief Psychiatric Rating Scale), 99, 191, 228, 307, 319
Bradykinesia, 309
Brain-derived neurotrophic factor (BDNF), 76, 119
Brain developmental abnormalities, 21, 69–79. *See also*
      Neurodevelopmental theories
Brain imaging. *See* Neuroimaging studies
Brain reward pathways, 223
Brain volumetric abnormalities, 71, 141, **142,** 143, 144, 171,
      176, **176,** 357, **357, 358**
Breast cancer, 312
Brief intermittent psychotic syndrome, 347–348
Brief Psychiatric Rating Scale (BPRS), 99, 191, 228, 307, 319
Brief psychotic disorder, 213
Bromocriptine, 318
   for hyperprolactinemia, 312
   for neuroleptic malignant syndrome, 310

Bronchitis, chronic, 388

Brown-Goodwin assessment for lifetime history of aggression, 209

BTSAS (Behavioral Therapy for Substance Abuse in Schizophrenia), 386

Bupropion
    interaction with clozapine, 317
    for smoking cessation, 226, 385

Buss-Durkee Hostility Inventory, 209

CAARMS (Comprehensive Assessment of At Risk Mental States), 344

Cabergoline, for hyperprolactinemia, 312

Calbindin, 155

Calgary Depression Rating Scale for Schizophrenia (CDSS), 210–211

Calgary Early Psychosis Program, 346

California Verbal Learning Test, 247

Calretinin, 155

CAMs (cell adhesion molecules), 76, 155

Cancer, 389

Candidate genes, **47,** 47–50, 75–76
    catechol-*O*-methyltransferase *(COMT),* 49, 56, **56,** 76, 93, 223, 297
    disrupted in schizophrenia 1 and 2 *(DISC1* and *DISC2),* 44, 49
    dopamine₃ receptor *(DRD3),* 50
    dystrobrevin binding protein 1 *(DTNBP1),* 48, 56, **56,** 76, 101
    G72 and *G30,* 48, 101
    neuregulin 1 *(NRG1),* 47–48, 56, **56,** 76, 101
    proline dehydrogenase *(PRODH),* 49
    regulator of G-protein signaling 4 *(RGS4),* 48–49, 76, 101, 102
    serotonin₂ₐ receptor *(HTR2A),* 49

Cannabinoid receptors, 126

Cannabis use, 29–30, 126, 212, 224, 296, 385

Canon (Avicenna), 6

Capgras syndrome, 12, 197

Carbamazepine, 318
    interaction with clozapine, 316, 318

Cardiovascular effects of antipsychotics, 312–313
    in elderly patients, 377
    hypotension, 304, **306,** 312–313, **376**
    QTc interval prolongation, **306,** 308
    tachycardia, 313

Case finding, 17

Case identification, 17

Case management, 334, 386

CASH (Comprehensive Assessment of Symptoms and History), 189

Caspase-3, 144

Catatonia Rating Scale, 373

Catatonic schizophrenia, 12, 189, 190, **192,** 194, 201, 214–215, 373–374

Catechol-*O*-methyltransferase gene *(COMT),* **47,** 49, 56, **56,** 76, 93, 223, 297

Caudate, 174–175

CBT. *See* Cognitive-behavioral therapy

CDSS (Calgary Depression Rating Scale for Schizophrenia), 210–211

Celiac disease, 28

Cell adhesion molecules (CAMs), 76, 155

Cellular membranes, 73, 118
    free radical–mediated damage of, 118, **120, 122,** 123–124
    phospholipid composition of, 117–129 (*See also* Phospholipids)

Celsus, Aulus Cornelius, 4

Cerebellar abnormalities, 171

Cerebral blood flow studies, 169. *See also* Positron emission tomography studies; Single photon emission computed tomography studies

Cerebrospinal fluid volume, 171

Cerebrovascular events, antipsychotic-induced, **376,** 377

CGI (Clinical Global Impression) score, 307

Charles VI of France, 7

Child raising by parents with schizophrenia, 280

Childhood developmental abnormalities, 21, 69–79. *See also* Neurodevelopmental theories

Children and adolescents at risk for schizophrenia, 353. *See also* Prenatal and perinatal risk factors
    cognitive deficits in, 249–250, 353–354
    impulse-control problems in, 276
    neurobiological changes in, 74
    panic attacks and psychoticism in, 231
    social impairments in, 275–276

Chlorpromazine, 88, 304, 307
    adverse effects of, 304, **306,** 311
        hepatotoxicity, 388
    dosage and half-life of, **305,** 315

Cholesterol levels, **306,** 312

Choreoathetosis, 310

CHRNA7 (α7 nicotinic acetylcholine receptor subunit gene), 40

Chromosomal abnormalities, 44–45, 223

Chronic obstructive pulmonary disease, 384, 386, 388, **389**

Chronic symptoms and disability, 21–22, 291–292, **293,** 297
    treatment of, 365–378 (*See also* Long-term treatment)

CIDI (Composite International Diagnostic Interview), 17

Circumstantiality, 207

Cirrhosis, 388

Clanging, 207

Clinical Antipsychotic Trials of Intervention Effectiveness Schizophrenia Trial, 314
Clinical Global Impression (CGI) score, 307
Clomipramine, for obsessive-compulsive disorder, 234
Clonazepam, **309**
Clothing of patient, 201
Clozapine, 305–307
    adverse effects of, 304, 305, **306**, 307, 311, 315
        agranulocytosis, 304, 305, 307, 316
        myocarditis, 316
        seizures, 307, 317
    augmentation of, 319, 368
        electroconvulsive therapy, 368
        lamotrigine, 368, 369
        other antipsychotics, 319, 368
    D$_2$ receptor occupancy of, 89
    discontinuation of, 316
    dosage and half-life of, **305**, 315–316
    drug interactions with
        bupropion, 317
        carbamazepine, 316, 318
        selective serotonin reuptake inhibitors, 316, 317
    effect on smoking, 385
    in elderly patients, **378**
    failure of, **368**
    high caloric diet and, 124
    history and development of, 304, 305
    implementing treatment with, 315–316
    laboratory tests before initiation of, 315
    maintenance treatment with, 316
    mechanism of action of, 89, 226
    NMDA agonists combined with, 100, **101**
    in patients with substance use disorders, 226
    pharmacological profile of, 226
    for polydipsia, 373, 388
    to reduce suicide risk, 230, 307, 359–360
    for tardive dyskinesia, 310
    therapeutic plasma concentration of, 368
    for treatment-refractory schizophrenia, 307, **368**, 368–369
Clubhouse model of psychosocial rehabilitation, 333
CMHCs. *See* Community mental health centers
Cocaine use, 226, 385–386
Cognitive-behavioral therapy (CBT), 329, 337
    for anxiety disorders
        obsessive-compulsive disorder, 235
        panic disorder, 231
        posttraumatic stress disorder, 233
        social phobia, 232
    to challenge veracity of delusions, 329
    compliance therapy, 329, 372
    coping strategy enhancement, 329

    effect on negative symptoms, 329
    efficacy in schizophrenia, 329
    problem-solving intervention, 329
    in prodromal period, 349, 350
Cognitive impairments, 99, 204–208, 245–256
    anatomical correlates of, 71
    attentional problems, 70, 205, 208, 246
    classification of, 205
    as core symptom, 245
    correlation with negative symptoms, 202
    definitions of, 205
    dopamine and, 86, 89
    effect of antipsychotics on, 251, 253–254, 316
    facial affect recognition deficit and, 269–270
    in first-episode patients, 358–359
    historical concepts of, **2**, 2–6
    measurement of thought disorder, 206
    mechanisms of thought disorder, 205–206
    natural history of, 248–251, **249**
        changes in patients recovering from acute exacerbation, 250
        in children at risk for schizophrenia, 249–250, 353–354
            follow-back studies, 249–250
            prodrome studies, 250
        in elderly patients, 251
        first-episode psychosis studies, 250
        longitudinal changes, 139, 250–251
    NMDA receptor dysfunction and, 102
    in premorbid and prodromal phases of illness, 139, **140**, 245, 250, 289–290, 353–354
    profile and magnitude of, 245–248
        immediate/working memory, 248
        reasoning and problem solving, 247
        severity, 246, **246**
        social cognition, 248
        speed of processing, 247
        verbal fluency, 247–248
        verbal learning and memory, 246–247
        vigilance and attention, 246
        visual learning and memory, 247
    prognostic significance of, 295
    relation to functional outcome, 139, 254–255
        costs, 255
        medical comorbidity, 255
        quality of life, 255
        relapse prevention, 255
        unemployment, 254–255
    relation to schizophrenia symptoms, 251–254
        cross-sectional studies of, 251–253
            affective symptoms, 253
            negative symptoms, 252

positive symptoms, 252
thought disorder, 253
longitudinal studies of, 253–254
impact of second-generation antipsychotics on, 253–254
pseudospecificity of, 251
residual, 359
social, 248, 261–270 (*See also* Social cognition)
theory-of-mind deficits and, 263–264
twin studies of, 245
types of thought disorder, 206–208
work performance and, 281
Cognitive remediation, 331, 332–333
Community functioning, 254, 279–280. *See also* Social functioning impairments; Vocational functioning impairments
Community Mental Health Center Amendments of 1975, 397
Community mental health centers (CMHCs), 397–398
best practices of, 398
legislation for development of, 397
practice guidelines for treatment in, 398
in rural areas, 397–398
services provided by, 397
target populations for, 397
Comorbidity, 383–391
bidirectional model of, 384, **384**
common factor model of, 384, **384**
definition of, 383
medical, 255, 292, 386–390 (*See also* Medical comorbidity)
nicotine dependence, 384–385
psychiatric, 223–235, **227**
anxiety symptoms and disorders, 211–212, 230–235
obsessive-compulsive disorder and symptoms, 233–235
panic attacks and panic disorder, 231
social phobia, 231–232
trauma and posttraumatic stress disorder, 232–233
depressive disorders, 209–211, 227–229
genetic factors and, 223
prevalence of, 223
suicide, 211, 229–230
secondary disorder model of, 383–384, **384**
secondary psychiatric disorder model of, 384, **384**
substance use disorders, 224–227, **225,** 385–386
Complexins I and II, 155
Compliance therapy, 329, 372
Composite International Diagnostic Interview (CIDI), 17
Comprehensive Assessment of At Risk Mental States (CAARMS), 344
Comprehensive Assessment of Symptoms and History (CASH), 189
Computed tomography (CT) studies, 167, 168

COMT (catechol-*O*-methyltransferase gene), **47,** 49, 56, **56,** 76, 93, 223, 297
Contextual difficulties, 205–206
Continuous Performance Test (CPT), 205, 246, 343
"AX" version of, 70, 100, 246
Coping mechanisms, 255
Coping skills training, 229
Coping strategy enhancement, 329
Cortical cytoarchitecture, 152
Cortical laminae, 152, **153**
Cortical thinning, 71–72
Corticosterone, prenatal exposure to, 63
Corticostriatothalamic circuitry, 157–158
Cortisol, 145
Costs of schizophrenia
cognitive deficits and, 255
unemployment and, 281
value of antipsychotic drug market, 303
Course of illness, 21–23, **22–23,** 290–294, **291,** 297, 354
chronic symptoms and disability, 21–22, 291–292, **293,** 297
death, 292
in elderly patients, 375
sustained recovery, 290–291, **292**
trends in outcome over time and place, 293–294, **294**
CPT (Continuous Performance Test), 205, 246, 343
"AX" version of, 70, 100, 246
Criminal justice system, 400–401
"Criminalization" of mental illness, 400
Critical period, 361
CT (computed tomography) studies, 167, 168
Cullen, William, 9
Cultural beliefs, 2
vs. delusions, 195–196
D-Cycloserine, 319, 359
actions at NMDA receptor, 100
dosage of, 100
therapeutic effect of, 100, **101**
Cytochrome P450 enzymes, 50
Cytogenetic abnormalities, 44–45, 223
Cytokines, inflammatory, 62

DA. *See* Dopamine
DAAO (D-amino acid oxidase), 101
Dantrolene, for neuroleptic malignant syndrome, 310
DAO, 48
Dartmouth Assessment of Lifestyle Instrument, 225
DAS (Disability Assessment Scale), 290, 292
De Anima Brutorum (Willis), 8
De Praestigiis Daemonum (Weyer), 7
Death, 292, 383. *See also* Suicidal behavior
Deficit schizophrenia, 203–204, **204**
Deinstitutionalization, 276

Delasiauve, Louis, 12
Délire, 10
Delirium, persecutory, 12
Delusional disorder vs. schizophrenia, 213
Delusional ideas, 196
Delusional mood, 196
Delusional perceptions, 196
Delusional states of consciousness, 196
Delusions, 2, 8, 9, 85, 167, **188**, 190, **192**, 194, **194**, 195–199
    of being controlled, 198
    bizarre, 196
    cognitive-behavioral therapy for, 329
    definition of, 195
    differential diagnosis of, 196–197
        affective disorder with psychotic features, 197
        Capgras syndrome, 197
        organic delusional syndrome, 197
        paranoid disorders, 196–197
    grandiose, 199
    vs. obsessions, 233–234
    paranoid, 196
    persecutory, 197–198
        self-esteem and, 267
        self-serving and personalizing biases associated with,
            265–267
    persistence of, 196
    primary delusional experience, 196
    of reference, 198
    religious, 199
    vs. religious or cultural beliefs, 195–196
    of sin or guilt, 198–199
    somatic, 199
    thought broadcasting, 198
    thought insertion, 198
    thought withdrawal, 198
Démence précoce, 1, 11
Dementia patients, use of antipsychotics in, 375, **376**
Dementia praecox, 1, 4, 11, 12–13, 69, 137, 214
Dementia praecox, oder die Gruppe der Schizophrenieen (Bleuler),
    13
Demonic possession, 6
Demoralization, 228
Dendritic abnormalities, 140, 141, 154, 159, 161
2-Deoxyglucose, 159
Department of Veterans Affairs services, 400
Depot antipsychotics, **314**, 314–315, 373
Depression, 209–211, **227**, 227–229
    attributional style in, 265
    detection of, 228
    in first-episode patients, 359
    gender distribution of, 227
    management of, 228–229

antidepressants, 229, 317
antipsychotics, 228–229
psychosocial interventions, 229
measurement of, 210–211
vs. negative symptoms, 210, 228, 253
postpsychotic, 210, 227, 228, 317, 359
prevalence of, 227
prognostic significance of, 209–210, 227–228
with psychotic features, 197, 346
relation of cognitive deficits to, 253
vs. schizoaffective disorder, 210
suicide and, 211, 229–230, 359
throughout course of illness, 209–210, 228
vegetative symptoms of, 228
Depressive disorder with psychotic features, 213
Derailment, 206
Descriptive epidemiology, 18–20
    incidence, **18–19**, 19–20, 117, 345
        by age and sex, 20, **20**
        by employment status, 23, **25**
        by marital status, 23, **24**
    prevalence, **18**, 18–19, 85, 345
"Designer drugs," 98
Desipramine, for patients with comorbid substance abuse, 226
Developing vs. developed countries, 294, 296
Developmental abnormalities. *See* Neurodevelopmental
    theories
Dextroamphetamine, 318
DHA. *See* Docosahexaenoic acid
Diabetes mellitus, 28, 387, **389**
    acute complications of, 387
    antipsychotic-induced, **306**, 311–312, 387
    chronic complications of, 387
    metabolic syndrome and, 387
    monitoring for, **311**, 312
    in pregnancy, **56**, 59
    prevalence in patients with schizophrenia, 311, 387
    risk factors for, 312, 387
    treatment implications of, 387
Diabetic ketoacidosis, 387
Diacylglycerol, 122
Diagnosis, 167, 177, 187–189, 212, 290, 354
    assessment tools for, 17, 189 (*See also* Assessment
        instruments)
    Bleuler's four As for, 13, 187
    DSM-IV-TR criteria for, 13, 188, 189, **190**, 275, 342
    in elderly patients, 374–375
    evolution of criteria for, 13, 187–188
    factors influencing concepts of, 187
    ICD-10 criteria for, 188–189, **191**
    implications for treatment, 366
    prognostic significance of, 295

Research Diagnostic Criteria for, 189, **193**

of schizophrenia subtypes, **192**

Schneider's first-rank symptoms for, 10, **10**, 13, 188, **188**, 195

symptom duration for, 188, 189

Washington University (Feighner) criteria for, 188, **189**

Diagnosis-related groups (DRGs), 396

Diagnostic and Statistical Manual of Mental Disorders (DSM-IV-TR)

criteria for schizophrenia in, 13, 188, 189, **190**, 275, 342

compared with ICD-10 criteria, **193**

organic delusional syndrome in, 197

posttraumatic stress disorder in, 232

schizoaffective disorder in, 210, 213

schizophrenia subtypes in, 189, **192**

schizophreniform disorder in, 212

schizotypal personality disorder in, 214

tardive dyskinesia in, 310

Diagnostic instruments, 17

Diagnostic Interview Schedule (DIS), 17, 189

Diazepam, 317

Diet

essential polyunsaturated fatty acids in, 122–123

outcomes related to, 126

supplementation of, 127–129

oxidative stress and, 124

supplementing antioxidants in, 127–129

Differential diagnosis

of aggressive behavior, 209

of anxiety symptoms, 230

of delusions, 196–197

affective disorder with psychotic features, 197

Capgras syndrome, 197

organic delusional syndrome, 197

paranoid disorders, 196–197

of schizophrenia, 212–214

affective disorders, 213

body dysmorphic disorder, 214

brief psychotic disorder, 213

delusional disorder, 213

obsessive-compulsive personality disorder, 213

in prodromal phase, 346–347

psychotic disorders due to medical conditions, 214

schizoaffective disorder, 212–213

schizophreniform disorder, 212

schizotypal personality disorder, 214

shared psychotic disorder, 213

substance-induced psychotic disorders, 214

Diffusion tensor imaging studies, 169, 180

Digit Symbol Test, 247

Diphenhydramine, 309, **309**

DIS (Diagnostic Interview Schedule), 17, 189

Disability Assessment Scale (DAS), 290, 292

DISC1 and *DISC2* (disrupted in schizophrenia 1 and 2), 44, **47**, 49

Disorganized (hebephrenic) schizophrenia, 189, **192**, 214–215

Disorganized speech, 188, 190, 194, 205

Disrupted in schizophrenia 1 and 2 (*DISC1* and *DISC2*), 44, **47**, 49

Dissociative anesthetics, 96, **96**. *See also* Phencyclidine

pharmacological effects of, 99–100

receptors for, 96, 97–98

Disulfiram, 226

Divalproex, 318, 369

Dizocilpine maleate (MK-801), 98, 105

Docosahexaenoic acid (DHA), 118–121, **120**, 125

antipsychotic effects on levels of, 123

defective conversion of n-3 fatty acids to, 123

dietary intake of, 122

neurodevelopmental effects of deficits of, 125

in peripheral tissues, 120–121

smoking effects on levels of, 124

supplementation of, 127–129

symptom severity and, 126

Documentation

of symptoms, 366

of treatments, 367

L-Dopa, 87, 318

Dopa decarboxylase, 90

Dopamine (DA), 72, 75, 76, 85–95, 156–157

actions of, 87

amphetamine-induced release of, 90–91, **91–92**

ketamine effects on, 104–106, **105**

baseline occupancy of striatal D_2 receptors by, 91–92

classification of receptors for, 86

decreased activity at cortical D_1 receptors, 86, 93–95, **93–95**, 157

dopamine–glutamate interactions, 86, 87, 106–107

in cortex, 106–107

in striatum, 106, **107**

endogenous sensitization to, 88

GABA-regulated production of, 179

glutamate–dopamine interactions, 86, 102–106

imaging studies of, 104–106, **105**

neuronal circuitry model of, 102–104, **103**

imbalance of subcortical to cortical levels of, 156

increased activity at striatal D_2 receptors, 85, 87–93, **91–93**, 157

limbic system levels of, 178

postmortem studies of, 89–90, 157

rate of synthesis of, 90

in working memory circuit, 161

Dopamine agonists, 93, 318

Dopamine D$_1$ receptor agonists, 93

Dopamine D$_1$ receptor antagonists, 93

Dopamine D$_1$ receptors, 86
    brain localization of, 86
    cortical, decreased dopamine activity at, 93–95, 157
        imaging evidence of, 94–95, **94–95**
        ketamine effects on, 106
        postmortem evidence of, 93–94
        preclinical evidence of, 93
        weight of evidence for, **93**
    gene for *(DRD1)*, 51
    postmortem studies of, 89, 93–94
    striatal, 90

Dopamine D$_2$ receptor antagonists, 85–86, 88–89, 156. *See also*
    Antipsychotics

Dopamine D$_2$ receptors, 86
    baseline dopamine occupancy of, 91–92
    brain localization of, 85, 86
    striatal, increased dopamine activity at, 87–93,
        156–157
        imaging evidence of, 90–92, **91–92**
        pharmacological evidence of, 87–89
            aversive effects, 87–88
            therapeutic effects, 88–89, 156, 304
        postmortem evidence of, 89–90
        weight of evidence for, 92–93, **93**

Dopamine D$_3$ receptors, 86, 157
    brain localization of, 86–87
    gene for *(DRD3)*, **47,** 50, 51
    postmortem studies of, 89

Dopamine D$_4$ receptors, 86, 157
    brain localization of, 87
    postmortem studies of, 90

Dopamine D$_5$ receptors, 86
    brain localization of, 86

Dopamine transporter
    imaging studies of, 90
    postmortem studies of, 90

Dorsal prefrontal cortex (DPFC). *See* Prefrontal cortex, dorsal

Downward drift, 395

DPFC (dorsal prefrontal cortex). *See* Prefrontal cortex, dorsal

DRD1 (dopamine$_1$ receptor gene), 51

DRD3 (dopamine$_3$ receptor gene), **47,** 50, 51

DRGs (diagnosis-related groups), 396

Drug Use Scale, 225

DSM-IV-TR. *See Diagnostic and Statistical Manual of Mental
    Disorders*

DTNBP1 (dystrobrevin binding protein 1 [dysbindin] gene),
    47, 48, 56, **56,** 76, 101

Dual-disorder patients. *See* Substance use disorders

Dyslexia, 127

Dyslipidemia, antipsychotic-induced, **306,** 312, **389**

Dysphagia, antipsychotic-induced, 309

Dysphoria, 228
    antipsychotic-induced, 313

Dystonias, 304, 309
    definition of, 309
    management of, 309, **309**
    prophylaxis for, 309
    tardive, 310
    time of onset of, 308, 309

Dystrobrevin binding protein 1 (dysbindin) gene *(DTNBP1),*
    47, 48, 56, **56,** 76, 101

Early developmental model, 74

Early Psychosis Prevention and Intervention Centre (EPPIC)
    (Australia), 356

Ebers papyrus, 3

Echolalia, 207

Echopraxia, 207–208

Edinburgh High-Risk Study, 70

Educational level, 281

Egyptians, ancient, 3

Eicosanoids, 126

Eicosapentaenoic acid (EPA), 121, 123
    supplementation of, 127–129

Eighteenth-century conceptions, 8–9

Einheitpsychose, 10

Ejaculatory disorders, 312

Elderly patients, 374–378
    antidepressants for, 378
    antipsychotics for, 375–378
        adverse effects of, 375–376, **376,** 377
        "black box" warning for, 375
        choice of, 375
        concomitant medications and, 378
        dosage of, 377, **378**
        first-generation drugs, 376
        second-generation drugs, 376–377
        switching between, 377–378
    baseline evaluation of, 375
    cognitive deficits in, 251, 255
    context of care in, 375
    course of illness in, 375
    diagnosis in, 374–375
    integrating pharmacological and psychosocial treatments in,
        378
    pharmacokinetics and pharmacodynamics in, 375
    tardive dyskinesia in, 310, 375, 376, 377

Electroconvulsive therapy, 328
    clozapine and, 368
    for neuroleptic malignant syndrome, 310

Emphysema, 388

Employment, 23, **25**, 254–255, 280–283, 333. *See also*
    Vocational functioning impairments
    supported, 281–283, 333–334 (*See also* Supported
        employment)
Endocannabinoids, 119, 126
Endophenotypes for schizophrenia, 40
Enlightenment period, 8–9
Environmental risk factors, 39, 76–77, 101
    prognostic significance of, 294, 295–296
EPA (eicosapentaenoic acid), 121, 123
    supplementation of, 127–129
Epidemiologic Catchment Area study, 224, 385
Epidemiology of schizophrenia, 17–33, 187, 345
    descriptive, 18–20
        incidence, **18–20**, 19–20, 345
        prevalence, **18**, 18–19, 85, 345
    genetic, 41–44
        adoption studies, 40, 41–42
        family studies, 41, **42**
        twin studies, 40, 41, 42–44, **43**, 55–56, 75,
            77
    methods in, 17–18
        case finding, 18
        case identification, 17
    natural history, 20–23, 289–298
        course of illness, 21–22, **22**, 290–294, **292**
        minor physical anomalies, 21, 70
        neurodevelopmental abnormalities, 21, 69–79
        onset, 20, **20**
        outcome, 22–23, **23–25**
        prognostic factors, 294–297
        stages of illness, 138, **138**, 289–290, 341–342, **342**,
            353–354
    risk factors, 23–33, 346
        autoimmune diseases, **28**, 28–29
        cannabis use, 29–30
        ethnicity, 29, **29**
        infections and immune system, 27–28, **56**, 60,
            61–62
        modernization, **31**, 31–32, **33**
        parental age, 25–27
        prenatal and perinatal factors, 23–25, **26–27**, 55–63, **57**,
            76, 295, 297
        urban residence, **30**, 30–31
Epigenetic dysregulation, 77
Epistles, 5
EPPIC (Early Psychosis Prevention and Intervention Centre)
    (Australia), 356
EPS. *See* Extrapyramidal side effects of antipsychotics
EPUFAs. *See* Essential polyunsaturated fatty acids
Erectile dysfunction, 312
Esquirol, Jean Etienne, 10, 11

Essential polyunsaturated fatty acids (EPUFAs), 118–121, **119,
    120**
    antipsychotic effects on levels of, 123
    in brain, 121
    decreased incorporation in phospholipids, 123
    dietary supplementation of, 127–129
        antioxidant supplementation and, 129
        factors affecting efficacy of, 127–128
    free radical–mediated damage of, **122**, 123–124
    low dietary intake of, 122–123
        outcomes related to, 126
    neurodevelopmental effects of deficits of, 125
    niacin-induced flushing and, 127
    pediatric behavioral, neurological, and language disorders
        and, 127
    in peripheral tissues, 119–121
    smoking effects on levels of, 124
    symptom severity and, 126
    tardive dyskinesia and, 126
Estrogen/progestogen replacement therapy, for
    hyperprolactinemia, 312
Ethnicity, 29, **29**
Euripides, 3
Evoked-response potentials, 75
Excitement symptoms, 208–209
"Executive center" of brain, 170
Executive function, 70, 100, 157, 177
    tests of, 70
    theory-of-mind deficits and, 264
Exercise, 229
Expressed emotion in families, 330
Extraction of the Stone of Madness (Bosch), 32
Extrapyramidal side effects (EPS) of antipsychotics, 304, **306**,
    308–310
    akathisia, 308–309
    dystonias, 309
    in elderly patients, 376, **376**
    monitoring for, 309, 310
    neuroleptic malignant syndrome, 309–310
    parkinsonism, 309
    pharmacological treatment of, **309**
    second-generation drugs, 307, 308
    tardive dyskinesia and other tardive syndromes, 310
    time of onset of, 308
    types of, 308
Ezekiel, 3

Facial affect perception deficit, 248, **262**, 268–270
    emotions included in, 268
    relationship with neurocognition and social functioning,
        269–270
    as result of specific vs. generalized impairment, 269

Facial affect perception deficit (continued)
    specificity of, 268
    stability over time, 268–269
    unanswered questions about, 270
Facial Emotion Identification Task, 270
Falloon project (England), 343
Falret, Jean-Pierre, 12
False beliefs, 262–263
Family studies, 41, **42**, 224
Family support, 296
Family therapy, 229, 330–331
    effect on relapse rate, 331
    maintenance antipsychotic treatment and, 330–331
    to reduced expressed emotion, 330
Fasting lipid profile, **311**
Fasting plasma glucose, **311**, 312, 387
Feighner (Washington University) criteria for schizophrenia, 188, **189**
Fetal growth restriction, **56**, 58, 61
First-episode psychosis, 250, 354–361
    maintenance treatment after, 360–361
        functional recovery and, 360
        model programs for, 361
        relapse prevention, 360
    treatment of, 355–360
        antipsychotic choice and dosing, 356–358, **357**
        delay before initiation of, **355**, 355–356
        median time to symptom remission, 358
        negative and cognitive symptoms, 358–359
        positive symptoms, 358
        principles of, 356
        residual symptoms, 359
        substance use disorders, 360
        suicide risk, 359–360
Five-factor model of schizophrenia, 194
Flashbacks, 200
Fluoxetine
    interaction with clozapine, 316, 317
    for obsessive-compulsive disorder, 234
Fluphenazine, 304
    adverse effects of, 304, 311
    dosage and half-life of, **305**
    long-acting injectable formulation of, 313, **314**, 314–315
Fluphenazine decanoate, 313, **314**, 314–315
Fluvoxamine
    interaction with clozapine, 316, 317
    for obsessive-compulsive disorder, 234
FMR1 (fragile X mental retardation–1 gene), 77
fMRI. *See* Magnetic resonance imaging studies, functional
Folie à deux, 196, 213
Folie à double forme, 12
Folie circulaire, 12

Folie lucide, 12
Folie raisonnante, 12
Forensic treatment settings, 400–401
Fountain House, 333
Four elements, 1, 3
Four humours, 3, 4, 5, 6, 8, 9
Four temperaments, 1, 3
Fragile X mental retardation-1 gene (*FMR1*), 77
Free radicals, 118, **120, 122**, 123–124
Frontal lobes. *See also* Prefrontal cortex
    abnormalities in persons at risk for schizophrenia, 171
    abnormalities in schizophrenia, 71, 171
    effects of damage to, 170–171
    gray matter volume reductions in, 71, 141, **142**, 143, 144, 171
    structural studies of, **170**, 170–171
Frontotemporal circuitry, 158–159, 178
Functional outcome, 138–139
    after first-episode psychosis, 360
    effect of cognitive deficits on, 139, 254–255
        costs, 255
        medical comorbidity, 255
        quality of life, 255
        relapse prevention, 255
        unemployment, 254–255
    negative symptoms and, 139
    related to duration of untreated psychosis, 143
    types of, 254

G proteins, 87
G30, **47**, 48
G72, **47**, 48, 101
GABA. *See* γ-Aminobutyric acid
GABA membrane transporter (GAT-1), 154, 155, 159
GAD (glutamic acid decarboxylase), 73, 155
GAF (Global Assessment of Functioning) Scale, 290, **293**, 343, 344
Galactorrhea, 312
Galen, 4–5, 6
GAP-43 (growth-associated protein–43), 125
GAS (Global Assessment Scale), 290
GAT-1 (GABA membrane transporter), 154, 155, 159
Gender differences
    in age at onset, 290
    in course and prognosis, 295
    in distribution of schizophrenia, 345
        by age, 20, **20**
        by employment status, 23, **25**
        by marital status, 23, **24**
Generalized anxiety disorder, 212, 230
Genetics of schizophrenia, 39–51, 75–76, 346
    genetic epidemiology, 41–44
        adoption studies, 40, 41–42

family studies, 41, **42**, 224
   twin studies, 40, 41, 42–44, **43**, 55–56, 75, 77, 224, 245
genomic approaches to etiology, 44–50
   association studies, 46
   candidate genes, **47**, 47–50, 75–76 (*See also* Candidate genes)
   chromosomal abnormalities, 44–45
   linkage studies, 45–46, **45–46**
   mode of transmission, 44
NMDA receptors and, 100–101
pharmacogenetics, 39, 50–51
phenotype, 40
prognosis and, 297
psychiatric comorbidity and, 223
single-gene disorders compared w/complex traits, 39–40, **40**
Genital self-mutilation, 211
Genome scan, 45–46, **45–46**
Geographic differences in prognosis, 294, 296
Georget, Étienne-Jean, 10
Geriatric patients. *See* Elderly patients
Glial fibrillary acidic protein (GFAP), 139, 152
Glial numbers and markers, 72, 139, 152–153
Global Assessment of Functioning (GAF) Scale, 290, **293**, 343, 344
Global Assessment Scale (GAS), 290
Glucocorticoid-induced stress, 145
Glucose abnormalities, antipsychotic-induced, **306**, 311–312
Glutamate (GLU), 72–73, 75, 76, 85, 86, 95–107
   brain concentrations of, 97
   dopamine–glutamate interactions, 86, 87, 106–107
      in cortex, 106–107
      in striatum, 106, **107**
   excitotoxicity of, 97, 144, 155
      neuropathology and, 144
   glutamate–dopamine interactions, 86, 102–106
      imaging studies of, 104–106, **105**
      neuronal circuitry model of, 102–104, **103**
   neurotransmitter function of, 97
      pyramidal neurons in, 152
   regulation of release of, 99
   role in schizophrenia, 99–102, 155–156
      genetic evidence of, 100–101
      history of models of, 95–96
      pharmacological evidence for, 99–100
         aversive effects, 99–100
         therapeutic effects, 100, **101**
      postmortem evidence of, 102, 156, **156**
      preclinical evidence of, 101–102
      weight of evidence for, **93**, 102
Glutamate receptors, 97–99, 155
   α-amino-3-hydroxy-5-methyl-4-isoxazolepropionic acid (AMPA), 97, 98–99, **156**

differential sensitivity of, 97
ionotropic, 97–99, 155
kainate, 97, **156**
metabotropic, 97, 99, 155
N-methyl-D-aspartate (NMDA), 97, 155, **156**
PCP, 96, 97–98, **98**
postmortem studies of, 156, **156**
Glutamatergic agents, 318–319
Glutamic acid decarboxylase (GAD), 73, 155
Glutamine, 97
Glutathione, 97, 101
Glycerol, 118
Glycine, 101, 319, 359
   actions at NMDA receptor, 97, 100
   dosage of, 100
   therapeutic effect of, 100, **101**
Glycine type-1 transporter (GLYT1), 97, 100, 102
Goals of treatment, 365
Graeco-Roman period, 1, 3–6
Grandiose delusions, 199
Gray matter volume reductions, 71, 141, **142**, 143, 144, 171, 176, **176**, 357, **357, 358**
Griesinger, Wilhelm, 1–2, 11–12
GRM3, 101
Grooming, 203
Group homes, 398
Growth-associated protein–43 (GAP-43), 125
Gynecomastia, 312

Hallucinations, 85, 167, **188**, 190, **192**, 194, **194**, 199–200
   alcohol-related, 214
   amphetamine-induced, 87
   anxiety associated with, 211–212
   auditory, 199–200
   definition of, 199
   Lilliputian, 200
   olfactory, 200
   vs. prehallucinatory experiences, 199
   somatic and tactile (haptic, kinesthetic), 200
   visual, 200
Hallucinogens, 73, 214
Haloperidol, 88, 304
   adverse effects of, 304–305, **306**, 309, 311
   dosage and half-life of, **305**
   effect on membrane phospholipids, 123
   in first-episode psychosis, 356–357, **357, 358**, 359
   long-acting injectable formulation of, 313, **314**, 315
   in patients with depressive symptoms, 228–229
Haloperidol decanoate, 313, **314**, 315
Haptic hallucinations, 200
Haslam, John, 1, 2, 10, 11
Health insurance, 396

Hebephrenia, 4, 12

Hebephrenic (disorganized) schizophrenia, 189, **192**, 214–215

Hebrews, ancient, 3

Hecker, Ewald, 12

Heidelberg school, 13

Helplessness, 228

Hemoglobin A_{1C}, 312

Henry VI of England, 7

Hepatitis, viral, 388, **389**
  risk reduction strategies for, 390

Hepatocellular carcinoma, 388

Herpes simplex virus infection during pregnancy, 27, 60

Hippocampus, 158, 172
  abnormalities in schizophrenia, 154, 155, 172, **172,** 173
  animal studies of lesions of, 158–159
  projections between prefrontal cortex and, 158
  synaptic markers in, 155

Hippocrates, 3–4, 6

Histopathology, 152–157. *See also* Neuropathology
  dopaminergic system, 156–157
  GABAergic system, 155
  glial numbers and markers, 72, 139, 152–153
  glutamatergic system, 155–156, **156**
  neuronal number and distribution, 140, 153–154
  neuronal soma, 155
  neuropil and synaptic markers, 140, **154,** 154–155

Historical concepts of schizophrenia, 1–14
  cognitive madness before Graeco-Roman period, 3
  cognitive madness in Graeco-Roman period, 3–6
  Islamic physicians of Medieval period, 6
  in Medieval and Renaissance Europe, 6–7
  modernization and, 31–32, **33**
  nineteenth century, 9–12
  seventeenth and eighteenth centuries, 8–9
  twentieth century, 12–14

HIV disease, 387–388, **389**
  risk reduction strategies for, 390

Holmes, Sherlock, 87

Homelessness, 233, 370

Homocysteine, 101

Homovanillic acid, 89

Hopelessness, 211, 228, 229

Horace, 5

Hormone replacement therapy, for hyperprolactinemia, 312

Hospitalization
  cognitive deficits and length of, 255
  indications for, 399
  in state psychiatric hospitals, 398–400 (*See also* State psychiatric hospitals)
  time to rehospitalization, 21–22, **22**

Hostility/aggression, 208–209, 399
  assessment of, 209
  causes of, 208–209
  differential diagnosis of, 209
  epidemiology of, 208
  substance abuse and, 209

HTR2A (serotonin$_{2A}$ receptor gene), **47,** 49, 51

Humoural theory, 3, 4, 5, 6, 8, 9

Huntington's disease, 175

Hygiene, 203

Hyperlipidemia, antipsychotic-induced, **306,** 312, **389**

Hyperprolactinemia, antipsychotic-induced, **306,** 312
  in elderly patients, **376**

Hypertension, pregnancy-related, 24, **56,** 59

Hyperthermia, in neuroleptic malignant syndrome, 309

Hyponatremia, 373, 388

Hypotension, antipsychotic-induced, 304, **306,** 312–313
  in elderly patients, **376,** 377

Hypoxia-ischemia, perinatal, **56,** 57–58, 61, 62, 101

Hysteria, historical conceptions of, 3

ICD-10. *See International Classification of Diseases*

Ideas of reference, 87

Ideler, Karl, 5, 11

IL-1β (interleukin-1β), 62

IL-6 (interleukin-6), 62

IL-8 (interleukin-8), 62

Illness Management and Recovery resource tool kit, 330

Illogicality, 207

Illustrations of Madness (Haslam), 1

Imipramine
  for obsessive-compulsive disorder, 234
  for panic disorder, 231
  for patients with comorbid substance abuse, 226

Immigrants, 29

Immune system, 27–29

Impersistence at work or school, 203

"Implementing Evidence-Based Practices for Severe Mental Illness Project," 328

Impulsivity, 230

Incidence of schizophrenia, **18–19,** 19–20, 117, 345
  by age and sex, 20, **20**
  by employment status, 23, **25**
  by marital status, 23, **24**

Incoherence, 207

Independent living, 279–280

Infections during pregnancy, 24, 27–28, **56,** 60, 61–62
  herpes simplex virus, 27, 60
  influenza, 24, 27, **56,** 60
  rubella, 27, 60
  toxoplasmosis, 27

Inositol 1,4,5-trisphosphate (1,4,5-IP$_3$), 122, 125
Inositol polyphosphate, 119
Insanity, historical conceptions of, 5, 11–12
Insanity defense, 401
Integrated Dual Disorder Treatment, 225
Integrated treatment
    pharmacological and psychosocial, 366, 374
        for elderly patients, 378
    psychological, 332
    for schizophrenia and substance use disorders, 225, **225**, 386
Integrative model of schizophrenia, 77–78, **78**
Intelligence. *See* Cognitive impairments
Interleukin-1β (IL-1β), 62
Interleukin-6 (IL-6), 62
Interleukin-8 (IL-8), 62
Internal, Personal, and Situational Attributions Questionnaire (IPSAQ), 265, 266
International Classification of Diseases, 10th Revision (ICD-10), 18
    criteria for schizophrenia in, 188–189, **191**, 275
        compared with DSM-IV-TR criteria, **193**
    postschizophrenic depression in, 210
    schizoaffective disorder in, 210
    schizophrenia subtypes in, 189, **192**
International Late-Onset Schizophrenia Group, 374
Interviews, 17. *See also* Assessment instruments
Intimate partnerships, 280
Involuntary commitment to state psychiatric hospitals, 399
Involuntary outpatient commitment, 335–336
Iowa Tests, 249
1,4,5-IP$_3$ (inositol 1,4,5-trisphosphate), 122, 125
IPSAQ (Internal, Personal, and Situational Attributions Questionnaire), 265, 266
Islamic physicians of Medieval period, 6

Jackson, Hughlings, 190
Jail treatment settings, 400–401

Kahlbaum, Karl Ludwig, 12
Kainate receptors, 97, 155, **156**
Kant, Immanuel, 2
Ketamine, 96, 158
    effects on amphetamine-induced dopamine release, 104–106, **105**
    pharmacological effects of, 99–100
    receptors for, 97–98
Kinesthetic hallucinations, 200
Korsakoff, Sergei, 12
Kraepelin, Emil, 1, 11, 12–13, 69, 137, 151, 167, 201, 214, 343
Kynurenic acid, 101

Lamotrigine, 368, 369
Langfeldt, Gabriel, 13

Language impairments, 70
Late developmental model, 74
Late-onset schizophrenia, 374–375. *See also* Elderly patients
Latent inhibition, 205
LDL (low-density lipoprotein), 312
LDT (lexical decision task), 205
Learning deficits, 99
    verbal, 246–247
    visual, 247
Least restrictive environment for treatment, 398
Legislation
    Americans with Disabilities Act, 398
    Community Mental Health Center Amendments of 1975, 397
    Mental Health Study Act of 1955, 397
    Mental Retardation Facilities and Community Mental Health Centers Construction Act of 1963, 397
Lexical decision task (LDT), 205
Libido, decreased, 312
Life expectancy, 383
Lifetime prevalence of schizophrenia, **18**, 19–20
Lilliputian hallucinations, 200
Limbic system, 178
Linkage studies, 45–46, **45–46**
Linoleic acid, 122–123
Lipid abnormalities, antipsychotic-induced, **306,** 312
Lithium, 318
Living arrangements, 279–280
Long-term potentiation, 97
Long-term treatment, 365–378
    acute patient characteristics influencing, 369–370
    adherence to, 371–373
    augmentation of antipsychotics, 369
    catatonia and, 373–374
    combination antipsychotics for, 369
    difficulties in conducting studies of, 365
    integrating pharmacotherapy and psychosocial therapies, 374
    long-term patient characteristics influencing, 370–371
    in older patients, 374–378
    options for antipsychotic treatment failures, 367–368, **368**
    polydipsia–hyponatremia and, 373
    principles of, 366–367
        context, 367
        diagnosis, 366
        documentation, 366
        integration of treatments, 366
        treatment plans, 366
        use of "effective" treatments, 366–367
    of treatment-refractory illness, 368–369
Loosening of associations, **2,** 188, 206
Lorazepam, **309**
"Lovesickness," 6

Low birth weight, **56,** 58
Low-density lipoprotein (LDL), 312
Loxapine
    adverse effects of, 304
    combined with clozapine, 319
    dosage and half-life of, **305**
LSD (lysergic acid diethylamide), 73, 214
LY354740, 99
Lycanthropy, 3, 5
Lysergic acid diethylamide (LSD), 73, 214

Mad Meg (Bruegel), **31,** 32
Magnetic resonance imaging (MRI) studies, 71, 141, 142, 167, 168–169
    diffusion tensor imaging, 169, 180
    functional (fMRI), 71, 167, 168–169, 177–180
        of corticostriatothalamic circuitry, 157
        of prefrontal cortex dysfunction, 177–178, **178**
        of prefrontal–anterior cingulate circuitry, 158
    structural, 167, 170–176
        of basal ganglia, 173–174
        of caudate, 174–175
        of frontal lobes, **170,** 170–171
        of temporal lobes, 171–173, **172, 174**
        of thalamus, 174
        of ventricular enlargement, **175,** 175–176
    technological aspects of, 168–169
Magnetic resonance spectroscopy (MRS) studies, 73, 79, 121, 141–142, 157
Magnetization transfer imaging (MTR), 180
Magnetoencephalography, 179
Maintenance treatment, 313
    after first-episode psychosis, 360–361
    with clozapine, 316
    family therapy and, 331
Malnutrition during pregnancy, **56,** 60, 62
Mania, historical descriptions of, 3, 5, 8, 10, 11, 12
Manic-depression, 2, **2**
Marcellus, 5
Marijuana use, 29–30, 126, 212, 224, 296, 385
Marital status, 23, **24,** 280
Mask of Sanity (Cleckley), 2
Maternal age, 25
Matthews, James Tilly, 1, 10, 11
MECP2, 77
Medicaid, 396
Medical comorbidity, 386–390
    barriers to health care for, 386
        reduction of, 390
    cognitive deficits and, 255
    conditions negatively associated with schizophrenia, 389
        cancer, 389

    rheumatoid arthritis, 28, **28,** 389
    diabetes mellitus, 387
    HIV/AIDS, 387–388
        risk reduction strategies for, 390
    mortality related to, 292
    osteoporosis, 388
    polydipsia–hyponatremia, 373, 388
    possible pathways to, **390**
    respiratory disease, 388
    state psychiatric hospital services for, 399–400
    viral hepatitis, 388
        risk reduction strategies for, 390
Medicare, 396
Medieval period, 6–7
Megalomania, 85
Melancholy, historical descriptions of, 3–6, 8, 12
Memory, 99, 100, 156–157
    prefrontal cortex dysfunction and, 177
    verbal, 246–247
    visual, 247
    working, 70, 72, 248
        cellular basis of working memory circuitry, 159–161, **160**
            dopaminergic afferents, 161
            GABA interneurons, 159
            thalamic projection neurons, 161
Meningitis, 27
Mental Health Study Act of 1955, 397
Mental Retardation Facilities and Community Mental Health Centers Construction Act of 1963, 397
Mental status changes, in neuroleptic malignant syndrome, 309
Mentis alienatio, 7
Mesocortical system, 86
Mesolimbic system, 86
Mesoridazine, **305**
Metabolic effects of antipsychotics, 310–312
    diabetes, 311–312, 387
    dyslipidemia, 312
    monitoring for, 311, **311, 389**
    prolactin elevation, 312
    weight gain, 311
Metabolic syndrome, 386, 387
Methamphetamine, 214
N-Methyl-D-aspartate (NMDA) receptor agonists, 97, 100, **101**
N-Methyl-D-aspartate (NMDA) receptor antagonists, 86, 96, 98, 144, 145
    effects on amphetamine-induced dopamine release, 104–106, **105**
    pharmacological effects of, 99–100
    receptors for, 96, 97–98, **98**

N-Methyl-D-aspartate (NMDA) receptors, 73, 76, 78, 86, 97
    alcohol effects at, 385
    in animal models, 101–102
    drug stimulation of neurotransmission at, 100, **101**
    functional properties of, 97
    genetic studies of, 100–101, 297
    glycine and D-serine effects at, 97, 100, **101**
    interaction with AMPA receptors, 98–99
    in long-term potentiation, 97
    pharmacological effects of blockade of, 99–100
    pharmacological effects of stimulation of, 100, **101**
    for phencyclidine, 96, 97–98, **98**
    postmortem studies of, 102, 156, **156**
    subunits of, 97
N-Methylglycine, 100
Methylphenidate, 87
Meyer, Ernst, 12
Midbrain functional deficits, 179
Milieu treatment, 328
Mind deficits, 263
Mini-Mental State Examination, 100
Minor physical anomalies (MPAs), 21, 70
MK-801 (dizocilpine maleate), 98, 105
Modernization, **31**, 31–32, **33**
Molindone
    adverse effects of, 304, 311
    dosage and half-life of, **305**
Monomania, 10, 11, 12
Mood stabilizers, 303, 318
Morel, Bénédict, 1, 11
Morositas, 4
Mortality, 292, 383. *See also* Suicidal behavior
Motor behavior, 70, 201, 252
    in akathisia, 308
    in catatonia, 201, 373
    in drug-induced parkinsonism, 309
    in dystonias, 309
    stereotyped movements, 201
    in tardive syndromes, 310
MPAs (minor physical anomalies), 21, 70
MRI (magnetic resonance imaging) studies, 71, 141
MRS (magnetic resonance spectroscopy) studies, 73, 79, 121, 141–142, 157
MTR (magnetization transfer imaging), 180
Myocarditis, clozapine-induced, 316

n-3 and n-6 fatty acids, 123–124
NAA (*N*-acetylaspartate), 73, 142, 157
Najab ud-din Unhammad, 6
Naltrexone, 226
Napier, Richard, 8
National Cholesterol Education Program, 312

National Comorbidity Study, 224, 227
National Psychiatric Hospitalization Case Registry (Israel), 249
Natural history of schizophrenia, 20–23, 289–298
    cognitive impairments, 248–251, **249**
    course of illness, 21–22, **22**, 290–294, **291**, 354
    minor physical anomalies, 21, 70
    neurodevelopmental abnormalities, 21, 69–79
    onset, 20, **20**
    outcome, 22–23, **23–25**
    prognostic factors, 294–297
    stages of illness, 138, **138**, 289–290, 341–342, **342**, 353–354
"Nature versus nurture," 39
NCAM (neural cell adhesion molecule), 155
Nebuchadnezzar, 3
Neologism, 207
Nerve growth factor, 119
Nervenzarzt (Schneider), 13
Neumann, Heinrich, 11
Neural cell adhesion molecule (NCAM), 155
Neuregulin 1 gene *(NRG1)*, **47**, 47–48, 56, **56**, 76, 101
Neuroanatomy, 167–180
    correlation with neurocognitive deficits, 71
    functional, 177–180
        abnormal connectivity hypothesis, 180
        deficits in limbic cortex and midbrain pathology, 178–179
        prefrontal cortex dysfunction, 177–178, **178, 179**
        temporal cortex dysfunction, 178
    imaging methods for study of, 168–169
    structural, 170–176
        basal ganglia, 173–174
        caudate, 174–175
        frontal lobes, **170**, 170–171
        temporal lobes, 171–173, **172, 174**
        thalamus, 174
        ventricular enlargement, 71, 141, 143, 171, **175**, 175–176
Neurochemical theories, 85–108. *See also specific neurotransmitters*
    dopamine receptors, 85–95, 156–157
    dopamine–glutamate interactions, 96, 106–107
    GABAergic system, 155
    glutamate and NMDA receptors, 86, 95–102, 155–156, **156**
    glutamate–dopamine interactions, 86, 102–106
    neurochemical sensitization, 75, 145
    weight of evidence for, 92–93, **93**
Neurocognitive impairments. *See* Cognitive impairments
Neurodegenerative disorders, 137–138, 153. *See also* Neuroprogressive theories
Neurodevelopmental theories, 21, 69–79, 137, 346
    anatomical correlations, 71
    animal models of, 79
    causes of brain abnormalities, 75–77
        environmental factors, 76–77

Neurodevelopmental theories (continued)
    causes of brain abnormalities (continued)
        epigenetic factors, 77
        genetic factors, 75–76
    disordered brain development and mediation of
        schizophrenia, 70
    evaluating strength of, 79
    membrane and neuronal integrity, 73
    membrane phospholipid deficits and, 125
    neuropathology and, 71–72, 137, 152
    neurotransmitter mechanisms, 72–73
    timing of pathophysiology, 73–75
        early developmental model, 74
        late developmental model, 74
        post-illness progression model, 74–75
    unitary genetic-developmental perspective, 77–78, **78**
Neuroimaging studies, 86, 141–142, 167–180, 346. See also
    Neuroanatomy; specific imaging modalities
    of cortical D_1 receptors, 94–95, **94–95**
    of corticostriatothalamic circuitry, 157–158
    of frontotemporal circuitry, 159
    functional and spectroscopic, 141–142, 177–180
    of glutamate–dopamine interactions, 104–106, **105**
    of prefrontal–anterior cingulate circuitry, 158
    principles and techniques of, 168–169
    of sensitization to effects of amphetamine, 88
    of striatal amphetamine-induced dopamine release, 90–91,
        91–92
    of striatal dopamine transmission, 90, 156
    structural, 141, 170–176
Neuroleptic dysphoria, 313
Neuroleptic malignant syndrome (NMS), 309–310
    clinical features of, 309
    risk factors for, 309
    treatment of, 310
Neuroleptics. See Antipsychotics
Neuromotor deviations, 70
Neuronal circuits, 157–159
    corticostriatothalamic, 157–158
    frontotemporal, 158–159
    prefrontal–anterior cingulate, 158
Neuronal glutaminase, 97
Neurons
    apoptosis of, 144, 154
    arrangement in cortical laminae, 152, **153**
    chandelier, 152, 155, 159
    cortical projections of, 152
    GABAergic, 152
    migrational deficits of, 154
    nonpyramidal (GABAergic), 152
    number and distribution of, 72, 140, 153–154
    proposed progression of abnormalities of, 141, **143**
    pyramidal, 152
    somal size of, 140, 155
    thalamic projection, in working memory circuits, 161
    of working memory circuitry, 159–161, **160**
Neuropathology, 71–72, 151–161, 346. See also Histopathology
    vs. Alzheimer's disease, 139
    cellular basis of working memory circuitry, 159–161, **160**
    correlation with psychopathology, 143
    dendritic deficits, 140, 141
    gray matter volume reductions, 71, 141, **142**, 143, 144, 171,
        176, **176**, 357, **357, 358**
    neuroimaging of, 141–142
    neuronal circuits, 157–159
    normal cortical cytoarchitecture and, 152
    postmortem studies of, 137, 139–141
    ventricular enlargement, 71, 141, 143, **175**, 175–176
Neuropil reductions, 140, **154**, 154–155
Neuroprogressive theories, 137–145, **138**
    cognitive deficits and, 139, 250–251
    neuroimaging pathology, 141–142
        functional and spectroscopic studies, 141–142, **142, 143**
        structural studies, 141
    neuropathology–psychopathology correlation, 143
    postmortem neuropathology, 137, 139–141, 152
    psychopathology and neurocognitive deficits, 138–139
    underlying mechanisms of, 143–145
        apoptosis, 144
        glutamate excitotoxicity, 144
        neurochemical sensitization, 75, 145
        oxidative stress, 144–145
Neuropsychological testing, 202, 346
Neurotrophins, 76, 119
New Freedom Commission on Mental Health, 366
New York High-Risk Project (NYHRP), 70, 354
Niacin-induced flushing, phospholipid levels and, 127
Nicotine dependence, 224, 384–385
Nicotine replacement therapies, 226, 385
α7 Nicotinic acetylcholine receptor subunit gene (CHRNA7), 40
Nigrostriatal system, 86
Nineteenth-century conceptions, 9–12
NMDA receptors. See N-Methyl-D-aspartate receptors
NMR (nuclear magnetic resonance). See Magnetic resonance
    imaging studies
NMS. See Neuroleptic malignant syndrome
Nonsteroidal anti-inflammatory drugs, 28
Norwegian Early Treatment and Intervention in Psychosis
    project, 356
NRG1 (neuregulin 1 gene), **47**, 47–48, 56, **56**, 76, 101
Nuclear magnetic resonance (NMR). See Magnetic resonance
    imaging studies
Nucleus accumbens, 153
NYHRP (New York High-Risk Project), 70, 354

Object-sorting tasks, 206

Obsessive-compulsive disorder (OCD) and symptoms, 9, 212, 213, **227**, 233–235, 347

  vs. delusions, 233–234

  detection of, 234

  etiology of, 234

  management of, 234–235

    cognitive-behavioral therapy, 235

    pharmacological, 234–235

  prevalence of, 233

  prognostic significance of, 234

Obsessive-compulsive personality disorder (OCPD), 213

Obstetrical complications, 24–25, **27**, **56–57**, 57–60, 76, 295, 297. *See also* Prenatal and perinatal risk factors

  diabetes in pregnancy, 59

  fetal growth restriction, 58, 61

  hypoxia-ischemia, 57–58, 61, 62, 101

  maternal malnutrition, 60, 62

  maternal stress, 60, 62–63

  mechanisms of, 61–63

  placental abruption and bleeding, 59

  preeclampsia and hypertension, 24, 59

  premature birth, 58–59

  premature rupture of membranes, 59

  prenatal exposure to maternal infection, 24, 27–28, 60, 61–62

  Rhesus factor incompatibility, 59–60

  season and place of birth, 23–24, **26**, 60

  uterine atony, 59

OCD. *See* Obsessive-compulsive disorder and symptoms

OCPD (obsessive-compulsive personality disorder), 213

Oculogyric crisis, antipsychotic-induced, 309

Olanzapine, 304, 307–308

  adverse effects of, **306**, 307–308, 311

  augmentation of

    divalproex, 369

    other antipsychotics, 319

  dosage and half-life of, **305**, 315

  efficacy studies of, 307

  in elderly patients, 377, **378**

  in first-episode psychosis, 356–357, **357**, **358**, 359

  high caloric diet and, 124

  history and development of, 307

  NMDA agonists combined with, 100, **101**

  in patients with depressive symptoms, 228

  in patients with substance use disorders, 226

  in prodromal period, 350

Olfactory hallucinations, 200

Oligodendroglial dysfunction, 121

Olmstead v. L. C., 398–399

Onset of schizophrenia, 20, 138, **138**, 187, **291**

  age at, 20, **20**, 85, 187, 353, 354

  in elderly persons, 374–375

  social and vocational impairments, 275–276

Opiate receptors, sigma, 97

Organic delusional syndrome, 197

Osmotic demyelination syndrome, 373

Osteoporosis, 388

Outcomes of schizophrenia, 22–23, **23–25**, 118, 290, **291**

  assertive community treatment and, 334–335, **335**

  chronic symptoms and disability, 21–22, 291–292, **293**, 297

  dietary fatty acid intake and, 126

  environmental factors affecting, 295–296

  genetic factors affecting, 297

  neuropathology and, 143

  prognostic factors affecting, 295–297

  strategies for characterization of, 290

  sustained recovery, 290–291

  treatment effect on, **294**, 296–297

  trends over time and place, 293–294, **294**

Outpatient commitment, involuntary, 335–336

Overt Aggression Scale, 209

Oxidative stress, 118, **120**, **122**, 123–124

  factors influencing, 124

    antipsychotics, 124

    dietary and other factors, 124

    smoking, 124

  membrane phospholipid peroxidation due to, 123

  neuroprogressive theory of schizophrenia and, 144–145

P50 evoked potential, 40

PACE (Personal Assessment and Crisis Evaluation) Clinic (Melbourne, Australia), 343, 344, 349

Pandysmaturation, 70

Panic attacks and panic disorder, **227**, 231

  detection of, 231

  management of, 231

  prevalence of, 231

  prognostic significance of, 231

PANSS (Positive and Negative Syndrome Scale), 99, 100, 194, **196**, 205, 206, 209, 231

Pappenheim, Else, 12

Paranoia, 196

  amphetamine-induced, 87

  historical conceptions of, 1, 3–4, 12

Paranoid disorder, 196–197, 213

Paranoid schizophrenia, 189, **192**, 214–215

Paraphrosune, 4

Parental age, 25–27

Parents with schizophrenia, 280

Parietal lobe abnormalities, 171

Parkinsonism, drug-induced, 304, 309

Parkinsonism, drug-induced *(continued)*
  clinical features of, 309
  management of, 309, **309**
  time of onset of, 308
Parkinson's disease, 93, 175
Parvalbumin (PV), 154, 155, 159, 161
Paternal age, 25–27
Paul of Aegina, 6
PCP. *See* Phencyclidine
Peer-assisted treatment approaches, 327, 333
Peer relationships, 203
Perphenazine, 304
  adverse effects of, 304, **306**
  dosage and half-life of, **305**
Persecutory delusions, 85, 197–198
  self-esteem and, 267
  self-serving and personalizing biases associated with,
    265–267
Perseverations, 247
Personal Assessment and Crisis Evaluation (PACE) Clinic
    (Melbourne, Australia), 343, 344, 349
Personal therapy, 328
Personalizing bias in attributional style, 266
Pervasive developmental disorder, 347
PET. *See* Positron emission tomography studies
PFC. *See* Prefrontal cortex
PGD_2 (prostaglandin D_2), 126
Pharmacogenetics, 39, 50–51
Pharmacological therapies, 303–319
  antidepressants, 317
  antipsychotics, 303–316
    polypharmacy with, 315, 319, 369
  benzodiazepines, 317
  carbamazepine, 318
  dopamine agonists, 318
  glutamatergic agents, 318–319
  ineffective use of, 367
  integration with psychosocial treatments, 374
  lithium, 318
  pharmacokinetics and pharmacodynamics in elderly
    patients, 375
  for polydipsia–hyponatremia, 373
  side effects of, 50–51
  in state psychiatric hospitals, 399
  therapeutic response to, 50–51
  valproate, 318
Phencyclidine (PCP), 73, 96, **96**, 144, 145, 155, 156, 214,
    318–319
  pharmacological effects of, 99, 105
  receptors for, 96, 97–98, **98**
Phenotype of schizophrenia, 40
Phonological fluency, 247, 253

Phosphatidylcholine, 118, 121
Phosphatidylethanolamine, 118, 120, 121
Phosphatidylinositol, 118, 125
Phosphatidylinositol 4,5-bisphosphate (PI-4,5-P_2), 122, 125
Phosphatidylserine, 118
Phosphodiesters, 73, 121, 142
Phospholipase A_2 (PLA$_2$), 121–122
Phospholipase C (PLC), 122
Phospholipases (PLAs), 121–122
Phospholipids, 117–129
  alterations in schizophrenia, 119–129
    in brain, 121
    clinical implications of, 126–127
    correlation between peripheral and central findings, 121
    mechanisms of altered metabolism, 121–123
      antipsychotics, 123
      decreased essential polyunsaturated fatty acid
        incorporation in phospholipids, 123
      increased degradation by phospholipases, 121–122
      increased free radical–mediated phospholipid
        degradation, **122**, 123
      low dietary intake of essential polyunsaturated fatty
        acids, 122–123
    oxidative stress and, **122**, 123–124
    pathophysiological significance of, 124–126
    in peripheral tissues, 119–121
    therapeutic implications of, 127–129
  factors affecting function and levels of, 118
  free radical–mediated peroxidation of, 118
  functions of, 118–119, **120**
  localization of, 118
  second messengers derived from, 119, **120**, 125
  structure and metabolism of, 118, **119**
Phosphomonoesters, 73, 121, 142
Phosphoric acid, 118
Phosphoserine, 119
Physical anergia, 203
Physical anomalies, minor, 21, 70
PI-4,5-P_2 (phosphatidylinositol 4,5-bisphosphate), 122, 125
Pieter Breughel the Elder, **31**, 32
PKC (protein kinase C), 122
PLA$_2$ (phospholipase A_2), 121–122
Placental abruption, **56**, 59
Planum temporale, 173
PLAs (phospholipases), 121–122
Platelet phospholipids, 119–120
Platter, Felix, 7
PLC (phospholipase C), 122
Point prevalence of schizophrenia, **18**, 18–19
Polydipsia, 312, 373, 388
Polypharmacy with antipsychotics, 315, 319, 369

Polyuria, 312

Posidonius of Apamea, 4

Positive and Negative Syndrome Scale (PANSS), 99, 100, 194, **196,** 205, 206, 209, 231

Positron emission tomography (PET) studies, 141–142, 168, 169

    of cortical D$_1$ receptors, 94–95, **94–95**

    of corticostriatothalamic circuitry, 157, 158

    of frontotemporal circuitry, 159

    of midbrain functional deficits, 179

    of prefrontal–anterior cingulate circuitry, 158

    of striatal dopamine receptors and transporters, 90

    technological aspects of, 169

Post-illness progression model, 74–75

Postpsychotic depression, 210, 227, 228, 317, 359

Posttraumatic stress disorder (PTSD), **227,** 232–233, 347

    detection of, 233

    management of, 233

    prevalence of, 232

    prognostic significance of, 232–233

Poverty of content of speech, 203

Poverty of speech, 85, 190, 194, 203, 252

"Practice Guideline for the Treatment of Patients With Schizophrenia," 313, 357, 360, 369

Preeclampsia, 24, **56,** 59

Prefrontal cortex (PFC), 177–178

    decreased dopamine activity at D$_1$ receptors in, 86, 93–95, **93–95**

    dopamine–glutamate interactions in, 106–107

    dorsal

        cellular basis of working memory circuitry, 159–161, **160**

        connectivity between striatum and, 157–158

        dysfunction of, 177–178, **178, 179**

        GABAergic system in, 152, 155

    glutamate–dopamine interactions in, 102–106, **103**

    neuronal number and distribution in, 153

    prefrontal–anterior cingulate circuitry, 158

Prehallucinatory experiences, 199

Premature birth, **56,** 58–59

Premature rupture of membranes, **56,** 59

Premorbid phase of illness, 138, **138,** 289, 341, **342**

    cognitive deficits in, 139, 289, 353–354

    functioning in, 70

    negative symptoms in, 195, 202

    primary prevention interventions in, 342

Prenatal and perinatal risk factors, 23–25, 55–63, 76, 295, 297

    environmental, 55–57, **56**

    interrelations between, 57, **57**

    mechanisms of, 61–63

    obstetrical complications, 24–25, **27, 56–57,** 57–60

        diabetes in pregnancy, 59

        fetal growth restriction, 58, 61

        hypoxia-ischemia, 57–58, 61, 62, 101

        maternal malnutrition, 60, 62

        maternal stress, 60, 62–63

        placental abruption and bleeding, 59

        preeclampsia and hypertension, 24, 59

        premature birth, 58–59

        premature rupture of membranes, 59

        prenatal exposure to maternal infection, 24, 27–28, 60, 61–62

        Rhesus factor incompatibility, 59–60

        season and place of birth, 23–24, **26,** 60

        uterine atony, 59

    parental age, 25–27

Present State Examination (PSE), 17, 18, 189

Prevalence of schizophrenia, **18,** 18–19, 85, 345

Prevention, 342–343

    primary, secondary, and tertiary, 342, 401

    public sector programs for, 401

Prevention Through Risk Identification, Management and Education (PRIME) Clinic (New Haven, CT), 344, 347, 349, 350

Primary prevention, 342, 401

PRIME (Prevention Through risk Identification, Management and Education) Clinic (New Haven, CT), 344, 347, 349, 350

Prison treatment settings, 400–401

Problem-solving deficits, 247

Problem-solving training, 229

Processing speed, 247

PRODH (proline dehydrogenase gene), **47,** 49

Prodromal phase of illness, 20, 138, **138,** 187, 289–290, 341–351, **342,** 354

    assessment instruments for use in, 344–345

    case detection in, 290, 343, 351

    case histories of, 347–348

    clinical features of, 343

    course of, 349

    definition of, 341

    diagnostic criteria for, 344, **345**

    differential diagnosis of, 346–347

    duration of, 341

    epidemiology of, 345

    family interviews about, 348–349

    history of clinical research on, 343

    natural history of, 343

    negative symptoms in, 201

    neurocognitive deficits in, 139, **140,** 250, 289

    patients' memory of, 342

    prognosis for, 349

    social impairments in, 276, 290

    treatment in, 349–351

        public sector programs for, 401

Prodromal phase of illness (continued)
    treatment in (continued)
        recommendations for, 350–351
        studies of, 349–350
Prodromal States Questionnaire, 345
Prognostic factors, 295–297
    cognitive impairments, 295
    comorbid conditions
        depression, 209–210, 227–228
        obsessive-compulsive disorder, 234
        panic disorder, 231
        posttraumatic stress disorder, 232–233
        social phobia, 231–232
        substance use disorders, 296, 383, 385
    diagnosis, 295
    environmental factors, 294, 295–296
    genetic factors, 297
    treatment delay, 356
    treatment effects, **294**, 296–297
Prolactin elevation, antipsychotic-induced, **306**, 312
    in elderly patients, **376**
Proline dehydrogenase gene (PRODH), **47**, 49
Propranolol, **309**
Prostaglandin D$_2$ (PGD$_2$), 126
Prostaglandins, 119, 126
Protein kinase C (PKC), 122
Proverb interpretation, 206
PSD95, 102
PSE (Present State Examination), 17, 18, 189
Pseudoneurotic schizophrenia, 187
Psilocybin, 73
Psychiatric rehabilitation, 276, 399
"Psychiatrically indigent" patients, 396
Psychiatry, origin of term, 10
Psychodynamic psychotherapy, 328
Psychoeducation, 329
Psychopathology, 187–215. See also Diagnosis; Symptoms
    anxiety, 211–212
    cognitive symptoms, 204–208
    deficit schizophrenia, 203–204, **204**
    depression, 209–211
    diagnosis, 187–189, **188–193**
    differential diagnosis, 212–214
    excitement symptoms, 208–209
    negative symptoms, 201–203
    positive symptoms, 195–201
    self-injury, 211, 399
    subtypes, 189, **192**, 214–215
    suicide, 211
    symptom rating scales, 191–194, **194–196**
    syndromal concept, 191–195, **197**

Psychopathy, 2, **2**
Psychosocial therapies, 297, 327–337
    assertive community treatment, 334–335, **335**, 337, 361,
        398
    emerging trends in, 337
    family treatment, 330–331
    to improve treatment adherence, 372
    individual, 328–330
        cognitive-behavioral therapy, 329
        Illness Management and Recovery resource tool kit,
            330
        personal therapy, 328
        psychodynamic psychotherapy, 328
        psychoeducational programs, 329
    integration with pharmacotherapy, 374
    involuntary outpatient commitment and related procedures,
        335–336
    optimizing patient preferences in choice of, 327
    in patients with depressive symptoms, 229
    social skills training, 277–278, **278**, 331–333
    in state psychiatric hospitals, 399
    supported employment, 281–283, 333–334
Psychostimulants
    long-term sensitization to, 88, 145
    psychosis induced by, 87–88
        in nonschizophrenic subjects, 87–88
        in patients with schizophrenia, 88
Psychotic depression, 8
Psychotic disorders due to medical conditions, 214
PTSD. See Posttraumatic stress disorder
Public sector treatment, 366, 395–401
    budget cuts for, 396–397
    definition of, 396–397
    systems of care and persons served by, 395, 397–401
        community mental health centers, 397–398
        Department of Veterans Affairs services, 400
        dual diagnosis patients, 401
        jail, prison, and forensic treatment settings,
            400–401
        prevention programs, 401
        state psychiatric hospitals, 398–400
Pupillary responses, 252
PV (parvalbumin), 154, 155, 159, 161

QTc interval prolongation, antipsychotic-induced, **306**, 308,
    377, **389**
Quality of life
    anticholinergic medications and, 255
    anxiety and, 212
    cognitive deficits and, 255
    facial affect recognition deficit and, 269

Quetiapine, 304, 308
adverse effects of, **306,** 308, 311
D$_2$ receptor occupancy of, 89
dosage and half-life of, **305,** 308
efficacy studies of, 308
in elderly patients, **378**
history and development of, 308
mechanism of action of, 89
in patients with substance use disorders, 226

Radiotracer imaging methods, 169. *See also* Positron emission
tomography studies; Single photon emission computed
tomography studies
Rapid neuroleptization, 315
Rating scales, 191–194, **194–196,** 206. *See also* Assessment
instruments
RBC (red blood cell) phospholipids, 119–120, 121, 123, 124,
126
RDC (Research Diagnostic Criteria), 189, **193**
Reactive oxygen species, 118, **120, 122,** 123–124
Reasoning deficits, 247
Recovery from schizophrenia, 290–291, **292**
Recovery-oriented treatments, 337
Recurrence of schizophrenia, 21–22
Red blood cell (RBC) phospholipids, 119–120, 121, 123, 124,
126
Reelin-deficient animal models, 73
Register method of case finding, 18
Regulator of G-protein signaling 4 gene *(RGS4)*, **47,** 48–49, 76,
101, 102
Rehabilitation services, 276, 399
vocational, 281–283
Reil, Johann, 10
Relapse of schizophrenia, 297
anxiety and, 212
depression and, 209–210, 228
due to treatment nonadherence, 371–373
effect of family therapy on, 331
maintenance antipsychotic therapy and, 304
rate after treatment discontinuation, 313
Relapse prevention
after first-episode psychosis, 360
effect of cognitive deficits on, 255
maintenance antipsychotic treatment for, 313
Religious beliefs, vs. delusions, 195–196
Religious delusions, 199
"Religious madness," 5
Remissions, 21
Renaissance period, 7
Renal failure, in neuroleptic malignant syndrome, 309
Research Diagnostic Criteria (RDC), 189, **193**
Residual schizophrenia, 189, **192,** 215

Respiratory disease, 384, 386, 388, **389**
Response latency, 203
Restlessness. *See* Akathisia
Rett's syndrome, 77
RGS4 (regulator of G-protein signaling 4 gene), **47,** 48–49, 76,
101, 102
Rhabdomyolysis, in neuroleptic malignant syndrome,
309
Rhapsodien (Reil), 10
Rhazes of Baghdad, 6
RHD gene, 60
Rhesus (Rh) factor incompatibility, **56,** 59–60
Rheumatoid arthritis, 28, **28,** 389
Rigidity
in drug-induced parkinsonism, 309
in neuroleptic malignant syndrome, 309
Risk factors for schizophrenia, 23–33, 346
autoimmune diseases, **28,** 28–29
cannabis use, 29–30
environmental, 39, 76–77
epigenetic dysregulation, 77
ethnicity, 29, **29**
genetic, 39–51, 75–76
infections and immune system, 27–28, 60, 61–62
modernization, **31,** 31–32, **33**
parental age, 25–27
prenatal and perinatal, 23–25, **26–27,** 55–63, **56–57,** 76,
295, 297
urban residence, **30,** 30–31
Risk prediction, 354
Risperidone, 304, 307
adverse effects of, **306,** 307, 311, 312
augmentation with divalproex, 369
combined with clozapine, 319
dosage and half-life of, **305,** 307
efficacy studies of, 307
in elderly patients, 376–377, **378**
history and development of, 307
long-acting injectable formulation of, **314,** 315
NMDA agonists combined with, 100, **101**
in patients with depressive symptoms, 228
in patients with obsessive-compulsive symptoms, 235
in patients with substance use disorders, 226
in prodromal period, 349–350
Risperidone microspheres, **314,** 315
Riverius, Lazarus, 8
Role functioning, 275, 277
Romantic relationships, 280
Romanticism period, 9–10
Rousseau, 8
Rubella during pregnancy, 27, 60
Rural treatment services, 397–398

SADS (Schedule for Affective Disorders and Schizophrenia), 189

"Sally–Anne" task to measure false beliefs, 262–263

SANS (Scale for the Assessment of Negative Symptoms), 191, 194, **195,** 206

SAPS (Scale for the Assessment of Positive Symptoms), 191, 194, **194,** 205, 206

Sarcosine, 100

Scale for the Assessment of Negative Symptoms (SANS), 191, 194, **195,** 206

Scale for the Assessment of Positive Symptoms (SAPS), 191, 194, **194,** 205, 206

Scale of Prodromal Symptoms (SOPS), 344

SCAN (Schedules for Clinical Assessment in Neuropsychiatry), 17, 18

Schedule for Affective Disorders and Schizophrenia (SADS), 189

Schedule for Deficit Syndromes, 204, **204**

Schedules for Clinical Assessment in Neuropsychiatry (SCAN), 17, 18

Schizoaffective disorder, 11, 40, 212–213, 290
  vs. depression in schizophrenia, 210

Schizoaffective schizophrenia, 187

Schizophrenia
  abnormal connectivity hypothesis of, 180
  acute psychotic exacerbations in, 370
  age at onset of, 20, **20,** 85, 187, 353, 354
  atypical, 11
  catatonic, 12, 189, 190, **192,** 194, 201, 214–215, 373–374
  chronic, 21–22, 291–292, **293,** 297
    treatment of, 365–378
  cognitive impairments in, 204–208, 245–256
  course of, 21–23, **22–23,** 290–294, **291,** 297, 354
  critical period of, 361
  deficit, 203–204, **204**
  diagnosis of, 10, **10,** 13, 167, 177, 187–189, **188–191**
  differential diagnosis of, 212–214
  disorganized (hebephrenic), 189, **192,** 214–215
  epidemiology of, 17–33, 187, 345
  first episode of, 354–361
  five-factor model of, 194
  genetics of, 39–51, 346
  goals of treatment for, 365
  good-prognosis, 187
  history of, 1–14
  incidence of, **18–20,** 19–20, 117
  integrative model of, 77–78, **78**
  life expectancy in, 383
  natural history of, 20–23, 289–298
  neurochemical theories of, 75, 85–108, 145
  neurodevelopmental theories of, 21, 69–79, 137, 346
  neuroimaging studies in, 86, 141–142, 167–180, 346

neuropathology of, 71–72, 151–161, 346
neuroprogressive theories of, 137–145, **138**
paranoid, 1, 189, **192,** 214–215
pharmacotherapies for, 303–319
phenotype of, 40
phospholipids in, 117–129
poor-prognosis, 295
premorbid phase of, 138, **138,** 289, 341, **342,** 353–354
prevalence of, **18,** 18–19, 85
prevention of, 342–343
prodromal phase of, 20, 138, **138,** 187, 289–290, 341–351, **342,** 354
prognostic factors for, 295–297
pseudoneurotic, 187
psychiatric comorbidity with, 223–235, **227**
psychopathology of, 187–215
psychosocial therapies for, 297, 327–337
psychotic phase of, 138, **138,** 342, **342**
recognizing early warning signs of, 343
reduced neuropil hypothesis of, 140, **154,** 154–155
relapse of, 297
  anxiety and, 212
  depression and, 209–210, 228
  due to treatment nonadherence, 371–373
  effect of family therapy on, 331
  maintenance antipsychotic therapy and, 304
  rate after treatment discontinuation, 313
remissions of, 21
residual, 189, **192,** 215
risk factors for, 23–33, 346
schizoaffective, 187
social cognitive impairments in, 248, 261–270
social functioning impairments in, 194, **195,** 202–203, 275–280
subtypes of, 189, **192,** 214–215
sustained recovery from, 290–291, **292**
symptoms of, 187–215
syndromal concept of, 190–195, **197**
treatment-refractory, 307, 368–369
type I and type II, 190
undifferentiated, 189, **192,** 215
vocational functioning impairments in, 275–276, 280–283

Schizophrenia Patient Outcomes Research Team, 313, 314, 357, 386

Schizophrenia spectrum disorders, 13–14, 40, 290

Schizophreniform disorder, 212, 290

Schizotypal personality disorder, 40, 195, 214, 346

Schneider, Kurt, 10, **10,** 13, 188, **188,** 195

Schumann, Robert, 13

SCID (Structured Clinical Interview for DSM-III-R), 17

SCID (Structured Clinical Interview for DSM-IV), 189

Season of birth, 23–24, **26, 56,** 60

Second messengers, phospholipid-derived, 119, **120,** 125

Secondary prevention, 342, 401

Sedation, antipsychotic-induced, 304, **306,** 312–313

  in elderly patients, **376**

Seizures, drug-induced

  bupropion, 317

  clozapine, 307, 317

Selective serotonin reuptake inhibitors

  interaction with clozapine, 316, 317

  for obsessive-compulsive disorder, 234–235

  for social phobia, 232

Self-discrepancy theory, 267

Self-esteem

  intimate partnerships and, 280

  persecutory delusions and, 267

Self-help programs, 333

Self-injurious behavior, 211, 399

Self-serving bias in attributional style, 265–266

Semantic fluency, 247–248, 253

Semantic priming, 253

Semistructured interviews, 17

Sensitive Beziehungswahn, 12

Sérieux, P., 12

D-Serine, 101, 319

  actions at NMDA receptor, 97, 100

  dosage of, 100

  therapeutic effect of, 100, **101**

Serotonin, 73

Serotonin$_{1A}$ receptor, 89

Serotonin$_{2A}$ receptor, 88, 89

  gene for *(HTR2A),* **47,** 49, 51

Sertraline, interaction with clozapine, 317

Seventeenth-century conceptions, 8

Sexual behavior, 201, 202

Sexual dysfunction, antipsychotic-induced, 312, **376**

Shakespeare, William, 31–32

Shared delusional (psychotic) disorder, 196, 213

Sheltered employment, 334

Ship of Fools (Bosch), 32

Signal transduction

  membrane receptor–mediated, 125–126

    eicosanoids, 126

    endocannabinoid system, 126

    hyperactivity of phosphoinositide pathways, 125–126

  phosphatidylinositol system in, 122

  phospholipid-derived second messengers in, 119, **120,** 125

Single nucleotide polymorphisms (SNPs), 48, 49

Single photon emission computed tomography (SPECT)

    studies, 169

  of striatal dopamine transmission, 90, 156

  technological aspects of, 169

SIPS (Structured Interview for Prodromal Syndromes), 344–345, 401

Smoking, 224, 384–385

  cessation of, 226, 385

    antipsychotics and, 226

    bupropion for, 226, 385

    clozapine for, 385

    nicotine replacement strategies for, 226, 385

  nicotine interaction with antipsychotics, 384

  oxidative stress and, 124

  in pregnancy, 384

  prevalence of, 384

  respiratory disease and, 384, 388

SNAP-25, 154, 155

Snell, Ludwig, 11

SNPs (single nucleotide polymorphisms), 48, 49

Social cognition, 248, 261–270

  definition of, 261

  domains of, 262, **262**

    attributional style, 265–267

    facial affect recognition, 268–270

    theory of mind, 248, 262–265

  independence from nonsocial cognition, 261–262

  neural network associated with, 261

Social functioning impairments, 69, 85, 194, **195,** 202–203, 275–280

  definitions related to, 276

  effect of antipsychotics on, 277, 327

  facial affect recognition deficit and, 269–270

  independent living and, 279–280

  intimate partnerships and, 280

  onset and course of deficits in, 275–276, 290

  outcome of, 292

  parenting and, 280

  predictors of, 278

  social perception, 276

  social skills, 276–278

  stability of, 276

  strategies for improvement of, 279–280

    antipsychotics, 279

    environmental modifications, 279

    social skills training, 278, 279

  substance use disorders and, 279

  suicidal behavior and, 211

  theory-of-mind deficits and, 264–265

Social phobia, 212, **227,** 231–232

  detection of, 232

  management of, 232

  prevalence of, 231

  prognostic significance of, 231–232

Social problem-solving model, 331, 332

Social skills, 276–278
  deficits in, 277
  definition of, 276
  effect of antipsychotics on, 277
  types of, 276–277
  work performance and, 281
Social skills training (SST), 277–278, **278**, 331–333
  basic model of, 331–332
  clubhouse model of, 333
  cognitive remediation model of, 332–333
  social problem-solving model of, 332
Socioeconomic status, 23, 395–396
  downward drift in, 395
  vocational functioning and, 280–281
Socrates, 4
Somatic delusions, 199
Somatic hallucinations, 200
Sophocles, 3
SOPS (Scale of Prodromal Symptoms), 344
SPECT. *See* Single photon emission computed tomography
  studies
Speed of processing, 247
Spiess, Christian, 11
SST. *See* Social skills training
Stages of illness, 138, **138**, 289–290, 341–342, **342**, 353–354
State psychiatric hospitals, 398–400
  downsizing of, 398
  indications for treatment in, 399
  involuntary commitment to, 399
  involuntary forced treatment in, 399
  legislation related to treatment in, 398–399
  medical services in, 399–400
  psychosocial therapies in, 399
  services provided in, 399
Stereotyped movements, 201
Stereotyped thinking, 203
Stigmatization, 280
Stoic theory, 4
Stoliditas, 7
Stress
  glucocorticoid-induced, 145
  during pregnancy, 60, 62–63
Stress-vulnerability model
  of schizophrenia, 328, 353
  of substance use disorders, 224
Striatum
  corticostriatothalamic circuitry, 157–158
  dopamine–glutamate interactions in, 106, **107**
  glutamate–dopamine interactions in, 104–105, **105**
  increased dopamine activity at D_2 receptors in, 85, 87–93,
    91–93
Stroop color-naming task, 70

Structured Clinical Interview for DSM-III-R (SCID), 17
Structured Clinical Interview for DSM-IV (SCID), 189
Structured diagnostic instruments, 17, 189
Structured Interview for Prodromal Syndromes (SIPS),
  344–345, 401
Subcortical abnormalities, 171
  basal ganglia, 173–174
Substance-induced psychotic disorders, 214
Substance use disorders, 224–227, **227**, 385–386. *See also*
  Alcohol use disorders; *specific substances of abuse*
  aggressive behavior and, 209
  anxiety and, 212
  benzodiazepines and, 226
  detection of, 225
  effect on treatment adherence, 372
  effects on illness course and treatment, 224
  etiology of, 224–225
  family history and risk of, 224
  among first-episode patients, 360
  management of, 225–227
    integrated treatment, 225, **225**, 386
    pharmacological, 225–227
    in public sector, 401
  neurobiological hypothesis of, 223, 224–225
  posttraumatic stress disorder and, 233
  prevalence of, 224, 385
  prognostic significance of, 296, 383, 385
  screening for, 225
  self-medication hypothesis of, 224
  social functioning and, 279
  stress-vulnerability model of, 224
  suicidal behavior and, 211, 229–230
Subtypes of schizophrenia, 189, **192**, 214–215
Suicidal behavior, 211, 229–230, 359–360
  assessing risk for, 370
  clinical variables associated with, 211, 229
  clozapine for reduction of, 230, 307
  detection of, 230
  in first-episode patients, 359–360
  management of, 230
    clozapine, 230, 307, 359–360
  prevalence and epidemiology of, 211, 229, 359
  risk factors for, 229–230
    akathisia, 309
    depression, 211, 229–230, 359
  substance use disorders and, 211, 229–230
Superior temporal gyrus, 173, **174**
Supported employment, 281–283, 333–334
  benefits of, 334
  case management and, 334
  definition of, 281–282
  individual placement and support approach to, 333–334

integration with clinical services, 282

purpose of, 282

research on efficacy of, 282–283, **283**

scope of, 282

vs. traditional vocational rehabilitation programs, 334

Supported housing, 279–280, 398

Supportive therapy

for patients with depressive symptoms, 229

in prodromal period, 350

Survey method of case finding, 18

Susceptibility genes. *See* Candidate genes

Symptoms, 187–215. *See also specific symptoms*

amphetamine-induced, 87–88

anxiety, 211–212

Bleuler's four As, 13, 187

chronicity of, 21–22, 291–292, **293,** 297

clusters of, 194

cognitive, **2,** 2–6, 71, 86, 204–208, 245–256

functional outcome and, **139**

depression, 209–211

diagnosis based on, 187–189, **188–191** (*See also* Diagnosis)

dimensional approach to, 194–195

dissociative anesthetic–induced, 73, 96, 99–100

documentation of, 366

duration of, 188, 189

effect of antipsychotic drugs on, 303, 304, 316

essential polyunsaturated fatty acid levels and severity of, 126

excitement, 208–209

five-factor model of, 194

functional decline and, 138

gradual emergence of, 354

heterogeneous presentation of, 190

negative, 85, 87, 138, 167, 190–194, **195, 196,** 201–203

affective flattening or blunting, 2, **2,** 12, 85, 167, 202

alogia, 203

avolition and apathy, 203

concept of, 201–202

deficit symptoms, 195, 201

vs. depression, 210, 228, 253

in first-episode patients, 358–359

frontal lobe gray matter loss and, 171

functional status and, 139

neurocognitive correlates of, 202

passive/apathetic social withdrawal, 202–203

poor rapport, 202

postpsychotic deterioration component of, 201

premorbid, 195, 202

primary, 195, 201

psychotic-phase, 201

relation of cognitive deficits to, 252

residual, 359

secondary, 195, 202

stability of, 139, 191, 202

stereotyped thinking, 203

positive, 85, 138–139, 167, 190–201, **194, 196**

attenuated positive symptoms syndrome, 347

bizarre behavior, 2, **2,** 190, **194,** 200–201

concept of, 195

delusions, 195–199

in first-episode patients, 358

hallucinations, 199–200

relation of cognitive deficits to, 252

residual, 359

Schneider's first-rank symptoms, 10, **10,** 13, 188, **188,** 195

prognostic significance of, 295

psychotic, 85

rating scales for, 191–194, **194, 195**

self-injury, 211

sequence of onset of, 343

in specific subtypes, **192**

suicide, 211

sustained recovery from, 290–291, **292**

syndromal domains of, 189

theory-of-mind deficits and, 263

treatment-refractory, **368,** 368–369

Synaptic abnormalities, 154–155

Synaptic apoptosis, 144

Synaptophysin, 63, 154–155

Syndromal concept of schizophrenia, 190–195, **197**

Tachycardia, antipsychotic-induced, 313

Tactile hallucinations, 200

Tangentiality, 206

Tardive akathisia, 310

Tardive dyskinesia (TD), 310

antipsychotics associated with, 310

cannabis use and, 385

clinical features of, 310

diagnostic criteria for, 310

DRD3 gene and, 51

in elderly patients, 310, 375, 376, 377

essential polyunsaturated fatty acid levels and, 126

management of, 310

vitamin E, 128, 310

prevalence of, 310

risk factors for, 310

vs. stereotyped movements, 201

time of onset of, 310

Tardive dystonia, 310

TCP (thienylcyclohexylpiperidine), 98

TD. *See* Tardive dyskinesia

Telemental health, 398

Temporal cortex dysfunction, 178
Temporal lobe structural studies, 171–173
    hippocampal abnormalities, 172, **172**
    planum temporale, 173
    superior temporal gyrus, 173, **174**
    volume reductions in, 173
Tertiary prevention, 342, 401
Testosterone replacement therapy, for hyperprolactinemia, 312
Δ-9-Tetrahydrocannabinol, 126
Thalamus
    dopamine receptors in, 178
    neuronal loss in, 153
    structural studies of, 174
    thalamocortical connectivity, 72
The Sacred Disease (Hippocrates), 3
Theory of mind (ToM), 248, **262**, 262–265
    definition of, 262
    development of abilities, 263
    first-order vs. second-order, 262–263
    in schizophrenia, 263–265
        cognitive abilities, 263–264
        mind deficits, 263
        social functioning and, 264–265
        as state or trait deficit, 264
    skills included in, 262
Thienylcyclohexylpiperidine (TCP), 98
Thioridazine, 304
    adverse effects of, 311
    dosage and half-life of, **305**
Thiothixene
    adverse effects of, 304
    dosage and half-life of, **305**
Thought blocking, 208
Thought broadcasting, 198
Thought disorder, 2, **2, 188, 194,** 204–208. *See also* Cognitive
    impairments
    classification of, 205
    definition of, 205
    measurement of, 206
    mechanisms of, 205–206
        attention impairment, 205
        contextual difficulties, 205–206
    relation of cognitive deficits to, 253
    types of, 206–208
        circumstantiality, 207
        clanging, 207
        derailment, 206
        difficulty in abstract thinking, 207
        echolalia and echopraxia, 207–208
        illogicality, 207
        incoherence, 207
        neologism, 207
        tangentiality, 206
        thought blocking, 208
Thought insertion, 198
Thought withdrawal, 198
Thyroid disorders, 28
TNF-α (tumor necrosis factor–α), 62
ToM. *See* Theory of mind
Torticollis, antipsychotic-induced, 309
Toxoplasmosis during pregnancy, 27
Trail Making Parts A and B tests, 255
Trauma, 232–233
Treatment
    acute patient characteristics influencing, 369–370
    adherence to, 367, 370, 371–373
        assessment of, 372
        in community mental health centers, 398
        compliance therapy and, 329, 372
        cutoff for, 371–372
        depot antipsychotics and, 314, 367, 373
        strategies for improvement of, 372–373
        among substance-abusing patients, 372
    of chronic schizophrenia, 365–378 (*See also* Long-term
        treatment)
    context of, 367
    documentation of, 367
    of elderly patients, 374–378
    of first-episode psychosis, 355–360
    goals of, 365
    guidelines and algorithms for, 367
    ineffective use of, 367
    integration of, 366, 374, 378
    in least restrictive environment, 398
    pharmacological, 303–319
    plan for, 366
    "Practice Guideline for the Treatment of Patients With
        Schizophrenia," 313, 357, 360, 369
    psychosocial, 297, 327–337
    in the public sector, 395–401
Treatment Strategies for Schizophrenia Study, 330
Tremor, parkinsonian, 309
Trifluoperazine, **305**
Trihexyphenidyl hydrochloride, **309**
Tumor necrosis factor–α (TNF-α), 62
Turner, Daniel, 8–9
Twentieth-century conceptions, 12–14
Twin studies, 40, 41, 42–44, **43,** 55–56, 75, 77, 224, 245, 346

U.K. National Child Development Study, 76
U.K. National Survey of Health and Development, 249
"Uncinate fits," 200

Undifferentiated schizophrenia, 189, **192**, 215
Unemployment, 23, **25**, 254–255, 280–283, 333, 395. *See also*
    Supported employment; Vocational functioning
    impairments
Uninsured/underinsured patients, 396
Unitary genetic-developmental model of schizophrenia, 77–78,
    78
Urban birth, **56**, 60
Urban residence, **30**, 30–31
Uterine atony, **56**, 59

VA (Veterans Affairs) medical centers, 400
Valproate, 77, 318, 369
Velocardiofacial syndrome (VCFS), 44–45, 223
Ventral tegmental area (VTA), 86, 102–104, **103**
Ventricular enlargement, 71, 141, 143, 171, **175**, 175–176
Verbal fluency, 247–248, 252
Verbal learning and memory, 246–247
Verbigeration, 12
Veterans Affairs (VA) medical centers, 400
Vigilance, 211, 246
Violent behavior. *See* Hostility/aggression
Visual hallucinations, 200
Visual learning and memory, 247
Vitamin C, 129
Vitamin E, for tardive dyskinesia, 128, 310
Vocational functioning impairments, 23, **25**, 254–255, 280–283
    correlates and predictors of work, 281
        cognitive impairment, 281
        educational level, 281
        social skills, 281
    onset and course of, 275–276, 290
    outcome of, 292
    prevalence of, 280
    self-esteem and, 281
    socioeconomic consequences of, 280–281
    stability of, 276

Vocational rehabilitation, 281–283, **283**, 333–334. *See also*
    Supported employment
Voltaire, 8
VTA (ventral tegmental area), 86, 102–104, **103**

Waldrop scale, 21
Washington University (Feighner) criteria for schizophrenia,
    188, **189**
Waxy flexibility, 201
WCST (Wisconsin Card Sorting Test), 70, 100, 202, 247, 252,
    254
Wechsler Adult Intelligence Scale, 247, 264
Weight gain, antipsychotic-induced, 304, **306**, 311, **389**
    in elderly patients, **376**
Weyer, Johann, 7
White matter volume, 71
Williams syndrome, 261–262
Willis, Thomas, 8
Wisconsin Card Sorting Test (WCST), 70, 100, 202, 247, 252,
    254
World Health Organization
    age- and sex-related onset of schizophrenia, 20, **20**
    International Pilot Study of Schizophrenia, 294, 297
    schizophrenia outcome study, 22, **23**
    studies of aggression in schizophrenia, 208
    studies of diet in schizophrenia, 122

Yale-Brown Obsessive Compulsive Scale, 234

Zeller, Ernst, 10, 11
Ziprasidone, 304, 308
    adverse effects of, **306**, 308, 311
    dosage and half-life of, **305**, 308
    history and development of, 308
    mechanism of action of, 89
    in patients with substance use disorders, 226